THE ROLE OF PHYTONUTRIENTS IN METABOLIC DISORDERS

THE ROLE OF PHYTONUTRIENTS IN METABOLIC DISORDERS

Edited by

HAROON KHAN

Department of Pharmacy, Abdul Wali Khan University Mardan, Mardan, Pakistan

ESRA KÜPELI AKKOL

Department of Pharmacognosy, Faculty of Pharmacy, Gazi University, Ankara, Turkey

MARIA DAGLIA

Department of Pharmacy, School of Medicine and Surgery, University of Naples Federico II, Naples, Italy

International Research Center for Food Nutrition and Safety, Jiangsu University, Zhenjiang, China

ELSEVIER

ACADEMIC PRESS

An imprint of Elsevier

Academic Press is an imprint of Elsevier
125 London Wall, London EC2Y 5AS, United Kingdom
525 B Street, Suite 1650, San Diego, CA 92101, United States
50 Hampshire Street, 5th Floor, Cambridge, MA 02139, United States
The Boulevard, Langford Lane, Kidlington, Oxford OX5 1GB, United Kingdom

ISBN 978-0-12-824356-5

For information on all Academic Press publications
visit our website at https://www.elsevier.com/books-and-journals

Publisher: Andre G. Wolff
Editorial Project Manager: Samantha Allard
Production Project Manager: Maria Bernard
Cover Designer: Mark Rogers

Typeset by STRAIVE, India

Contents

Section B

Contributors

Imad Ahmad
Department of Pharmacy, Abdul Wali Khan University Mardan, Mardan; Department of Pharmacy, Abasyn University Peshawar, Peshawar, Pakistan

Esra Küpeli Akkol
Department of Pharmacognosy, Faculty of Pharmacy, Gazi University, Ankara, Turkey

Waqas Alam
Department of Pharmacy, Abdul Wali Khan University Mardan, Mardan, Pakistan

Ahmed Al-Harrasi
Natural and Medical Sciences Research Centre, University of Nizwa, Nizwa, Oman

Reem Hasaballah Alhasani
Department of Biology, Faculty of Applied Science, Umm Al-Qura University, Makkah, Saudi Arabia

Ifat Alsharif
Department of Biology, Jamoum University College, Umm Al-Qura University, Makkah, Saudi Arabia

Norah A. Althobaiti
Department of Biology, College of Science and Humanities, Shaqra University, Al-Quwaiiyah, Saudi Arabia

Giuseppe Annunziata
Department of Pharmacy, University of Naples Federico II, Naples, Italy

Michael Aschner
Department of Molecular Pharmacognosy, Albert Einstein College of Medicine, Bronx, NY, United States

Amira Yasmine Benmelouka
Faculty of Medicine, University of Algiers, Algiers, Algeria

Shabana Bibi
Department of Biosciences, Shifa Tameer-e-Millat University, Islamabad, Pakistan; Yunnan Herbal Laboratory, School of Ecology and Environmental Sciences; Research Center for Sustainable Utilization of Cordyceps Bioresources in China and Southeast Asia, Yunnan University, Kunming, China

Partha Biswas
Department of Genetic Engineering and Biotechnology, Faculty of Biological Science and Technology, Jashore University of Science and Technology (JUST), Jashore, Bangladesh

Shazia Anwer Bukhari
Department of Biochemistry, Government College University, Faisalabad, Pakistan

Gul Bushra
Department of Bioinformatics and Biotechnology, Faculty of Life Sciences, Government College University, Faisalabad, Pakistan

Maria Daglia
Department of Pharmacy, School of Medicine and Surgery, University of Naples Federico II, Naples, Italy; International Research Center for Food Nutrition and Safety, Jiangsu University, Zhenjiang, China

Alaa Ahmed Elshanbary
Faculty of Medicine, Alexandria University, Alexandria, Egypt

Sajad Fakhri
Pharmaceutical Sciences Research Center, Health Institute, Kermanshah University of Medical Sciences, Kermanshah, Iran

Mohammad Mehedi Hasan
Department of Biochemistry and Molecular Biology, Mawlana Bhashani Science and Technology University, Tangail, Bangladesh

Yaseen Hussain
Laboratory of Controlled Release and Drug Delivery System, College of Pharmaceutical Sciences, Soochow University, Suzhou, China; Department of Pharmacy, Bashir Institute of Health Sciences, Islamabad, Pakistan

Shabnoor Iqbal
Department of Zoology, Faculty of Life Sciences, Government College University, Faisalabad, Pakistan

Muhammad Irfan
Department of Pharmaceutics, Government College University, Faisalabad, Pakistan

Nazia Kanwal
Department of Life Sciences, Khwaja Fareed University of Engineering and Information Technology, Rahim Yar Khan, Pakistan

Abdul Haleem Khan
Department of Pharmacy, Forman Christian College (A Chartered University), Lahore, Pakistan

Ajmal Khan
Natural and Medical Sciences Research Centre, University of Nizwa, Nizwa, Oman

Haroon Khan
Department of Pharmacy, Abdul Wali Khan University Mardan, Mardan, Pakistan

Mostafa Meshref
Department of Neurology, Al-Azhar University, Cairo, Egypt

Sana Piri
Pharmaceutical Sciences Research Center, Health Institute, Kermanshah University of Medical Sciences, Kermanshah, Iran

Shafiq Ur Rahman
Department of Pharmacy, Shaheed Benazir Bhutto University, Sheringal, Dir Upper, Pakistan

Azhar Rasul
Department of Life Sciences, Khwaja Fareed University of Engineering and Information Technology, Rahim Yar Khan; Department of Zoology, Faculty of Life Sciences, Government College University, Faisalabad, Pakistan

Ammara Riaz
Department of Life Sciences, Khwaja Fareed University of Engineering and Information Technology, Rahim Yar Khan, Pakistan

Ayesha Sadiqa
Department of Life Sciences, Khwaja Fareed University of Engineering and Information Technology, Rahim Yar Khan, Pakistan

Uzma Saleem
Department of Pharmacology, Faculty of Pharmaceutical Sciences, Government College University, Faisalabad, Pakistan

Iqra Sarfraz
Department of Life Sciences, Khwaja Fareed University of Engineering and Information Technology, Rahim Yar Khan, Pakistan

Gökçe Şeker Karatoprak
Department of Pharmacognosy, Faculty of Pharmacy, Erciyes University, Kayseri, Turkey

Ghulam Mujtaba Shah
Department of Pharmacy; Department of Botany, Hazara University, Mansehra, Pakistan

Muhammad Ajmal Shah
Department of Pharmacy, Hazara University, Mansehra; Department of Pharmacognosy, Faculty of Pharmaceutical Sciences, Government College University, Faisalabad, Pakistan

Shahid Shah
Department of Pharmacy Practice, Faculty of Pharmaceutical Sciences, Government College University, Faisalabad, Pakistan

Farzana Shareef
Department of Life Sciences, Khwaja Fareed University of Engineering and Information Technology, Rahim Yar Khan, Pakistan

Anastasiia Shkodina
Poltava State Medical University, Poltava, Ukraine

Antoni Sureda
Research Group on Community Nutrition and Oxidative Stress (NUCOX), Department of Fundamental Biology and Health Sciences, Health Research Institute of the Balearic Islands (IdISBa), and CIBEROBN (Physiopathology of Obesity and Nutrition CB12/03/30038), University of the Balearic Islands, Palma, Spain

Silvia Tejada
Laboratory of Neurophysiology, Department of Biology, Health Research Institute of the Balearic Islands (IdISBa), and CIBEROBN (Physiopathology of Obesity and Nutrition CB12/03/30038), University of the Balearic Islands, Palma, Spain

Gian Carlo Tenore
Department of Pharmacy, University of Naples Federico II, Naples, Italy

Ilknur Ucak
Nigde Omer Halisdemir University, Nigde, Turkey

Hammad Ullah
Department of Pharmacy, School of Medicine and Surgery, University of Naples Federico II, Naples, Italy

Çiğdem Yücel
Department of Pharmaceutical Technology, Faculty of Pharmacy, Erciyes University, Kayseri, Turkey

Rabia Zara
Department of Life Sciences, Khwaja Fareed University of Engineering and Information Technology, Rahim Yar Khan, Pakistan

SECTION A

CHAPTER 1

An overview on metabolic disorders and current therapy

Esra Küpeli Akkol[a] and Michael Aschner[b]
[a]Department of Pharmacognosy, Faculty of Pharmacy, Gazi University, Ankara, Turkey
[b]Department of Molecular Pharmacognosy, Albert Einstein College of Medicine, Bronx, NY, United States

1. Introduction

Metabolism is a process involving the transformation of metabolites, the biochemical pathways in which this transformation takes place, and the mechanisms that regulate metabolite flow in the pathways. Any disease or disorder that disrupts normal metabolism, the process of converting food into energy at the cellular level, is referred to as a metabolic disease. Thousands of enzymes that participate in numerous interconnected metabolic pathways play a role in this process [1]. Metabolic diseases affect the cell's ability to perform critical biochemical reactions involving the processing or transport of carbohydrates (sugars and starches), proteins (amino acids), or lipids (fatty acids).

While metabolic diseases are typically inherited, most individuals affected by them may appear healthy for days, months, or even years. Symptoms usually occur when the body's metabolism undergoes extensive stress, such as prolonged starvation or a febrile illness [2]. Detection of some metabolic disorders is possible with prenatal diagnostic screening [3]. This type of analysis is often offered to families who have a previous child with a metabolic disease or who belong to a defined ethnic group. If a metabolic disorder is detected in a baby soon after birth, appropriate treatment can be initiated early, resulting in an improved prognosis. Early initiation of treatment responds very well in some metabolic disorders [4]. However, others have no effective therapy and cause severe problems, despite the early diagnosis. Symptoms of inherited and acquired metabolic disorders are presented in Table 1.

Metabolic diseases are very rare when considered individually, but relatively common when considered as a group. Specific metabolic disorders have incidences ranging from approximately 1 in 500 to less than 1 in 1,000,000. When metabolic disorders are considered as a whole, they are

The Role of Phytonutrients in Metabolic Disorders
https://doi.org/10.1016/B978-0-12-824356-5.00004-7

Table 1 Symptoms of inherited and acquired metabolic disorders.

Symptoms of inherited metabolic disorders	Symptoms of acquired metabolic disorders
Body fluids that have a maple smell	Chronic or persistent diarrhea
Bone abnormalities such as osteoporosis (thinning and weakening of the bones)	Fatigue
Difficulty with memory, thinking, talking, comprehension, writing or reading	Headache
Enlarged liver, heart, kidney, or spleen	Irritability and mood changes
Failure to thrive in infants and children	Muscle cramping
Frequent infections	Nausea with or without vomiting
Hypoglycemia (low blood sugar)	Rapid breathing (tachypnea) or shortness of breath
Loss of vision or changes in vision	Bluish coloration of the lips or fingernails
Muscle twitching, spasms, or seizures	Change in mental status or sudden behavior change, such as confusion, delirium, lethargy, hallucinations, and delusions
Muscle weakness	Respiratory or breathing problems, such as shortness of breath, difficulty breathing, labored breathing, wheezing, not breathing, choking
Paralysis	Seizure

estimated to affect approximately 1 in 1000 people [5]. Certain chronic medical conditions, such as lung or kidney disease (includes any type of kidney problem, such as kidney stones, kidney failure, and kidney anomalies), family history of genetic metabolic disorder and HIV/AIDS are the risk factors for metabolic disorders [6].

The treatment approach for metabolic disorders depends on the specific disorder. Inherited metabolic disorders are often treated with nutritional counseling and support, periodic assessment, physical therapy, and other supportive care options. Acquired metabolic disorder treatment includes normalizing the metabolic balance by both reversing the cause and administering medications [7,8].

In this chapter, origins of metabolic diseases, types of metabolic disorders, and present status and new trends on the treatment of metabolic disorders are presented.

2. Origins of metabolic disease

2.1 Metabolic pathways

Foods are broken down into products of different biochemical structures in a series of steps by means of cellular enzymes. Then these products become a substrate for the next enzyme in a metabolic pathway [9]. In this process, if there is an enzyme deficiency or a decrease in enzyme activity, the pathway becomes blocked and the formation of the final product is insufficient, causing disease [10,11]. Low activity of an enzyme may cause subsequent accumulation of the enzyme substrate, which can be toxic at high levels. Furthermore, minor metabolic pathways that generally lie dormant may be activated when a substrate accumulates, probably forming atypical, potentially toxic, products. Each cell contains many metabolic pathways, all of which are interlinked to some extent, so that a single blockage may affect a plethora of biochemical processes [12,13].

Serious problems can arise as a result of metabolic imbalance. Depending on which enzyme is dysfunctional, blindness, deafness, seizures, mental disability, decreased muscle tone and organ failure may occur [14]. In recent years, it has been determined that even some conditions associated with multiple congenital anomalies such as Smith-Lemli-Opitz syndrome are caused by an underlying metabolic cause.

2.2 Inheritance

The inheritance of inborn errors of metabolism is most frequently *autosomal recessive*, the importance that two mutant genes are essential to produce the symptoms and signs of disease [15]. The parents of an affected child are most often asymptomatic carriers since 50% of normal enzyme activity is adequate to maintain necessary *health* [16]. When two carriers of a *deleterious* trait produce offspring, there is a 25% chance of having an affected child, a 25% chance of having a child without the mutant allele, and a 50% chance of having a child who is similarly a carrier (Fig. 1). In genetic terms, the carrier of an autosomal recessive situation has only one mutant gene (heterozygous), whereas an affected individual has two mutant genes (homozygous) [17]. All human beings have about six recessive mutant alleles in their genomes, however, it is relatively rare for an individual to mate with someone who carries a mutation in the same gene [18]. Conversely, in cases of parental *consanguinity*, there is an increased risk of having a child with an autosomal recessive situation, since a common genetic background is shared [19].

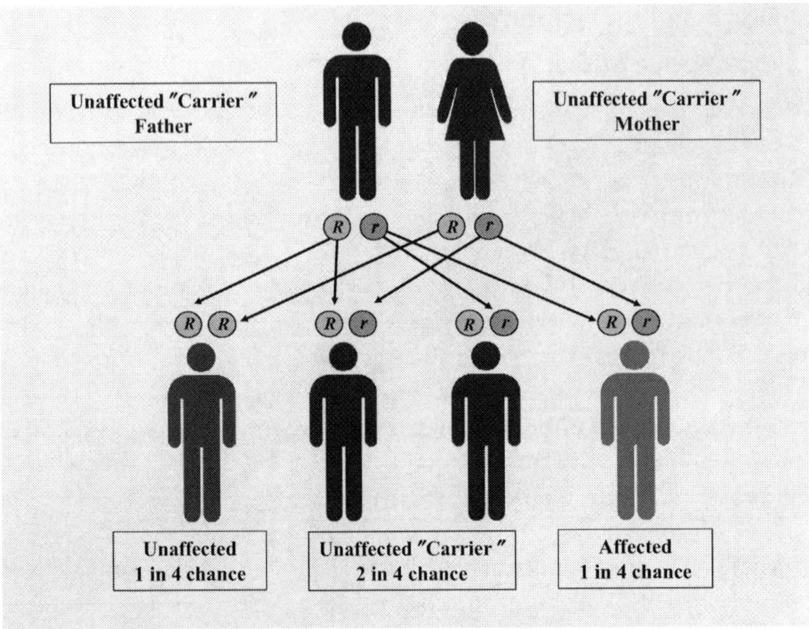

Fig. 1 Autosomal recessive inheritance (*r*: patient allele, *red*, *R*: healthy allele, *blue*).

In contrast to autosomal recessive diseases, *autosomal dominant* diseases are expressed when only one mutant gene is present. These disorders display a strong family history, except for the condition arising from a new spontaneous mutation in an individual ([20]). A heterozygous individual has a 50% chance of passing the disorder to his offspring. Individuals with autosomal dominant disorders display a wide spectrum of disease severity, and carriers of a *dominant trait* may even seem asymptomatic.

If a mutant gene is part of the X chromosome, the resulting disease is called X-linked. All male offsprings who inherit an X-linked mutation are affected, since the Y chromosome of the XY pair does not have a compensating normal gene. As the mutation is on the X chromosome and males transmit only the Y chromosome to their sons through fertilization, fathers do not transmit the disease to their sons. They can, however, transmit the carrier state to their daughters. A heterozygous female carrier, meanwhile, has a 50% chance of producing a carrier daughter or affected son [21,22].

X-linked inheritance is complicated by the process of X chromosome inactivation in females. While females carry two X chromosomes, early in embryonic development one of the X chromosomes is inactivated in each cell. The process of X chromosome inactivation is generally random, resulting in the formation of two cell lines in a given female who carries an X-linked disease mutation; one cell line has an inactivated normal X chromosome, and the other has an inactivated abnormal X chromosome [23]. Though, it is likely that a higher proportion of normal X chromosomes will be inactivated in a given individual, with the resultant appearance of symptoms of disease in several degrees. Such females are known as *manifesting heterozygotes*. X-linked disorders include *Lesch-Nyhan syndrome* (a disorder of purine metabolism that is characterized by the excretion of large amounts of *uric acid* in the urine, neurological disturbances, and self-mutilation), *X-linked adrenoleukodystrophy* (a disorder that is characterized by progressive mental and physical deterioration and adrenal insufficiency), and *ornithine transcarbamylase deficiency* (an enzyme deficiency resulting in high blood levels of ammonia and impaired urea formation) [24,25].

Maternal (mitochondrial) inheritance is the transmission of genes that are located in mitochondria. Mitochondrial DNA (*mtDNA*), while much smaller than nuclear DNA, is serious in cellular metabolism [26]. Most of the energy essential for a cell to drive its metabolism is produced in mitochondria by proteins in a series of electron donor-acceptor reactions that make up the respiratory or electron-transport chain (ETC) [27]. Mitochondria are located in the cytoplasm of the ova and are inherited from the mother. Spermatozoa similarly have mitochondria; however, these do not become incorporated into the developing embryo. After a cell divides, the mitochondria are casually distributed to daughter cells. Each mitochondrion contains 2–10 copies of mtDNA, and each cell contains several mitochondria. In a given cell of a person with a *mitochondrial disorder*, the number of normal mitochondria could be greater than the number of abnormal mitochondria, and the cell may function well [28]. Conversely, if a cell contains an important percentage of abnormal mitochondria, this cell and any tissue containing many such cells will display impaired function. Affected children may exhibit a spectrum of abnormalities, from appearing normal or mildly affected to being severely compromised, depending on the degree of mitochondrial dysfunction and the extent of tissue involvement [29].

3. Metabolic disorders

3.1 Amino acid metabolism disorders

A total of 20 amino acids play a role in metabolism, including nine amino acids that cannot be synthesized in humans and must be obtained through food. Amino acids function as important molecules in the body, such as hormones, oxygen-carrying molecules, neurotransmitters, and pigments, or these are synthesized within molecules. Each amino acid is further broken down into water, carbon dioxide, and ammonia [30,31]. Disorders such as phenylketonuria, homocystinuria, tyrosinemia, maple syrup urine disease, nonketotic hyperglycinemia are among the disorders in the metabolism of amino acids. These disorders are autosomal recessive and all can be diagnosed by analysis of amino acid concentrations in body fluids.

Phenylketonuria (PKU) is caused by a decrease in the activity of phenylalanine hydroxylase (PAH), an enzyme that converts the amino acid phenylalanine to tyrosine, a precursor of several important hormones and skin, hair, and eye pigments [32]. Due to the decreased PAH activity, there is a decrease in phenylalanine accumulation and the amount of tyrosine and other metabolites [33]. Persistent elevation in blood phenylalanine levels results in a small head circumference, progressive developmental delay, behavioral disturbances, and seizures [34]. Because of the decreased amount of melanin, people with PKU tend to have milder features such as blond hair and blue eyes than other family members without the disease [35]. Treatment with special formulas and foods low in protein and phenylalanine can reduce phenylalanine levels to normal. However, rare cases of PKU resulting from impaired metabolism of biopterin, which is an important cofactor in the phenylalanine hydroxylase reaction, may not respond consistently to treatment [36].

Classical tyrosinemia is a disease caused by a deficiency of fumarylacetoacetate hydrolase (FAH), the last enzyme in tyrosine catabolism. Characteristics of classical tyrosinemia include severe inadequate weight gain, liver disease, peripheral nerve disease, and kidney defects [37,38]. Approximately 40% of people will develop liver cancer if the disease is not treated until the age of 5 years [39]. Treatment with 2-(2-nitro-4-trifluoromethylbenzoyl)-1,3-cyclohexanedione (NTBC), a potent inhibitor of the tyrosine catabolic pathway, inhibits the production of toxic metabolites. Although this improves liver, kidney, and neurological symptoms, the occurrence of liver cancer may not be prevented [40]. Liver transplantation may be required in case of severe liver disease or cancer development. There is also a benign, transient neonatal form of tyrosinemia that responds to protein restriction and vitamin C therapy [41].

Homocystinuria is a disease caused by the defect of cystathionine β-synthase, an enzyme that plays a role in methionine metabolism and leads to homocysteine accumulation [42]. The most prominent symptoms are reddening of the cheeks, a thin-elongated rim, lens dislocation, vascular disease, and osteoporosis. However, psychiatric disorders and mental disabilities may develop [43]. About 50% of patients with homocystinuria respond to pyridoxine therapy, and these individuals tend to have a better intellectual prognosis. Betaine, folic acid, dietary protein, and methionine intake and treatment with aspirin also give positive results [44].

Nonketotic hyperglycinemia is a condition characterized by breath-holding, hiccups, low muscle tone, seizures, and severe developmental impairment [45]. It develops as a result of the increase in the neurotransmitter glycine levels in the central nervous system due to defects in the enzymes responsible for the breakdown of glycine [46]. Drugs such as dextromethorphan, sodium benzoate, and a low-protein diet can provide symptom relief, but there is no cure for this disease [47].

3.1.1 Urea cycle defects

Liver cells play a serious role in disposing of nitrogenous waste by forming the urea through the action of the urea cycle. Once an amino acid is degraded, the ammonia nitrogen at one end of the molecule is split off, incorporated into urea, and excreted in the urine [48]. A defect in any of the enzymes in the urea cycle leads to a toxic accumulation of ammonia in the blood. This, in turn, causes poor feeding, lethargy, vomiting, and probably coma in the first two or three days of life [49].

Urea cycle defects are autosomal recessive. However, X-linked ornithine transcarbamylase (OTC) deficiency is an exceptional case [50]. However, OTC deficiency may also affect females who are "manifesting heterozygotes," presenting with severe disease through infancy or later in life during times of metabolic stress—such as, during childbirth or viral illness [51]. People with urea cycle disorders have recurrent seizures due to high ammonia levels, especially at times of infection; untreated or repeated episodes of high ammonia levels can lead to intellectual disability and developmental impairment [52]. In the urea cycle disorders, hemodialysis is first applied to use intravenous ammonia scavenging drugs and to reduce the blood ammonia level [53]. Long-term therapy includes a low-protein diet, providing deficient nutrients, and the use of drugs such as phenylbutyrate or benzoate [54].

3.1.2 Amino acid transport disorders

Energy is required to transfer several amino acids from the intestinal tract into the blood or to reclaim them from the urine through special cells in the kidney. This transport of amino acids does not include enzymes in metabolic pathways but reasonably transport proteins embedded in cellular or intracellular organelle membranes. Mutant proteins with reduced transport activities can interfere with the absorption of dietary amino acids or cause their loss in the urine [55].

Cystinosis is a condition characterized by a defect in cystine output due to a defect in the carrier cystinosis. People with this disorder develop corneal deposits and kidney disease [56]. Defective membrane transport of arginine, lysine, and ornithine in the intestines causes lysinuric protein intolerance (LPI), a disorder characterized by rash, insufficient weight gain, diarrhea, protein intolerance, and osteoporosis [57,58]. Advanced complications of LPI include lung and kidney diseases. Hartnup disease is characterized by symptoms of ataxia, a photosensitive rash, and mental abnormalities, and is a disorder in amino acid transport in the intestines and kidneys [59,60].

3.2 Organic acidemias

Organic acidemias are conditions characterized by the accumulation of organic acids known as carbon-based compounds in body fluids (especially in urine) and tissues, which appear at abnormally high levels when metabolic pathways involving specific enzymes are blocked. The most common of these disorders are autosomal recessive conditions involving the metabolism of leucine, isoleucine, and valine [61]. Organic acidemias share many traits, including acidemia, hypoglycemia, neutropenia, poor growth, and varying degrees of mental impairment. These disorders can occur in infancy or later in childhood [62].

Propionic acidemia is a condition characterized by propionic acid accumulation due to the deficiency of the propionyl-CoA carboxylase enzyme. It is usually a life-threatening disease in early infancy. Dehydration, acidemia, low white blood cell count, low muscle tone, and lethargy progressing to coma are typical features [63,64]. The ammonia level in the blood can also be high, as abnormal metabolites prevent the urea cycle from working properly. Treatment includes restriction of branched-chain amino acids with diet, carnitine supplementation, and severe treatment of metabolic crises with glucose, bicarbonate, and intravenous fluids [65,66].

Classical methylmalonic acidemia (MMA) is a disease caused by a defect in the methylmalonyl-CoA mutase enzyme, with symptoms similar to individuals with propionic acidemia, but with long-term complications of kidney failure [67]. In the case of severe kidney disease, combined liver-kidney transplantation may be beneficial. One form of classical MMA responds to treatment with vitamin B12. Other forms are caused by defects in the processing of vitamin B12 and frequently current advanced in childhood with progressive neurological impairment [68].

Maple syrup urinary disease (MSUD) is a branched-chain amino acid metabolism disorder that causes the accumulation of leucine, isoleucine, valine, and their corresponding oxoacids in body fluids [69,70]. The classic form of MSUD presents with drowsiness and progressive neurological deterioration, characterized by seizures and coma in infancy. Unlike most organic acidemias, significant acidemia is rare in this disease [71]. Restriction of proteins and nutrition with formulas lacking in branched-chain amino acids is an important element in treatment. People with MSUD may be mentally disabled despite therapy, but early diagnosis and correct treatment can provide normal mental development [72]. Milder forms of MSUD are treatable with simple protein restriction or thiamine administration [73].

3.3 Carbohydrate metabolism disorders

The metabolism of the carbohydrates glucose, galactose, and fructose is complicatedly linked through interactions among different enzymatic pathways, and disorders that affect these pathways may have symptoms extending from mild to severe or even life-threatening [74]. Clinical features include several combinations of liver enlargement, hypoglycemia, and muscle pain. Most of these disorders can be treated, or at least controlled, with precise dietary involvements.

3.3.1 Galactose and fructose disorders

Galactosemia naturally is caused by a defective constituent of the second major phase in the metabolism of the sugar galactose [75]. When galactose is ingested, as in milk, clinical signs of galactosemia appear when milk feeding begins, due to the accumulation of galactose-1-phosphate [76]. If feeding is continued, babies with this disorder develop jaundice, weight loss, lethargy, progressive liver dysfunction, and kidney disease [77,78]. However, these individuals are particularly susceptible to severe bacterial infections caused by *Escherichia coli*. Most babies with galactosemia will develop mental disabilities if the disorder is not treated or treatment is delayed [79]. Removing galactose from the diet in treatment allows the symptoms to be reversed [80]. Most children with this disease have normal intelligence, but learning difficulties and some degree of intellectual disability are also present despite early treatment [81].

Hereditary fructose intolerance (HFI) is a disease that occurs in the case of a deficiency of fructose-1-phosphate aldolase, one of the liver enzymes [82]. Symptoms of HFI seem later the ingestion of fructose and therefore present later in life than do those of galactosemia [83]. Symptoms are manifested by vomiting, inadequate weight gain, liver dysfunction, hypoglycemia, and kidney defects. Children with HFI tend to avoid sugary foods and might have teeth prominent for the absence of caries [84,85].

Fructose 1,6-diphosphatase deficiency is a condition associated with impaired glucose-forming ability during gluconeogenesis. Symptoms include starvation intolerance, severe hypoglycemia, and liver enlargement. Rapid treatment of hypoglycemic episodes with intravenous fluids containing glucose and avoidance of fasting are the mainstay of treatment [86]. Some patients need continuous overnight drip feeds or a time to a retire dose of cornstarch to control their tendency to develop hypoglycemia. Fructose- and sucrose-deficient diets in children with the disorder contribute greatly to efficacious treatment success [87].

3.3.2 Glycogen storage disorders

Red blood cells, brain, and adrenal medulla function depend on a constant quantity of glucose for their metabolic functions. Transport proteins mediate the uptake of glucose into cells lining the gut. Next, glucose, which enters the bloodstream, passes to the liver and is stored as glycogen [88]. When hunger, fasting, or when the body needs a sudden energy source, glycogen is broken down into glucose and released into the blood [89]. However, muscle tissue has its own glycogen stores that can be broken down during exercise. Several conditions known as glycogen storage disorders (GSD) can occur if the enzymes responsible for glycogen degradation are blocked so that glycogen remains in the liver or muscle. Depending on which enzyme is affected, these conditions can affect the muscles, the liver, or both. In von Gierke disease (GSD type I), the last step in glucose release from the liver is defective, resulting in hypoglycemia [90]. Continuous supply of glucose to the digestive system in infancy and early childhood is an important factor in treatment. There is improvement in symptoms as the child grows [91]. Adequate glucose is provided by frequent carbohydrate feeding and slow-release glucose before bed. Liver transplantation can also be curative, but this drastic measure applies to a small percentage of patients who do not respond to normal treatment or develop liver cancer [92]. For the muscle forms of the disease, avoiding strenuous exercise is the common treatment method. Defects in previous steps in glycogen breakdown in the liver cause GSD types III, IV, VI, and IX, which typically lead to slighter versions of type I disease [93].

In the case of phosphoenolpyruvate carboxylinases, carboxylase, and fructose-1,6-diphosphatase defects, which play a role as a key enzyme in the gluconeogenic pathway, people develop conditions such as fasting hypoglycemia, lactic acidemia, and liver enlargement. Therefore, gluconeogenesis disorders may be difficult to differentiate from glycogen storage disorders at first appearance [87].

3.3.3 Congenital glycosylation disorders

Congenital disorders of glycosylation (CDG) are recently described diseases that affect the brain and many other organs. The principal biochemical defects of CDG are in the N-glycosylation pathway that occurs in the endoplasmic reticulum and cytoplasm, cellular organelles involved in the synthesis of lipids and proteins [94]. A defect that develops in the phosphomannomutase 2 enzyme causes the most common form, CDG-type I. Although other enzymatic defects have been identified, the biochemical basis of some CDG subtypes has not yet been determined [95]. CDG-type Ia is a condition characterized by brain abnormalities, severe developmental delay, and low muscle tone seen in infancy [96]. Children with type Ia have inverted nipples and an unusual distribution of fat, especially in the hips and suprapubic region [97]. However, retinal damage, stroke-like episodes, seizures, hypoglycemia, impaired heart contraction, liver disease, vomiting, diarrhea, and bleeding tendency are present [98]. There is no effective treatment for CDG, except for type Ib disease, which is characterized by a rare phosphomannose isomerase deficiency, where oral administration of mannose can in some cases reverse symptoms [2].

3.3.4 Lipid metabolism disorders

Lipids are large, water-insoluble molecules that have a diversity of biological functions, storing energy and serving as constituents of cellular membranes and lipoproteins. Cells that line the small intestine absorb dietary lipids and process them into lipoprotein particles that enter the circulation through the lymphatic system for the last uptake by the liver. Cholesterol, triglycerides, and fat-soluble vitamins are transported through the blood via these lipoprotein particles [99].

3.3.5 Lipoprotein disorders

Defects affecting lipid metabolism can be caused by defects in the structural proteins of lipoprotein particles, cell receptors that recognize various lipoprotein types, or enzymes that breakdown fat. As a result of such defects, lipids can accumulate on the walls of blood vessels, which can lead to atherosclerosis [100].

Familial hypercholesterolemia is an autosomal dominant disease caused by a deficiency of the LDL receptor in cells in the liver and other organs and characterized by the inability of cholesterol to be transported into cells. Normally, when there is enough cholesterol in the cell, feedback mechanisms signal enzymes to stop cholesterol synthesis [101]. In familial hypercholesterolemia, these enzymes are released of feedback inhibition, consequently inducing the production of still more cholesterol [102]. The disease is characterized by fat accumulation in tendons, early coronary vascular disease, and paralysis [103]. Blood cholesterol levels are very high from birth, and LDL cholesterol is also raised. Treatment is with a low-cholesterol diet and drugs that inhibit cholesterol synthesis or increase its excretion in the gastrointestinal tract [104].

If a person with familial hypercholesterolemia is homozygous for this condition, the severe vascular disease begins in early childhood and heart attacks are typical by the age of 20. Similar symptoms are present in familial dysbetalipoproteinemia (hyperlipoproteinemia type III), which can be inherited as an autosomal dominant or autosomal recessive condition [105]. In this disorder, which occurs in adulthood, there is an increase in blood cholesterol and triglyceride levels due to an abnormality in a component of lipoproteins called apoprotein E. Treatment is similar to that required for familial hypercholesterolemia [106].

A deficiency of microsomal transfer protein reasons abetalipoproteinemia, an autosomal recessive disorder characterized by the virtual absence ofVLDL and LDL. Triglycerides accumulate in the liver and gastrointestinal tract, and there are low blood levels of cholesterol, triglycerides, and HDL cholesterol [107]. People with abetalipoproteinemia have severe fat malabsorption and improve neurological symptoms with retinal defects, unsteady gait, and nerve damage owing to the deficiency of vitamin E [108].

3.3.6 Fatty acid oxidation disorders

Through prolonged starvation, the metabolism of fats deposited in adipose tissue is necessary for energy production. When the glycogen stores are exhausted, both gluconeogenesis and the production of ketone bodies by liver fatty acid beta-oxidation are vital for as long as energy for the brain [109,110]. The oxidation of fatty acids for energy occurs in the mitochondria of liver cells and needs a carrier molecule, carnitine, which is synthesized in the body and is similarly obtained from the dietary intake of animal products such as milk, meat, and eggs [111]. Some fatty acid oxidation disorders arise through dysfunction of carnitine transport enzymes, while most of these circumstances are caused through fat-degrading enzymes directly involved in the beta-oxidation cycle itself [112]. In individuals with inherited disorders of carnitine transport, a deficiency of carnitine might cause severe heart, liver, and brain damage. Treatment with carnitine is moderately effective [113]. Fatty acid oxidation disorders are comparatively mutual and as a group may account for about 5%–10% of cases of sudden infant death syndrome (SIDS). The disorders usually manifest with liver disease, hypoglycemia, cardiomyopathy, and decreased muscle tone [114].

Children with *medium-chain acyl-CoA dehydrogenase deficiency (MCAD)* appear completely normal unless they face other metabolically stressful situations such as severe viral illness or starving for an extended period of time [115]. During periods of metabolic stress, vomiting, drowsiness, hypoglycemia, seizures, and liver dysfunction may develop in affected individuals. If intravenous hydration and glucose administration are not done immediately at the appropriate time, the disease can be fatal [116]. However, with proper hydration and nutrition, children with MCAD lead a relatively normal life. Carnitine administration and excessive fat intake should be avoided in treatment. Although other fatty acid oxidation disorders may respond to similar treatment, their prognosis is not generally as good [117,118].

Long-chain 3-hydroxy-acyl-CoA dehydrogenase (LCHAD) deficiency may present with retinal pigment changes, hypoglycemia, heart failure, and multiorgan system failure [119]. A fetus with LCHAD deficiency may induce the liver disease through pregnancy in a mother who is a heterozygous carrier for the disorder since a combination of the metabolic demands of pregnancy, the lack of enzyme activity in the fetus, and the reduced activity of the enzyme in the mother, causing enough of an imbalance in the usual energy pathways to result in the storage of fat in the maternal liver [120,121]. The present dietary treatment of LCHAD is effective and based on clinical experience. It is difficult to perform double-blind studies in fatty acid oxidation disorders, looking at prevention of cardiomyopathy, muscle weakness, and/or rhabdomyolysis. A diet has been suggested that replaces dietary medium-even-chain fatty acids with medium-odd-chain fatty acids [122], which are precursors of acetyl-CoA and anaplerotic propionyl-CoA, to reinstate energy production and improve cardiac and skeletal muscle function. It performed effectively in three children with very long-chain acylCoA dehydrogenase (VLCAD) deficiency.

3.4 Mitochondrial disorders

The mitochondrial ETC consists of five multisubunit protein complexes that produce the majority of energy driving cellular responses. Respiratory chain dysfunction causes a decrease in energy production and an increase in the production of toxic reactive oxygen species. However, damaged mitochondria release apoptotic factors that act as signals to trigger cell death [123]. Respiratory chain proteins are formed by the coordinated actions of both mitochondrial and nuclear genes. Therefore, mitochondrial disorders may be inherited in a Mendelian or maternal fashion, as mutations can occur in the nuclear or mitochondrial genome [124,125].

The signs and symptoms of mitochondrial disorders depend on the percentage of dysfunctional mitochondria, the severity of the mutation, and the energy requirements of the affected tissues. Patients with mitochondrial disorders present with a bewildering array of symptoms, as any tissue in the body can be affected in any way. However, pronounced involvement of the nervous and muscular systems is common, as these tissues are highly dependent on mitochondrial metabolism [126]. Patients frequently have biochemical markers of primary disease, but some patients have totally normal metabolic screens. Frequently the diagnosis of mitochondrial disorders involves demonstration of respiratory chain dysfunction through the measurement of complex activities in muscle tissue obtained from a biopsy [127].The so-called muscle ragged red fibers may be seen on microscopic investigation and are suggestive of mitochondrial disease, however frequently are not present and may be seen in further muscle disorders [128]. Occasionally a diagnosis can be made by identifying an mtDNA mutation through molecular diagnostic techniques [129]. Conversely, not all mutations are known, and it is unreasonable to perform a widespread analysis of an individual's mtDNA [130]. Moreover, since some mitochondrial disorders may be caused by mutations inherent to the nuclear DNA, screening of nuclear genes that code for mitochondrial respiratory gene subunits eventually may be essential to pinpoint the underlying cause of a patient's symptoms; though, such a comprehensive examination is not useful [131].

Intramitochondrial metal homeostasis, transmembrane carrier proteins, and defective mitochondrial membrane ion transporters can also cause mitochondrial disorders. Neurodegenerative disorders, including Wilson's disease and Friedreich's ataxia, have been associated with abnormal mitochondrial metal metabolism; while copper metabolism is abnormal in Wilson's disease, impaired iron homeostasis is present in Friedreich's ataxia

[132,133]. In these conditions, the respiratory chain is affected secondarily. It has been theorized that mitochondrial respiratory chain dysfunction plays a role in normal aging as well as in more common neurodegenerative diseases such as Huntington's disease, Alzheimer's disease, Parkinson's disease, and amyotrophic lateral sclerosis (ALS) [134]. There is no proven therapy for patients with respiratory chain disorders, however, several dietary supplements and cofactors have been tried, and investigations have been initiated in the area of gene therapy.

3.5 Lysosomal storage disorders

Macromolecules normally degraded by lysosomes accumulate if lysosomal enzymes are deficient, their activity is reduced, or enzymes are not correctly targeted to lysosomes, encoded by nuclear DNA, and targeted to lysosomes by specific recognition markers. Thus, various complex compounds such as oligosaccharides, glycosaminoglycans, glycoproteins, and glycolipids are stored abnormally [135]. Lysosomal storage disorders are autosomal recessive, except for X-linked Fabry disease and Hunter syndrome. Abnormal macromolecule storage causes a variety of signs and symptoms depending on where the storage occurs [136]. Some diseases, such as Gaucher disease type I usually only affect peripheral tissues such as spleen, liver, or bone, diseases such as Tay-Sachs disease affect only the central nervous system, and diseases such as Niemann-Pick disease affect both the brain and systemic organs [137].

Most of the lysosomal storage disorders include eye abnormalities, coarsening of facial features, enlarged spleen, and liver and bone disease. As a group, these disorders cause severe neurological impairment, frequently starting in infancy [138]. Conversely, each disease often has a spectrum of severity depending on the degree of enzymatic compromise such as Tay-Sachs disease is usually fatal in early childhood, although some forms do not occur until adulthood [139]. Many lysosomal storage disorders have no treatment other than supportive care. The struggle with most therapies is that they do not enter the brain, due to the presence of the so-called blood-brain barrier [140]. Although bone marrow transplantation has been tried in individuals with lysosomal storage disorders, the results have been disappointing [141]. On the other hand, enzyme replacement therapy was responded to in disorders without central nervous system involvement such as Gaucher disease type I, that is, frequent intravenous infusions of the specific enzyme that is missing in the disorder and encouraging results have been informed in Pompe disease and Fabry disease [142].

3.6 Peroxisomal disorders

Peroxisomes, cytoplasmic organelles that play a central role in the catabolism of very long-chain fatty acids and other compounds during the beta-oxidation process, are critical in the biosynthesis of plasmalogens, cholesterol, and bile acids. Peroxisomes do not contain DNA, unlike mitochondria, so all components of enzyme systems and membrane proteins are encoded by the nucleus [143]. Several peroxisomal disorders are autosomal recessive inheritance, except for the X-linked form of adrenoleukodystrophy. They typically present with severe neurological compromise, but other organ systems such as kidneys and bone may similarly be affected [144]. No specific treatment exists for these disorders, and approximately all are fatal early in their course.

In some disorders, there is a decrease or complete absence of peroxisomes. This results in a severely suppressed activity of peroxisomal functions and affects the functions of many enzymes [145]. Such disorders include Zellweger syndrome with the cerebrohepatorenal disease, hyperpipecholic acidemia, neonatal adrenoleukodystrophy, and infantile Refsum disease [146]. Patients can have severely reduced hypotonia, seizures, cerebral malformations, and an enlarged liver during infancy. Many develop eye abnormalities, particularly a defect in the retinal pigment. In addition, patients with Zellweger syndrome may have cranial abnormalities and small kidney cysts [147].

In *X-linked adrenoleukodystrophy (X-ALD)*, an insidious disorder in which affected individuals develop normally early, peroxisomes seem normal, with decreased activity of only a single enzyme [148,149]. Affected boys between the ages of 4–8 have behavioral problems such as poor school performance, aggression, and hyperactivity. Children often lose their memory skills, speech, and walking abilities, and seizures occur later in the disease. The skin may have a brownish color due to adrenal insufficiency [150]. Other forms of X-ALD may not involve neurological disease, or neurological complications may be mild, as in adrenomyeloneuropathy [151]. Classical severe X-ALD and adrenomyeloneuropathy can coexist in the same family. Lorenzo oil, a mixture of trioleate and thieroate oils that improve or completely correct the elevation of very long-chain fatty acids in the blood, unfortunately, has no effect on neurological progression as it is effective but does not cross the blood-brain barrier [152]. Some success has been reported in patients treated with bone marrow transplant in the early stages of the disease [153–155].

3.7 Purine and pyrimidine disorders

Purine and pyrimidine disorders have a wide range of signs and symptoms, including susceptibility to infections, autism, severe mental disability, and kidney stones [7,8,156]. Symptoms can occur from infancy to old age. Most metabolic screening tests do not give results in the detection of purine or pyrimidine metabolism disorders, so special analyzes are required [157,158].

Adenosine deaminase (ADA) deficiency causes the accumulation of 2′-deoxyadenosine in circulating lymphocytes, leading to a decrease in lymphocyte count and severe combined immunodeficiency (SCID) [159]. In this case, while bone marrow transplantation and gene therapy can be curative, enzyme replacement therapy is the standard treatment [160,161]. Lesch-Nyhan syndrome is an X-linked condition caused by a deficiency in the hypoxanthine-guanine phosphoribosyltransferase enzyme. In this disease, the nervous system is affected and results in writhing movements in the first year of life after a normal development period. A principally worrying feature is the occurrence of self-mutilation [162,163]. Mental disability also occurs commonly. Most individuals with Lesch-Nyhan syndrome secrete large amounts of uric acid in their urine, causing conditions such as gout, kidney stones, and possible kidney failure. Although high fluid intake and allopurinol help treat joint and kidney problems, it has no effect on severe mental disability [164,165].

3.8 Porphyrin metabolism disorders

Porphyrias are inherited disorders caused by mutations in genes that direct the synthesis of enzymes involved in "heme" biosynthesis [166]. Porphyrias are a group of diseases characterized by the impairment of heme (porphyrin) synthesis and excessive accumulation of heme precursors before the defective step as a result of a partial deficiency of enzymes in the synthesis of "heme" [167]. Coproporphyrin and urporphyrin increase in the blood and are excreted in the urine in these diseases [168]. As with many hereditary defects, clinical manifestations are related to the accumulation of nonmetabolized substances as a result of enzyme defects [169]. Therefore, in some porphyrias, neuropsychiatric symptoms and abdominal pain can be seen in the abdominal nerves or central nervous system due to the toxic effects of porphyrins. These neuropathic findings are observed in each type of porphyria where the synthesis of aminolevulinic acid (ALA), which is neurotoxic, is increased [170]. In addition, photosensitivity is observed as a result of the accumulation of porphyrins in tissues, due to their characteristic absorbance at 300nm. Porphyrias are uncommon, but should not be ignored when abdominal pain and neuropsychic disorders are present in the anamnesis. Photosensitivity can cause nocturnal activities and a "werewolf" appearance. In congenital erythropoietic porphyria, urine, teeth, and bones can take on colors ranging from dark red, which can make the "werewolf" or "vampire" appearance even more realistic [171,172].

4. Present status and new trends on the treatment of metabolic disorders

4.1 Reducing the load on the affected pathway

Substrate reduction by dietary restriction: Substrate reduction therapy addresses the disease pathology associated with toxic accumulation of metabolites, by down-regulating the enzymatic step(s) involved in the biosynthesis of the metabolites. Dietary treatment is often considered the first original application of substrate reduction therapy, albeit not a pharmaceutical. Disorders in which the defective enzyme's substrate might be efficiently partial in the diet and in which substrate levels in the body may be monitored, such as MSUD or PKU [69,173].

Substrate reduction by inhibition of enzymes within the pathway: NTBC treatment in tyrosinaemia type 1 shows great efficacy. Inhibition of 4-hydroxyphenylpyruvate dioxygenase by NTBC prevents the production of fumarylacetoacetate, maleylacetoacetate, and succinylacetone, compounds that are the main toxic agents in this disease [174,175].

4.2 Correcting product deficiency

Replenishing depleted products: Where the deficiency of an enzyme's product is significant in the cause of clinical disease, replacement with the depleted product, such as the administration of carbohydrate in glycogen storage disease (GSD), citrulline or arginine in urea cycle disorders, may be efficacious [176].

Increasing substrate supply: Giving pharmacological quantities of the substrate may be effective mainly in inborn errors of membrane transport proteins, such as ornithine in triple H syndrome and L-carnitine in carnitine transporter deficiency [177].

Providing alternative substrates: In GLUT1 deficiency there is a failure of glucose to be transported through the blood-brain barrier. The ketogenic diet provides another fuel for the brain [178,179].

4.3 Decreasing metabolite toxicity

Removing toxic metabolites: Many medications are used to hasten the removal of normal metabolites that accumulate to toxic levels in particular inborn errors, such as sodium benzoate for hyperammonaemia caused by urea cycle disorders [180,181].

Blocking the effects of toxic metabolites: Disorders in which the clinical manifestation is associated with metabolites binding to receptors may be amenable to treatments that block this effect [182,183].

4.3.1 Stimulating residual enzyme

Co-enzyme treatment: Some metabolic disorders are secondary to mutations that affect the metabolism or binding of a cofactor or coenzyme, essential for normal enzyme activity. Treatment with the coenzyme may cause a comprehensive reversal of the clinical manifestations, such as biotin in biotinidase deficiency [184,185]. Other disorders may have limited advances (B12 responsive), or struggle in getting the co-enzyme to the appropriate location (disorders of biopterin synthesis). Several single enzyme disorders are owing to mutations that prevent any enzyme production and cannot consequently progress with coenzyme therapy [186].

4.3.2 Transplantation

Stem cell transfer: Hematopoetic stem cell transfer (HSCT) modifies the enzyme deficiencies related to peroxisomal and lysosomal disorders at least in cells of hematopoetic origin [187,188]. The first disorder treated by this method was mucopolysaccharidosis (MPS) type I, most qualified [189]. An effective bone marrow transplantation (BMT) in MPS I changes the natural history of the disease, however, there are considerable problems principally with joint disease and spinal deformity. Furthermore, BMT must be performed initially if neurological progress is to be prevented [190,191].

Other organ transplantation: Liver transplantation has been used as an effective treatment for a number of inborn errors of metabolism such as urea cycle disorders, organic acidaemias, homozygous familial hypercholesterolemia, severe forms of GSD [192,193].

5. Pharmacologic enzyme replacement therapy (ERT)

Enzyme replacement therapy is an interesting field of management, unfortunately, it is not yet successful for all disorders [194]. The following disorders have useful results with ERT are Gaucher Disease, Fabry Disease,

Mucopolysaccharidosis Type I, Mucopolysaccharidosis Type VI, and Pompe Disease [195–197].

5.1 Gene therapy

Gene transfer: Successful therapy for metabolic disorders must combine proper disease targeting with an effective delivery system that ensures long-term appearance with no toxicity [198]. More success has been realized in hematological disorders and gene therapy for adenosine deaminase deficiency has progressed from early trials of feasibility and safety to more current studies reporting on efficacy and clinical benefit [199].

Pharmacological gene therapy: Stimulating the expression of endogenous genes by pharmacological mediators may be responsible for treatment [200]. In hemoglobinopathies, the production of fetal hemoglobin may be stimulated by several agents such as 5-azacytidine, hydroxyurea, and sodium phenylbutyrate. Also, sodium phenylbutyrate increases CTFR gene expression in cystic fibrosis [201].

6 Conclusions

Metabolic disorders can be problematic to understand owing to their rarity and the multiplicity of conditions. Disorders of energy sources can principally be screened for by a few simple tests. Amino acidopathies can be assessed via urine organic acids (UOA) and plasma acylcarnitine (PAA) analysis; organic acidemias via urine ketones, electrolytes, UOA analysis, and PAC profile; urea cycle disorders via PAA and UOA analysis and ammonia; and fatty acid oxidation disorders (FAOD) via UOA, PAC profile, urine ketones, plasma carnitine, and blood glucose. In addition, newborn screening (NBS) allows for the early recognition of many, but not all of these disorders.

The management of patients with many metabolic disorders needs a multi-disciplinary approach that combines both nutritional and medical management. In these disorders, nutritional therapy is a serious constituent of the management to prevent acute complications, for example, metabolic decompensation, and/or to prevent long-term complications of the given disorder. Such nutritional therapy is modified for the specific disorder and individualized for each patient to support compliance. Moreover, nutritional therapy for patient with several metabolic disorders is lifelong.

References

[1] S. Lazzer, G. Bedogni, C.L. Lafortuna, N. Marazzi, C. Busti, R. Galli, A. De Col, F. Agosti, A. Sartorio, Relationship between basal metabolic rate, gender, age, and body composition in 8,780 white obese subjects, Obesity 18 (3) (2010) 71–78.

[2] J. Jaeken, R. Peanne, What is new in CDG? J. Inherit. Metab. Dis. 40 (2017) 569–586.

[3] E. Gilbert-Barness, P.M. Farrell, Approach to diagnosis of metabolic diseases, Transl. Sci. Rare Dis. 1 (2016) 3–22.

[4] J.F. Clark, K.M. Cecil, Diagnostic methods and recommendations for the cerebral creatine deficiency syndromes, Pediatr. Res. 77 (2015) 398–405.

[5] L.P. Palaniappan, E.C. Wong, J.J. Shin, S.P. Fortmann, D.S. Lauderdale, Asian Americans have greater prevalence of metabolic syndrome despite lower body mass index, Int. J. Obes. 35 (2017) 393–400.

[6] D. Frankenfield, L. Roth-Yousey, C. Compher, Comparison of predictive equations for resting metabolic rate in healthy nonobese and obese adults: a systematic review, J. Am. Diet. Assoc. 105 (5) (2005) 775–789.

[7] C.R. Scriver, A.L. Beaudet, W.S. Sly, D. Valle (Eds.), Purines and pyrimidines, in: The Metabolic and Molecular Bases of Inherited Disease, eighth ed., McGraw-Hill, New York, 2001, pp. 2512–2702.

[8] C.R. Scriver, A.L. Beaudet, W.S. Sly, D. Valle, The Metabolic and Molecular Basis of Inherited Disease, McGraw Hill, New York, 2001.

[9] A. Garrod, Inborn Errors of Metabolism, Oxford University Press, 1923.

[10] F.H. Einstein, S. Fishman, J. Bauman, R.F. Thompson, D.M. Huffman, G. Atzmon, N. Barzi, R.H. Muzumdar, Enhanced activation of a "nutrient-sensing" pathway with age contributes to insulin resistance, FASEB J. 22 (2008) 3450–3457.

[11] J.E. Morley, Diabetes and aging: epidemiologic overview, Clin. Geriatr. Med. 24 (2008) 395–405.

[12] K.F. Petersen, D. Befroy, S. Dufour, J. Dziura, C. Ariyan, D.L. Rothman, L. DiPietro, G.W. Cline, G.I. Shulman, Mitochondrial dysfunction in the elderly: possible role in insulin resistance, Science 300 (2003) 1140–1142.

[13] M. Rincon, R. Muzumdar, G. Atzmon, N. Barzilai, The paradox of the insulin/IGF-1 signaling pathway in longevity, Mech. Ageing Dev. 125 (2004) 397–403.

[14] D.L. Smith, C.F. Elam, J.A. Mattison, A.E. Lane, G.S. Roth, D.K. Ingram, D.B. Allison, Metformin supplementation and life span in Fischer-344 rats, J. Gerontol. A Biol. Sci. Med. Sci. 65 (2010) 468–474.

[15] S.H. Korman, Inborn errors of isoleucine degradation: a review, Mol. Genet. Metab. 89 (2006) 289–299.

[16] H. Ogier de Baulny, Management and emergency treatments of neonates with a suspicion of inborn errors of metabolism, Semin. Neonatol. 7 (2002) 17–26.

[17] J.M. Saudubray, A. Garcia-Cazorla, Inborn errors of metabolism overview: pathophysiology, manifestations, evaluation, and management, Pediatr. Clin. N. Am. 65 (2018) 179–208.

[18] A. Tebani, C. Afonso, S. Marret, S. Bekri, Omics-based strategies in precision medicine: toward a paradigm shift in inborn errors of metabolism investigations, Int. J. Mol. Sci. 2016 (2016) 17.

[19] R. Bonilla-Guerrero, K. Karen, D. Salazar, R. Sharma, The porphyrias, in: K. Sarafloglou (Ed.), Pediatric Endocrinology and Inborn Errors of Metabolism, second ed., McGraw Hill, New York, 2017.

[20] R.J. Wanders, Metabolic and molecular basis of peroxisomal disorders: a review, Am. J. Med. Genet. A 126A (2004) 355–375.

[21] E.J. Gardner, M.J. Simmons, D.P. Snustad, Principles of Genetics, eighth ed., Wiley, India, 2008.

[22] D.P. Snustad, M.J. Simmons, Principles of Genetics, fifth ed., John Wiley & Sons, 2009.
[23] D.L. Nelson, M.M. Cox, Lehninger, Principles of Biochemistry, fourth ed., 2008.
[24] J. Calvin, S. Hogg, Biochemical investigation for inborn errors of metabolism in adults presenting with neurological disorders, Adv. Clin. Neurosci. Rehabil. 9 (2010) 12–16.
[25] M. Pasquali, G. Monsen, L. Richardson, M. Alston, N. Longo, Biochemical findings in common inborn errors of metabolism, Am. J. Med. Genet. C: Semin. Med. Genet. 142*C* (2006) 64–76.
[26] M. Kompare, W.B. Rizzo, Mitochondrial fatty acid oxidation disorders, Semin. Pediatr. Neurol. 15 (2008) 140–149.
[27] J. Vockley, R.H. Singh, D.A. Whiteman, Diagnosis and management of defects of mitochondrial beta-oxidation, Curr. Opin. Clin. Nutr. Metab. Care 5 (2002) 601–609.
[28] J. Finsterer, S. Zarrouk-Mahjoub, Biomarkers for detecting mitochondrial disorders, J. Clin. Med. 7 (2) (2018) 16.
[29] R.H. Haas, S. Parikh, M.J. Falk, R.P. Saneto, N.I. Wolf, N. Darin, L.-J. Wong, B.H. Cohen, R.K. Naviaux, The in-depth evaluation of suspected mitochondrial disease, Mol. Genet. Metab. 94 (2008) 16–37.
[30] G.W. Beadle, E.L. Tatum, Genetic control of biochemical reactions in neurospora, Proc. Natl. Acad. Sci. U. S. A. 27 (1941) 499–506.
[31] A. Garrod, The incidence of Alkaptonuria: a study in chemical individuality, Lancet 160 (1902) 1616–1620.
[32] R.C. Eisensmith, S.L. Woo, Phenylketonuria and the phenyl-alanine hydroxylase gene, Mol. Biol. Med. 8 (1991) 3–10.
[33] P. Guldberg, H.L. Levy, W.B. Hanley, R. Koch, R. Matalon, B.M. Rouse, F. Trefz, F. de la Cruz, K.F. Henriksen, F. Güttler, Phenylalanine hydroxylase gene mutations in the United States: report from the Maternal PKU Collaborative Study, Am. J. Hum. Genet. 59 (1996) 84–94.
[34] S. Cedarbaum, Phenylketonuria: an update, Curr. Opin. Pediatr. 14 (2002) 702–706.
[35] J. Vockley, H.C. Andersson, K.M. Antshel, N.E. Braverman, B.K. Burton, D.M. Frazier, J. Mitchell, W.E. Smith, B.H. Thompson, S.A. Berry, American College of Medical Genetics and Genomics Therapeutics Committee, Phenylalanine hydroxylase deficiency: diagnosis and management guideline, Genet. Med. 16 (2014) 188–200.
[36] R. Koch, K.D. Moseley, S. Yano, M. Nelson, R.A. Moats, Large neutral amino acid therapy and phenylketonuria: a promising approach to treatment, Mol. Genet. Metab. 79 (2003) 110–113.
[37] C.J. Ellaway, E. Holme, S. Standing, M.A. Preece, A. Green, E. Ploechl, M. Ugarte, F.K. Trefz, J.V. Leonard, Outcome of tyrosinaemia type III, J. Inherit. Metab. Dis. 24 (2001) 824–832.
[38] H.L. Levy, V.E. Shih, P.M. Madigan, R.A. MacCready, Transient tyrosinemia in full-term infants, JAMA 209 (1969) 249.
[39] T. Kitagawa, Hepatorenal tyrosinemia, Proc. Jpn. Acad. Ser. B 88 (2012) 192–200.
[40] J.M. Chinsky, R. Singh, C. Ficicioglu, C.D.M. van Karnebeek, M. Grompe, G. Mitchell, S.E. Waisbren, M. Gucsavas-Calikoglu, M.P. Wasserstein, K. Coakley, C.R. Scott, Diagnosis and treatment of tyrosinemia type I: a US and Canadian consensus group review and recommendations, Genet. Med. 19 (12) (2017).
[41] G.A. Mitchell, M. Grompe, M. Lambert, R.M. Tanguay, Hypertyrosinemia, in: A.L. Beaudet, B. Vogelstein, K.W. Kinzler, et al. (Eds.), The Online Metabolic and Molecular Bases of Inherited Disease, The McGraw-Hill Companies, Inc, New York, NY, 2014.
[42] N.P. Dudman, X.W. Guo, R.B. Gordon, P.A. Dawson, D.E. Wilcken, Human homocysteine catabolism: three major pathways and their relevance to development of arterial occlusive disease, J. Nutr. 126 (Suppl. 4) (1996) 295s–300s.

[43] L.A. Kluijtmans, G.H. Boers, E.M. Stevens, W.O. Renier, J.P. Kraus, F.J. Trijbels, L.P. van den Heuvel, H.J. Blom, Defective cystathionine beta-synthase regulation by S-adenosyl-methionine in a partially pyridoxine responsive homocystinuria patient, J. Clin. Invest. 98 (1996) 285–289.

[44] J.P. Kraus, Molecular basis of phenotype expression in homocystinuria. Komrower lecture, J. Inherit. Metab. Dis. 17 (1994) 383–390.

[45] A. Hamosh, M.V. Johnston, Nonketotic hyperglycinemia, in: A.L. Beaudet, B. Vogelstein, K.M. Gibson, et al. (Eds.), The Online Metabolic and Molecular Bases of Inherited Disease, The McGraw-Hill Companies, Inc, New York, NY, 2014.

[46] R.D. Steiner, D.A. Sweetser, J.R. Rohrbaugh, S.B. Dowton, J.R. Toone, D.A. Applegarth, Nonketotic hyperglycinemia: atypical clinical and biochemical manifestations, J. Pediatr. 128 (1996) 243–246.

[47] J.L. Van Hove, P. Kishnani, J. Muenzer, R.J. Wenstrup, M.L. Summar, M.R. Brummond, A.M. Lachiewicz, Benzoate therapy and carnitine deficiency in non-ketotic hyperglycinemia, Am. J. Med. Genet. 59 (1995) 444–453.

[48] J. Häberle, Clinical and biochemical aspects of primary and secondary hyperammonemic disorders, Arch. Biochem. Biophys. 536 (2013) 101–108.

[49] R.H. Singh, W.J. Rhead, W. Smith, B. Lee, L.S. King, M. Summar, Nutritional management of urea cycle disorders, Crit. Care Clin. 21 (2005) S27–S35.

[50] N.E. Maestri, S.W. Brusilow, D.B. Clissold, S.S. Bassett, Long-term treatment of girls with ornithine transcarbamylase deficiency, N. Engl. J. Med. 335 (1996) 855–859.

[51] H. Ogier de Baulny, M. Schiff, C. Dionisi-Vici, Lysinuric protein intolerance (LPI): a multi organ disease by far more complex than a classic urea cycle disorder, Mol. Genet. Metab. 106 (2012) 12–17.

[52] H. Iyer, M. Sen, C. Prasad, C.A. Rupar, R.M. Lindsay, Coma, hyperammonemia, metabolic acidosis, and mutation: lessons learned in the acute management of late onset urea cycle disorders, Hemodial. Int. 16 (2012) 95–100.

[53] A. Auron, P.D. Brophy, Hyperammonemia in review: pathophysiology, diagnosis, and treatment, Pediatr. Nephrol. 27 (2012) 207–222.

[54] V. Walker, Ammonia toxicity and its prevention in inherited defects of the urea cycle, Diabetes. Obes. Metab. 11 (2009) 823–835.

[55] B.A. Buehler, Inherited disorders of amino acid transport in relation to the kidney, Ann. Clin. Lab. Sci. 11 (3) (1981) 274–278.

[56] W.A. Gahl, J.G. Thoene, J.A. Schneider, Cystinosis, N. Engl. J. Med. 347 (2002) 111–121.

[57] B. Liu, H. Du, R. Rutkowski, A. Gartner, X. Wang, LAAT-1 is the lysosomal lysine/arginine transporter that maintains amino acid homeostasis, Science 337 (2012) 351–354.

[58] J.M. Saudubray, D. Rabier, Biomarkers identified in inborn errors for lysine, arginine, and ornithine, J. Nutr. 137 (2007) 1669S–1672S.

[59] A. Jézégou, E. Llinares, C. Anne, C. Kieffer-Jaquinod, S. O'Regan, J. Aupetit, A. Chabli, C. Sagné, C. Debacker, B. Chadefaux-Vekemans, A. Journet, B. André, B. Gasnier, Heptahelical protein PQLC2 is a lysosomal cationic amino acid exporter underlying the action of cysteamine in cystinosis therapy, Proc. Natl. Acad. Sci. U. S. A. 109 (2012) E3434–E3443.

[60] G. Nesterova, W.A. Gahl, Cystinosis: the evolution of a treatable disease, Pediatr. Nephrol. 28 (2013) 51–59.

[61] K. Vaidyanathan, M.P. Narayanan, D.M. Vasudevan, Organic acidurias: an updated review, Indian J. Clin. Biochem. 26 (2011) 319–325.

[62] H. Ogier de Baulny, J.M. Saudubray, Branched-chain organic acidurias, Semin. Neonatol. 7 (2002) 65–74.

[63] G. Touati, V. Valayannopoulos, K. Mention, Methylmalonic and propionic acidurias: management without or with a few supplements of specific amino acid mixture, J. Inherit. Metab. Dis. 29 (2006) 288–298.
[64] B. Wolf, Y.E. Hsia, L. Sweetman, R. Gravel, D.J. Harris, W.L. Nyhan, Propionic acidemia: a clinical update, J. Pediatr. 99 (1981) 835–846.
[65] W. Lehnert, W. Sperl, T. Suormala, E.R. Baumgartner, Propionic acidaemia: clinical, biochemical and therapeutic aspects. Experience in 30 patients, Eur. J. Pediatr. 153 (1994) 68–80.
[66] L. Pena, J. Franks, K.A. Chapman, A. Gropman, N. Ah Mew, A. Chakrapani, E. Island, E. MacLeod, D. Matern, B. Smith, K. Stagni, V.R. Sutton, K. Ueda, T. Urv, C. Venditti, G.M. Enns, M.L. Summar, Natural history of propionic acidemia, Mol. Genet. Metab. 105 (2012) 5–9.
[67] A.T. Tuncel, N. Boy, M.A. Morath, F. Hörster, U. Mütze, S. Kölker, Organic acidurias in adults: late complications and management, J. Inherit. Metab. Dis. 41 (5) (2018) 765–776.
[68] M.R. Baumgartner, F. Hörster, C. Dionisi-Vici, G. Haliloglu, D. Karall, K.A. Chapman, M. Huemer, M. Hochuli, M. Assoun, D. Ballhausen, A. Burlina, B. Fowler, S.C. Grünert, S. Grünewald, T. Honzik, B. Merinero, C. Pérez-Cerdá, S. Scholl-Bürgi, F. Skovby, F. Wijburg, A. MacDonald, D. Martinelli, J.O. Sass, V. Valayannopoulos, A. Chakrapani, Proposed guidelines for the diagnosis and management of methylmalonic and propionic acidemia, Orphanet J. Rare Dis. 9 (2014) 130–138.
[69] D.M. Frazier, C. Allgeier, C. Homer, B.J. Marriage, B. Ogata, F. Rohr, P.L. Splett, A. Stembridge, R.H. Singh, Nutrition management guideline for maple syrup urine disease: an evidence- and consensus-based approach, Mol. Genet. Metab. 112 (2014) 210–217.
[70] D.H. Morton, K.A. Strauss, D.L. Robinson, E.G. Puffenberger, R.I. Kelley, Diagnosis and treatment of maple syrup dis-ease: a study of 36 patients, Pediatrics 109 (2002) 999–1008.
[71] D.T. Chuang, J.R. Davie, R.M. Wynn, J.L. Chuang, H. Koyatam, R.P. Cox, Molecular basis of maple syrup urine disease and stable correction by retroviral gene transfer, J. Nutr. 125 (1995) 1766S–1772S.
[72] D.T. Chuang, J.L. Chuang, R.M. Wynn, Lessons from genetic disorders of branched-chain amino acidmetabolism, J. Nutr. 136 (1 Suppl) (2006) 243S–249S.
[73] G. Novarino, P. El-Fishawy, H. Kayserili, N.A. Meguid, E.M. Scott, J. Schroth, J.L. Silhavy, M. Kara, R.O. Khalil, T. Ben-Omran, A.G. Ercan-Sencicek, A.F. Hashish, S.J. Sanders, A.R. Gupta, H.S. Hashem, D. Matern, S. Gabriel, L. Sweetman, Y. Rahimi, R.A. Harris, M.W. State, J.G. Gleeson, Mutations in BCKD-kinase lead to a potentially treatable form of autism with epilepsy, Science 338 (2012) 394–397.
[74] B. Pérez, C. Medrano, M.J. Ecay, et al., A novel congenital disorder of glycosylation type without central nervous system involvement caused by mutations in the phosphoglucomutase 1 gene, J. Inherit. Metab. Dis. 36 (2013) 535–542.
[75] N.D. Leslie, Insights into the pathogenesis of galactosemia, Annu. Rev. Nutr. 23 (2003) 59–80.
[76] S.E. Waisbren, N.L. Potter, C.M. Gordon, R.C. Green, P. Greenstein, C.S. Gubbels, E. Rubio-Gozalbo, D. Schomer, C. Welt, A. Wessl, B.-L. Wu, H. Levy, L. Elsas, G.T. Berry, The adult galactosemic phenotype, J. Inherit. Metab. Dis. 35 (2012) 279–286.
[77] R.B. Canani, V. Pezzella, A. Amoroso, T. Cozzolino, C. Di Scala, A. Passariell, Diagnosing and treating intolerance to carbohydrates in children, Nutrients 8 (3) (2016) 157.
[78] J.B. Holton, J.H. Walter, L.A. Tyfield, Galactosemia, in: W.S. Sly, D. Valle, C.R. Scriver (Eds.), The Metabolic and Molecular Bases of Inherited Disease, McGraw-Hill, New York, 2001, pp. 1553–1587.
[79] D.J. Timson, The molecular basis of galactosemia—past, present and future, Gene 589 (2) (2016) 133–141.

[80] P.P. Jumbo-Lucioni, K. Garber, J. Kiel, I. Baric, G.T. Berry, A. Bosch, A. Burlina, A. Chiesa, M.C. Pico, S.C. Estrada, H. Henderson, N. Leslie, N. Longo, A.A.M. Morris, C. Ramirez-Farias, S. Schweitzer-Krantz, C.L.T. Silao, M. Vela-Amieva, S. Waisbren, J.L. Fridovich-Keil, Diversity of approaches to classic galactosemia around the world: a comparison of diagnosis, intervention, and outcomes, J. Inherit. Metab. Dis. 35 (2012) 1037–1049.

[81] G.T. Berrry, J.H. Walter, Disorders of galactose metabolism, in: J. Fernandes, J.M. Saudubray, G. van den Berghe, J.H. Walter (Eds.), Inborn Metabolic Diseases, fifth ed., Springer, Heidelberg, 2012, pp. 141–150.

[82] I.M. Yasawy, U.R. Folsch, W.E. Schmidt, M. Schwend, Adult hereditary fructose intolerance, World J. Gastroenterol. 15 (19) (2009) 2412–2413.

[83] H. Li, H.M. Byers, A. Diaz-Kuan, M.B. Vos, P.L. Hall, S. Tortorelli, R. Singh, M.B. Wallenstein, M. Allain, D.P. Dimmock, R.M. Farrell, S. McCandless, M.J. Gambello, Acute liver failure in neonates with undiagnosed hereditary fructose intolerance due to exposure from widely available infant formulas, Mol. Genet. Metab. 123 (2018) 428–432.

[84] N. Bouteldja, D.J. Timson, The biochemical basis of hereditary fructose intolerance, J. Inherit. Metab. Dis. 33 (2010) 105–112.

[85] R. Santer, J. Rischewski, M. von Weihe, M. Niederhaus, S. Schneppenheim, K. Baerlocher, A. Kohlschütter, A. Muntau, H.-G. Posselt, B. Steinmann, The spectrum of aldolase B (ALDOB) mutations and the prevalence of hereditary fructose intolerance in Central Europe, Hum. Mutat. 25 (2005) 594.

[86] B. Steinmann, R. Santer, Disorders of fructose metabolism, in: J. Fernandes, J.M. Saudubray, G. van den Berghe, J.H. Walter (Eds.), Inborn Metabolic Diseases, fourth ed., Springer, Heidelberg, 2012, pp. 101–112.

[87] H.H. Huidekoper, G. Visser, M.T. Ackermans, H.P. Sauerwein, F.A. Wijburg, A potential role for muscle in glucose homeostasis: in vivo kinetic studies in glycogen storage disease type 1a and fructose-1,6-bisphosphatase deficiency, J. Inherit. Metab. Dis. 33 (2010) 25–31.

[88] M.W. Kilimann, A. Oldfors, Glycogen pathways in disease: new developments in a classical field of medical genetics, J. Inherit. Metab. Dis. 38 (2015) 483–487.

[89] Y.T. Chen, Glycogen storage diseases, in: C.R. Scriver, A. Beaudet, W.S. Sly, D. Valle (Eds.), The Metabolic and Molecular Bases of Inherited Disease, McGraw-Hill, New York, 2001, pp. 1521–1551.

[90] W.G. Leen, J. Klepper, M.M. Verbeek, M. Leferink, T. Hofste, B.G. van Engelen, R.A. Wevers, T. Arthur, N. Bahi-Buisson, D. Ballhausen, J. Bekhof, P. van Bogaert, I. Carrilho, B. Chabrol, M.P. Champion, J. Coldwell, P. Clayton, E. Donner, A. Evangeliou, F. Ebinger, K. Farrell, R.J. Forsyth, C. de Goede, S. Gross, S. Grunewald, H. Scheffer, M.A. Willemsen, Glucose transporter-1 deficiency syndrome: the expanding clinical and genetic spectrum of a treatable disorder, Brain 133 (2010) 655–670.

[91] M. Adeva-Andany, M. González-Lucán, C. Donapetry-García, C. Fernández-Fernández, E. Ameneiros-Rodríguez, Glycogen metabolism in humans, BBA Clin. 5 (2016) 85–100.

[92] M.K. Davis, D.A. Weinstein, Liver transplantation in children with glycogen storage disease: controversies and evaluation of the risk/benefit of this procedure, Pediatr. Transplant. 12 (2008) 137–145.

[93] J.Y. Chou, N. Raben, Glycogen storage diseases (GSDs), Curr. Mol. Med. 2 (2002) 101–227.

[94] B. Cylwik, M. Naklicki, L. Chrostek, E. Gruszewska, Congenital disorders of glycosylation. Part I. Defects of protein N-glycosylation, Acta Biochim. Pol. 60 (2013) 151–161.

[95] J. Jaeken, G. Matthijs, Congenital disorders of glycosylation: a rapidly expanding disease family, Annu. Rev. Genomics Hum. Genet. 8 (2007) 261–278.

[96] P. de Lonlay, N. Seta, S. Barrot, B. Chabrol, V. Drouin, B.M. Gabriel, H. Journel, M. Kretz, J. Laurent, M. Le Merrer, A. Leroy, D. Pedespan, P. Sarda, N. Villeneuve, J. Schmitz, E. van Schaftingen, G. Matthijs, J. Jaeken, C. Korner, A. Munnich, J.M. Saudubray, V. Cormier-Daire, A broad spectrum of clinical presentations in congenital disorders of glycosylation I: a series of 26 cases, J. Med. Genet. 38 (2001) 14–19.
[97] E. Schollen, S. Kjaergaard, E. Legius, M. Schwartz, G. Matthijs, Lack of Hardy-Weinberg equilibrium for the most prevalent PMM2 mutation in CDG-Ia (congenital disorders of glycosylation type Ia), Eur. J. Hum. Genet. 8 (2000) 367–371.
[98] J. Jaeken, G. Matthijs, Congenital disorders of glycosylation, Annu. Rev. Genomics Hum. Genet. 2 (2001) 129–151.
[99] D.J. Rader, J.M. Hoeg, H.B. Brewer, Quantitation of plasma apolipoproteins in the primary and secondary prevention of coronary artery disease, Ann. Intern. Med. 120 (12) (1994) 1012–1025.
[100] M.C. Orngreen, R. Ejstrup, J. Vissing, Effect of diet on exercise tolerance in carnitine palmitoyltransferase II deficiency, Neurology 61 (2003) 559–561.
[101] S. Ishibashi, M.S. Brown, J.L. Goldstein, R.D. Gerard, R.E. Hammer, J. Herz, Hypercholesterolemia in low density lipoprotein receptor knockout mice and its reversal by adenovirus-mediated gene delivery, J. Clin. Investig. 92 (2) (1993) 883–893.
[102] J.A. Shaw, A. Bobik, A. Murphy, P. Kanellakis, P. Blombery, N. Mukhamedova, K. Woollard, S. Lyon, D. Sviridov, A.M. Dart, Infusion of reconstituted highdensity lipoprotein leads to acute changes in human atherosclerotic plaque, Circ. Res. 103 (2008) 1084–1091.
[103] H.H. Hobbs, D.W. Russell, M.S. Brown, J.L. Goldstein, The LDL receptor locus in familial hypercholesterolemia: mutational analysis of a membrane protein, Annu. Rev. Genet. 24 (1990) 133–170.
[104] A.C. Goldberg, P.N. Hopkins, P.P. Toth, C.M. Ballantyne, D.J. Rader, J.G. Robinson, S.R. Daniels, S.S. Gidding, S.D. de Ferranti, M.K. Ito, M.P. McGowan, P.M. Moriarty, W.C. Cromwell, J.L. Ross, P.E. Ziajka, National Lipid Association Expert Panel on Familial Hypercholesterolemia, Familial hypercholesterolemia: Screening, diagnosis and management of pediatric and adult patients: clinical guidance from the National Lipid Association Expert Panel on Familial Hypercholesterolemia, J. Clin. Lipidol. 5 (3 Suppl) (2011) S1–S8.
[105] A. Wiegman, B.A. Hutten, E. de Groot, J. Rodenburg, H.D. Bakker, H.R. Büller, E.J.G. Sijbrands, J.J.P. Kastelein, Efficacy and safety of statin therapy in children with familial hypercholesterolemia: a randomized controlled trial, JAMA 292 (2004) 331–337.
[106] S.R. Daniels, F.R. Greer, Committee on Nutrition., Lipid screening and cardiovascular health in childhood, Pediatrics 122 (2008) 198–208.
[107] M. Soufi, B. Kurt, H. Schweer, A.M. Sattler, G. Klaus, J. Zschocke, J.R. Schaefer, Genetics and kinetics of familial hypercholesterolemia, with the special focus on FH-(Marburg) p.W556R, Atheroscler. Suppl. 10 (2009) 5–11.
[108] K.K. Buhman, M. Accad, S. Novak, R.S. Choi, J.S. Wong, R.L. Hamilton, S. Turley, R.V. Farese, Resistance to diet-induced hypercholesterolemia and gallstone formation in ACAT2-deficient mice, Nat. Med. 6 (12) (2000) 1341–1347.
[109] J.O. Sass, T. Fukao, G.A. Mitchell, Inborn errors of ketone body metabolism and transport: an update for the clinic and for clinical laboratories, J. Inborn Erros Metab. 6 (2018) 1–7.
[110] R.C. Wüst, G. Visser, R.J. Wanders, R.H. Houtkooper, Ketones and inborn errors of metabolism: old friends revisited, J. Inherit. Metab. Dis. 40 (2017) 3–4.
[111] M.B. Gillingham, Nutrition studies in long-chain fatty acid oxidation disorders: diet composition and monitoring, in: Nutrition Management of Inherited Metabolic Diseases, Springer International Publishing, Switzerland, 2015.
[112] J.P. Bonnefont, J. Bastin, A. Behin, F. Djouadi, Bezafibrate for an inborn mitochondrial beta-oxidation defect, N. Engl. J. Med. 360 (2009) 838–840.

[113] V.A. Zammit, R.R. Ramsay, M. Bonomini, A. Arduini, Carnitine, mitochondrial function and therapy, Adv. Drug Deliv. Rev. 61 (2009) 1353–1362.
[114] E. Wraige, M.P. Champion, C. Turner, R.N. Dalton, Fat oxidation defect presenting with overwhelming ketonuria, Arch. Dis. Child. 87 (2002) 428–429.
[115] J.S. Patel, J.V. Leonard, Ketonuria and medium-chain acylCoA dehydrogenase deficiency, J. Inherit. Metab. Dis. 18 (1995) 98–99.
[116] J.M. Saudubray, D. Martin, P. de Lonlay, G. Touati, F. Poggi-Travert, D. Bonnet, P. Jouvet, M. Boutron, A. Slama, C. Vianey-Saban, J.P. Bonnefont, D. Rabier, P. Kamoun, M. Brivet, Recognition and management of fatty acid oxidation defects: a series of 107 patients, J. Inherit. Metab. Dis. 22 (1999) 488–502.
[117] L. Aksglaede, M. Christensen, J.H. Olesen, M. Duno, R.K. Olsen, B.S. Andresen, D.M. Hougaard, A.M. Lund, Abnormal newborn screening in a healthy infant of a mother with undiagnosed medium-chain Acyl-CoA dehydrogenase deficiency, JIMD Rep. 23 (2015) 67–70.
[118] K.B. Leydiker, J.A. Neidich, F. Lorey, E.M. Barr, R.L. Puckett, R.M. Lobo, J.E. Abdenur, Maternal medium-chain acyl-CoA dehydrogenase deficiency identified by newborn screening, Mol. Genet. Metab. 103 (2011) 92–95.
[119] M.J. Bennett, M.J. Weinberger, J.A. Kobori, P. Rinaldo, A.B. Burlina, Mitochondrial short-chain L-3-hydroxyacyl-coenzyme A dehydrogenase deficiency: a new defect of fatty acid oxidation, Pediatr. Res. 39 (1996) 185–188.
[120] M.B. Gillingham, D. Matern, C.O. Harding, Effect of feeding, exercise and genotype on plasma 3-hydroxyacylcarnitines in children with LCHAD deficiency, Top. Clin. Nutr. 24 (2009) 359–365.
[121] M.B. Gillingham, B. Scott, D. Elliott, C.O. Harding, Metabolic control during exercise with and without medium-chain triglycerides (MCT) in children with long-chain 3-hydroxy acyl-CoA dehydrogenase (LCHAD) or trifunctional protein (TFP) deficiency, Mol. Genet. Metab. 89 (2006) 58–63.
[122] C.R. Roe, L. Sweetman, D.S. Roe, F. David, H. Brunengraber, Treatment of cardiomyopathy and rhabdomyolysis in long-chain fat oxidation disorders using an anaplerotic odd-chain triglyceride, J. Clin. Investig. 110 (2002) 259–269.
[123] D.R. Thorburn, H.H. Dahl, Mitochondrial disorders: genetics, counseling, prenatal diagnosis and reproductive options, Am. J. Med. Genet. 106 (2001) 102–114.
[124] P. Chinnery, K. Majamaa, D. Turnbull, D. Thorburn, Treatment for mitochondrial disorders, Cochrane Database Syst. Rev. 1 (2006) CD004426.
[125] P.F. Chinnery, D.M. Turnbull, Epidemiology and treatment of mitochondrial disorders, Am. J. Med. Genet. 106 (2001) 94–101.
[126] I. Nelson, M.G. Hanna, N. Alsanjari, F. Scaravilli, J.A. Morgan-Hughes, A.E. Harding, A new mitochondrial DNA mutation associated with progressive dementia and chorea: a clinical, pathological, and molecular genetic study, Ann. Neurol. 37 (1995) 400–403.
[127] R.W. Taylor, A. Pyle, H. Griffin, E.L. Blakely, J. Duff, L. He, T. Smertenko, C.L. Alston, V.C. Neeve, A. Best, J.W. Yarham, J. Kirschner, U. Schara, B. Talim, H. Topaloglu, I. Baric, E. Holinski-Feder, A. Abicht, B. Czermin, S. Kleinle, A.A. Morris, G. Vassallo, G.S. Gorman, V. Ramesh, D.M. Turnbull, M. Santibanez-Koref, R. McFarland, R. Horvath, P.F. Chinnery, Use of whole-exome sequencing to determine the genetic basis of multiple mitochondrial respiratory chain complex deficiencies, JAMA 312 (2014) 68–77.
[128] J. Arpa, A. Cruz-Martinez, Y. Campos, M. Gutierrez-Molina, F. Garcia-Rio, C. Perez-Conde, M.A. Martin, J.C. Rubio, P. Del Hoyo, A. Arpa-Fernandez, J. Arenas, Prevalence and progression of mitochondrial diseases: a study of 50 patients, Muscle Nerve 28 (2003) 690–695.
[129] N.G. Larsson, D.A. Clayton, Molecular genetic aspects of human mitochondrial disorders, Annu. Rev. Genet. 29 (1995) 151–178.

[130] S. Di Mauro, E.A. Schon, Mitochondrial DNA mutations in human disease, Am. J. Med. Genet. 106 (2001) 18–26.
[131] A. Munnich, P. Rustin, Clinical spectrum and diagnosis of mitochondrial disorders, Am. J. Med. Genet. 106 (2001) 4–17.
[132] J.V. Leonard, A.V.H. Schapira, Mitochondrial respiratory chain disorders II: neurodegenerative disorders and nuclear gene defects, Lancet 355 (2000) 389–394.
[133] A. Rötig, P. de Lonlay, D. Chretien, F. Foury, M. Koenig, D. Sidi, A. Munnich, P. Rustin, Aconitase and mitochondrial iron-sulphur protein deficiency in Friedreich ataxia, Nat. Genet. 17 (1997) 215–217.
[134] S. Lutsenko, M.J. Cooper, Localization of the Wilson's disease protein product to mitochondria, Proc. Natl. Acad. Sci. U. S. A. 95 (1998) 6004–6009.
[135] J.E. Wraith, Lysosomal disorders, Semin. Neonatol. 7 (2002) 75–83.
[136] B.A. Heese, Current strategies in the management of lysosomal storage diseases, Semin. Pediatr. Neurol. 15 (2008) 119–126.
[137] M. Ries, E. Schaefer, T. Lührs, L. Mani, J. Kuhn, M.T. Vanier, F. Krummenauer, A. Gal, M. Beck, E. Mengel, Critical assessment of chitotriosidase analysis in the rational laboratory diagnosis of children with Gaucher disease and NiemannPick disease type A/B and C, J. Inherit. Metab. Dis. 29 (2006) 647–652.
[138] A.W.N. Garcia-Cazorla, G.F. Hoffman, Neurological disease, in: G.F. Hoffman, J. Zschocke, W.L. Nyhan (Eds.), Inherited Metabolic Diseases: A Clinical Approach, 2010, pp. 127–159.
[139] B. Winchester, Lysosomal diseases: diagnostic update, J. Inherit. Metab. Dis. 37 (2014) 599–608.
[140] S. Elliott, N. Buroker, J.J. Cournoyer, A.M. Potier, J.D. Trometer, C. Elbin, M.J. Schermer, J. Kantola, A. Boyce, F. Turecek, M.H. Gelb, C.R. Scott, Pilot study of newborn screening for six lysosomal storage diseases using Tandem Mass Spectrometry, Mol. Genet. Metab. 118 (2016) 304–309.
[141] P. Tanpaiboon, G. Lopez, Lysosomal storage disorders and epilepsy, in: P.L. Pearl (Ed.), Inherited Metabolic Epilepsies, second ed., Demos Medical Publishing, LLC, New York, 2017.
[142] B.A. Johnson, A. Dajnoki, O. Bodamer, Diagnosis of lysosomal storage disorders: Gaucher disease, Curr. Protoc. Human Genet. 82 (2014) 1–6.
[143] B.M. Goldman, G. Blobel, Biogenesis of peroxisomes: intracellular site of synthesis of catalase and uricase, Proc. Natl. Acad. Sci. U. S. A. 75 (1978) 5066–5070.
[144] S. Steinberg, G. Dodt, G. Raymond, N. Braverman, A. Moser, H. Moser, Peroxisome biogenesis disorders, Biochim. Biophys. Acta (BBA)–Mol. Cell Res. 1763 (12) (2006) 1733.
[145] G.V. Raymond, P. Watkins, S. Steinberg, J. Powers, Peroxisomal disorders, in: Handbook of Neurochemistry and Molecular Neurobiology, 2009, pp. 631–670.
[146] H.S.A. Heymans, R.B.H. Schutgens, R. Tan, H. van den Bosch, P. Borst, Severe plasmalogen deficiency in tissues of infants without peroxisomes (Zellweger syndrome), Nature 306 (1983) 69–70.
[147] W.Y. Yik, S.J. Steinberg, A.B. Moser, H.W. Moser, J.G. Hacia, Identification of novel mutations and sequence variation in the Zellweger syndrome spectrum of peroxisome biogenesis disorders, Hum. Mutat. 30 (3) (2009) E467–E480.
[148] B.R. Migeon, H.W. Moser, A.B. Moser, J. Axelman, D. Sillence, R.A. Norum, Adrenoleukodystrophy: evidence for X linkage, inactivation, and selection favoring the mutant allele in heterozygous cells, Proc. Natl. Acad. Sci. U. S. A. 78 (8) (1981) 5066–5070.
[149] J. Mosser, Y. Lutz, M.E. Stoeckel, C.O. Sarde, C. Kretz, A.M. Douar, L. Lopez, P. Aubourg, J.L. Mandel, The gene responsible for adrenoleukodystrophy encodes a peroxisomal membrane protein, Hum. Mol. Genet. 3 (2) (1994) 265–271.

[150] P. Dubey, G.V. Raymond, A.B. Moser, S. Kharkar, L. Bezman, H.W. Moser, Adrenal insufficiency in asymptomatic adrenoleukodystrophy patients identified by very long-chain fatty acid screening, J. Pediatr. 146 (4) (2005) 528–532.
[151] M. Engelen, S. Kemp, M. de Visser, B.M. van Geel, R.J. Wanders, P. Aubourg, B.T. Poll-The, X-linked adrenoleukodystrophy (X-ALD): clinical presentation and guidelines for diagnosis, follow-up and management, Orphanet J. Rare Dis. 7 (2012) 51.
[152] B.M. van Geel, J. Assies, E.B. Haverkort, J.H. Koelman, B. Verbeeten, R.J. Wanders, P.G. Barth, Progression of abnormalities in adrenomyeloneuropathy and neurologically asymptomatic Xlinked adrenoleukodystrophy despite treatment with "Lorenzo's oil", J. Neurol. Neurosurg. Psychiatry 67 (3) (1999) 290–299.
[153] N. Cartier, S. Hacein-Bey-Abina, C.C. Bartholomae, G. Veres, M. Schmidt, I. Kutschera, M. Vidaud, U. Abel, L. Dal-Cortivo, L. Caccavelli, N. Mahlaoui, V. Kiermer, D. Mittelstaedt, C. Bellesme, N. Lahlou, F. Lefrère, S. Blanche, M. Audit, E. Payen, P. Leboulch, B. L'Homme, P. Bougnères, C.V. Kalle, A. Fischer, M. Cavazzana-Calvo, P. Aubourg, Hematopoietic stem cell gene therapy with a lentiviral vector in X-linked adrenoleukodystrophy, Science 326 (5954) (2009) 818–823.
[154] S. Hein, P. Schonfeld, S. Kahlert, G. Reiser, Toxic effects of X-linked adrenoleukodystrophy-associated, very long chain fatty acids on glial cells and neurons from rat hippocampus in culture, Hum. Mol. Genet. 17 (12) (2008) 1750–1761.
[155] S. Kemp, J. Berger, P. Aubourg, X-linked adrenoleukodystrophy: clinical, metabolic, genetic and pathophysiological aspects, Biochim. Biophys. Acta 1822 (9) (2012) 1465–1474.
[156] M. Loffler, L.D. Fairbanks, E. Zameitat, A.M. Marinaki, H.A. Simmonds, Pyrimidine pathways in health and disease, Trends Mol. Med. 11 (2005) 430–437.
[157] G.M. Enns, A.J. Barkovich, A.B. Van Kuilenburg, M. Manning, T. Sanger, D.R. Witt, A.H. van Gennip, Head imaging abnormalities in dihydropyrimidine dehydrogenase deficiency, J. Inherit. Metab. Dis. 27 (2004) 513–522.
[158] W.L. Nyhan, Disorders of purine and pyrimidine metabolism, Mol. Genet. Metab. 86 (2005) 25–33.
[159] D. Valik, J. Jones, Hereditary disorders of purine and pyrimidine metabolism: identification of their biochemical phenotypes in the clinical laboratory, Mayo Clin. Proc. 72 (1997) 719–725.
[160] H.D. Ochs, J.E. Yount, E.R. Giblett, S.H. Chen, C.R. Scott, R.J. Wedgwood, Adenosine-deaminase deficiency and severe combined immunodeficiency syndrome, Lancet 301 (7816) (1973) 1393–1394.
[161] G. Rijksen, W. Kuis, S.K. Wadman, L.J. Spaapen, M. Duran, B.S. Voorbrood, G.E. Staal, J.W. Stoop, B.J. Zegers, A new case of purine nucleoside phosphorylase deficiency: enzymologic, clinical, and immunologic characteristics, Pediatr. Res. 21 (1987) 137–141.
[162] A.H. Van Gennip, Defects in metabolism of purines and pyrimidines, Ned. Tijdsch. Klin. Chem. 24 (1999) 171–175.
[163] S.K. Wadman, P.K. de Bree, A.H. van Gennip, J.W. Stoop, B.J. Zegers, G.E. Staal, L.H. Siegenbeek, Urinary purines in a patients with severely defective T cell immunity and purine nucleoside phosphorylase deficiency, Adv. Exp. Med. Biol. 76A (1977) 471–476.
[164] J. Clarke, Laboratory investigations and treatment, in: J. Clarke (Ed.), A Clinical Guide to Inherited Metabolic Diseases, Cambridge University Press, Port Chester, NY, 2006, pp. 241–321.
[165] G.J. Peters, A.B. Van Kuileburg, R.A. Abreu, Purine and pyrimidine metabolism: new challenges, Nucleosides Nucleotides Nucleic Acids 23 (2004) 1077–1079.
[166] P. Poblete-Gutierrez, S. Badeloe, T. Wiederholt, H.F. Merk, J. Frank, Dual porphyrias revisited, Exp. Dermatol. 15 (9) (2006) 685–691.

[167] K. Furuyama, K. Kaneko, P.D. Vargas, Heme as a magnificent molecule with multiple missions: heme determines its own fate and governs cellular homeostasis, Tohoku J. Exp. Med. 213 (1) (2007) 1–16.
[168] D.S. Lee, E. Flachsova, M. Bodnarova, B. Demeler, P. Martásek, C.S. Raman, Structural basis of hereditary coproporphyria, Proc. Natl. Acad. Sci. U. S. A. 102 (40) (2005) 14232–14237.
[169] G.H. Elder, R.J. Hift, P.N. Meissner, The acute porphyrias, Lancet 349 (9065) (1997) 1613–1617.
[170] C. Canavese, D. Gabrielli, C. Guida, M.D. Cappellini, Nephrologists and porphyrias, G. Ital. Nefrol. 19 (4) (2002) 393–412.
[171] R.W. Hedger, W.H. Wehrmacher, A.V. French, Porphyria syndrome associated with diabetic nephrosclerosis and erythropoietin, Compr. Therapy 32 (3) (2006) 163–171.
[172] D.J. Todd, Erythropoietic protoporphyria, Br. J. Dermatol. 131 (6) (1994) 751–766.
[173] S.C. van Calcar, E.L. MacLeod, S.T. Gleason, M.R. Etzel, M.K. Clayton, J.A. Wolff, D.M. Ney, Improved nutritional management of phenylketonuria by using a diet containing glycomacropeptide compared with amino acids, Am. J. Clin. Nutr. 89 (4) (2009) 1068–1077.
[174] A.M. Bosch, Classic galactosemia: dietary dilemmas, J. Inherit. Metab. Dis. 34 (2) (2011) 257–260.
[175] A.M. Bosch, Classical galactosaemia revisited, J. Inherit. Metab. Dis. 29 (4) (2010) 516–525.
[176] S.W. Boyer, L.J. Barclay, L.C. Burrage, Inherited metabolic disorders: aspects of chronic nutritional management, Nutr. Clin. Pract. 30 (4) (2015) 502–510.
[177] N. Longo, A. di San, C. Filippo, M. Pasquali, Disorders of carnitine transport and the carnitine cycle, Am. J. Med. Genet. C: Semin. Med. Genet. 142C (2006) 77–85.
[178] A.I. Amaral, Effects of hypoglycaemia on neuronal metabolism in the adult brain: role of alternative substrates to Glucose, J. Inherit. Metab. Dis. 36 (4) (2013) 621–634.
[179] M.G. Bischof, A. Brehm, E. Bernroider, M. Krssák, V. Mlynárik, M. Krebs, M. Roden, Cerebral glutamate metabolism during hypoglycaemia in healthy and type 1 diabetic humans, Eur. J. Clin. Investig. 36 (3) (2006) 164–169.
[180] G.M. Enns, S.A. Berry, G.T. Berry, W.J. Rhead, S.W. Brusilow, A. Hamosh, Survival after treatment with phenylacetate and benzoate for urea-cycle disorders, N. Engl. J. Med. 356 (22) (2007) 2282–2292.
[181] M.J. Miller, A.D. Kennedy, A.D. Eckhart, L.C. Burrage, J.E. Wuff, L.A.D. Miller, M.V. Milburn, J.A. Ryals, A.L. Beaudet, Q. Sun, V.R. Sutton, S.H. Elsea, Untargeted metabolomic analysis for the clinical screening of inborn errors of metabolism, J. Inherit. Metab. Dis. 38 (2015) 1029–1039.
[182] A.S. Clay, B.E. Hainline, Hyperammonemia in the ICU, Chest 132 (2007) 1368–1378.
[183] N.E. Maestri, D. Clissold, S.W. Brusilow, Neonatal onset ornithine transcarbamylase deficiency: a retrospective analysis, J. Pediatr. 134 (1999) 268–272.
[184] J. Fernanddes, J.M. Saudubray, G. Van den Berghe, Inborn Metabolic Diseases, third ed., Springer, Berlin, Heidelberg, New York, 2000.
[185] E. Treacy, D. Valle, C.R. Scriver, The treatment of genetic diseases, in: C.R. Scriver, et al. (Eds.), The Metabolic and Molecular Bases of Inherited Diseases, eighth ed., McGraw Hill, New York, 2001, pp. 175–191.
[186] C.A. Stanley, Carnitine deficiency disorders in children, Ann. N. Y. Acad. Sci. 1033 (2004) 42–51.
[187] M.R. Alison, R. Poulsom, R. Jeffery, A.P. Dhillon, A. Quaglia, J. Jacob, M. Novelli, G. Prentice, J. Williamson, N.A. Wright, Hepatocytes from non-hepatic adult stem cells, Nature 406 (6793) (2000) 257.

[188] K. Overturf, M. Al-Dhalimy, K. Manning, C.N. Ou, M. Finegold, M. Grompe, Ex vivo hepatic gene therapy of a mouse model of Hereditary Tyrosinemia Type I, Hum. Gene Ther. 9 (3) (1998) 295–304.
[189] R. Arnon, N. Kerkar, M.K. Davis, R. Anand, W. Yin, R.P. González-Peralta, SPLIT Research Group, Liver transplantation in children with metabolic diseases: the studies of pediatric liver transplantation experience, Pediatr. Transplant. 14 (6) (2010) 796–805.
[190] M.Z. Ratajczak, M. Kucia, R. Reca, M. Majka, A. Janowska-Wieczorek, J. Ratajczak, Stem cell plasticity revisited: CXCR4-positive cells expressing mRNA for early muscle, liver and neural cells 'hide out' in the bone marrow, Leukemia 18 (1) (2004) 29–40.
[191] S. Terai, I. Sakaida, H. Nishina, K. Okita, Lesson from the GFP/CCl4 model—translational research project: the development of cell therapy using autologous bone marrow cells in patients with liver cirrhosis, J. Hepato-Biliary-Pancreatic Sci. 12 (3) (2005) 203–207.
[192] R. Jaffe, Liver transplant pathology in pediatric metabolic disorders, Pediatr. Dev. Pathol. 1 (2) (1998) 102–117.
[193] T.E. Starzl, Liver transplantation, Johns Hopkins Med. J. 143 (3) (1978) 73–83.
[194] K.A. Strauss, D.L. Robinson, H.J. Vreman, E.G. Puffenberger, G. Hart, D.H. Morton, Management of hyperbilirubinemia and prevention of kernicterus in 20 patients with Crigler-Najjar disease, Eur. J. Pediatr. 165 (5) (2006) 306–319.
[195] A. Aynsley-Green, K. Hussain, J. Hall, J.M. Saudubray, C. Nihoul-Fékété, P. De Lonlay-Debeney, F. Brunelle, T. Otonkoski, P. Thornton, K.J. Lindley, Practical management of hyperinsulinism in infancy, Arch. Dis. Child. Fetal Neonatal Ed. 82 (2) (2000) F98–F107.
[196] K. Hussain, A. Aynsley-Green, C.A. Stanley, Medications used in the treatment of hypoglycemia due to congenital hyperinsulinism of infancy (HI), Pediatr. Endocrinol. Rev. 1 (2004) 163–167.
[197] F.F. Yan, Y.W. Lin, C. MacMullen, A. Ganguly, C.A. Stanley, S.L. Shyng, Congenital hyperinsulinism associated ABCC8 mutations that cause defective trafficking of ATP-sensitive K+ channels: identification and rescue, Diabetes 56 (9) (2007) 2339–2348.
[198] D.J. Weiss, T. Beckett, L. Bonneau, J. Young, J.K. Kolls, G. Wang, Transient increase in lung epithelial tight junction permeability: an additional mechanism for enhancement of lung transgene expression by perfluorochemical liquids, Mol. Ther. 8 (6) (2003) 927–935.
[199] U. Griesenbach, S. Ferrari, D.M. Geddes, E.W.F.W. Alton, Gene therapy progress and prospects: cystic fibrosis, Gene Ther. 9 (20) (2002) 1344–1350.
[200] J.C. Davies, E.W. Alton, Gene therapy for cystic fibrosis, Proc. Am. Thorac. Soc. 7 (6) (2010) 408–414.
[201] T.J. Burneyi, J.C. Davies, Gene therapy for the treatment of cystic fibrosis, Appl. Clin. Genet. 5 (2012) 29–36.

CHAPTER 2

Effects of phytonutrients in various metabolic pathways

Yaseen Hussain
Laboratory of Controlled Release and Drug Delivery System, College of Pharmaceutical Sciences, Soochow University, Suzhou, China
Department of Pharmacy, Bashir Institute of Health Sciences, Islamabad, Pakistan

1. Introduction

Metabolism is a Greek terminology that means "to change," and it involves a series of biochemical reactions that produces energy for various activities within the biological system. The substrate precursors highly rich in energy are converted into complex energy storage molecule through a process known as anabolism. In contrast, the degradation of such complex molecules into usable energy form within the body is termed as catabolism [1]. Such a biosynthesis and degradation process inside the cell or tissue is led by enzyme-mediated biochemical reactions termed as metabolic pathways. Aerobic respiration involves the Krebs cycle and glycolysis metabolic pathways that lead to the production of primary metabolite (ATP), whereas other metabolic pathways produce secondary metabolites [2]. The production of energy (ATP) and then its utilization to operate the bioenvironment is, of course, too essential. However, to support functional changes, there is keen interest in the regulation of metabolic pathways. Metabolic pathways have a significant role associated with human health. Any disturbance in these pathways leads to abnormal consequences within the living system. Therefore, its regulation and modulation is of vital importance [3]. Phytochemicals are bioactive nutrients from a plant source that, apart from its desirable intrinsic protecting value in plants, provide health benefits by preventing the body from chronic pathological conditions. More than 8000 phytochemicals have been discovered yet and are under investigation. The main phytochemical includes primary metabolites such as carbohydrate, proteins, and lipids and secondary metabolites such as alkaloids, glycosides, polyphenols, phytosterols, terpenes, etc. Many years ago, plants were used to prevent and treat certain diseases. The new research era has

The Role of Phytonutrients in Metabolic Disorders
https://doi.org/10.1016/B978-0-12-824356-5.00009-6

now proven the existence of phytochemicals in those plants. Phytonutrients are not recommended as nutritional agents such as proteins, minerals, etc.; however, they can be used as protecting weapons by humans and plants as well. After scratching the surface of phytochemicals, it was identified that it significantly contributes toward protection against multiple pathological progressions. It is the beauty of plants that they are replacing pills. So, it offers a positive lead for nutraceutical and pharmaceutical industries for its formulation in supplement form [4–6]. Metabolic syndrome is a cluster of pathological conditions that include obesity, diabetes, hypercholesterolemia, hypertension, neurodegenerative disorders, cancer, and inflammatory cascades. Insulin resistance with excessive fatty acid flux is the main factor for metabolic syndrome. Metabolic pathways within the body continue with a normal rhythm. Any deviation from the normal pathway leads to pathological conditions. In such a circumstance, phytonutrients are the versatile class of chemicals that interfere to overwhelm such conditions. In addition, diet, physical activity, and lifestyle have a great effect on metabolic syndrome. When all these factors are unable to overcome metabolic syndrome, then treatment is carried out following pharmacological aspects. However, improvement can also be achieved via phytochemicals. Such nutrients from a plant source have diverse biological activities against metabolic syndrome, i.e., saponins reduce chronic metabolic diseases by lowering the cholesterol level. Phytic acid exhibits potential cytotoxic effects. Similarly, glucosinolates are considered potential phytonutrients for reducing the risk of metabolic disorder-associated inflammation, neurodegenerative disorders, and cardiovascular diseases. Cinnamon phytochemicals play a key role in reducing the glucose level in metabolic disorders. In a nutshell, phytochemicals have a significant and potential role in treating metabolism-related disorders, especially metabolic syndrome contributing toward health benefits [7–9]. This chapter focuses on the background of primary phytochemical metabolism and its concerned metabolic pathways. How various secondary phytochemicals (phytonutrients) affect these metabolic pathways and help to control multiple pathological conditions concerned with these pathways has been discussed.

1.1 Carbohydrates

Carbohydrate is a major source of calories required for healthy life. It is found in a variety of healthy and unhealthy foods. Carbohydrates are available in a wide array of forms; however, the major forms of its existence are fibers, sugars, and starches [10]. Carbohydrates are mainly composed of hexoses and pentoses that play an important role in the vital activities. The hexoses are comprised of table sugar (sucrose), milk sugar (lactose), products of starch hydrolysis (maltose), and fermented product derivatives (galactose). The pentoses are composed of arabinose and xylose, which are abundant in fruits [11]. Ptyalin in saliva acts on α-1,4 linkage of amylum (starch) and hydrolyzes it into maltose. Then the remaining 60% of starches are digested in the small intestine by amylopsin (pancreatic amylase), while the six-carbon carbohydrates are digested by the epithelial cell enzymes in the small intestine [12]. In the same way, lactase, sucrase, and maltase digest lactose, sucrose, and maltose, respectively. Arabinoses and xyloses do not need any degradation process and they directly diffused and absorbed into intestinal cells [13]. Absorption of carbohydrates, especially six-carbon, takes place by two main mechanisms, i.e., active and passive transport system. In the passive transport system, glucose or galactose (carbohydrates) in intestinal cells is phosphorylated into glucose-6-phosphate and galactose-6-phosphate. The resultant G6P and Gal6P due to its phosphorylation gets transferred to the circulation. These forms are then dephosphorylated and enter the liver. In contrast, the active diffusion system utilizes a carrier protein—coupled with sodium/potassium pump—to enter enterocytes against the gradient. During this process, the sodium/potassium (Na^+/K^+) pump utilizes adenosine triphosphate (ATP) to exchange three molecules of Na^+ with three molecules of K^+ [14]. Inside the liver, fructose and galactose are converted into glucose. The product obtained is further used in various sorts of metabolic pathways, including blood sugar stability in the management of hypoglycemic state, provision of energy to peripheral tissues, glycogen storage in liver and skeletal muscles, energy storage in adipose tissues, and regulation of body temperature [15–17].

1.1.1 Metabolic pathways of carbohydrates

A carbohydrate undergoes various pathways for its metabolism. Numerous phytochemicals have a tremendous effect on these metabolic pathways which leads to regulation thereof. Consequently, it has great effect on the human physiology. Among these phytochemicals, alkaloids such as nitensidine B affect the glycolytic pathway, underexpressing aldolase A, α-enolase, G3P dehydrogenase, and pyruvate kinase. As a result, the glycolysis is decreased. Similarly, norditerpenoid alkaloids improve carbohydrate metabolism through improvement of glucose consumption, hexokinase activity, and glycogen contents. In the same way, polyphenols modulate gluconeogenesis at the hepatic level along with other genes that contribute in maintaining human health. Gossypol is a polyphenol that increases glycolysis and the pentose phosphate pathway, that causes increase glucose consumption due to its anticancer effect. Epigallocatechin increases the glycogen synthesis pathway as compared to insulin alone. Flavonoids reduce the glucose metabolic pathways and play a key role in treating hyperglycemia. Phytosterols affect the pathway of the electron transport chain resulting in the regulation of the body's physiological activities. Apart from that, phytosterols also reduce the activity of the phosphoenol pyruvate carboxykinase enzyme during hepatic gluconeogenesis, treating diabetes mellitus. Betulinic acid belongs to the phytochemical class of terpenes. It inhibits aerobic glycolysis following the mechanism of hampering lactate production, glucose uptake, and lactate dehydrogenase A leading to anticancer activity [18–23]. Although glucose is a major source of energy, cells also use fructose as a source of energy because of the high consumption of glucose. Muscles, kidneys, and adipose tissues contain an enzyme-hexokinase that acts to convert phosphorylate fructose into fructose-6-phosphate that is further used in the glycolysis pathway. On the other hand, the fructose used in the glycolysis pathway must be converted into glucose. Therefore, the glucokinase present in the liver first causes phosphorylation of fructose and then produces interconvertible intermediates (three-carbon glycolysis intermediates), i.e., dihydroxyacetone phosphate and glyceraldehyde. The produced glyceraldehyde is phosphorylated into glyceraldehyde-3-phosphate (GA3P). The GA3P recombines with dihydroxyacetone phosphate (DHAD) to form fructose 1,6-bisphosphate (F1,6BP). This double-phosphorylated conjugate is dephosphorylated by phosphatase into fructose-6-phosphate (F6P). This resultant product is used in two ways, either as a substrate for the glycolysis pathway or acted by an isomerase and converted to glucose-6-phosphate (G6P). G6P further either loses its attached phosphate group entering the circulation or through the action of the mutase enzyme is converted to G1P (glucose-1-phosphate) that is next used as a substrate for the synthesis of glycogen [24,25] (Fig. 1).

The consumption of milk sugar or lactose leads to the entrance of galactose and glucose into the body. The brush border of the small intestine is composed of lactase enzyme that acts on the entered galactose and converts it into its consecutive constituents. After systemic absorption, galactose enters into enterocytes followed by ingress into the liver through the portal vein and metabolized to glucose which is further used as a source of energy for vital activities. Mechanistically, galactose is phosphorylated and is converted to galactose-1-phosphate and then to galactose-1-phosphate

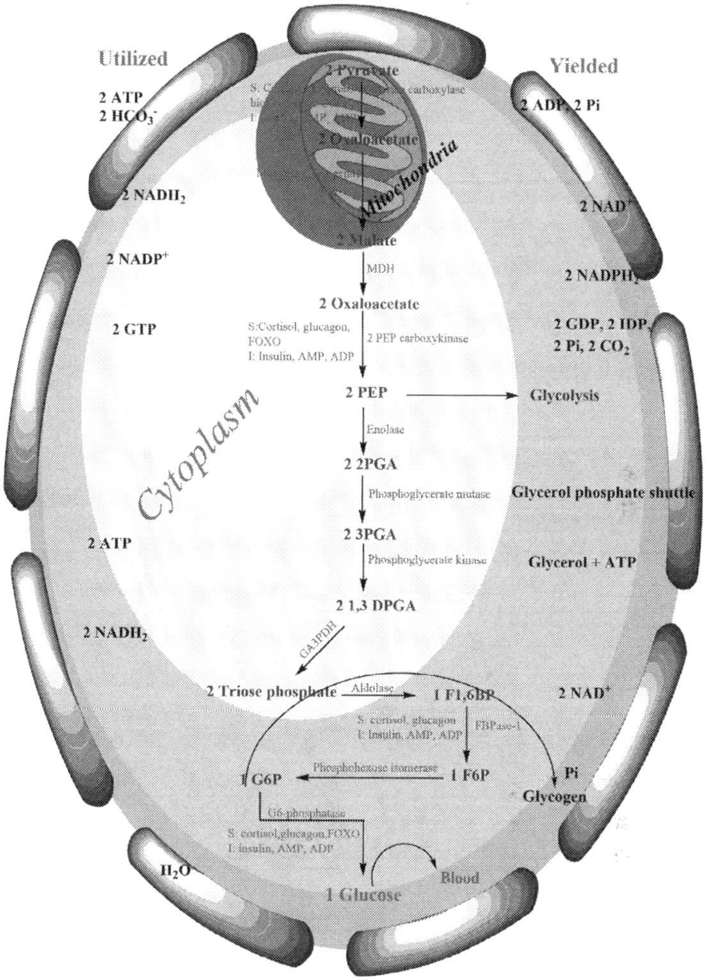

Fig. 1 Fructose metabolism. In hepatocytes, fructose is phosphorylated to F1P which is cleaved to DHAP. A glycolytic intermediate GA3P is formed after phosphorylation of glyceraldehyde. DHAP and GA3P obtained from fructose have multiple metabolic fates in the metabolic pool. ATP, adenosine triphosphate; ADP, adenosine diphosphate; F1P, fructose1phosphate; DHAP, dihydroxyacetone phosphate; GA3P, glyceraldehyde-3-phosphate; F1,6BP, fructose-1,6-bisphosphate; F6P, fructose-6-phosphate; G6P, glucose-6-phosphate; G1P, glucose-1-Phosphate.

uridylyl transferase (GALT). Finally, GALT and its concerned coenzyme-uridine diphosphate glucose (UDPG) replace the galactose of galactose-1-phosphate by glucose evolving uridine diphosphate galactose (UDPgal). The uridine diphosphate galactose-4-epimerase activity transforms the uridine diphosphate galactose (UDPgal) to uridine diphosphate glucose (UDPG) [26] (Fig. 2).

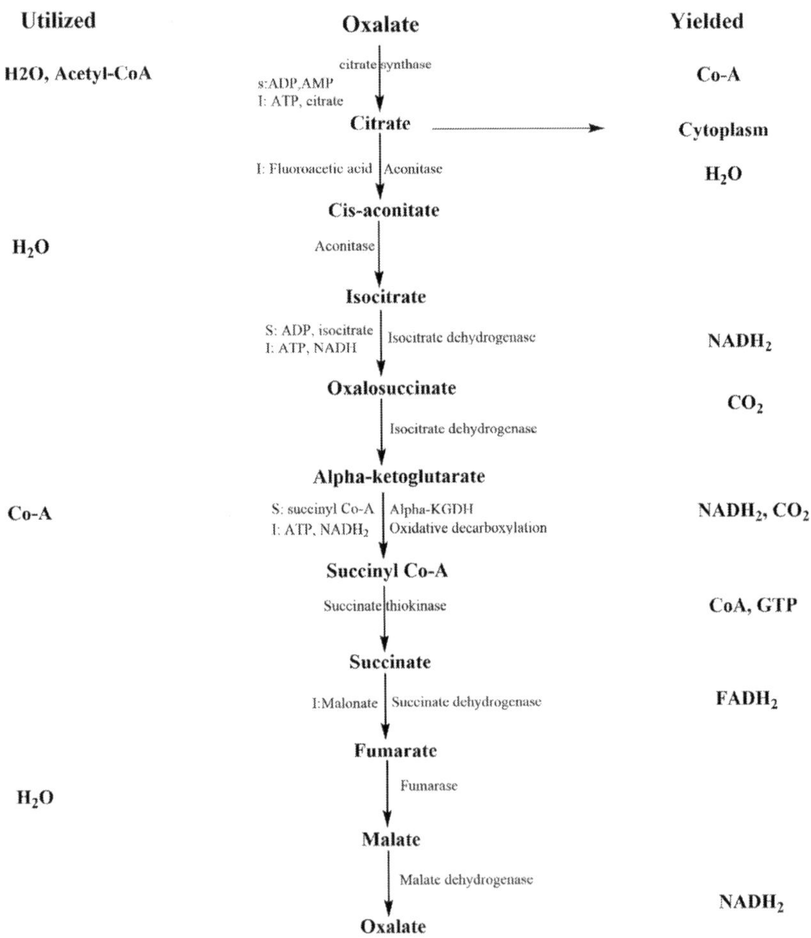

Fig. 2 Galactose metabolism. Galactose is also used by cells as an energy source. It is converted to G6P next substrate for glycolysis and G1P for glycogenesis. Gal1P, galactose-1-phosphate; UDPG, uridine diphosphate glucose; UDPgal, uridine diphosphate galactose; DHAP, dihydroxyacetone phosphate; G1P, glucose-1-phosphate; G6P, glucose-6-phosphate. Glucose metabolism is governed by oxidative and nonoxidative pathways.

Glycolysis

Glycolysis is also known as pyruvate fermentation or anaerobic respiration which takes place in the cytoplasm. It involves partial glucose oxidation with the production of pyruvic acid. During heavy exercise or in case of those cells having no mitochondria, the produced pyruvate is converted to lactate. This conversion occurs through a bilateral way, i.e., the reaction is catalyzed through the lactate dehydrogenase enzyme with the consumption of one molecule of $NADH_2$ [27] (Fig. 3).

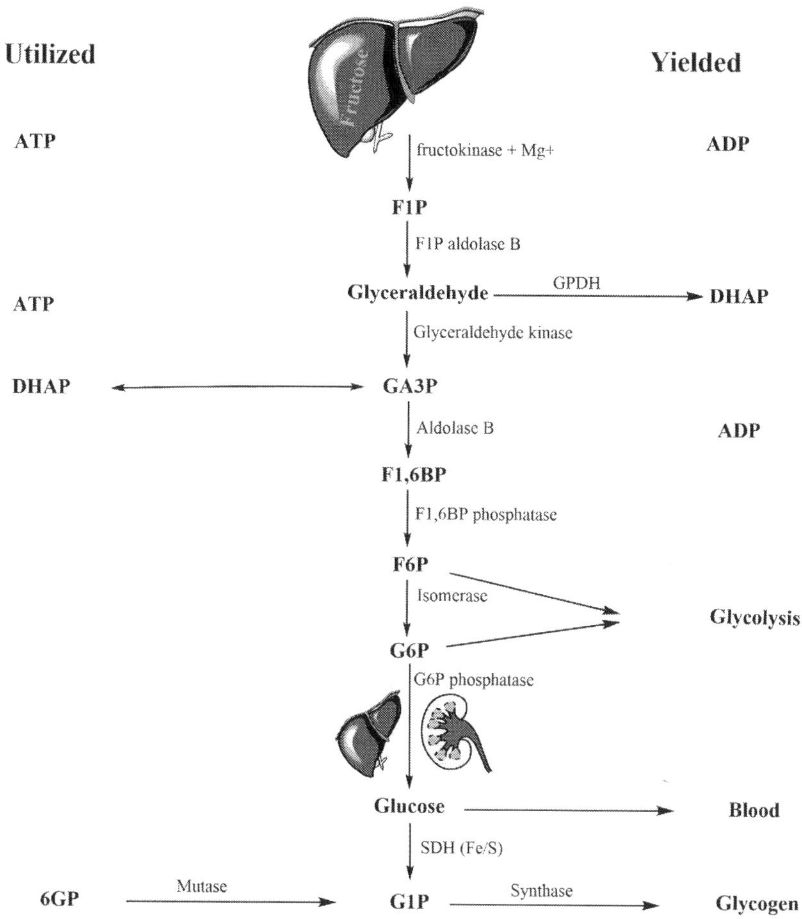

Fig. 3 Glycolysis pathway. It is a nonoxidative pathway that yields 2 pyruvates from glucose. The high energy is further utilized to form ATP and $NADH_2$. PGA, phosphor glyceric acid; DHAP, dihydroxyacetone phosphate; GA3P, glyceraldehyde-3-phosphate; $NADH_2$, nicotinamide adenine dinucleotide; G6P, glucose-6-phosphate; F6P, fructose-6-phosphate; F1,6BP, fructose-1,6-bisphosphate.

Krebs cycle and electron transport chain

Krebs cycle is an oxidative and aerobic pathway that takes place in the mitochondrion. During the Krebs cycle, the output of glycolysis (2 pyruvate) are break down evolving energy in the form of guanosine triphosphate (2GTP), nicotinamide adenine dinucleotide in reduced form (6 $NADH_2$), and flavin adenine dinucleotide in reduced form (2 $FADH_2$). The resultant energy is then utilized in the electron transport chain. $NADH_2$ and $FADH_2$ liberate their proton, which in turn produces water after combining with oxygen at the end of the whole process. The protons of the reduced coenzymes are in an excited state of energy, lose their energy during transfer to oxygen, and a proton gradient is established across the intermembrane space. Thus, the reverse flow of protons to the mitochondrion releases energy which is utilized in the production of ATP. The electron transport chain provides 3ATP from $NADH_2$ and 2ATP from $FADH_2$ with carbon dioxide and water as an end product. In a nutshell, the electron transport chain produces most of the energy through aerobic respiration [28] (Fig. 4).

Glycogenesis and glycogenolysis

Glucose is stored in the liver and skeletal muscles in the form of glycogen—a glucose polymer linked by α-1,4 and α-1,6 glyosidic linkages. The synthesis of glycogen is termed as glycogenesis. During glycogenesis, glycogen through the α-1,4 bond gets bound to glucose and glucose-1-phosphate (G1P) is converted to uridine diphosphate glucose (UDPG-active form of glucose) through an enzyme Glucosyl-1-phosphate uridylyl-transferase and uridine triphosphate. Then in the presence of glycogen synthase, the glycogen approaches the active glucose by binding through α-1,4 linkage. During this process, uridine diphosphate (UDP) is released after binding of carbon-1 of glucose and carbon-4 of glycogen. As the binding of glucose to glycogen proceeds up to 12 glucose molecules, the amylo-α-1,4 to 1,6-trans glycosylase enzyme picks up 7 glucose molecules and forms a new branch of glycogen by using an α-1,6 linkage [29] (Fig. 5).

In contrast, the process of breakdown of glycogen is known as glycogenolysis. The process of glycogenolysis occurs in the kidney and liver that produce glucose, which in turn stabilizes the sugar level in the blood. In addition, glycogenolysis in the muscles produces glucose-6-phosphate used as a source of energy by the muscle cells. Glycogenolysis produces glucose-1-phosphate by hydrolysis of glyosidic linkage (α-1,4) of glycogen by the action of an enzyme glycogen phosphorylase using the

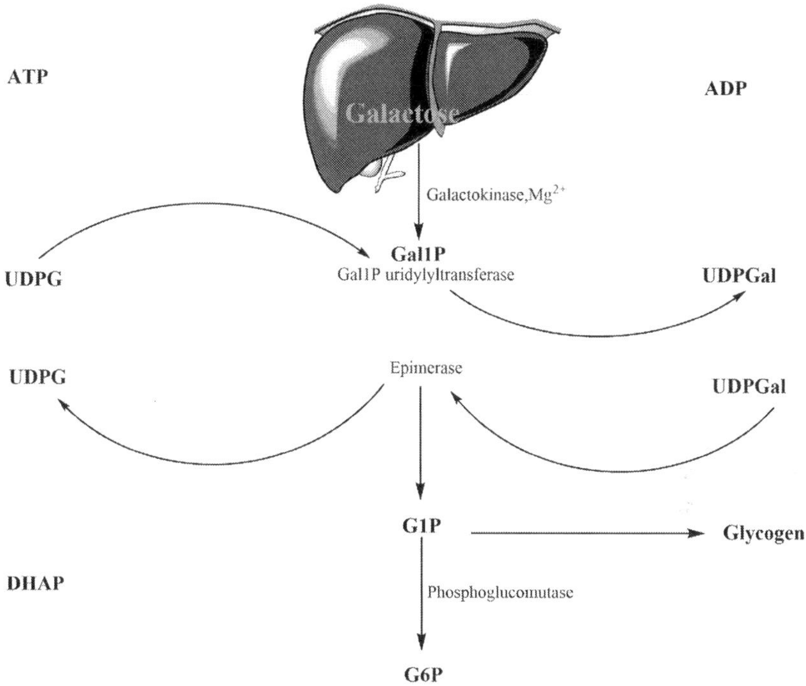

Fig. 4 Krebs Cycle. Pyruvate, ATP, and NADH are produced by glycolysis. Pyruvate then undergoes decarboxylation via pyruvate decarboxylase into acetyl-CoA that enters into the Krebs cycle. This cycle then primarily yields GTP, $FADH_2$, $NADH_2$ but also produces certain molecules that are in/exit to cycle on demand. For example, α-ketoglutarate and succinate which when leave the cycle are converted into amino acid and haem, respectively. ADP, adenosine diphosphate; ATP, adenosine triphosphate; AMP, adenosine monophosphate; $FADH_2$, flavin adenine dinucleotide; $NADH_2$, nicotinamide adenine dinucleotide.

phosphate group (Pi-inorganic). The resultant glucose-1-phosphate in the liver and kidneys is converted to glucose-6-phosphate using glucose-6-phosphatase enzyme (G6Pase). As skeletal muscles are devoid of the glucose-6-phosphatase enzyme, so glucose-6-phosphate is converted to fructose-6-phosphate which is further used in glycolysis. The α-1,4 linkage is continuously acted by the phosphorylase enzyme and break until four molecules of glucose remain on the branch. Here, another three glucose molecules are shifted to the concerned branch of glucose through the action of the glucan transferase enzyme, while the terminal glucose molecule of the α-1,6 linkage is broken down through amylo-α-1,6-glucosidase activity [30] (Fig. 6).

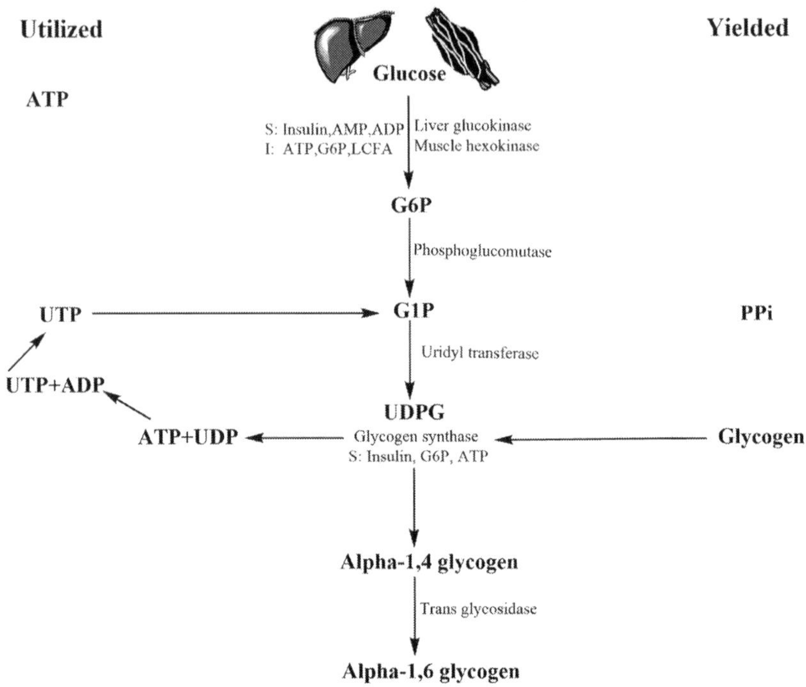

Fig. 5 Glycogenesis pathway. Uridine diphosphate is used as a substrate in this pathway while glucose is converted to glycogen. During synthesis of glycogen, each glucose molecule requires one ATP for incorporation into the polymeric and branched glycogen structure. UDP, uridine diphosphate; UTP, uridine triphosphate; PPi, pyrophosphate; UDPG, uridine diphosphate glucose; G6P, glucose-6-phosphate, G1P, glucose-1-phosphate; LCFA, long-chain fatty acid.

Gluconeogenesis

It is the process of production of glucose in the liver, kidneys, testes, brain, and red blood cells from noncarbohydrate sources, i.e., lactate, glycerol, pyruvate, and glutamine. It happens in the cytoplasm and is contrary to the process of glycolysis. This process is used especially in the case of chronic starvation and in diabetic patients. During gluconeogenesis, the pyruvate is converted to oxalate in the presence of pyruvate carboxylase and biotin coenzymes inside the mitochondrion. The cytoplasm needs oxalate, so it must be shifted to the mitochondrion, but due to the nondiffusible nature of the mitochondrial membrane the transport may occur through one of the following ways. Oxalate is converted to phosphoenol pyruvate through phosphoenol pyruvate carboxy kinase (mitochondrial isoform). The transamination of oxalate to aspartate-diffusible form take place. In addition, reduction of oxalate to malate through $NADPH_2$ is reconverted in cytoplasm to oxaloacetate [31,32] (Fig. 7).

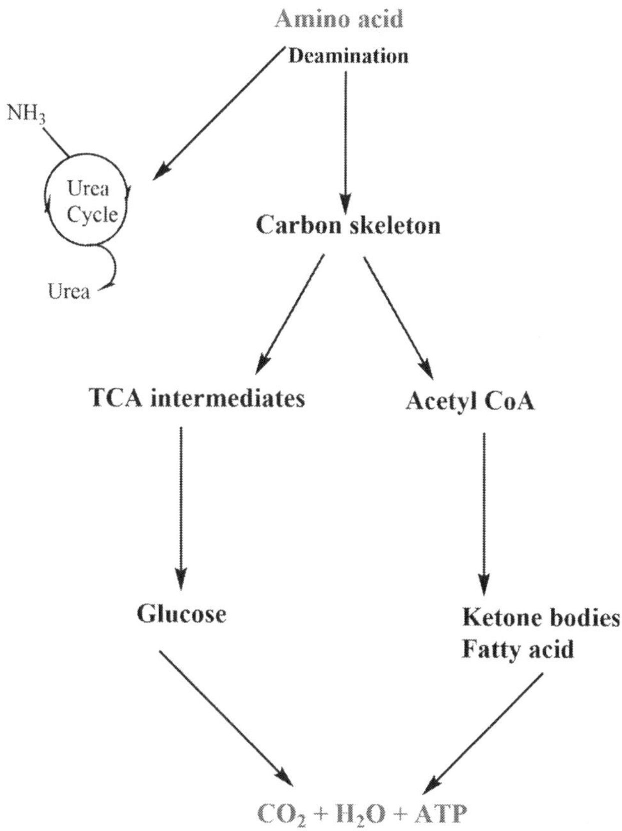

Fig. 6 Glycogenolysis pathway. It yields free glucose which enters the blood to restore the glucose level, whereas the G6P is again taken by the glycolysis pathway where glucose is cleaved to free energy in the form of ATP. G1P, glucose-1-phosphate; G6P, glucose-6-phosphate; F6P, fructose-6-phosphate.

The high level of blood glucose stimulates the β cells of the pancreas to release insulin, which in response stimulates glycogenesis and glycolysis. Thus, insulin acts as an anabolic signal for lowering the blood glucose level. On the other hand, catabolic pathways such as gluconeogenesis and glycogenolysis are inhibited by insulin. In case of carbohydrate catabolism, glucagon is a major stimulating signal that elevates the blood glucose level.

1.2 Lipids and alcohols

In relation to the metabolic pathways of carbohydrates, phytochemicals also pose effects on lipid and alcohol metabolic pathways. As a consequence, they play a vital role in the management of multiple pathological conditions that arise from metabolic disturbances. Piperine, pipernonaline, and

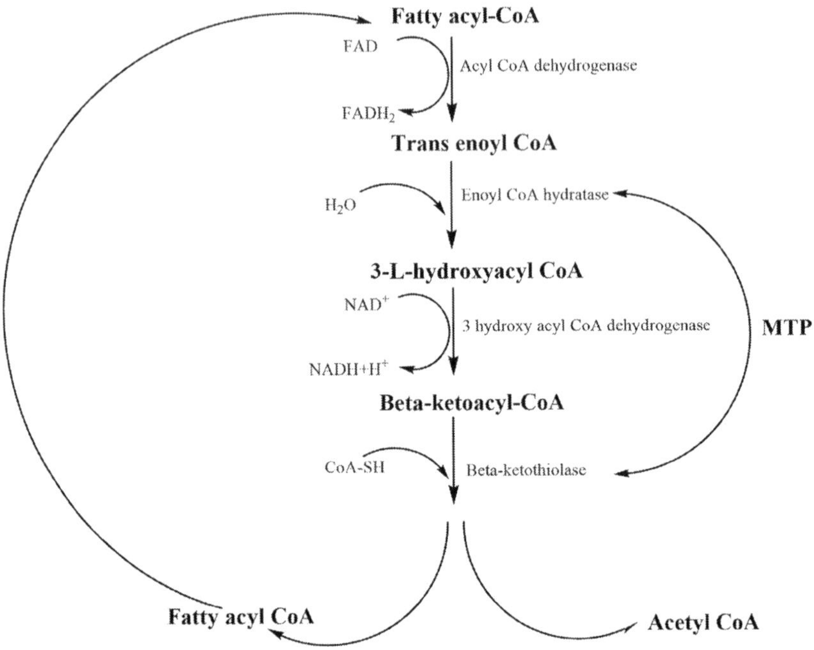

Fig. 7 Gluconeogenesis mitochondrial-cytoplasmic metabolic pathway. Glucose is produced from non-carbohydrate precursors, i.e., amino acid, lipid, pyruvate, glycerol, etc., where high energy is consumed in the form of ATP and GTP. Fructose 1,6-bis phosphatase is the rate-limiting enzyme for the process. Insulin inhibits the pathway while glucagon stimulates the process. $NADH_2$, nicotinamide adenine dinucleotide; NADP, nicotinamide adenine dinucleotide phosphate; MDH, malate dehydrogenase; GDP, guanosine diphosphate; GTP, guanosine triphosphate; PEP, phosphoenolpyruvate; PGA, phosphoglyceric acid; FOXO, forkhead box protein. GA3PDH, glyceraldehyde-3-phosphate dehydrogenase.

dehydropipernonaline are piperidine alkaloids that act on the peroxisome proliferator activated receptor pathway and activate AMP activated protein kinase that leads to antiobesity effect in a mice model. Similarly, berberine reduces the expression of convertase subtilisin/kexin type 9 modulation and increases the hepatic LDL receptor expression, leading to enhanced lipid metabolism behaving as an antihyperlipidemic agent. Increased excretion of bile acid during lipid metabolism by polyphenols results in a reduction of the cholesterol level. Mouse model experiments have shown that flavonoids through the suppression of atherogenesis cause improved metabolic parameters. Phytosterols downregulate the lipid metabolic pathway via stimulation of the MAPK pathway [33–35]. The building blocks of lipid—fatty acid are utilized in oxidative tissue for energy production. Their plasma concentration is maintained up to 0.5 mM being toxic and they are transported in bound form with albumin. During stress conditions such as fasting and heavy exercise, the lipids are mobilized and stored in adipose tissues (~15 kg triglyceride). These triglycerides are degraded by lipase enzymes into fatty acid and glycerol. The released components in the circulation are used where required. Fatty acids are used by oxidative tissues for energy production while the glycerol is used in hepatic gluconeogenesis [36]. The passive diffusion system and specific transporters are the main mechanisms for the absorption of fatty acid. CD36 is a fatty acid transporter that is located in the villi of the small intestine and is responsible for uptake by intestinal cells. A mice study on lipid absorption reveals that in case of absence of the CD36 transporter, the distal intestine is the absorption site for fatty acids [37]. The absorbed fatty acid along with its coenzyme (FA-Co-A) undergoes oxidation in mitochondria. During this β-oxidation, the fatty acid chain β carbon is attacked and released in the form of acetyl Co-A. β-oxidation is repeated again and again until the whole chain of fatty acid is degraded and many acetyl Co-A along with NADH, $FADH_2$ are produced. Next, in the electron transport chain, NADH and $FADH_2$ are oxidized giving a huge amount of energy (ATP). In addition, the acetyl Co-A generated by β-oxidation is used in ketogenesis within the hepatocytes. The resultant ketone bodies from ketogenesis, along with other hydrophilic transportable forms of acetyl Co-A, i.e., acetoacetate, β-hydroxybutyrate, are used by the brain as an economical glucose-fuel [38]. Within adipose tissue and liver cytosol, the acetyl Co-A generated from amino acids and carbohydrates congregates to the fatty acid for lipogenesis. Where acetyl Co-A carboxylase acts on acetyl Co-A to form malonyl Co-A, the malonyl group in malonyl Co-A acts as a donor for an enzyme fatty acid synthetase—a polypeptide with multicatalytic properties that extends the two-carbon chain of fatty acid using NADPH as an energy source. Then the fatty acids (three in number) are esterified to glycerol phosphate forming triacyl glyceride which is stored in adipose tissue. The transport of triacyl glyceride is carried out by lipoprotein. Insulin is the signaling agent for the anabolic state of lipids. Lipogenesis in the liver, cholesterol, and triacyl glyceride synthesis are signaled by insulin while inhibiting ketogenesis. Insulin also stimulates lipoprotein lipase in adipose tissue, improving the uptake of triglyceride from triglyceride-rich lipoproteins in plasma by avoiding triglyceride lipolysis. This ultimately leads to a low level of nonesterified fatty acid. In contrast, the catabolic state is regulated by certain hormones and signals that mimic the breakdown and mobilization of lipids. These include catecholamines (enhancing sympathetic activity) and

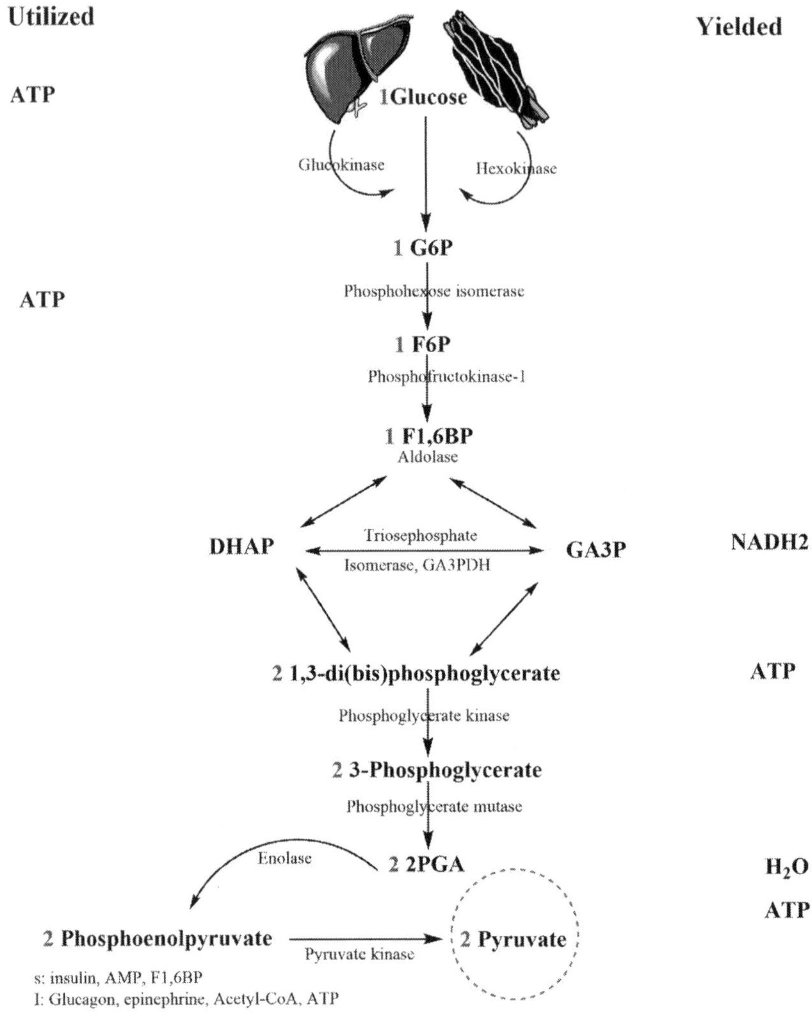

Fig. 8 Lipid metabolism pathway. Lipid metabolism produces 1 $FADH_2$, 1$NADH_2$ which moves into the electron transport chain. It also yields 1 acetyl CoA which enters into the citric acid cycle and produces 3NADH, 1GTP, AND 1$FADH_2$, from each cycle about 14 ATP are yielded. MTP, microsomal triglyceride transfer protein; $FADH_2$, flavin adenine dinucleotide; NAD, nicotinamide dinucleotide.

adrenocorticotrophic hormone (lipolysis in adipose tissue and increase level of nonesterified fatty acid) [39,40] (Fig. 8).

The metabolism of ingested alcohol by human (ethanol) has numerous effects on redox-potential, i.e., ratio of NAD^+ to NADH. The ingested ethanol undergoes oxidation in the liver and is converted to acetaldehyde through alcohol dehydrogenase. The resultant acetaldehyde in the presence of the aldehyde dehydrogenase enzyme follows the oxidation process and is converted to acetate. The resultant acetate from oxidation of acetaldehyde is converted to acetyl Co-A, which can be used as a plentiful source of energy. During oxidation of acetaldehyde, NADH is produced. However, the high level of NADH results in inhibition of lactate oxidation to pyruvate. Consequently, it affects gluconeogenesis and leads to metabolic lactic acidosis and hypoglycemia. In addition, oxidation of fatty acid is inhibited that leads to a fatty liver [41].

1.3 Proteins

Amino acids are the building blocks of protein which can be derived from endogenous proteins. Amino acids absorbed into portal circulation are obtained from dietary proteins. The usual uptake of proteins by the body from a routine diet is approximately 100 g per day, whereas the whole turnover of 10-kg body proteins is approximately 3% (300 g per day). Unlike lipids and carbohydrates, amino acids are composed of an amino group (nitrogen) which needs deamination (removal of amino group) before the metabolism of 2-oxoacid in the structure of amino acid. The removal of the amino group results in the production of ammonia which is toxic and must be removed from the body through the kidney or must be converted to non-toxic moieties by the ornithine cycle in the liver [42]. Phytochemicals affect various steps of the protein metabolic pathways, consequently preventing the body from various pathological progressions. The disposal of nitrogen is carried out by various reactions. One among them is transamination during which the amino group of one amino acid (α-amino group) is shifted to the carbon skeleton of another amino acid containing 2-oxoacid. Among all those amino acids which are exposed to deamination, α-ketoglutarate act as an amino acid receptor. Apart from that, α-ketoglutarate also directs the flow of amino acid to glutamates. Similarly, alanine amino transferase (ALT) is an enzyme that acts on the amino group of alanine and shifts it toward α-ketoglutarate resulting in the production of glutamate and pyruvate. Like ALT, aspartate aminotransferase is another enzyme that acts on aspartate and shifts the amino group toward α-ketoglutarate, leading to the production of oxaloacetate and glutamate. In addition to transamination, another reaction responsible for nitrogen disposal is oxidative deamination. This reaction involves the action of glutamate dehydrogenase on glutamate, ultimately resulting in the reformation of α-ketoglutarate and ammonia. Next, in the urea cycle, ammonia is detoxified to urea while α-ketoglutarate undergoes an intermediate metabolism [43]. The intermediary metabolism of amino acid yields seven products. Including pyruvate, succinyl-CoA, α-ketoglutarate, oxaloacetate, acetyl CoA, fumarate, and acetoacetyl-CoA. Proteins have the capability to act as a carbohydrate reserve. This fact can be justified by the statement that pyruvate, α-ketoglutarate, succinyl-CoA, fumarate, and oxaloacetate producing amino acid are glucogenic and can be effectively used in glucose synthesis. Because all these products constitute three-carbons while the other two—acetyl CoA and acetoacetyl-CoA—constitute two carbons that cannot take part in glucose synthesis, rather they can be directly used in lipogenesis or ketogenesis. Both amino acid metabolism and carbon skeleton metabolism are carried out in the liver that eventually results in the removal of dietary amino acid from portal circulation. In case of inter-tissue flux, amino acid in the form of alanine generated by transamination reaction is transported by muscles to the liver. In the liver, alanine undergoes transamination reaction forming pyruvate, which in turn produces glucose. The produced glucose is retransported to muscles. In the same way, muscles also provide glutamine (containing two amino groups). Within the kidney, glutamine is acted on by the glutaminase enzyme that breaks the side chain of amino groups producing glutamate and ammonia. The toxic ammonia is then removed by the urinary system [44]. In case of amino acid, approximately one-third of the body is comprised of valine, leucine, and isoleucine. These amino acids are a three-branched chain and are found in high concentration in the blood due to its lack of clearance by the liver from portal circulation. Therefore, they are metabolized in muscles and being a significant source of nitrogen, they keep the alanine, glutamate, and glutamine pool at the optimal level. These amino acids are degraded by aminotransferases to 2-oxoacids followed by oxidative decarboxylation through α-ketoacid dehydrogenase [45]. Protein metabolism is regulated by insulin. It acts as a main anabolic signal that stimulates protein synthesis and inhibits proteolysis. In addition to insulin, growth factors, anabolic steroids, and growth hormones are also the signaling agents that activate protein anabolism. Controversially, thyroid hormones and cortisol are stimulatory agents for protein catabolism [46] (Fig. 9).

2. Significance of metabolic pathways in health and diseases

Metabolic syndrome is a disease cluster that includes obesity, hypertension, hyperglycemia, and hyperlipidemia. These conditions sequentially lead toward cardiac problems, cerebrovascular incidents, and diabetes mellitus [47]. The World Health Organization Report reveals that obesity is found in

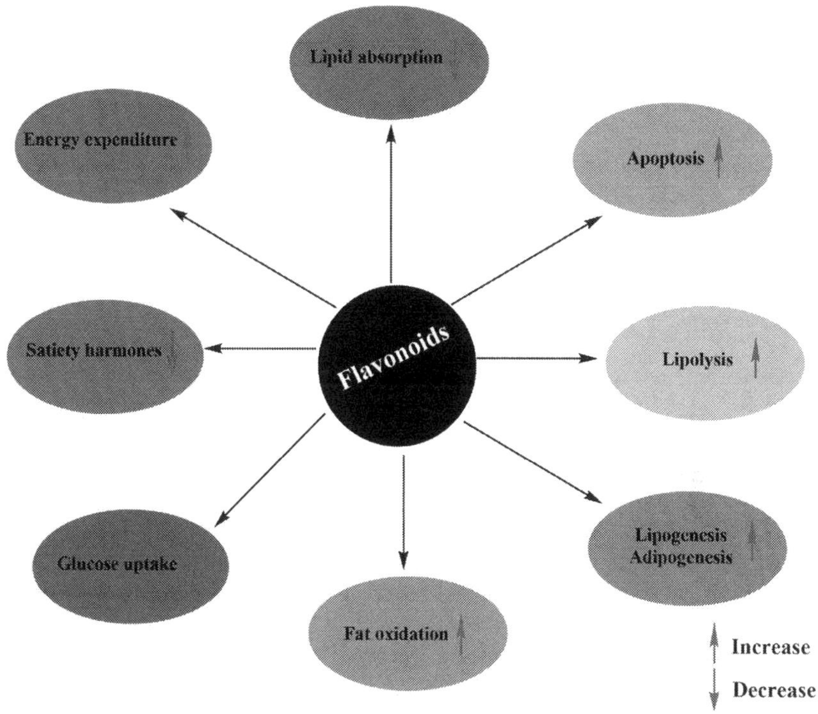

Fig. 9 Protein metabolic pathway. Here the amino group is removed from the amino acid and produces ammonia and keto acid. It is then converted to urea using 3ATP while keto acid enters into the Krebs cycle forming ATP. Deamination of glutamate in kidney also produces urea, but it is excreted in the urine without entering the urea cycle.

about 650 million people, 422 million people live with diabetes mellitus, and 1.13 million people are suffering from hypertension.

2.1 Obesity

Obesity is the accumulation of fats in the adipose tissue of the body with adverse alterations, including macrophages accumulation and low lipid turnover [48]. Adipose tissues have negative consequences on metabolic pathways, especially on the insulin signaling pathway. Thus, they provide directions toward obesity pathogenesis and metabolic syndromes [49]. According to WHO, criteria for obesity include BMI greater than 30 or waist-to-hip ratio greater than 0.9 for male and 0.85 for female. Insulin resistance presents the most accepted hypothesis toward the pathophysiology of metabolic syndrome. Insulin resistance is a defect in the action of insulin that leads to various pathological consequences and acts as a framework that corelates abnormal biological events with pathophysiological conditions. Adipose tissues in the body release fatty acid into the bloodstream and an excessive release at this point contributes toward insulin resistance, because the uptake of glucose by insulin is blocked by free fatty acid in muscles that results in reduced insulin sensitivity. Also, inhibition of glucose uptake by insulin results in elevated blood glucose concentration, which triggers secretion of insulin from the pancreas and eventually leads to hyperinsulinemia. Free fatty acid in the liver mimics glucose, triglyceride, and VLDL production. This ultimately results in inhibition of glucose conversion to glycogen.

2.2 Diabetes

Certain amino acids such as leucine, arginine, and glucose in the blood are detected by the beta cells of the pancreas. A higher concentration of these agents leads to nutrient repletion and trigger the release of insulin. The action of insulin as an anabolic signal is opposed by catabolic signals which leads to insulin deficiency and other worst metabolic consequences. The beta cells of the pancreas are completely destroyed in type-I diabetes mellitus and no sensing mechanism for glucose exists. Here the peripheral tissues become catabolic due to the lack of insulin with depletion in the energy reservoir. The liver shows this low level of insulin in the form of hypoglycemia and to cope with this condition it improve gluconeogenesis and glycogenolysis. In order to provide more substrate for the mentioned metabolic pathways, both carbohydrates and proteins are consumed. Apart from this hepatic glucose production, glycolysis and glycogenesis are decreased peripherally, which results in glucose sparing. As the patient's diet intake is continuous, the glucose level rises in blood and leads to hyperglycemia. When the tubular reabsorption exceeds the maximum, then glucose approaches toward urine causing glycosuria and water are excreted resulting in thirst, polyurea, polydipsia, dehydration, etc. Lipid metabolism also contributes to such a consequence. The low level of insulin is detected by adipose tissues, which in turn stimulate the lipolysis of triacyl glyceride. Nonesterified fatty acids are released to bloodstream which are utilized by liver in ketogenesis and by muscles so further decreases glucose. Further, the consequence leads to metabolic ketoacidosis [1].

2.3 Hypercholesterolemia

Hypercholesterolemia is related to metabolic syndrome characterized by an irregular lipid profile. This abnormal lipid profile includes elevated levels of triglycerides, low-density lipoprotein, and very low-density lipoprotein.

Hypercholesterolemia has a risky contribution toward atherosclerosis that further leads to vascular damage, especially is obese and diabetic patients [50]. Abnormalities in lipoprotein metabolism mostly account for the hypercholesterolemia [51].

2.4 Cancer

Hypermetabolism contributes toward cancer in humans. Tumors are considered to increase glucose up take with a high rate of glycolysis. Such a consequence is due to abnormal functions of the mitochondria and overexpression of type II hexokinase or various oncogenes. Also, the hypoxic environment of tumor affects glucose metabolism. Through the Cori-cycle, the excess of lactate is converted to glucose in the liver. The disturbance in the Cori-cycle of cancer patients leads to weight loss variations; however, the gluconeogenesis and glycogenolysis are increased in such patients. In addition, alanine or glycerol gluconeogenesis has no significant role in energy drain [52]. Lipid loss is excessive in cancer patients either due to the inhibited lipogenesis (due to inflammatory cytokines) or enhanced lipolysis. Insulin activates phatidyl inositol kinase which further stimulates phosphodiesterase and results in production of adenosine mono phosphate. It indicates that fat atrophy is the main effect of lipolysis in cancer patients.

2.5 Inflammation cascade

Inflammatory cascades due to disturbance in metabolic pathways are the hallmark for metabolic syndrome. It reduces the life span of humans by increasing cardiovascular consequences. Misregulation of metabolic pathways elevates the TNF-α and IL-6 levels in circulation which are responsible for chronic inflammations [46]. Macrophages living in adipose tissues upon activation cause the expression of TNF-α and IL-6. These macrophages, along with adipocytes in conditions such as hyperglycemia, dyslipidemia, and hyperinsulinemia, result in endothelial dysfunction. Consequently, it leads to high morbidity and mortality rates due to metabolic syndrome [53].

3. Phytonutrients

Natural products affect various metabolic and epigenetic pathways leading to an effective treatment of certain disorders. The main classes of natural products and their effects on metabolic pathways are discussed below.

3.1 Alkaloids

These are organic natural products obtained from plants, animals, and microorganisms. Alkaloids contain nitrogen as their basic structural moiety and present the most versatile class with biological activities. They are further categorized as tropane, quinolone, pyridine-piperidine, indole, isoquinolone, imidazole, steroidal and ergot alkaloids. Defects in carbohydrate, lipid, and lipoprotein metabolism lead to diabetes and its other complications pertaining to either insulin deficiency or resistance. Various cell functions such as gene expression, glucose transport, receptor translocation, and synthesis of fatty acid are targeted by insulin in the body. All these mentioned effects are mediated through special signaling pathways and adapter molecules such as G-protein, lipid, and tyrosine kinase. Alterations in such pathways or molecules result in abnormal cell response in diabetic patients [53]. Increased glucose production with reduced utilization, high level of fatty acid and lipolysis leads to insulin resistance resulting in hyperglycemia and irregular beta-cell functions as well. Lately, the alkaloids have gotten extra consideration because of their likely role in the treatment of diabetes and diabetes-related complications (Fig. 10).

Oriciacridone C and Oriciacridone F from Vepris glaberrima inhibit α-glucosidase with IC_{50} values of 56 and 34 μM, respectively. Similarly, vasicine do the same inhibition with 125 and 250 μM IC_{50} values. Similarly, Chelerythrine and sanguinarine from *Sanguinaria canadensis* are α-amylase inhibitors that show 100% inhibition with IC_{50} value of 250 μM. A well-known alkaloid-berberine from Berberis aristata poses an insulinotropic effect in rat pancreatic islets via hepatic nuclear factor 4-α modulation [56]. Betanin from *Beta vulgaris* regulates plasma glucose, glycosylated Hb, insulin, and levels of hemoglobin by elevating the glycolytic enzyme activity, G6P dehydrogenase and decreasing gluconeogenic enzymes. This contributes to enhanced glycogen contents in the liver of diabetics [57]. YS-51(6,7-dihydroxy-1-(β-naphthylmethyl)-1,2,3,4 tetrahydroisoquinoline) is an alkaloid that has a significant antiobese effect through suppression of lipogenesis. Also, in the liver, it expresses proteins and AMPK through boosting up the NAD^+/NADH ratio followed by phosphorylation. This eventually improves glucose tolerance and insulin resistance [58]. Because of their lipolytic and antilipase activity, alkaloids from *Nelumbo nucifera* help in many metabolic disorders, including obesity, hypercholesterolemia, and insulin resistance [59]. Bouchardatine from Bouchardatia neurococca has a significant effect on metabolic disorders, especially obesity and hypercholesterolemia, through activation of the SIRT1–LKB1–AMPK signaling pathway [60,61].

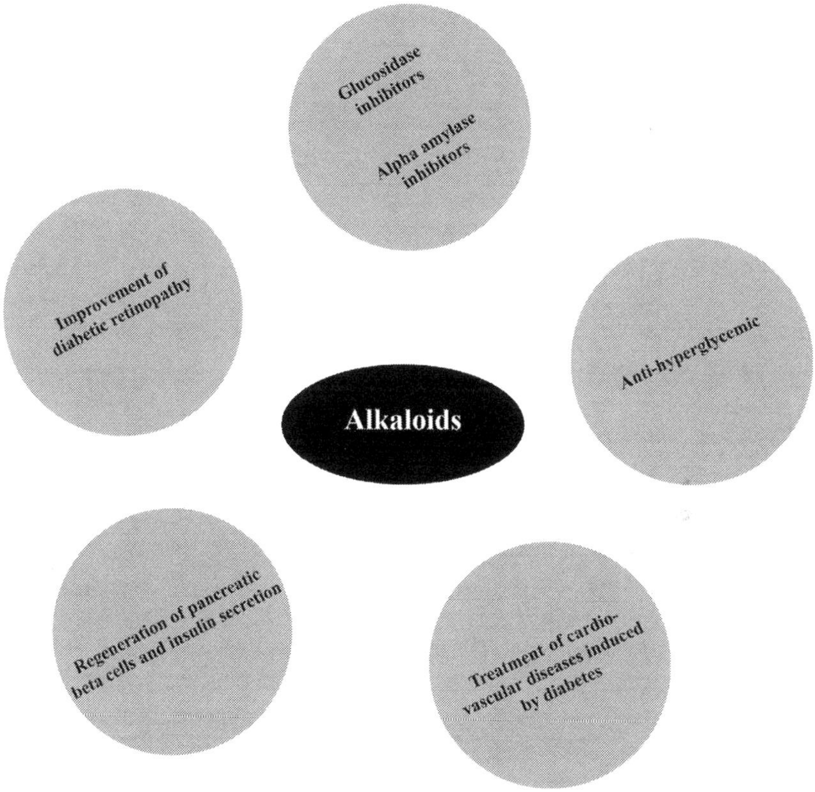

Fig. 10 Various activities of alkaloids against diabetes and its complications Complex carbohydrates such as starches are converted into glucose by α-glucosidase in the small intestine. Certain α-glucosidase inhibitors such as miglitol and acarbose prevent such conversion. Such an inhibition causes glycemic control. The American Association of Clinical Endocrinologists and International Diabetes Federation recommend these inhibitors as first-line therapy in diabetes [54,55].

3.2 Phenols

Flavonoids are an important class of phytonutrients with multiple biological activities belonging to the class of phenols. A couple of lines of assessment recommend that flavonoids supplementation is beneficial for the treatment of obesity, diabetes, hypertension, and metabolic issue. The total daily consumptions of flavonoids vary from ~20 mg/d to more than 70 mg/d depending on cultures and nations [62]. Flavonoids from lemon (polyphenols) act as antiobese agents following the mechanism of mRNA upregulation enzymes, mainly those involved in β-oxidation. Such enzymes include hepatic fatty acid synthase, acyl-coA oxidase, and peroxisome proliferator activated receptor α [63]. Flavonoids such as catechins, quercetin, and rutin inhibit adipogenesis by suppressing adipocyte differentiation, which leads to activation of the AMPK signal pathway and downregulation of adipogenic transcription factor expression. Naringin is a citrus flavonoid that has antihyperlipidemic activity through reduction of the Hepatic 3-hydroxy-3-methyl CoA (HMG-CoA) reductase activity [64] (Fig. 11).

Flavonoids enhance diabetes pathogenesis and its complications by regulating the metabolism of glucose, function of hepatic enzymes, and a lipid profile. Catechins reduce the accumulation of intracellular lipids significantly; thus, the glycerol-3-phosphate dehydrogenase activity is responsible for lipid synthesis. Quercetin's antidiabetic activity includes the reduction of lipid peroxidation, glucose absorption by GLUT2, and the inhibition of insulin-dependent phosphoinositide 3-kinase activation. Rutin administration stimulates liver enzymes that are active in the gluconeogenic and lipid metabolic cycle, such as hexokinase. Rutin therapy has demonstrated antiapoptotic activity by increasing the level of activity of B-cell lymphoma 2 (Bcl-2) and decreasing the level of caspase-3 in the diabetic retina. Kaempferol has many antidiabetic effects, such as enhancing the expression and activation of cellular protein regulated by AMP, decreasing cell apoptosis by suppressing caspase 3 activities, and increasing insulin output and secretion from β-cells. In addition, kaempferol increases the absorption of glucose by cells through protein kinase C and PI3 K pathways, and the synthesis of new glucose transporters [66]. As metabolic disorders are associated with inflammatory cascades, flavonoids are considered as strong antiinflammatory agents for such inflammatory consequences. The mechanistic approach behind such a scenario is the normalization of a high level of tissue necrosis factor-α (TNF α). In addition, flavonoids also normalize the invasion of macrophage infiltration exhibiting antiinflammatory action concerned with metabolic disorders. Cancer from metabolic disorders is also modulated by flavonoids, i.e., the JAK/STAT pathway is mainly responsible for breast cancer which is modulated by flavonoids. Apart from it, the PI3K/AKT/mTOR pathway is responsible for multiple features of cancer such as proliferation, differentiation, cell cycles, metabolism, and genetic stability. So all these characteristics can be controlled by flavonoids [67]. In fat tissues, curcumin hinders macrophage invasion and activation of nuclear factors, avoiding inflammatory cascades. Apart from it, curcumin also inhibits the expression of potent proinflammatory adipokines tumor necrosis factor-α and plasminogen activator inhibitor type-1. Through all these diverse mechanisms, curcumin

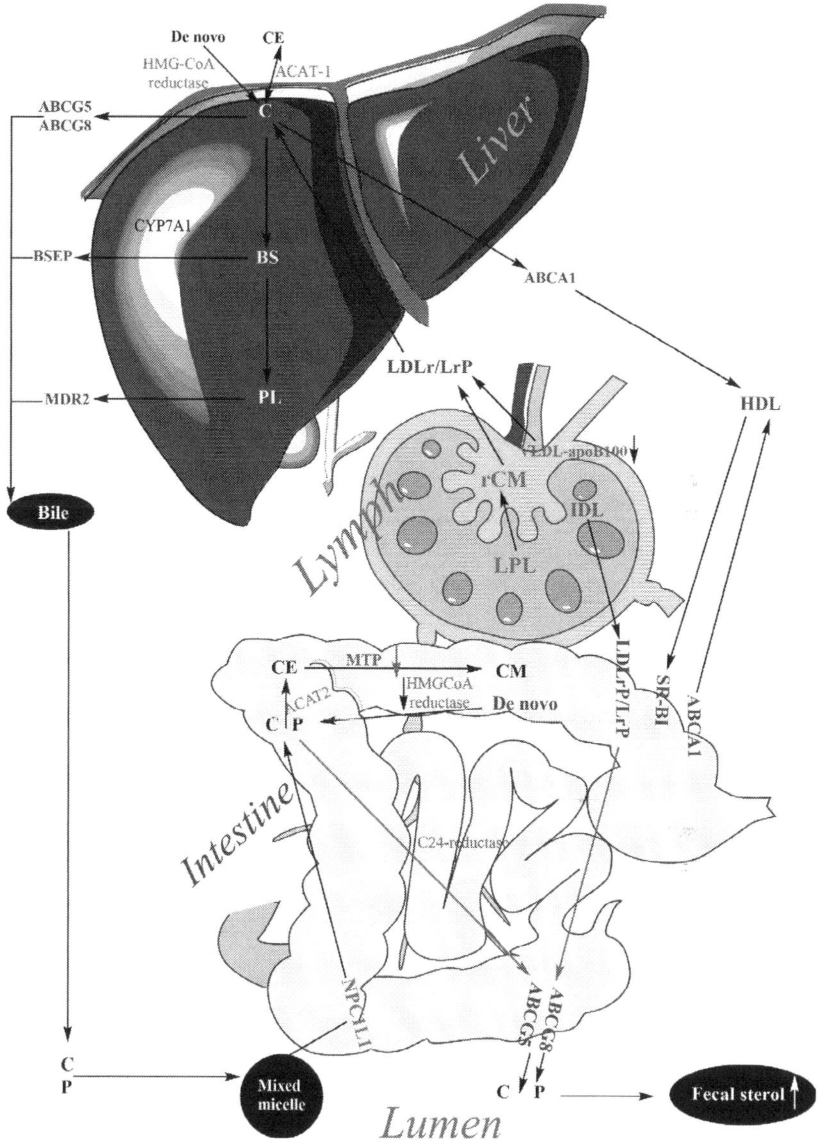

Fig. 11 The antiobesity mechanism of action of flavonoids Naringin in the kidney and liver reduces the activities of glucose-6-phosphatase and fructose-1,6-bisphosphatase contributing toward antidiabetic activity [65].

plays a vital role as an antiobese agent healing the inflammatory cascades. The expression of PPAR-γ and C/EBP induces adipo- and lipogenesis. Curcumin regulates such an expression leading to the cure of metabolic disorders [68]. Isoflavones upregulate the expression of the glutathione peroxidase enzyme leading to its anticancer activity. Cyanidin inhibits metastasis and proliferation by improving the apoptosis caspase-independent pathway. Chalcones contribute toward anticancer activity due to their antiproliferative action [69]. The HMG-CoA reductase enzyme plays an important role in the synthesis of cholesterol. The inhibition of that enzyme by sophoraflavanone G results in an antihypercholesterolemic effect [70].

3.3 Phytosterols

Phytosterol are the essential components of the plant cell membrane and plant steroid compounds in nature. Stigmasterol, β-sitosterol, and campesterol are the most abundant existing phytosterols. The dietary average intake of phytosterol is approximately 250 mg. Phytosterols are mainly considered for the management of hypercholesterolemia. The well-established study for phytosterol is based on the reduction of the cholesterol and LDL level. In general, phytosterol is thought to minimize the cholesterol levels by competitively inhibiting the absorption of cholesterol and modulating the genes involved in enterocyte and hepatocyte metabolism [71]. The antihypercholesterolemic effect of phytosterol as a whole is summarized in Fig. 12.

Cholesterol lowering by phytosterol is mainly due to the implication of the intestinal membrane transport proteins, ABCG5, ABCG8, and NPC1L1. In addition to it, the upregulation of lipoprotein lipase in skeletal muscles also contributes to the reduction in plasma triglyceride concentration [72]. Phytosterols have a key effect on various metabolic pathways leading to the maintenance of abnormal body state. β-Sitosterol and campesterol together with triterpene alcohol prevent obesity by increasing muscle fatty acid oxidation and decreasing liver fatty acid synthesis by glucose-polypeptide-dependent mechanisms. Saringosterol isolated from *Sargassum muticum* decreases the obesity dose dependently by inhibiting the differentiation of adipocytes and the expression of marker genes such as adipocyte fatty acid-binding protein, adiponectin, resistin, and fatty acid synthase. Similarly, Fecosterol—a novel phytosterol that treat obesity by minimizing the accumulation of lipid following the downregulation of insulin-triggered phosphoinositide 3 kinase/Akt and the extracellular signal regulated kinase pathway. In addition to it, fucosterol also reduces the lipid accumulation by suppression of PPAR-α. It is quite interesting that obesity-associated

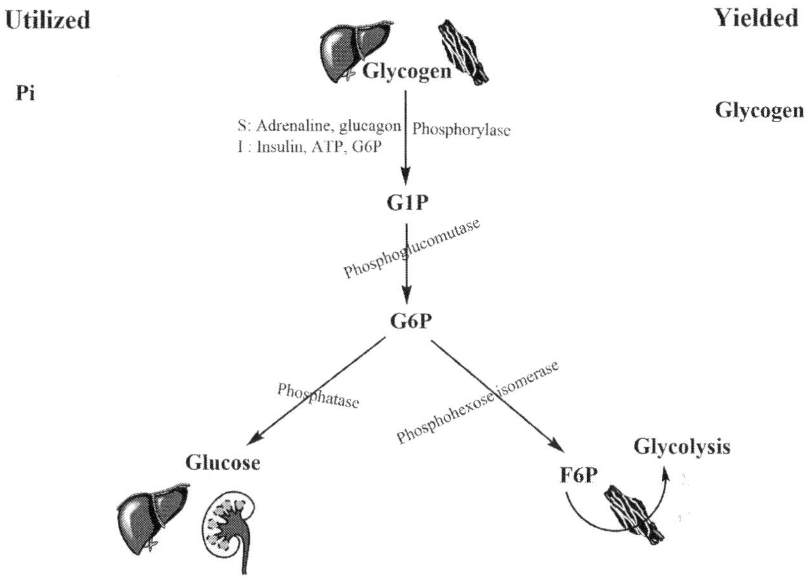

Fig. 12 Mechanism of antihypercholesterolemic effect of phytosterol. C, cholesterol; BSEP, bile salt export pump; BS, bile salt; MDR2, multidrug resistance protein; CE, cholesterol ester; ABCA1, ATP-binding cassette transporter A1; ABCG, ATP-binding cassette subfamily G; NPC1L1, Niemann-Pick C1-Like 1; HMG-CoA, hydroxy methyl glutaryl CoA; LDLrP, low-density lipoprotein receptor; LPL, lipoprotein lipase; CM, chylomicron; IDL, intermediate density lipoproteins.

inflammation is also healed by certain phytosterols such as sitosterol by inhibition of circulating interleukin-6 and TNF-α [73]. The alpha-glucosidase enzyme in the brush border of the small intestine triggers diabetes due to the breakdown of starches into glucose. Antcin a novel phytosterol from *Antrodia cinnamomea* has α-glucosidase inhibitory action that leads to antidiabetic activity [74]. Diabetes concerned with obesity is major health problem of the world. From the metabolic point of view, a disturbance in lipid metabolism leads to diabetes, while other features include hyperglycemia, insulin secretion abnormalities, and insulin sensitivity proceeding to resistance. Plant-sterols are considered as a vital glucose metabolism modulator acting through activation of AMP activated kinase or alternatively through the peroxisome proliferator activated receptor regulation pathway. Activation of AMP-kinase leads to a reduction in production of glucose, fatty acid synthesis inhibition, and glycolysis. It indicates that phytosterols are the regulator of carbohydrates and lipid metabolism [75]. Inflammation is usually concerned with metabolic disorder mediated by the invasion of macrophages or mast cells. Ergosterol has an antiinflammatory activity following the downregulation of expression of the low-density lipoprotein receptor. Another antiinflammatory pathway associated with phytosterol is suppression of NF-kB and reduction of TNF-α [76]. Phytosterols also exhibit potent activity in cancer risk. The anticancer activity of plant-sterol is governed by various mechanisms such as cholesterol synthesis downregulation, cell cycle progression inhibition, cell migration, cell adhesion, cell invasion, immune function stimulation, and cell apoptosis. Apart from it, β-sitosterol involves the protein kinase-C pathway and sphingomyelin cycle [77]. The phytosterol anticancer mechanisms involving signal pathways and molecular targets are summarized in the following figure.

3.4 Terpenes

Terpenes are a diverse group of organic aromatic compounds abundantly found in conifers. They are classified as Hemiterpenes, Monoterpenes, Sesquiterpenes, Diterpenes, Sesterterpenes, Triterpenes, and Carotenoids. Therapeutically, they are used in numerous pathological conditions, i.e., autoimmune diseases. In addition to it, terpenes are used as traditional medicine and fragrance materials in perfumes. Just like other phytonutrients, terpenes also affect various metabolic pathways and deal with certain pathological conditions (metabolic disorders). Diterpene carnosic acid from *Salvia officinalis* exhibits diverse antiobesity properties. Because of its pancreatic lipase inhibitory activity, it causes suppression of fats [78]. Peroxisome proliferator-activated receptor-gamma (PPARγ) are lipid sensors responsible for energy homeostasis and metabolic disorders. Geranylgeraniol, farnesol, and geraniol terpenoids actively stimulate the PPARγ pathway that leads to suppression of obesity. Similarly, within the adipocytes, the transcription of PPARγ is regulated by auraptene, which in turn inhibits MCP-1 via adiponectin expression. As a result, auraptene heals the inflammatory cascade associated with obesity. Abscisic acid is a sesquiterpene that is effective in diabetic- and obesity-related inflammation. Because of its proinflammatory endogenous cytokine nature, abscisic acid stimulates β-cells of the pancreas secreting insulin and thus plays a key role as an antidiabetic agent. Carotene causes the inhibition of the inflammatory gene expression pathway leading to eradication of atherosclerosis and obesity-related inflammation [79]. Apart from antiobesity effect, terpenes also play a potential role as antidiabetic agents by regulating metabolic pathways. Cucurbitane, cycloartane, and dammarane are triterpenes that exhibit antidiabetic activity following the α-glucosidase inhibitory pathway. Banaba regulates glucose metabolism owing to antidiabetic activity. It improves glucose cellular uptake and insulin sensitivity. Oleanolic acid poses antidiabetic activity through glucose level modulation and lipid metabolism regulation. Additionally, it also improves gluconeogenesis and insulin signal transduction. Sundaresan et al. demonstrated that ursolic acid at a concentration of 5 mg/kg induces the downregulation of lipogenesis and upregulation of fatty acid oxidative genes leading to reduced accumulation of hepatic lipids. It is obvious that insulin resistance is initiated in adipose tissues due to overexpression of TNF-α. In such a circumstance, the terpene stimulated PPARγ mimic lipid and glucose uptake followed by increasing glucose oxidation, decreasing insulin resistance and accumulation of fatty acid [80]. Terpenes also play a key role as an anticancer agent by modulating metabolic pathways. This type of activity is carried out through inhibition of PI3K-AKT and RAS-MAPK/ERK pathways. Limonene shows antiinflammatory activity through inhibition of the mitogen-activated kinase pathway. Similarly, α-pinene is another terpene which exhibits antiinflammatory activity by regulating the metabolic pathways. The mechanistic pathway approach is inhibition of NF-kB signals and caspase-activation inside the mast cells. β-caryophyllene is a sesquiterpene that ameliorates the proinflammatory cytokine expression resulting in an antiinflammatory effect [81].

4. Conclusions

The current chapter focuses on some of the major phytonutrients that affect the metabolic pathways within the living system that ultimately provides benefits to human health. The intake of such phytonutrients, either alone or in combination, modulates and regulates the metabolic pathways, thus overwhelming the chronic pathological progressions associated with metabolism, i.e., obesity, diabetes, hypercholesterolemia, inflammatory cascades, and cancer. The application of such phytonutrients has a positive impact at the industrial level. However, certain pathways and their mechanism carried out by phytonutrients are still unknown which need deep insight and investigation to make them expose for next generation of therapies.

References

[1] R.D. Evans, L.C. Heather, et al., Metabolic pathways and abnormalities, Surgery (Oxford) 34 (6) (2016) 266–272.

[2] I. Marin-Valencia, S.K. Cho, D. Rakheja, K.J. Hatanpaa, P. Kapur, T. Mashimo, A. Jindal, V. Vemireddy, L.B. Good, J. Raisanen, X. Sun, et al., Glucose metabolism via the pentose phosphate pathway, glycolysis and Krebs cycle in an orthotopic mouse model of human brain tumors, NMR Biomed. 25 (10) (2012) 1177–1186.

[3] E.L. Pearce, E.J. Pearce, et al., Metabolic pathways in immune cell activation and quiescence, Immunity 38 (4) (2013) 633–643.
[4] C.J. Dillard, J.B. German, et al., Phytochemicals: nutraceuticals and human health, J. Sci. Food Agric. 80 (12) (2000) 1744–1756.
[5] E. Idehen, Y. Tang, S. Sang, et al., Bioactive phytochemicals in barley, J. Food Drug Anal. 25 (1) (2017) 148–161.
[6] R.H. Vasanthi, N. ShriShriMal, K.D. Das, et al., Phytochemicals from plants to combat cardiovascular disease, Curr. Med. Chem. 19 (14) (2012) 2242–2251.
[7] A.F. Cicero, A. Colletti, et al., Role of phytochemicals in the management of metabolic syndrome, Phytomedicine 23 (11) (2016) 1134–1144.
[8] P.H. Mattila, J.M. Pihlava, J. Hellström, M. Nurmi, M. Eurola, S. Mäkinen, T. Jalava, A. Pihlanto, et al., Contents of phytochemicals and antinutritional factors in commercial protein-rich plant products, Food Qual. Saf. 2 (4) (2018) 213–219.
[9] R.H. Eckel, S.M. Grundy, P.Z. Zimmet, et al., The metabolic syndrome, Lancet 365 (9468) (2005) 1415–1428.
[10] K.E.B. Knudsen, H.N. Lærke, H. Jørgensen, et al., Carbohydrates and carbohydrate utilization in swine, in: K.E.B. Knudsen (Ed.), Sustainable Swine Nutrition, Wiley Online Library, 2013, pp. 109–137.
[11] N.S. Rosensweig, R.H. Herman, et al., Control of jejunal sucrase and maltase activity by dietary sucrose of fructose in man: a model for the study of enzyme regulation in man, J. Clin. Invest. 47 (10) (1968) 2253–2262.
[12] H.P. HAURI, B. SANDER, H. NAIM, et al., Induction of lactase biosynthesis in the human intestinal epithelial cell line Caco-2, Eur. J. Biochem. 219 (1–2) (1994) 539–546.
[13] O. Mac Donal, J.G. Chediack, E. Caviedes-Vidal, et al., Isolation of epithelial cells, villi and crypts from small intestine of pigeons (Columba livia), Biocell 32 (3) (2008) 219.
[14] A. Gupta, et al., Digestion and absorption of carbohydrates, in: A. Gupta (Ed.), Comprehensive Biochemistry for Dentistry, Springer, 2019, pp. 395–401.
[15] N. Charrière, J.P. Montani, A.G. Dulloo, et al., Postprandial thermogenesis and respiratory quotient in response to galactose: comparison with glucose and fructose in healthy young adults, J. Nutr. Sci. 5 (2016).
[16] S. Saisree, B.S. Rao, G. Sudhakara, P. Mallaiah, D. Saralakumari, et al., Screening ethanolic extract of Aerva lanata for α-amylase inhibition and in vitro uptake of glucose in adipose tissue and psoas muscle of male Sprague Dawley rats, Int. J. Pharm. Sci. Drug Res. 11 (6) (2019) 354–357.
[17] H.M. Rooijackers, E.C. Wiegers, C.J. Tack, M. van der Graaf, B.E. de Galan, et al., Brain glucose metabolism during hypoglycemia in type 1 diabetes: insights from functional and metabolic neuroimaging studies, Cell. Mol. Life Sci. 73 (4) (2016) 705–722.
[18] D. Tang, Q.B. Chen, X.L. Xin, H.A. Aisa, et al., Anti-diabetic effect of three new norditerpenoid alkaloids in vitro and potential mechanism via PI3K/Akt signaling pathway, Biomed. Pharmacother. 87 (2017) 145–152.
[19] S.F. de Oliveira, J.M. Sorbo, L.O. Regasini, B.V. da Silva, J.C. Rosa, C.É. da Silva, V. Valente, T.F. Moreira, G. Navegante, B.C. Fernandes, C.P. Soares, et al., Nitensidine B affects proteins of the glycolytic pathway and induces apoptosis in cervical carcinoma cells immortalized by HPV16, Phytomedicine 48 (2018) 179–186.
[20] G.G. Kang, N. Francis, R. Hill, D. Waters, C. Blanchard, A.B. Santhakumar, et al., Dietary polyphenols and gene expression in molecular pathways associated with type 2 diabetes mellitus: a review, Int. J. Mol. Sci. 21 (1) (2020) 140.
[21] E. Keating, F. Martel, et al., Antimetabolic effects of polyphenols in breast cancer cells: focus on glucose uptake and metabolism, Front. Nutr. 5 (2018) 25.

[22] L.H. Cazarolli, L. Zanatta, E.H. Alberton, M.S. Reis Bonorino Figueiredo, P. Folador, R.G. Damazio, M.G. Pizzolatti, F.R. Mena Barreto Silva, et al., Flavonoids: cellular and molecular mechanism of action in glucose homeostasis, Mini Rev. Med. Chem. 8 (10) (2008) 1032–1038.
[23] L. Jiao, S. Wang, Y. Zheng, N. Wang, B. Yang, D. Wang, D. Yang, W. Mei, Z. Zhao, Z. Wang, et al., Betulinic acid suppresses breast cancer aerobic glycolysis via caveolin-1/NF-κB/c-Myc pathway, Biochem. Pharmacol. 161 (2019) 149–162.
[24] S.A. Hannou, D.E. Haslam, N.M. McKeown, M.A. Herman, et al., Fructose metabolism and metabolic disease, J. Clin. Invest. 128 (2) (2018) 545–555.
[25] M.M. Adeva-Andany, N. Pérez-Felpete, C. Fernández-Fernández, C. Donapetry-García, C. Pazos-García, et al., Liver glucose metabolism in humans, Biosci. Rep. 36 (6) (2016), e00416.
[26] C.F. Iskandar, C. Cailliez-Grimal, F. Borges, A.M. Revol-Junelles, et al., Review of lactose and galactose metabolism in lactic acid bacteria dedicated to expert genomic annotation, Trends Food Sci. Technol. 88 (2019) 121–132.
[27] M. Dashty, et al., A quick look at biochemistry: carbohydrate metabolism, Clin. Biochem. 46 (15) (2013) 1339–1352.
[28] K. Shil, S.U. Pal, et al., Hexavalent chromium induced alteration of carbohydrate bioenergetics: a dose-dependent study, Asian J. Pharm. Clin. Res. 10 (2) (2017) 410–417.
[29] S.C. Patino, S.S. Mohiuddin, et al., Biochemistry, Glycogenesis, StatPearls Publishing LLC, 2019.
[30] J.P. Wynn, A.A. Hamid, Y. Li, C. Ratledge, et al., Biochemical events leading to the diversion of carbon into storage lipids in the oleaginous fungi Mucor circinelloides and Mortierella alpina, Microbiology 147 (10) (2001) 2857–2864.
[31] R.J. Perry, D. Zhang, M.T. Guerra, A.L. Brill, L. Goedeke, A.R. Nasiri, A. Rabin-Court, Y. Wang, L. Peng, S. Dufour, Y. Zhang, et al., Glucagon stimulates gluconeogenesis by INSP3R1-mediated hepatic lipolysis, Nature 579 (7798) (2020) 279–283.
[32] M. Lafontan, D. Langin, et al., Lipolysis and lipid mobilization in human adipose tissue, Prog. Lipid Res. 48 (5) (2009) 275–297.
[33] A. Pirillo, A.L. Catapano, et al., Berberine, a plant alkaloid with lipid-and glucose-lowering properties: from in vitro evidence to clinical studies, Atherosclerosis 243 (2) (2015) 449–461.
[34] J.M. Assini, E.E. Mulvihill, M.W. Huff, et al., Citrus flavonoids and lipid metabolism, Curr. Opin. Lipidol. 24 (1) (2013) 34–40.
[35] A.B. Awad, H. Williams, C.S. Fink, et al., Effect of phytosterols on cholesterol metabolism and MAP kinase in MDA-MB-231 human breast cancer cells, J. Nutr. Biochem. 14 (2) (2003) 111–119.
[36] K.R. Feingold, C. Grunfeld, et al., Introduction to lipids and lipoproteins, in: K.R. Feingold (Ed.), Endotext, MDText. com, Inc., 2018 Feb 2 (internet).
[37] R.J. Wanders, S. Ferdinandusse, P. Brites, S. Kemp, et al., Peroxisomes, lipid metabolism and lipotoxicity, Biochim. Biophys. Acta Mol. Cell Biol. Lipids 1801 (3) (2010) 272–280.
[38] Y. Li-Beisson, B. Shorrosh, F. Beisson, M.X. Andersson, V. Arondel, P.D. Bates, S. Baud, D. Bird, A. DeBono, T.P. Durrett, R.B. Franke, et al., Acyl-lipid metabolism, Arabidopsis Book 11 (2013).
[39] T.C. Walther, R.V. Farese Jr., et al., Lipid droplets and cellular lipid metabolism, Annu. Rev. Biochem. 81 (2012) 687–714.
[40] S. Zakhari, et al., Alcohol metabolism and epigenetics changes, Alcohol Res. Curr. Rev. 35 (1) (2013) 6.
[41] S.M. Phillips, R.N. Dickerson, F.A. Moore, D. Paddon-Jones, P.J. Weijs, et al., Protein turnover and metabolism in the elderly intensive care unit patient, Nutr. Clin. Pract. 32 (2017) 112S–120S.

[42] D.A. Bender, et al., Amino Acid Metabolism, John Wiley & Sons, 2012 Jul 2.
[43] C.R. Green, M. Wallace, A.S. Divakaruni, S.A. Phillips, A.N. Murphy, T.P. Ciaraldi, C.M. Metallo, et al., Branched-chain amino acid catabolism fuels adipocyte differentiation and lipogenesis, Nat. Chem. Biol. 12 (1) (2016 Jan) 15–21.
[44] C.J. Lynch, S.H. Adams, et al., Branched-chain amino acids in metabolic signalling and insulin resistance, Nat. Rev. Endocrinol. 10 (12) (2014) 723.
[45] P. Xi, Z. Jiang, C. Zheng, Y. Lin, G. Wu, et al., Regulation of protein metabolism by glutamine: implications for nutrition and health, Front. Biosci. 16 (1) (2011) 578–597.
[46] E. McCracken, M. Monaghan, S. Sreenivasan, et al., Pathophysiology of the metabolic syndrome, Clin. Dermatol. 36 (1) (2018) 14–20.
[47] S. Sam, T. Mazzone, et al., Adipose tissue changes in obesity and the impact on metabolic function, Transl. Res. 164 (4) (2014) 284–292.
[48] M. Fasshauer, S. Kralisch, M. Klier, U. Lossner, M. Bluher, J. Klein, R. Paschke, et al., Adiponectin gene expression and secretion is inhibited by interleukin-6 in 3T3-L1 adipocytes, Biochem. Biophys. Res. Commun. 301 (4) (2003) 1045–1050.
[49] S.C. Chan, C.H. Yeh, T.C. Yen, S.H. Ng, J.T.C. Chang, C.Y. Lin, T. Yen-Ming, K.H. Fan, B.S. Huang, C.L. Hsu, K.P. Chang, et al., Clinical utility of simultaneous whole-body 18 F-FDG PET/MRI as a single-step imaging modality in the staging of primary nasopharyngeal carcinoma, Eur. J. Nucl. Med. Mol. Imaging 45 (8) (2018) 1297–1308.
[50] M. Mbikay, et al., Therapeutic potential of Moringa oleifera leaves in chronic hyperglycemia and dyslipidemia: a review, Front. Pharmacol. 3 (2012) 24.
[51] K.C. Fearon, D.J. Glass, D.C. Guttridge, et al., Cancer cachexia: mediators, signaling, and metabolic pathways, Cell Metab. 16 (2) (2012) 153–166.
[52] A.J. Beijers, J.L. Jongen, G. Vreugdenhil, et al., Chemotherapy-induced neurotoxicity: the value of neuroprotective strategies, Neth. J. Med. 70 (1) (2012) 18–25.
[53] B.R. Clapp, A.D. Hingorani, R.K. Kharbanda, V. Mohamed-Ali, J.W. Stephens, P. Vallance, R.J. MacAllister, et al., Inflammation-induced endothelial dysfunction involves reduced nitric oxide bioavailability and increased oxidant stress, Cardiovasc. Res. 64 (1) (2004) 172–178.
[54] P. Aschner, et al., New IDF clinical practice recommendations for managing type 2 diabetes in primary care, Diabetes Res. Clin. Pract. 132 (2017) 169–170.
[55] A.J. Garber, M.J. Abrahamson, J.I. Barzilay, L. Blonde, Z.T. Bloomgarden, M.A. Bush, S. Dagogo-Jack, R.A. DeFronzo, D. Einhorn, V.A. Fonseca, J.R. Garber, W.T. Garvey, G. Grunberger, Y. Handelsman, I.B. Hirsch, P.S. Jellinger, J.B. McGill, J.I. Mechanick, P.D. Rosenblit, G.E. Umpierrez, et al., Consensus statement by the American Association of Clinical Endocrinologists and American College of Endocrinology on the comprehensive type 2 diabetes management algorithm—2018 executive summary, Endocr. Pract. 24 (1) (2018) 91–120.
[56] Z.Q. Wang, F.E. Lu, S.H. Leng, X.S. Fang, G. Chen, Z.S. Wang, L.P. Dong, Z.Q. Yan, et al., Facilitating effects of berberine on rat pancreatic islets through modulating hepatic nuclear factor 4 alpha expression and glucokinase activity, World J Gastroenterol: WJG 14 (39) (2008) 6004.
[57] A. Kumar, S. Aswal, R.B. Semwal, A. Chauhan, S.K. Joshi, D.K. Semwal, et al., Role of plant-derived alkaloids against diabetes and diabetes-related complications: a mechanism-based approach, Phytochem. Rev. 18 (5) (2019) 1277–1298.
[58] E.J. Park, Y.M. Kim, H.J. Kim, S.Y. Jang, M.H. Oh, D.H. Lee, K.C. Chang, et al., (S) YS-51, a novel isoquinoline alkaloid, attenuates obesity-associated non-alcoholic fatty liver disease in mice by suppressing lipogenesis, inflammation and coagulation, Eur. J. Pharmacol. 788 (2016) 200–209.
[59] C.C. Velusami, A. Agarwal, V. Mookambeswaran, et al., Effect of Nelumbo nucifera petal extracts on lipase, adipogenesis, adipolysis, and central receptors of obesity, Evid. Based Complement. Alternat. Med. 2013 (2013).

[60] Y. Rao, H.Yu, L. Gao,Y.T. Lu, Z. Xu, H. Liu, L.Q. Gu, J.M.Ye, Z.S. Huang, et al., Natural alkaloid bouchardatine ameliorates metabolic disorders in high-fat diet-fed mice by stimulating the sirtuin 1/liver kinase B-1/AMPK axis, Br. J. Pharmacol. 174 (15) (2017) 2457–2470.
[61] P.G. Bradford, et al., Curcumin and obesity, Biofactors 39 (1) (2013) 78–87.
[62] G.R. Beecher, et al., Overview of dietary flavonoids: nomenclature, occurrence and intake, J. Nutr. 133 (Suppl) (2003) 3248S–3254S.
[63] M.A. Alam, N. Subhan, M.M. Rahman, S.J. Uddin, H.M. Reza, S.D. Sarker, et al., Effect of citrus flavonoids, naringin and naringenin, on metabolic syndrome and their mechanisms of action, Adv. Nutr. 5 (4) (2014) 404–417.
[64] W.L. Li, H.C. Zheng, J. Bukuru, N. De Kimpe, et al., Natural medicines used in the traditional Chinese medical system for therapy of diabetes mellitus, J. Ethnopharmacol. 92 (1) (2004) 1–21.
[65] V.R. Punithavathi, R. Anuthama, P.S. Prince, et al., Combined treatment with naringin and vitamin C ameliorates streptozotocin-induced diabetes in male Wistar rats, J. Appl. Toxicol. Int. J. 28 (6) (2008) 806–813.
[66] R.K. AL-Ishaq, M. Abotaleb, P. Kubatka, K. Kajo, D. Büsselberg, et al., Flavonoids and their anti-diabetic effects: cellular mechanisms and effects to improve blood sugar levels, Biomol. Ther. 9 (9) (2019) 430.
[67] O.P. Martínez-Rodríguez, M.D. Thompson-Bonilla, M.E. Jaramillo-Flores, et al., Association between obesity and breast cancer: molecular bases and the effect of flavonoids in signaling pathways, Crit. Rev. Food Sci. Nutr. 2 (2020) 1–23.
[68] M. Abotaleb, S.M. Samuel, E.Varghese, S.Varghese, P. Kubatka, A. Liskova, D. Büsselberg, et al., Flavonoids in cancer and apoptosis, Cancer 11 (1) (2019) 28.
[69] K.H. Son, J.Y. Lee, J.S. Lee, S.S. Kang, H.Y. Sohn, C.S. Kwon, et al., Screening of flavonoid compounds with HMG-CoA reductase inhibitory activities, J. Life Sci. 28 (2) (2018) 247–256.
[70] C.A. Vanstone, M. Racini-Sarjaz, P.J. Jones, et al., Injected phytosterols/stanols suppress plasma cholesterol levels in hamsters, J. Nutr. Biochem. 12 (10) (2001) 565–574.
[71] C.P. Marinangeli, K.A. Varady, P.J. Jones, et al., Plant sterols combined with exercise for the treatment of hypercholesterolemia: overview of independent and synergistic mechanisms of action, J. Nutr. Biochem. 17 (4) (2006) 217–224.
[72] S. Feng, T. Belwal, L. Li, J. Limwachiranon, X. Liu, Z. Luo, et al., Phytosterols and their derivatives: potential health-promoting uses against lipid metabolism and associated diseases, mechanism, and safety issues, Compr. Rev. Food Sci. Food Saf. 19 (2020) 1243–1267.
[73] K.S. Kumar, M.G.Vani, C.Y. Chen, W.W. Hsiao, J. Li, Z.X. Lin, F.H. Chu, G.C.Yen, S.Y. Wang, et al., A mechanistic and empirical review of antcins, a new class of phytosterols of formosan fungi origin, J. Food Drug Anal. 28 (1) (2020) 38–59.
[74] M. Zakłos-Szyda, et al., Phytosterols in type 2 diabetes and obesity—molecular mechanisms of action, in: M. Zakłos-Szyda (Ed.), Plant Lipids Science, Technology, Nutritional Value and Benefits to Human Health, Research Signpost, Kerala, India, 2015, pp. 201–219.
[75] L. Yuan, F. Zhang, M. Shen, S. Jia, J. Xie, et al., Phytosterols suppress phagocytosis and inhibit inflammatory mediators via ERK pathway on LPS-triggered inflammatory responses in RAW264. 7 macrophages and the correlation with their structure, Foods 8 (11) (2019) 582.
[76] L. Jiang, X. Zhao, J. Xu, C. Li, Y. Yu, W. Wang, L. Zhu, et al., The protective effect of dietary phytosterols on cancer risk: a systematic meta-analysis, J. Oncol. 2019 (2019).
[77] M. Marrelli, F. Conforti, F. Araniti, G.A. Statti, et al., Effects of saponins on lipid metabolism: a review of potential health benefits in the treatment of obesity, Molecules 21 (10) (2016) 1404.

[78] M. González-Castejón, A. Rodriguez-Casado, et al., Dietary phytochemicals and their potential effects on obesity: a review, Pharmacol. Res. 64 (5) (2011) 438–455.
[79] H. Teng, B. Yuan, S. Gothai, P. Arulselvan, X. Song, L. Chen, et al., Dietary triterpenes in the treatment of type 2 diabetes: to date, Trends Food Sci. Technol. 72 (2018) 34–44.
[80] E.J. Downer, et al., Anti-inflammatory potential of terpenes present in Cannabis sativa L, ACS Chem. Nerosci. 11 (5) (2020) 659–662.
[81] F. Guesmi, S. Prasad, A.K. Tyagi, A. Landoulsi, et al., Antinflammatory and anticancer effects of terpenes from oily fractions of Teucruim alopecurus, blocker of IκBα kinase, through downregulation of NF-κB activation, potentiation of apoptosis and suppression of NF-κB-regulated gene expression, Biomed. Pharmacother. 95 (2017) 1876–1885.

CHAPTER 3

Nanotechnology and phytonutrients

Çiğdem Yücel[a] and Gökçe Şeker Karatoprak[b]
[a]Department of Pharmaceutical Technology, Faculty of Pharmacy, Erciyes University, Kayseri, Turkey
[b]Department of Pharmacognosy, Faculty of Pharmacy, Erciyes University, Kayseri, Turkey

1. Introduction

Nanotechnology has proven to be a promising area that can alleviate difficulties by increasing bioavailability and allowing targeting of the drug, providing continuous drug release, and reducing the required drug dose [1]. Conventional dosage forms have had limited success, demonstrating the difficulties encountered in developing an effective formulation. Nanotechnology-based formulations are seen as a new method for improving the targetability, pharmacokinetic properties, and bioavailability of bioactive molecules [2]. Nanodrug delivery systems including polymeric nanoparticles, liposomes, niosomes, nanomicelles, dendrimers, nanoemulsion/suspension, metallic nanoparticles, and nanostructured carriers are intelligent approaches that have been found to achieve great success in terms of stability, bioavailability, biodistribution, drug release, and efficiency compared to traditional drug delivery systems (Fig. 1) [2].

Phytonutrients are plant-based compounds that can modulate metabolic processes. Various classes of secondary metabolites are derived from phytonutrients, among which terpenoids, flavonoids, and alkaloids are the most studied groups, with their widespread distribution and different biological activities, and multiple chemical structures [3]. Studies on phytonutrients have shown that these compounds can be therapeutic and protective agents against diseases such as inflammation, oxidative stress, dyslipidemia, and insulin resistance. However, due to low bioavailability, their success in clinical trials is low as they have difficulty reproducing. Nanotechnology has played a vital role in providing new directions for the prevention and treatment of different diseases. Nanotechnology has shown the ability to deliver traditional natural products that have low solubility or short half-lives to target specific sites in the body and regulate the release of drugs [4].

The Role of Phytonutrients in Metabolic Disorders
https://doi.org/10.1016/B978-0-12-824356-5.00008-4

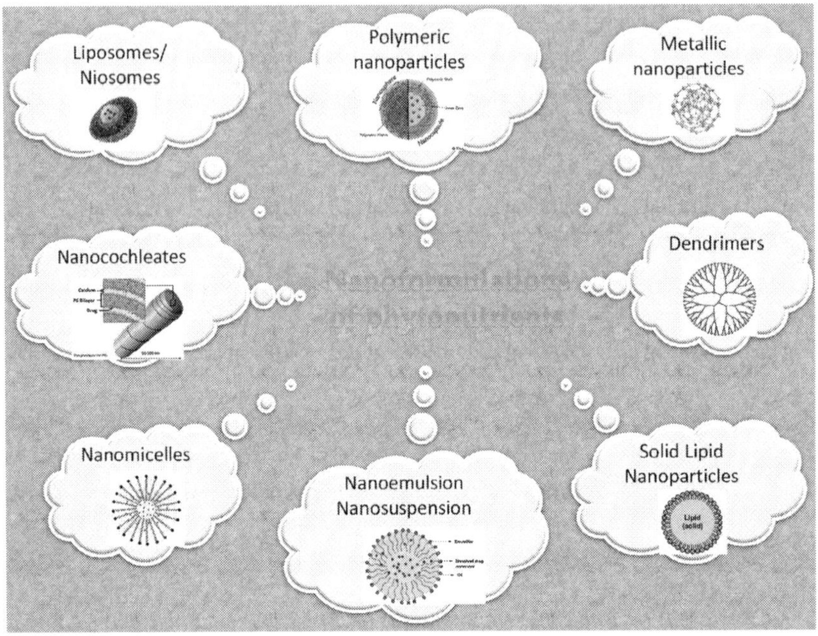

Fig. 1 Types of phytonutrient-based nanosized drug delivery systems.

According to the literature, loading polyphenols into nanocarriers has proven effective in increasing the solubility, chemical stability, and bioavailability of bioactive compounds associated with metabolic disorders [5].

Metabolic syndrome (MetS) is characterized by visceral fat accumulation associated with the combination of metabolic and pathophysiological cardiovascular risk factors, including impaired glucose tolerance or type 2 diabetes mellitus (T2DM), dyslipidemia, and hypertension, which is largely triggered by dietary excess. Lifestyle modifications mainly associated with drug therapy are effective in therapeutic approaches to MetS [6].

In this section, studies investigating the effectiveness of nanoformulations of natural compounds such as resveratrol, emodin, berberine, curcumin, and quercetin in metabolic syndrome and increasing their clinical potential are reviewed. Apart from these secondary metabolites, compounds with different flavonoid, anthocyanin, alkaloid, carotenoid, anthraquinone, and phenolic acid structures are also included.

2. Resveratrol

Resveratrol (3,a-trihydroxy-trans-stilbene) is a polyphenol phytoalexin (Fig. 2) found in grapes and red wine that has generally recognized as safe

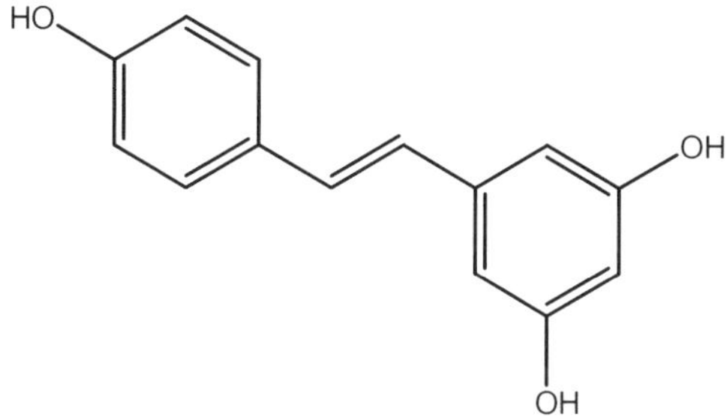

Fig. 2 Resveratrol.

(GRAS) compound status by the Food and Drug Administration [7] and has a wide range of pharmacological activities including antiinflammatory, antioxidant, antiplatelet, analgesic, neuroprotective, cardioprotective, and antiaging. It is a well-known and exclusive polyphenol encapsulated or conjugated with nanotechnology-based carriers to enhance its positive effects on glucose metabolism and oxidative damage [8–10].

In our previous study, we evaluated the efficacy of resveratrol-loaded nanoliposomes on diabetes in streptozocin-induced diabetic pancreatic β-TC cells, as well as the inhibitory effects of LPs on diabetes-related oxidative stress using superoxide dismutase (SOD) and glutathione peroxidase (GSH-Px) enzyme assays. At the end of the study, enhancement in the expression of ROS-inactivating enzymes such as GSH-Px and SOD with the extended release of resveratrol in diabetic pancreatic β-TC cells by liposomes was found. When all results were evaluated together, these newly developed liposomal formulations significantly decreased high glucose levels in diabetic cell groups synchronized with increased insulin levels, and long-term antioxidant activity against oxidative stress was observed compared to free resveratrol [11].

Nanocochleates, a new drug delivery system, are prepared using liposomes and attracted attention due to their more stable structure, which was developed with resveratrol for the assessment of antidiabetic effects by our workgroup. Similar results in diabetic β-TC cells were obtained with resveratrol-loaded nanocochleates, which may be an active formulation in the treatment of T2DM and related microvascular diseases [12].

In another study, a liposomal resveratrol formulation was designed to determine the antiobesity efficacy by local administration of resveratrol liposomes in subcutaneous white adipose tissue because resveratrol may cause the formation of beige adipocytes in subcutaneous white adipose tissue. Mice were fed a high-fat diet to determine antiobesity activity. Liposomal formulation increased the water solubility of resveratrol and improved its sustained release. The antiobesity activity of liposomes was higher relative to free resveratrol, which is associated with increased beige marker expression in inguinal white adipose tissue of mice. Browning subcutaneous white adipose tissue using liposomal resveratrol can provide an innovative and efficient approach to combating obesity [13].

In a similar study, it was aimed to apply resveratrol liposomes directly to inguinal white adipose tissue in mice and to maximize antiobesity effectiveness while minimizing side effects and toxicity. The lowest body weight, body fat mass, and body fat percentage as well as the lowest area under the curve in the glucose tolerance test at the fourth week of treatment with liposomal resveratrol treatment were determined [14].

For the same purpose, Zu et al. encapsulated resveratrol to improve its low aqueous solubility, stability, and poor bioavailability. Lipid nanocarriers and liposomes increased the water solubility and stability of resveratrol, leading to increased cellular resveratrol content and browning of 3T3-L1 white adipocytes. The findings of this study showed that using resveratrol nanoencapsulation to achieve improved own efficacy with minimal side effects is a novel strategy. While both formulations are promising for combating obesity and associated metabolic disorders, their different properties need to be taken into account and more research should be done in the treatment of obesity [15].

Mohseni et al. investigated the effect of resveratrol-loaded solid lipid nanoparticles (R-SLNs) on fasting blood glucose, insulin, and oxidative stress parameters with oral treatment in rats with T2DM. In addition, the effect of resveratrol nanoformulation on the gene expression of synaptosomal-associated protein 23 (Snap23), syntaxin-4 (Stx4), and vesicle-associated membrane protein 2 (Varnp2), which are the main elements of the SNAP-receptor (SNARE) protein complex that accelerates insulin resistance by downregulation was investigated in adipose and muscle tissues. They concluded that R-SLNs, which were developed to enhance the therapeutic effect of oral resveratrol therapy against insulin resistance by improving the hypoglycemic effect and increasing Snap23, Stx4, and Vamp2 expression, could be a promising delivery system. Besides, with the induction of diabetes, a decrease in antioxidant indicators and an increase in oxidant indicators are observed. R-SLN therapy inhibited serum total antioxidant capacity (TAC) level and increased malondialdehyde (MDA) [16]. The reason for this, thanks to R-SLNs, is that a better modulation is achieved with increased circulation time of resveratrol. However, studies are needed to elucidate the in vivo biodistribution and pharmacokinetic properties of this nanosystem will be required.

The antigestational diabetes mellitus activity of the resveratrol-zinc oxide (ZnO-RS) complex, encapsulated with chitosan (CS-ZnO-RS), was investigated by Du et al. For in vitro analyses, α-glucosidase and α-amylase inhibitory activities were measured and it was found that these activities were closely related to the CS-ZnO-RS concentration. CS-ZnO-RS treatment significantly reduced blood glucose levels caused by gestational diabetes mellitus in rats [17].

Shahraki et al. synthesized resveratrol nanocapsules as an efficient tool with $99.54 \pm 1.02\%$ encapsulation efficiency and assessed the effect of capsulated resveratrol in mice with metabolic syndrome by fat diet. For the diagnosis of insulin resistance on metabolic syndrome induction in mice by quantitative insulin sensitivity check index (QUICKI), which is the main index of insulin resistance and is derived directly from glucose and insulin values during metabolic syndrome, induction time was used. The validity and reproducibility of the QUICKI have been determined and there was a significant difference between the high-fat diet group and the control group. The resveratrol nanocapsule formulation proved its high efficiency and success by controlling the related insulin and glucose content and the QUICKI to normal lets. The results show that the obtained in vivo stability increase was related to the effectiveness of resveratrol nanocapsule formulation [18].

Insulin resistance and overweight have been associated with important risk factors for cardiovascular diseases such as blood pressure. In a previous study by the same research group, resveratrol-loaded nanocapsules were prepared and the effect of this nanoformulation on blood pressure was determined in mice with metabolic syndrome which was inducted by high-fat diet and blood pressure. A decrease in blood pressure was observed which was associated with weight reduction and increased QUICKI. Treatment with resveratrol nanocapsules regulated systolic and diastolic blood pressure in contrast to the control group [19]. It can be said that nanocapsules for effective resveratrol administration not only help in increasing stability in vivo, but also assist in regulating the patient's blood pressure with minimal treatment cost.

Teng et al. conducted a study with hepatic-targeted lysozyme micelles coated with D-(+) galactose conjugated oxidized starch natural biopolymer containing resveratrol to relieve diet-induced nonalcoholic fatty liver disease, which is the early stage of many metabolic syndromes. It was concluded that resveratrol-loaded hepatically targeted nanocarrier could potentially serve as a safe and promising platform to reverse nonalcoholic fatty liver disease and other liver-related diseases at an early stage [20].

For a similar purpose, Wan et al. prepared resveratrol-loaded poly (D, L-lactide-co-glycolide acid) (PLGA)nanoparticles (R-NPs) to overcome the bioavailability problem of resveratrol and to alleviate and reverse nonalcoholic fatty liver disease. The high stability of R-NPs, slow and prolonged release of resveratrol, and their inhibitory effect on hepatocellular proliferation and lipid accumulation compared to unformulated resveratrol have shown that they had the promising pharmacological potential to treat nonalcoholic fatty liver disease [21].

Oxidative stress plays a key role in diabetic pathogenesis and complications. Al-Bishri planned to evaluate the effect of neutralizing oxidative stress and the hypoglycemic effect of nanoresveratrol, which was purchased as a nanoemulsion, in neutralizing oxidative stress in streptozocin-induced diabetic rats. It was reported that nanoresveratrol provides glycemic control and has beneficial effects in reducing oxidative stress due to hyperglycemia and in reducing changes in antioxidant defense mechanisms [22]. Biochemical effects of nanoformulated resveratrol in metabolic disorders are summarized in Table 1.

3. Emodin

Emodin (1,3,8-trihydroxy-6-methylanthraquinone) is a naturally occurring anthraquinone derivative (Fig. 3) and an active ingredient in many herbs that have been widely used as traditional medicines. It is reported to have a wide range of pharmacological effects, such as antibacterial, antiviral, antiallergic, antiosteoporotic, antidiabetic, immunosuppressive, neuroprotective, and hepatoprotective activities [23]. It is known that emodin has an effective therapeutic effect in diabetes-associated diseases [24].

A novel strategy for obesity treatment, antiobesity drugs are targeted to adipocytes. Emodin was chosen as one of these in this study and polyethylene glycol (PEG)ylated PLGA nanoparticles were formulated with emodin and a combined targeting agent aptamer to target white adipose tissue, and in vitro delivery efficiency and lipid-lowering effects were investigated. The findings show that emodin PEGylated PLGA nanoparticles could not only selectively bind adipocytes, but also effectively reduce lipid droplets in adipocytes [25].

In terms of skin penetration and retention of the drug in the skin, nanotransfersomes are flexible in comparison to liposomes of similar structure,

Table 1 Resveratrol-based nanosized drug carriers for the management of metabolic syndrome

Nanoformulation	Metabolic disorder	In vitro/cellular/ animal model	Outcomes/mechanism	Reference
Nanoliposome	Diabetes Mellitus	Diabetic pancreatic β-TC cells	✓ Increased levels of GSH-Px and SOD ✓ Prolonged antioxidant activity against oxidative stress	[11]
Liposome	Obesity	Mice	✓ Enhanced water solubility ✓ Improved sustained release ✓ Increased antiobesity activity	[13]
Liposome	Obesity	Mice	✓ Increased antiobesity activity ✓ Minimized side effects and toxicity ✓ Decreased glucose tolerance	[14]
Nanocochleate	Diabetes mellitus	Diabetic pancreatic β-TC cells	✓ Increased levels of GSH-Px and SOD ✓ Prolonged antioxidant activity against oxidative stress	[12]
Solid lipid nanoparticles	Diabetes Mellitus	Rat	✓ Improved hypoglycemic effect of oral resveratrol against insulin resistance ✓ Increased SNAP-Receptor (SNARE) protein complex elements (Snap23, Stx4, and Vamp2) expression ✓ Inhibited serum TAC and MDA levels	[16]
Zinc oxide-chitosan complex	Gestational diabetes mellitus	In vitro Rat	✓ Inhibited α-glucosidase and α-amylase activities (in vitro) ✓ Reduced blood glucose level	[17]
Nanocapsule	Obesity	Mice	✓ Increased in vivo stability ✓ Reduced insulin resistance	[18]
Nanocapsule	Obesity	Mice	✓ Regulated the patient's blood pressure ✓ Reduced insulin resistance	[19]
Hepatically targeted micelles	Diet-induced nonalcoholic fatty liver	HepG2 cells	✓ Regulated the patient's blood pressure ✓ Reduced insulin resistance	[20]
PLGA nanoparticles	Nonalcoholic fatty liver	HepG2 cells	✓ Increased resveratrol stability ✓ Slow and prolonged resveratrol release ✓ Inhibited hepatocellular proliferation	[21]
Nanoemulsion	Diabetes Mellitus	Rat	✓ Reduced oxidative stress due to hyperglycemia ✓ Decreased in changes in antioxidant defense mechanisms	[22]

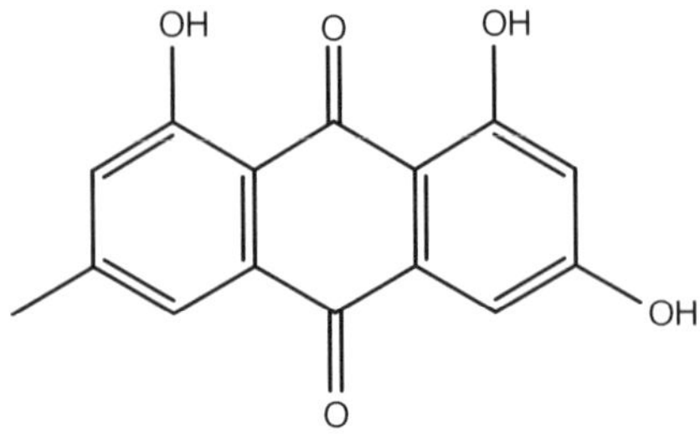

Fig. 3 Emodin.

expanding the therapeutic index of the drug and reducing the potential negative impact [26].The effect of emodin-loaded nanotransfersome, which can effectively penetrate the skin due to its elasticity, was assessed against obesity that causes T2DM. In the high-fat diet-induced obesity rat model, emodin-loaded nanotransfersomes were administrated through external friction massage for enhanced transdermal drug delivery. A relatively higher effect in terms of antiobesity activity was obtained by measuring body weight, adipocyte size, fasting blood glucose, and serum lipid levels [27].

For the treatment of angiogenesis associated with diabetic retinopathy, emodin-loaded magnesium hollow silicate nanocarriers were developed and higher efficacy at delivery of emodin and greater protective properties were obtained against angiogenesis [28].

Several other nanodelivery approaches have also been applied to improve the oral stability of emodin. The effect of emodin was improved with the developed emodin-loaded nanoemulsion, which shows sustained release in vitro [29]. Based on these data, there may be an alternative delivery approach for emodin, a functional compound, to improve bioavailability and bioactivity in the treatment of metabolic syndrome. Biochemical effects of nanoformulated emodin in metabolic disorders are summarized in Table 2.

4. Berberine

Berberine is an isoquinoline alkaloid derivative (Fig. 4) found in various species of plants (most frequently *Berberis vulgaris*) [31], which has many therapeutic effects (antiviral, antimicrobial, antidiabetic, antidiarrheal, anti-inflammatory, and antitumor). It has poor water solubility, which is classified as a class IV drug and has limitations in clinical practice due to its poor absorption and bioavailability by the gastrointestinal tract [32].

Table 2 Emodin-based nanosized drug carriers for the management of metabolic syndrome.

Nanoformulation	Metabolic disorder	In vitro/cellular/animal model	Outcomes/mechanism	Reference
PEGylated PLGA nanoparticles	Obesity	In vitro	✓ Inability to bind only selectively to adipocytes ✓ Reduced lipid droplets effectively in adipocytes	[25]
Nanoparticle	Diabetic neuropathic pain	Rat	✓ Decreased upregulation of P2X3 receptor, TNF-α protein, and the phosphorylation of ERK1/2 type II diabetes mellitus dorsal root ganglia	[30]
Nanotransfersomes	Obesity by high-fat food	Rat	✓ Enhanced transdermal drug delivery ✓ Reduced body weight, adipocyte size, fasting blood glucose, and serum lipid levels	[27]
Magnesium hollow silicate nanocarrier	Angiogenesis-associated diabetic retinopathy	In vitro	✓ Higher efficacy at emodin delivery ✓ Greater protective properties against angiogenesis	[28]

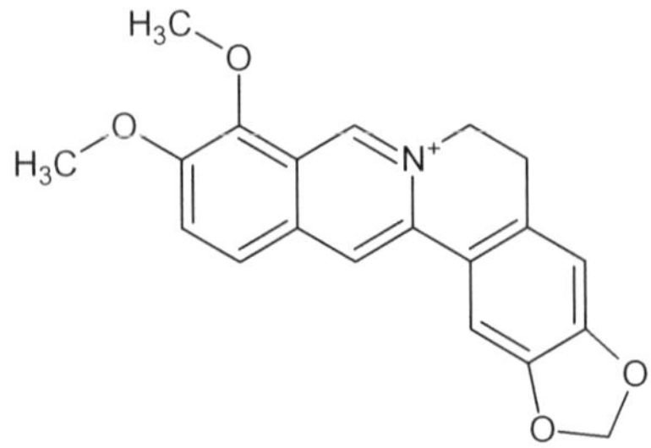

Fig. 4 Berberine.

A few reports were notified focusing on the development of new dosage forms containing berberine for oral bioavailability enhancement [33,34]. One of these solid lipid nanoparticles (SLNs) was designed by Xue et al. to advance bioavailability and obtain prolonged effect as well as investigate their pharmacokinetic properties and antidiabetic effects. It has been shown that by encapsulation into SLNs the absorption and antidiabetic effect of the berberine were effectively increased [35].

In another study, berberine nanosuspension reduced glucose, total cholesterol, and body weight compared to metformin and unformulated berberine, was equivalent in hypoglycemic effect, and established superiority in diabetic C57BL/6 mice [36,37].

In addition, antihyperlipidemic effect, tolerability, and safety supported compound berberine with numerous clinical trials was first discovered by Guo et al. They focused on the selective liver drug deposition strategy to increase the effectiveness of the berberine. Modified carrier cross-linked D-n-tocopheryl-PEG-thiol succinamide micellar structure was formulated with berberine. Berberine accumulation in the liver is increased by 248.8% with the help of micelles. A series of upregulation on energy-related genes could be detected in HepG2 cells and in vivo. The micellar intervention significantly improves metabolic profiles and reduces aortic arch plate formation in mice fed a high-fat diet [31]. Results support that the new micellar system is suitable for a liver targeting strategy to reveal the healing effect of berberine.

In a study by Yin et al., berberine-loaded selenium-coated nanostructured lipid carriers (SeNLCs) were formulated which had nanometer size and high loading efficiency compared to free berberine and exhibited better sustained release and had a stronger hypoglycemic effect compared to nonselenium coated nanoparticles [38]. Biochemical effects of nanoformulated berberine in metabolic disorders are summarized in Table 3.

Table 3 Berberine-based nanosized drug carriers for the management of metabolic syndrome.

Nanoformulation	Metabolic disorder	In vitro/cellular/ animal model	Outcomes/mechanism	Reference
Solid lipid nanoparticles	Diabetes Mellitus	Diabetic pancreatic β-TC cells	✓ Enhanced absorption and antidiabetic effect	[35]
Nanosuspension	Diabetes mellitus	diabetic C57BL/6 mice	✓ Reduced glucose and total cholesterol level and body weight	[36,37]
Modified carrier (micellar)	Hyperlipidemi	HepG2 cells Mice	✓ Improved metabolic profiles ✓ Reduced aortic arch plate formation ✓ Increased berberine accumulation in the liver	[31]
Selenium-coated nanostructured lipid carriers	Diabetes mellitus	Rat	✓ Sustained berberine release ✓ Increased oral bioavailability and hypoglycemic effect	[38]

5. Curcumin

Curcumin, (1E,6E)-1,7-bis (4-hydroxy-3-methoxyphenyl)-1,6-heptadiene-3,5-dione (Fig. 5), is an important secondary metabolite isolated from the rhizomes of *Curcuma longa* (Zingiberaceae). In the first researches, it was found that curcumin has antiinflammatory, cholesterol-lowering, antidiabetic, and antioxidant properties. Although it is a compound with many pharmacological activities, its poor solubility in water and stability poses a problem. Among many approaches, nanoformulation-based delivery systems are suitable to overcome this problem, and studies support this [39,40].

Curcumin-loaded nanoparticles accustomed with a modified emulsion-diffusion-evaporation method were tested in rats with diabetes induced by streptozocin (STZ). Nanocurcumin (15 mg/5 mL/kg bw) was given orally to the rats for 3 weeks. According to the results, treatment with nanocurcumin caused a reduction in glucose and insulin levels and also expression levels of insulin genes in liver and pancreas tissues [41]. More recently, Shamsi-Goushki et al. reported the effects of nanocurcumin on serum levels of fasting blood glucose (FBG), apelin, and lipid profile in STZ-induced diabetic rats. Nanocurcumin at 100 mg/kg concentration was found to be more potent than curcumin alone in decreasing lipid profile [42]. In a similar study, biodegradable curcumin nanoparticles prepared using PLGA were investigated in terms of their effectiveness in STZ-induced type 1 diabetes. When nonfasting rats were administered 10 and 50 mg/kg nanocurcumin 6 h before STZ loading, glucose levels decreased by 34% and 37%, respectively, the curcumin solution provided a 12% reduction at the 50 mg/kg dose. Islet or beta-cell death was also diminished with nanocurcumin treatment. Both nanocurcumin and curcumin solution reduced the amounts of inflammatory cytokines (IL-1α, G-CSF, IL-10, IL-17A, IL-1 β, IL-6, TNF-α, IL-4, GM-CSF, IFN-γ, IL-2, IL-5, IL-13, and IL-12) in pancreatic

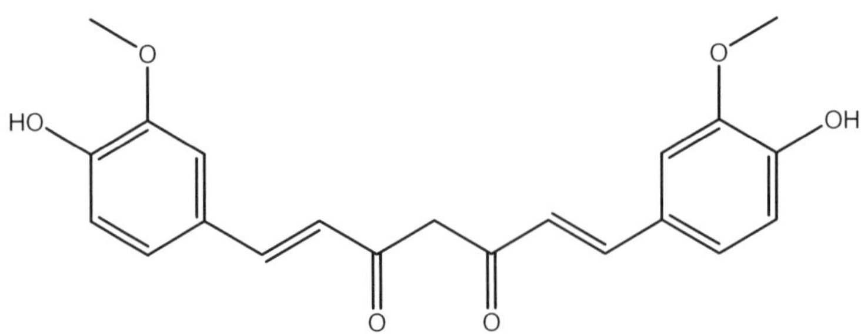

Fig. 5 Curcumin.

tissue homogenates. Only nanocurcumin pretreatment demonstrated the ability to reduce 8-oxo-20-deoxyguanosine, a critical biomarker of ROS-stimulated DNA injury in the pancreas [43]. In a study in which curcumin was stacked into polylactide-poly (ethylene glycol) (PLA-PEG) copolymer nanoparticles, STZ-induced diabetic rats were used to evaluate the antidiabetic potential of encapsulated curcumin. Compared to curcumin alone, encapsulated curcumin showed a dramatic decrease in serum glucose levels. In encapsulated curcumin-treated diabetic rats, GSH decreased, MDA increased, and NO levels were also found to approach control group levels. At the same time, NF-κB, COX-2, and TGF-β levels decreased gradually through the upregulation of PPARγ expression after treatment [44]. Chauhan et al. designed a research based on curcumin-loaded chitosan nanoparticles. The antihyperglycemic activity was investigated by measuring the level of GLUT-4 at the plasma membrane in L6myc myotubes and also the antiinflammatory potential was measured. The activity of nanocurcumin is more pronounced than that of curcumin solution, which causes a significant increase in GLUT-4 translocation to the cell surface in L6 skeletal muscle cells. This effect has been linked with enhanced phosphorylation of AKT (Ser-473) and its downstream target GSK-3β (Ser-9) [45]. Abdel Mageid et al. reported that curcumin nanosuspension has antidiabetic activity in STZ-induced rats just like nanoparticles. According to the results of the research, curcumin nanosuspension reversed the metabolic disorders induced by STZ by its antiinflammatory and antihypolipidemic effects. However, contrary to previous studies, the significant effect of curcumin nanosuspension on serum glucose and insulin levels could not be determined [46]. In insulin-resistant *ob/ob* mice liposome formulation of curcumin exerted therapeutic effect via decreasing NF-κB/RelA DNA binding activity and TNF-α levels, and increasing interleukin-4 levels. Besides, increased peripheral insulin resistance is among the parameters determined after treatment [47]. In a recent study, nanocurcumin reduced insulin resistance in rats with polycystic ovary syndrome and positively affected inflammatory and oxidative stress markers [48].

Success in in vitro studies has also been reflected in clinical trials, with several clinical studies indicating that curcumin nanoformulations exhibit improved bioavailability and pharmacokinetic properties, and high therapeutic potential. In a double-blind, placebo-controlled trial with diabetes on hemodialysis ($n = 60$), fasting plasma glucose and serum insulin levels decreased significantly by 80 mg/day nanocurcumin treatment [49]. In a different clinical trial with 35 type 2 diabetic patients, a significant reduction in FBG, glycosylated hemoglobin, low-density lipoprotein (LDL) cholesterol, triglycerides, and body mass index levels was found after treatment with 80 mg/day curcumin nanomicelles compared to placebo control patients [50]. In a pilot trial, 25 diabetic patients were administered lecithinized formulation of curcumin (Meriva) two tablets a day for 4 weeks. Microcirculation and clinical evaluations showed a decrease in skin flux at the surface of the foot, which is a diagnostic sign of an improvement in microangiopathy. Reduction in the edema score and enhancement in the venoarteriolar response were also reported [51]. Asadi et al. [52] reported the efficacy of nanocurcumin in their double-blind randomized, placebo-controlled trial. A significant reduction in glycated hemoglobin (HbA1c), FBG, total score of neuropathy, and total reflex score were recorded after nanocurcumin treatment in patients with type 2 diabetes mellitus ($n = 40$) compared with the control group. Nanocurcumin (80 mg/daily) in metabolic syndrome patients, similar to previous studies, caused a reduction in fasting plasma glucose, insulin, homeostatic model assessment of insulin resistance, and afamine levels [53].

The relationship between Proteobacteria found in the human intestine and obesity and metabolic diseases has been elucidated by the studies. In an in vitro study, Chen et al. explained the effect of nano-bubble curcumin on gut microbiota and exercise performance. Raw curcumin was soaked in nano-bubble water prepared with high pressure based on high-speed grinding. For 6 weeks the mice were administered 15.375 gkg/day (1X and 5X) of nano-bubble curcumin extract. When the results were evaluated, it was found that the application of nano-bubble curcumin changed the gut microbiota composition and helped to overcome physical fatigue. In the treatment group, the amount of tissue glycogen, which is an important energy supply for exercise, increased significantly with a longer comprehensive swimming time and higher relative forelimb grip strength compared to the control group [54]. Other studies on the efficacy of curcumin formulations on obesity were clinical studies and were evaluated in terms of their effects on obese patients. The first of these studies was conducted by Panahi et al. In this randomized controlled trial phytosomal curcumin was reported to decrease body mass index and waist circumference as well as serum enzyme levels of aspartate aminotransferase and alanine aminotransferase [55]. In a similar study nano-curcumin was evaluated for its effect on appetite in obese patients with nonalcoholic fatty liver disease (NAFLD). In this double-blind controlled trial, patients ($n = 42$) received nanocurcumin with meals at a dose of 80 mg/day for 3 months. A significant decrease in appetite on obese patients with nanocurcumin treatment has been reported [56]. In a different study, 40 mg of nanocurcumin capsule was administered to obese patients with nonalcoholic fatty liver disease ($n=42$) for 3 months after meals. In obese patients, nanocurcumin supplementation improved some markers of obesity and NAFLD, including nesfatin, quantitative insulin sensitivity control index, fatty liver grade, waist circumference, glucose indices, lipids, inflammation, and liver transaminases. However, the effects of nanocurcumin on weight, body mass index, systolic blood pressure, and diastolic blood pressure were not found prominent [57]. In a quasi-experimental study, 80 mg of nanocurcumin capsule treatment daily for 6 weeks in overweight girls, body mass index and waist-to-hip ratio, low-density lipoprotein, total cholesterol, triglyceride, and high-density lipoprotein, and CRP levels were not significantly affected [58]. Another previous study by the same research team evaluated the effects of nanocurcumin administration on the antioxidant defense system and lipid peroxidation in overweight girls. Serum glutathione, superoxide dismutase, and catalase indexes were significantly increased and MDA levels were reduced in the nanocurcumin treated group [59]. A double-blind, placebo-controlled clinical trial evaluated the efficacy of nanomicelle curcumin (80 mg capsule) in coronary elective angioplasty against curcumin given alone (500 mg capsule). Significant alterations were recorded in the total cholesterol, triglyceride, and low-density lipoprotein in the treatment groups compared to the placebo group. Also, enhancement in plasma levels of total antioxidant capacity, MDA, SOD, GPx, IL-1β, and TNF-α were reported compared to baseline measurements. When nanocurcumin and curcumin groups were compared, these changes were greater in the nanocurcumin group [60]. In female metabolic syndrome patients ($n=44$), nanocurcumin treatment caused a decrease in malondialdehyde and hs-CRP, and an increase in brain-derived neurotrophic factor (BDNF), interleukin-10, and total antioxidant capacity [61].

Low dose (5 mg/kg/day) and high dose (100 mg/kg/day) of curcumin PLGA nanoparticles were administered to rats with metabolic syndrome for 16 weeks. Low-dose and high-dose curcumin showed a significant improvement in systolic blood pressure, left ventricular diastolic stiffness, and liver fat deposition compared to the control group. In the study, low-dose curcumin was at least as effective as the high dose, but no effect on glucose tolerance was observed in both groups [62]. In a study based on the anti-inflammatory properties of curcumin, curcumin nanoparticles (50 mg/kg i.p.) applied to rats reduced the mRNA expressions of TNF-α and IL-1β. The decreased inflammatory status also led to a decrease in right ventricular hypertrophy [63]. The effect of curcumin magnetic hydrogel nanocomposite in the treatment of heart hypertrophy was also shown in an in vitro study. In this study, the effect of nanocomposite curcumin on heart failure and hypertension has been associated with an increase in antioxidant GPx and SOD enzymes and a decrease in atrial natriuretic peptide, B-type natriuretic peptide, and beta major histocompatibility complex [64].

The β-diketone moiety in curcumin, although is the main reason for its instability and poor pharmacokinetics, nanoformulations synthesized to overcome this problem and increased the solubility and stability [65–67]. Studies show that new distribution strategies such as nanoparticles, liposomes, and phospholipid complexes have been assigned to increase the effectiveness of curcumin. These nanoscale formulations prepared using different methods have proven to be effective in diabetes, obesity, hypertension, and dyslipidemia. Although some contradictory results are encountered when the research results are examined, the effectiveness of the appropriate curcumin nanoformulation will be revealed with large-scale and long-term clinical studies. Biochemical effects of nanoformulated curcumin in metabolic disorders are summarized in Table 4.

6. Quercetin

Quercetin is a flavonoid (Fig. 6) that has caught the attention of researchers due to its pharmacological activities and its widespread accessibility in the diet. Quercetin (3,3′,4′,5,7-pentahydroxyflavone) is abundant in fruits, vegetables, seeds, nuts, tea, and red wine as a glycoside and present in the form of quercetin aglycone conjugated to glucose or rutinose like sugar moieties [68,69]. Studies that take into account the instability, low water solubility, and low bioavailability of quercetin have managed to overcome this problem with carrier systems such as nanosphere, nanomicelle, nanorod, and nanoparticle [1,70].

One of the first studies to develop quercetin nanoformulation was carried out by Chitkara et al. According to the results of the pharmacokinetic study, the oral bioavailability of quercetin-loaded PLGA nanoparticles increased by 523% compared to quercetin suspension, so the dose could be reduced by using nanoparticles. Quercetin suspension (150 mg/kg, daily) and quercetin-loaded PLGA nanoparticles (150 mg/kg, every 5th day) were administered to STZ-induced rats. An increase in catalase and SOD levels as well as a decrease in blood sugar level were detected. In this study, the nanoparticle given every 5 days was compared with the suspension given every day and it was proved that the nanoparticle carrier system could

Table 4 Curcumin-based nanosized drug carriers for the management of metabolic syndrome.

Nanoformulation	Metabolic disorder	Invitro/cellular/animal model/clinical trial	Outcomes/mechanism	Reference
Nanoparticles	Diabetes mellitus	Rat	✓ Reduction in glucose and insulin levels ✓ Decreased expression levels of insulin genes	[41]
Nanomicelle	Diabetes mellitus	Rat	✓ Decreased the lipid profile ✓ Decreased insulin resistance	[42]
Nanoparticles	Diabetes mellitus	Rat	✓ Decreased Islet/ beta-cell death ✓ Reduced amounts of inflammatory cytokines ✓ Reduced 8-oxo-20-deoxyguanosine biomarker	[43]
Nanoparticles	Diabetes mellitus	Rat	✓ Decreased serum glucose level ✓ Increased GSH ✓ Decreased MDA, NO, NF-κB, COX-2, and TGF-β levels ✓ Upregulation of PPARγ expression	[44]
Chitosan nanoparticles	Diabetes mellitus	L6 skeletal muscle cells	✓ Stimulated GLUT-4myc translocation ✓ Increased phosphorylation of AKT ✓ Inhibition of GSK-3β ✓ Decrease in TNF-α, IL-6, MCP-1 levels	[45]
Nanoparticles	Diabetes mellitus	Rat	✓ Decreased serum CK-MB, LDH and AST levels ✓ Decreased serum triacylglycerol level ✓ No change in serum glucose, insulin, and total cholesterol levels	[46]
Liposome	Diabetes mellitus	Insulin-resistant *ob/ob* mice	✓ Decreased NF-κB/RelA DNA-binding activity ✓ Decreased TNF-α, increased IL-4 levels ✓ Enhanced peripheral insulin resistance	[47]
Nanoparticles	Polycystic ovarian syndrome	Rat (polycystic ovary syndrome)	✓ Decreased fasting blood glucose (FBG) and insulin level ✓ Improved β cells function ✓ Increased GSH and SOD ✓ Decreased MDA and TNF-α levels ✓ Attenuated PI3K/AKT/mTOR pathway inhibition	[48]

Continued

Table 4 Curcumin-based nanosized drug carriers for the management of metabolic syndrome—cont'd

Nanoformulation	Metabolic disorder	Invitro/cellular/animal model/clinical trial	Outcomes/mechanism	Reference
Nanomicelle	Diabetes mellitus	Double-blind, placebo-controlled clinical trial	✓ Decreased FBG ✓ Decreased serum insulin level ✓ Reduction in serum CRP and plasma MDA ✓ Reduction in triglycerides, VLDL-cholesterol, and total cholesterol ✓ Increase in plasma total antioxidant capacity	[49]
Nanomicelle	Diabetes mellitus	Double-blind, placebo-controlled clinical trial	✓ Decreased FBG, glycosylated hemoglobin, low-density lipoprotein ✓ Reduction in (LDL)-cholesterol, triglycerides, and body mass index	[50]
Phytosome	Diabetes mellitus	Pilot trial	✓ Decreased edema score ✓ Enhanced venoarteriolar response ✓ An improvement in microangiopathy	[51]
Nanomicelle	Diabetes mellitus	Double-blind, placebo-controlled clinical trial	✓ Decreased glycated hemoglobin, and FBG ✓ Reduction in total score of neuropathy and total reflex score	[52]
Nanomicelle	Metabolic syndrome	Clinical trial	✓ Reduction in FBG, insulin ✓ Decreased HOMA-IR and afamin levels	[53]
Nano-bubble	Obesity	Mice	✓ Improvement in gut microbiota composition ✓ Increased tissue glycogen ✓ Longer swimming time	[54]
Phytosome	Obesity	Randomized placebo-controlled clinical trial	✓ Decreased body mass index ✓ Decreased waist circumference ✓ Reduction in AST and ALT	[55]
Nanomicelle	Obesity with NAFLD	Double-blind, placebo-controlled clinical trial	✓ Decrease in appetite	[56]

Nanomicelle	Obesity with NAFLD	Double-blind, placebo-controlled clinical trial	✓ Increase in HDL, QUICKI, and nesfatin ✓ Reduction in FBS, FBI, HOMA-IR, TNF-α, and IL-6	[57]
Nanomicelle	Obesity	Quasi-experimental study	✓ No pronounced influence on anthropometric indicators, CRP level, and lipid profile	[58]
Nanomicelle	Obesity	Semiexperimental study.	In the training supplement group: ✓ Increase in CAT, GSH, SOD, GPx ✓ Decrease in MDA	[59]
Nanomicelle	Coronary elective angioplasty	Double-blind, placebo-controlled clinical trial	✓ Decrease in total cholesterol, triglyceride, and LDL ✓ Increase in plasma total antioxidant capacity, SOD, GPx ✓ Decrease in IL-1β, TNF-α, and MDA	[60]
Submicron particle	Metabolic syndrome	Double-blind, placebo-controlled, and semiexperimental study	✓ Reduction in MDA and hs-CRP ✓ Increase in BDNF, IL-10, total antioxidant capacity	[61]
Nanoparticles	Metabolic syndrome	Rat	✓ Improvement in systolic blood pressure, left ventricular diastolic stiffness and liver fat accumulation ✓ No effect on glucose tolerance	[62]
Nanoparticles	Hypertension	Rat	✓ Decrease in the mRNA expressions of TNF-α and IL-1β ✓ Decrease in right ventricular hypertrophy	[63]
Hydrogel nanocomposite	Heart hypertrophy	Rat	✓ Enhanced levels of GPX and SOD ✓ Decrease in atrial natriuretic peptide, B-type natriuretic peptide, and beta major histocompatibility complex	([64]

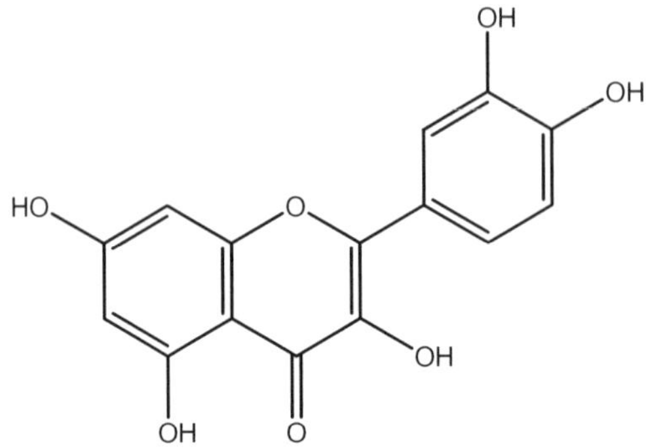

Fig. 6 Quercetin.

reduce the dose and dosing interval [71]. In alloxan-induced diabetic mice, quercetin nanorod treatment (20 mg/kg bw) for 4 weeks caused a decrease in FBG, lipid peroxidation, and protein carbonylation, and an increase in SOD, GSH, and catalase levels [72]. In 2017, two different studies evaluated the activity of quercetin nanoparticle on diabetes. Abd El-Rahman et al. reported that quercetin nanoparticle (20 mg/kg bw/day) exhibited its protective role on the pancreas and the liver in STZ-induced diabetic rats by reducing lipid profile, hepatic enzymes, and oxidative stress. As in previous studies, it has been proven in this study that the levels of SOD and GSH enzymes increased hence MDA levels decreased [73]. In a research by Tong et al. PEG-b-(PELG-g-PZLL) quercetin nanoparticle was evaluated against quercetin suspension. Quercetin suspension was administered at a dose of 10 mg/kg every day, while quercetin nanoparticle was administered at a dose of 10 mg/kg every 5 days to STZ-induced rats. Both quercetin suspension and quercetin nanoparticles improved pathological damage to the kidney as well as decreased neutrophil adhesion, kidney oxidative stress injury, and ICAM-1 expression. Decreased blood glucose levels are also the findings of the research. In comparison, it was emphasized that all these effects were more significant in the group treated with nanoparticles [74].

Quercetin-conjugated superparamagnetic iron oxide nanoparticles, which were tested in diabetic rats, increased memory performance and reduced blood glucose levels [75]. The same research group also reported that quercetin-conjugated superparamagnetic iron oxide nanoparticles in diabetic rats exhibited antioxidant activity by increasing the expression of Nrf2, SOD, and CAT, reduced the expression of NF-κB, and then normalized the expression rate of BACE1, AβPP, and Bax/Bcl-2, thus preventing memory loss [76,77].

Singh et al. investigated the effect of nano-spherical quercetin-loaded Soluplus micelles in STZ-induced diabetic rats. In the study, quercetin suspension and quercetin formulation were administered at a dose of 50 mg/kg for 15 days. Blood glucose levels, body weight change, SOD, and CAT levels were determined. It was stated that quercetin nanoformulation shows statistically more significant results than quercetin suspension in all the parameters evaluated [78]. In an analogous study, the antidiabetic activity of quercetin-succinylated chitosan-alginate core-shell nanoparticles was reported. For 28 days, rats received quercetin suspension and quercetin-loaded core-shell nanoparticles orally at a dose of 100 mg/kg. The results of this study show that the prepared nanoformulation was found to be more potent in lowering the levels of blood glucose, cholesterol, and triglyceride compared to the quercetin suspension. Besides, after the treatment in the group where quercetin nanoparticles were applied, significant improvement and regeneration in Langerhans cells were investigated [79].

Water soluble form of quercetin and liposomal quercetin administered at a dose of 10 mg/kg were compared in a research for their antidiabetic efficiency in obese, type 1, and type 2 diabetic rats. While liposomal quercetin significantly lowered blood glucose and glycosylated hemoglobin levels, it also showed antiinflammatory properties by affecting IL-6 and IL-4 levels [80].

Liquid crystalline nanoparticles containing insulin and quercetin were evaluated in diabetic rats at an equivalent dose of 50 IU/kg insulin. While the combined nanoparticles formulation did not show a significant difference in blood glucose levels compared to the nanoparticle containing insulin alone, they reduced it by 60% in 6 h. Insulin and quercetin nanoparticles exerted a significant decrease in MDA levels than the free quercetin group [81]. Polymeric microspheres containing quercetin delayed the progression of aging in the pancreatic islets both in vitro and in vivo, and also enhanced glycemic control in diabetic mice was observed after treatment with quercetin microspheres [82]. More recently, in a study conducted with pegylated liposomes loaded with quercetin (200 mg/kg), free quercetin (50 mg/kg) was also studied to compare efficacy in diabetic rats. The data of the study show that this formulation delayed the progression of diabetic nephropathy by decreasing oxidative stress and AGE expression and had renal preventive activity in the rat model of STZ-induced diabetic nephropathy [83].

The efficiency of gold-quercetin nanoparticles was evaluated in a model of chronic kidney disease caused by metabolic syndrome associated with high-fat diet and subsequent intestinal endotoxemia. As a result of high-fat diet in mice, TLR4/NF-κB and Nrf2 pathways were upregulated, SOD decreased, $O_2^{\bullet-}$ and (superoxide radical), H_2O_2, MDA, XO, XDH, and XO/XDH, were increased. The results of the study show that gold-quercetin nanoparticles can reverse these changes and correct metabolic disorders caused by a high-fat diet [84].

A preventive effect against oxidative damage induced by ischemia/reperfusion in young and old rats after oral treatment of quercetin-loaded PLGA nanoparticles was observed [85]. In a study by Wang et al., the PLGA layers applied on superparamagnetic SiN to control the drug discharge profile were assigned as a passage protective layer to direct drug discharge from the SiN. According to the outcomes of the study, the SiN @ quercetin-PLGA nanobio-composite formulation improved practical similarity to the local myocardium by allowing cell participation, binding, expansion, and articulation of heart proteins that can be used in the anticipation of atherosclerosis and other cardiovascular diseases [86,87]. In a different study, quercetin-loaded polymeric PLGA nanoparticle prepared via electrohydrodynamic atomization process has been reported to have significant potential to prevent atherosclerosis and other related cardiovascular diseases [88]. Biochemical effects of nanoformulated quercetin in metabolic disorders are summarized in Table 5.

7. Other phytonutrients

Many studies have proven that phytonutrients have various pharmacological activities. This approach has also been reflected in studies on the prevention and treatment of metabolic syndrome. The high risk of morbidity and mortality from metabolic and cardiovascular disorders has led to the discovery of new effective and nontoxic compounds for use in therapy. Many herbs find use traditionally among the public because they are considered more reliable in treatment [89]. Based on traditional usage, the efficacy of both herbal extracts and active ingredients against metabolic syndrome is still being evaluated today. In recent years, the application of these active substances, especially through nanocarrier systems, has brought many advantages. Studies of plant-derived compounds in this context are summarized in Table 6. When the studies are examined, antiinflammatory activity, improvement in blood lipid profile and insulin sensitivity, decrease in blood glucose level, and normalization in oxidative stress parameters come to the fore.

Table 5 Quercetin-based nanosized drug carriers for the management of metabolic syndrome.

Nanoformulation	Metabolic disorder	In vitro/cellular/ animal model	Outcomes/mechanism	Reference
Nanoparticles	Diabetes mellitus	Rat	✓ Reduction in glucose levels ✓ Increase in CAT and SOD	[71]
Nanorod	Diabetes mellitus	Mice	✓ Reduction in FBG, lipid peroxidation, and protein carbonylation ✓ Enhanced SOD, GSH, and CAT levels	[72]
Nanoparticles	Diabetes mellitus	Rat	✓ Reduction in lipid profile, hepatic enzymes, and oxidative stress ✓ Increase in SOD and GSH levels ✓ Decrease in MDA levels	[73]
Nanoparticles	Diabetes mellitus	Rat	✓ Decrease in neutrophil adhesion, oxidative stress injury, and ICAM-1 expression ✓ Reduction in blood glucose level	[74]
Quercetin conjugated superparamagnetic iron oxide nanoparticles	Diabetes mellitus	Rat	✓ Increase in memory performance ✓ Reduction in blood glucose levels	[75]
Quercetin conjugated superparamagnetic iron oxide nanoparticles	Diabetes mellitus	Rat	✓ Increase in expression of Nrf2, SOD, and CAT expressions ✓ Reduction in NF-κB expression ✓ Normalized BACE1, AβPP, and Bax/Bcl-2 expressions	[76] [77]
Nano-spherical micelles	Diabetes mellitus	Rat	✓ Decreased blood glucose levels ✓ Increase in SOD and CAT levels	[78]

Continued

Table 5 Quercetin-based nanosized drug carriers for the management of metabolic syndrome—cont'd

Nanoformulation	Metabolic disorder	In vitro/cellular/ animal model	Outcomes/mechanism	Reference
Nanoparticles	Diabetes mellitus	Rat	✓ Decreased blood glucose, cholesterol, and triglyceride levels ✓ Regeneration in Langerhans cells	[79]
Liposome	Diabetes mellitus	Rat	✓ Decreased blood glucose and HbA1C levels ✓ Reduction in IL-6 levels ✓ Increase in IL-4 levels	[80]
Nanoparticles	Diabetes mellitus	Rat	✓ Decrease in MDA levels ✓ Reduction in blood glucose	[81]
Microspheres	Diabetes mellitus	Mice	✓ Regeneration of pancreatic islets ✓ Enhanced glycemic control	[82]
Pegylated liposome	Diabetes mellitus	Rat	✓ Reduction in FBG ✓ Reduction in urinary protein level ✓ Reduction in BUN, Scr, TNF-α, IL-1β, AGEs, and MDA ✓ Increase in SOD and GSH-Px	[83]
Gold-quercetin nanoparticles	Kidney disease caused by metabolic syndrome associated with high-fat diet	Mice	✓ Downregulated TLR4/NF-κB and Nrf2 pathways ✓ Increase in SOD levels ✓ Decrease in MDA levels	[84]

Table 6 Phytonutrients-based nanosized drug carriers for the management of metabolic syndrome.

Compound	Nanoformulation	Metabolic disorder	Invitro/cellular/ animal model	Outcomes/mechanism	Reference
Naringenin	Nanoparticles (alginate coated)	Diabetes mellitus	Rat	✓ Improved hypoglycemic effect ✓ No toxicity	[90]
Naringenin	Nanoparticle	Diabetes mellitus	Rat	✓ Reduction in blood glucose levels and HbA1C ✓ Decreased total cholesterol, and total triglyceride ✓ Decreased levels of MDA ✓ Increase levels of GSH	[91]
Apigenin	Liposome	Diabetic cardiomyopathy	Rat	✓ Decrease in myocardial cell apoptosis ✓ Increase in Bcl-2, decrease in Bax	[92]
Apigenin	Nanoparticle	Diabetic nephropathy	Rat	✓ Decrease in NF-κB expression ✓ Decrease in MDA levels ✓ Increase in SOD and CAT levels ✓ Decreased blood glucose level ✓ Increased levels of insulin ✓ Downregulated IL-6, TNF-α, IL-1β expressions	[93]
Crocetin	Nanoparticle	Diabetic nephropathy	Rat	✓ Downregulated IL-6, TNF-α, IL-1β and MCP1 expressions ✓ Downregulated PKC and in NF-κB expressions ✓ Increase in plasma insulin	[94]
Gymnemic acid	Nanosuspension	Diabetes mellitus	Rat	✓ Decreased blood glucose concentration ✓ Improved antihyperglycemic activity	[95]

Continued

Table 6 Phytonutrients-based nanosized drug carriers for the management of metabolic syndrome—cont'd

Compound	Nanoformulation	Metabolic disorder	Invitro/cellular/ animal model	Outcomes/mechanism	Reference
Rhein	Liponanoparticle	Diabetic nephropathy	Mice	✓ Reduction in urea nitrogen, and serum creatinine ✓ Suppresive effect on fibronectin and TGF-β1 ✓ Increase in urinary creatinine levels and the creatinine clearance	[86,87]
Rhein	Nanoparticle	Diabetic nephropathy	Mice	✓ Decrease in FBG ✓ Increase in body weight ✓ Protective effect against renal dysfunctions	[96]
Baicalin	Nanostructured lipid carriers	Diabetes mellitus	Rat	✓ Decreased total cholesterol, total triglyceride, fasting blood glucose and HbA1C	[97]
Scutellarin	Nanoparticle	Diabetic retinopathy	Caco-2 cells Rat	✓ Enhanced bioavailability and cellular uptake efficiency ✓ Inhibited retinal neovascularization by preventing expression of angiogenesis proteins	[98]
Gallic acid	Nanoparticle	Diabetes Mellitus	In vitro	✓ Inhibition of α-glucosidase	[99]
Gallic acid + Insulin	Nanoparticle	Diabetes mellitus	Rat	✓ Decreased FBG ✓ Promotive effect on glycogen storage	[100]
Silybin	Nanoparticles	Diabetes mellitus	Rat	✓ Reduction in serum cholesterol, triglyceride, glycated hemoglobin levels, and restorated of liver glycogen content ✓ Increased regenerative effect on beta cell's membrane permeability	[101]

Stevioside	Nanoparticles	Diabetes mellitus	In vitro	✓ Increased intestinal absorption and bioavailability	[102]
Myricitrin	Solid lipid nanoparticles	Diabetes mellitus	Hyperglycemic myotube cells Diabetic mouse	✓ Reduced diabetes and hyperglycemia complications (hyperglycemia, insulin resistance, and pancreas apoptosis and lipid peroxidation)	[103]
Alpha-eleosteric acid	Nanoemulsion	Diabetes mellitus	Rat	✓ Reduced oxidative stress associated with diabetes by increasing the level GPx, CAT, and SOD	[104]
Capsicum oleoresin	Nanoemulsion	Obesity	3T3-L1 adipocyte cells Rat	✓ Increased lipolytic activity ✓ Decreased the body weight, adipose tissue mass and mRNA levels of adipogenic genes ✓ Increased AMP-activated protein kinase (AMPK) activity	[105]
Capsicum oleoresin	Nanoemulsion	Obesity	Rat	✓ Reduction in adipogenic gene expression ✓ Enhanced expression of PPAR-α, UCP2, and CPT-1α	[106]
Capsaicin	Microsphere	Obesity	Rat	✓ Better effect in controlling body weight, body mass index, organ index, body fat, fat to body weight ratio and serum lipids ✓ Upregulated PPARα, PPARγ, UCP2 expressions, and adiponectin ✓ Downregulated leptin expression.	[107]

Continued

Table 6 Phytonutrients-based nanosized drug carriers for the management of metabolic syndrome—cont'd

Compound	Nanoformulation	Metabolic disorder	Invitro/cellular/ animal model	Outcomes/mechanism	Reference
Pelargonidin	Nanoparticle	Diabetes mellitus	Rat	✓ Reduction in blood glucose level ✓ Increase in GHb level ✓ Decreased levels of hypercholesterolemia and triglycerides ✓ Increase in SOD and CAT levels	[108]
Pelargonidin	Nanoparticle	Diabetes mellitus	L6 cells	✓ Protective effect against DNA damage ✓ Inhibited glucose uptake ✓ Decreased ROS generation ✓ Increase in GLUT-4 and p-53	[109]
Pelargonidin	Nanoparticle	Diabetes mellitus	L6 cells	✓ Increase in GLUT-4 and GK ✓ Decrease in Cyt-c release	[109]
Trans-cinnamic acid	SNEEDS	Diabetes mellitus	Rat	✓ Increased body weight ✓ Decreased serum blood glucose, total cholesterol, and triglyceride levels ✓ Decreased ALT and AST	[36,37]
Trigonellin	Nanoparticle	Diabetes mellitus	Mice	✓ Increase in SOD, CAT, and GPx levels ✓ Decrease in blood glucose levels ✓ Decrease in lipid peroxidation	[110]
Fisetin	Nanoparticle	Diabetes mellitus	In vitro	✓ Inhibition on α-glucosidase activity ✓ DPPH and ABTS radical scavenging	[111]
Lycopene	Niosome	Diabetes mellitus	Rat	✓ Decrease in blood glucose levels ✓ Decrease in total cholesterol, LDL and VLDL	[112]

8. Conclusions

While phytochemicals have the potency to address metabolic syndromes, their low bioavailability and high levels of metabolism limit their activity. These phytochemicals are much less bioavailable due to their weak solubility and stability, and also due to additional agents such as the intestinal wall barrier, active flux in enterocytes and microbiota, and degradation and metabolism by intestinal and hepatic enzymes. Besides, after oral administration, their concentrations in blood and adipose tissue are very low. They are excreted as metabolites in urine and bile. Low bioavailability and rapid metabolism significantly limit their bioactivity, so it is very important that nanocarrier systems exceed and increase these constraints [113]. In many studies examined in this review, phytochemical-containing nanoformulations were compared with free phytochemicals and the formulations were found to be significantly more effective. For this reason, nanoformulations appear to be a promising solution for compounds with poor bioavailability and low stability.

References

[1] F.T. Rambaran, Nanopolyphenols: a review of their encapsulation and anti-diabetic effects, SN Appl. Sci. 2 (2020), 1335.

[2] S. Dewanjee, P. Chakraborty, B. Mukherjee, V. De Feo, Plant-based antidiabetic nanoforrnulations: the emerging paradigm for effective therapy, Int. J. Mol. Sci. 21 (6) (2020) 2217.

[3] K. Niaz, M.A. Shah, F. Khan, U. Saleem, C. Vargas, P. Panichayupakaranant, Bioavailability and safety of phytonutrients, in: Phytonutrients in Food: From Traditional to Rational Usage, Elsevier, 2019, pp. 117–136, https://doi.org/10.1016/B978-0-12-815354-3.00003-4.

[4] U.I. Salman, M.B. Ahmed, U.I. Mazhar, A. Shehzad, Y.S. Lee, Switching from conventional to nano-natural phytochemicals to prevent and treat cancers: special emphasis on resveratrol, Curr. Pharm. Des. 25 (34) (2019) 3620–3632.

[5] C. Bonechi, S. Martini, L. Ciani, S. Lamponi, H. Rebmann, C. Rossi, S. Ristori, Using liposomes as carriers for polyphenolic compounds: the case of Trans-resveratrol, PLoS One 7 (8) (2012), e41438.

[6] K. Fujitaka, H. Otani, F. Jo, H. Jo, E. Nomura, M. Iwasaki, M. Nishikawa, T. Iwasaka, D.K. Das, Modified resveratrol Longevinex improves endothelial function in adults with metabolic syndrome receiving standard treatment, Nutr. Res. 31 (11) (2011) 842–847.

[7] A. Brotons-Canto, C.J. Gonzalez-Navarro, J. Gurrea, C. González-Ferrero, J.M. Irache, Zein nanoparticles improve the oral bioavailability of resveratrol in humans, J. Drug Deliv. Sci. Technol. 57 (2020), 101704.

[8] D. Arora, S. Jaglan, Therapeutic applications of resveratrol nanoformulations, Environ. Chem. Lett. 16 (1) (2018) 35–41.

[9] J. Ruivo, C. Francisco, R. Oliveira, A. Figueiras, The main potentialities of resveratrol for drug delivery systems, Brazilian J. Pharm. Sci. 51 (3) (2015) 499–513.

[10] A.C. Santos, I. Pereira, M. Pereira-Silva, L. Ferreira, M. Caldas, M. Collado-González, M. Magalhães, A. Figueiras, A.J. Ribeiro, F. Veiga, Nanotechnology-based formulations for resveratrol delivery: effects on resveratrol in vivo bioavailability and bioactivity, Colloids Surf. B: Biointerfaces 180 (2019) 127–140.
[11] Ç. Yücel, G. Şeker Karatoprak, Y. Aktaş, Nanoliposomal resveratrol as a novel approach to treatment of diabetes mellitus, J. Nanosci. Nanotechnol. 18 (6) (2018) 3856–3864.
[12] Ç. Yücel, G. Şeker Karatoprak, A. Atmar, Novel resveratrol-loaded nanocochleates and effectiveness in the treatment of diabetes, Fabad J. Pharm. Sci. 43 (2) (2018) 35–44.
[13] Y. Zu, S. Wang, Resveratrol-loaded liposomes: browning subcutaneous white adipose tissue for combating obesity in C57BL/6 mice, Curr. Dev. Nutr. 4 (2) (2020) 1709.
[14] M. Khan, L. Hao, S. Wang, The anti-obesity effects of direct delivery of resveratrol-encapsulated liposomes to inguinal white adipose tissue in male APOE*3Leiden.CETP transgenic mice (P21-006-19), Curr. Dev. Nutr. Suppl 1 (2019). nzz041.P21-006-19.
[15] Y. Zu, H. Overby, G. Ren, Z. Fan, L. Zhao, S. Wang, Resveratrol liposomes and lipid nanocarriers: comparison of characteristics and inducing browning of white adipocytes, Colloids Surf. B: Biointerfaces 164 (2018) 414–423.
[16] R. Mohseni, Z. ArabSadeghabadi, N. Ziamajidi, R. Abbasalipourkabir, A. RezaeiFarimani, Oral administration of resveratrol-loaded solid lipid nanoparticle improves insulin resistance through targeting expression of snare proteins in adipose and muscle tissue in rats with type 2 diabetes, Nanoscale Res. Lett. 14 (1) (2019) 227.
[17] S. Du, Y. Lv, N. Li, X. Huang, X. Liu, H. Li, C. Wang, Y.F. Jia, Biological investigations on therapeutic effect of chitosan encapsulated nano resveratrol against gestational diabetes mellitus rats induced by streptozotocin, Drug Deliv. 27 (1) (2020) 953–963.
[18] A. Shahraki, S. Bahadorikhalili, M. Hashemzaei, J. Shahraki, O. Tajrobekar, Effects of resveratrol nanocapsules on the quantitative insulin sensitivity check index in insulin resistance: a study on metabolic syndrome induce mice, SN Appl. Sci. 2 (2020) 962, https://doi.org/10.1007/s42452-020-2759-3.
[19] A. Shahraki, S. Bahadorikhalili, M. Hashemzaei, M. Hajinezhad, A. Afsharimoghaddain, F. Sarani, O. Tajrobekar, Resveratrol nano-capsule as an efficient tool for blood pressure regulation: a study on metabolic syndrome induced mice, Biosci. Biotechnol. Res. Commun. 10 (4) (2017) 623–630.
[20] W. Teng, L. Zhao, S. Yang, C. Zhang, M. Liu, J. Luo, J. Jin, M. Zhang, C. Bao, D. Li, W. Xiong, Y. Li, F. Ren, The hepatic-targeted, resveratrol loaded nanoparticles for relief of high fat diet-induced nonalcoholic fatty liver disease, J. Control. Release 307 (2019) 139–149.
[21] S. Wan, L. Zhang, Y. Quan, K. Wei, Resveratrol-loaded PLGA nanoparticles: enhanced stability, solubility and bioactivity of resveratrol for non-alcoholic fatty liver disease therapy, R. Soc. Open Sci. 5 (2018), 181457.
[22] W.M. Al-Bishri, Attenuating impacts of chromium and nano resveratrol against hyperglycemia induced oxidative stress in diabetic rats, Int. J. Pharm. Res. Allied Sci. 6 (2) (2017) 61–69.
[23] X. Dong, J. Fu, X. Yin, S. Cao, X. Li, L. Lin, J. Ni, Emodin: a review of its pharmacology, toxicity and pharmacokinetics, Phytother. Res. 30 (8) (2016) 1207–1218.
[24] P. Ganesan, P. Arulselvan, D.K. Choi, Phytobioactive compound-based nanodelivery systems for the treatment of type 2 diabetes mellitus—current status, Int. J. Nanomedicine 12 (2017) 1097–1111.
[25] B. Yu, Y. Pu, J. Liu, J. Liao, K. Chen, J. Zhang, W. Zhong, Y. Hu, X.Q. Wang, B. Liu, H. Liu, W. Tan, Targeted delivery of emodin to adipocytes by aptamer-functionalized PEG-PLGA nanoparticles in vitro, J. Drug Deliv. Sci. Technol. 57 (2020), 101739.
[26] F.A. Moawad, A.A. Ali, H.F. Salem, Nanotransfersomes-loaded thermosensitive in situ gel as a rectal delivery system of tizanidine HCL: preparation, in vitro and in vivo performance, Drug Deliv. 24 (1) (2017) 252–260.

[27] K. Lu, S. Xie, S. Han, J. Zhang, X. Chang, J. Chao, Q. Huang, Q. Yuan, H. Lin, L. Xu, C. Shen, M. Tan, S. Qu, C. Wang, X. Song, Preparation of a nano emodin transfersome and study on its anti-obesity mechanism in adipose tissue of diet-induced obese rats, J. Transl. Med. 12 (2014) 72.
[28] H. Ren, C. Zhu, Z. Li, W. Yang, E. Song, Emodin-loaded magnesium silicate hollow nanocarriers for anti-angiogenesis treatment through inhibiting VEGF, Int. J. Mol. Sci. 15 (9) (2014) 16936–16948.
[29] Y. Shi, H. Li, J. Li, D. Zhi, X. Zhang, H. Liu, H. Wang, H. Li, Development, optimization and evaluation of emodin loaded nanoemulsion prepared by ultrasonic emulsification, J. Drug Deliv. Sci. Technol. 27 (2015) 46–55.
[30] L. Li, X. Sheng, S. Zhao, L. Zou, X. Han, Y. Gong, H. Yuan, L. Shi, L. Guo, T. Jia, S. Liu, B. Wu, Z. Yi, H. Liu, Y. Gao, G. Li, G. Li, C. Zhang, H. Xu, S. Liang, Nanoparticle-encapsulated emodin decreases diabetic neuropathic pain probably via a mechanism involving P2X3 receptor in the dorsal root ganglia, Purinergic Signal 13 (4) (2017) 559–568.
[31] H.H. Guo, C.L. Feng, W.X. Zhang, Z.G. Luo, H.J. Zhang, T.T. Zhang, C. Ma, Y. Zhan, R. Li, S. Wu, Z. Abliz, C. Li, X.L. Li, X.L. Ma, L.L. Wang, W.S. Zheng, Y.X. Han, J.D. Jiang, Liver-target nanotechnology facilitates berberine to ameliorate cardio-metabolic diseases, Nat. Commun. 10 (1) (2019), 1981.
[32] E. Mirhadi, M. Rezaee, B. Malaekeh-Nikouei, Nano strategies for berberine delivery, a natural alkaloid of Berberis, Biomed. Pharmacother. 104 (2018) 465–473.
[33] Y. Chen, Y. Wang, J. Zhang, C. Sun, A. Lopez, Berberine improves glucose homeostasis in streptozotocin-induced diabetic rats in association with multiple factors of insulin resistance, ISRN Endocrinol. 2011 (2011), 519371.
[34] J.X. Zhu, D. Tang, L. Feng, Z.G. Zheng, R.S. Wang, A.G. Wu, T.T. Duan, B. He, Q. Zhu, Development of self-microemulsifying drug delivery system for oral bioavailability enhancement of berberine hydrochloride, Drug Dev. Ind. Pharm. 39 (3) (2013) 499–506.
[35] M. Xue, M.X. Yang, W. Zhang, X.M. Li, D.H. Gao, Z.M. Ou, Z.P. Li, S.H. Liu, X.J. Li, S.Y. Yang, Characterization, pharmacokinetics, and hypoglycemic effect of berberine loaded solid lipid nanoparticles, Int. J. Nanomedicine 8 (2013) 4677–4687.
[36] H. Wang, Q. Li, W. Deng, E. Omari-Siaw, Q. Wang, S. Wang, S. Wang, X. Cao, X. Xu, J. Yu, Self-nanoemulsifying drug delivery system of trans-cinnamic acid: formulation development and pharmacodynamic evaluation in alloxan-induced type 2 diabetic rat model, Drug Dev. Res. 76 (2) (2015) 82–93.
[37] Z. Wang, J. Wu, Q. Zhou, Y. Wang, T. Chen, Berberine nanosuspension enhances hypoglycemic efficacy on streptozotocin induced diabetic C57BL/6 mice, Evid. Based Complement. Alternat. Med. 2015 (2015), 239749.
[38] J. Yin, Y. Hou, Y. Yin, X. Song, Selenium-coated nanostructured lipid carriers used for oral delivery of berberine to accomplish a synergic hypoglycemic effect, Int. J. Nanomedicine 12 (2017) 8671–8680.
[39] A. Karthikeyan, N. Senthil, T. Min, Nanocurcumin: a promising candidate for therapeutic applications, Front. Pharmacol. 11 (2020) 487.
[40] J. Nath, B. Kalıta, G. Das, Curcumin and its nanoformulations: a comprehensive overview for the management of diabetes complications, Int. J. Curr. Pharm. Res. 11 (4) (2019) 18–21.
[41] W. Gouda, N.A. Hafiz, L. Mageed, A.S. Alazzouni, W.K.B. Khalil, M. Afify, M.D.E. Abdelmaksoud, Effects of nano-curcumin on gene expression of insulin and insulin receptor, Bull. Natl. Res. Cent. 43 (2019) 128.
[42] A. Shamsi-Goushki, Z. Mortazavi, M.A. Mirshekar, M. Mohammadi, N. Moradi-Kor, S. Jafari-Maskouni, M. Shahraki, Comparative effects of curcumin versus nano-curcumin on insulin resistance, serum levels of apelin and lipid profile in type 2 diabetic rats, Diabetes Metab. Syndr. Obes. 13 (2020) 2337–2346.

[43] R. Ganugula, M. Arora, P. Jaisamut, R. Wiwattanapatapee, H.G. Jørgensen, V.P. Venkatpurwar, B. Zhou, A. Rodrigues Hoffmann, R. Basu, S. Guo, N.V.R.K. Majeti, Nano-curcumin safely prevents streptozotocin-induced inflammation and apoptosis in pancreatic beta cells for effective management of type 1 diabetes mellitus, Br. J. Pharmacol. 174 (13) (2017) 2074–2084.

[44] M.E. El-Naggar, F. Al-Joufi, M. Anwar, M.F. Attia, M.A. El-Bana, Curcumin-loaded PLA-PEG copolymer nanoparticles for treatment of liver inflammation in streptozotocin-induced diabetic rats, Colloids Surf. B: Biointerfaces 177 (2019) 389–398.

[45] P. Chauhan, A.K. Tamrakar, S. Mahajan, G.B.K.S. Prasad, Chitosan encapsulated nanocurcumin induces GLUT-4 translocation and exhibits enhanced anti-hyperglycemic function, Life Sci. 213 (2018) 226–235.

[46] A.D. Abdel Mageid, M.E. Abou Salem, N. Salaam, The biochemical role of curcumin nano-suspension in the metabolism of experimentally induced diabetic rats, Benha Veterinary Med. J. 33 (2) (2017) 396–401.

[47] S.K. Yekollu, R. Thomas, B. O'Sullivan, Targeting curcusomes to inflammatory dendritic cells inhibits NF-κB and improves insulin resistance in obese mice, Diabetes 60 (11) (2011) 2928–2938.

[48] N.Z. Abuelezz, M.E. Shabana, H.M. Abdel-Mageed, L. Rashed, G.N.B. Morcos, Nanocurcumin alleviates insulin resistance and pancreatic deficits in polycystic ovary syndrome rats: insights on PI3K/AkT/mTOR and TNF-α modulations, Life Sci. 256 (2020), 118003.

[49] R. Shafabakhsh, Z. Asemi, Ž. Reiner, A. Soleimani, E. Aghadavod, F. Bahmani, The effects of nano-curcumin on metabolic status in patients with diabetes on hemodialysis, a randomized, double blind, placebo-controlled trial, Iran. J. Kidney Dis. 14 (4) (2020) 290–299.

[50] H.R. Rahimi, A.H. Mohammadpour, M. Dastani, M.R. Jaafari, K. Abnous, Mobarhan, & Oskuee., The effect of nano-curcumin on HbA1c, fasting blood glucose, and lipid profile in diabetic subjects: a randomized clinical trial, Avicenna J. Phytomed. 6 (5) (2016) 567–577.

[51] G. Appendino, G. Belcaro, U. Cornelli, R. Luzzi, S. Togni, M. Dugall, M.R. Cesarone, B. Feragalli, E. Ippolito, B.M. Errichi, L. Pellegrini, A. Ledda, A. Ricci, P. Bavera, M. Hosoi, S. Stuard, M. Corsi, S. Errichi, G. Gizzi, Potential role of curcumin phytosome (Meriva) in controlling the evolution of diabetic microangiopathy. A pilot study, Panminerva Med. 53 (3 Suppl 1) (2011) 43–49.

[52] S. Asadi, M.S. Gholami, F. Siassi, M. Qorbani, K. Khamoshian, G. Sotoudeh, Nano curcumin supplementation reduced the severity of diabetic sensorimotor polyneuropathy in patients with type 2 diabetes mellitus: a randomized double-blind placebo-controlled clinical trial, Complement. Ther. Med. 43 (2019) 253–260.

[53] N. Kheiripour, Z. Khodamoradi, A. Ranjbar, S. Borzouei, The positive effect of short-term nano-curcumin therapy on insulin resistance and serum levels of afamin in patients with metabolic syndrome, Avicenna J. Phytomed. 11 (2) (2020) 146–153.

[54] Y.M. Chen, W.C. Chiu, Y.S. Chiu, T. Li, H.C. Sung, C.Y. Hsiao, Supplementation of nano-bubble curcumin extract improves gut microbiota composition and exercise performance in mice, Food Funct. 11 (4) (2020) 3574–3584.

[55] Y. Panahi, P. Kianpour, R. Mohtashami, R. Jafari, L.E. Simental-Mendía, A. Sahebkar, Efficacy and safety of phytosomal curcumin in non-alcoholic fatty liver disease: a randomized controlled trial, Drug Res. 67 (4) (2017) 244–251.

[56] S.A. Jazayeri-Tehrani, S.M. Rezayat, S. Mansouri, M. Qorbani, S.M. Alavian, M. Daneshi-Maskooni, M.J. Hosseinzadeh-Attar, The nanocurcumin reduces appetite in obese patients with non-alcoholic fatty liver disease (NAFLD): a double-blind randomized placebo-controlled clinical trial, Nanomed. J. 5 (2) (2018) 67–76.

[57] S.A. Jazayeri-Tehrani, S.M. Rezayat, S. Mansouri, M. Qorbani, S.M. Alavian, M. Daneshi-Maskooni, M.J. Hosseinzadeh-Attar, Nano-curcumin improves glucose

indices, lipids, inflammation, and Nesfatin in overweight and obese patients with non-alcoholic fatty liver disease (NAFLD): a double-blind randomized placebo-controlled clinical trial, Nutr. Metabol. 16 (8) (2019) 8.

[58] F. Fakhri, S. Fakhri, S. Shakeryan, A. Alizadeh, The effect of short-term nanocurcumin supplementation on the anthropometric indices, lipid profile and C-reactive protein of overweight girls (Persian), Complement. Med. J. 10 (1) (2020) 94–105.

[59] S. Fakhri, S. Shakeryan, A. Alizadeh, A. Shahryari, Effect of 6 weeks of high intensity interval training with nano-curcumin supplement on antioxidant defense and lipid peroxidation in overweight girls- clinical trial, Iran. J. Diabet. Obes. 11 (3) (2019) 173–180.

[60] H. Bijan, G. Hadis, K. Maria, H. Habib, H.S. Kianoosh, H.H. Khadem, Curcumin nanomicelle improves lipid profile, stress oxidative factors and inflammatory markers in patients undergoing coronary elective angioplasty; a randomized clinical trial, Endocr Metab Immune Disord Drug Targets 21 (2021), https://doi.org/10.2174/1871530321666210104145231.

[61] A. Osali, Aerobic exercise and nano-curcumin supplementation improve inflammation in elderly females with metabolic syndrome, Diabetol. Metab. Syndr. 12 (1) (2020) 1–7.

[62] R. du Preez, J. Pahl, M. Arora, M. Ravi Kumar, L. Brown, S.K. Panchal, Low-dose curcumin nanoparticles normalise blood pressure in male Wistar rats with diet-induced metabolic syndrome, Nutrients 11 (7) (2019) 1542.

[63] K.M. Rice, N.D.P.K. Manne, M.B. Kolli, P.S. Wehner, L. Dornon, R. Arvapalli, V. Selvaraj, A. Kumar, E.R. Blough, Curcumin nanoparticles attenuate cardiac remodeling due to pulmonary arterial hypertension, Artif. Cells Nanomed. Biotechnol. 44 (8) (2016) 1909–1916.

[64] M. Namdari, A. Eatemadi, Cardioprotective effects of curcumin-loaded magnetic hydrogel nanocomposite (nanocurcumin) against doxorubicin-induced cardiac toxicity in rat cardiomyocyte cell lines, Artif. Cells Nanomed. Biotechnol. 45 (4) (2017) 731–739.

[65] A. Mukerjee, J.K. Vishwanatha, Formulation, characterization and evaluation of curcumin-loaded PLGA nanospheres for cancer therapy, Anticancer Res. 29 (10) (2009) 3867–3875.

[66] A.P. Ranjan, A. Mukerjee, L. Helson, J.K. Vishwanatha, Scale up, optimization and stability analysis of Curcumin C3 complex-loaded nanoparticles for cancer therapy, J. Nanobiotechnol. 10 (2012), 38.

[67] D.E. Said, L.M. ElSamad, Y.M. Gohar, Validity of silver, chitosan, and curcumin nanoparticles as anti-Giardia agents, Parasitol. Res. 111 (2) (2012) 545–554.

[68] M. Bule, A. Abdurahman, S. Nikfar, M. Abdollahi, M. Amini, Antidiabetic effect of quercetin: a systematic review and meta-analysis of animal studies, Food Chem. Toxicol. 125 (2019) 494–502.

[69] G. Oboh, A.O. Ademosun, O.B. Ogunsuyi, Quercetin and its role in chronic diseases, Adv. Exp. Med. Biol. 929 (2016) 377–387.

[70] X. Li, Y. Liu, Y. Yu, W. Chen, Y. Liu, H. Yu, Nanoformulations of quercetin and cellulose nanofibers as healthcare supplements with sustained antioxidant activity, Carbohydr. Polym. 207 (2019) 160–168.

[71] D. Chitkara, S.K. Nikalaje, A. Mittal, M. Chand, N. Kumar, Development of quercetin nanoformulation and in vivo evaluation using streptozotocin induced diabetic rat model, Drug Deliv. Transl. Res. 2 (2) (2012) 112–123.

[72] M.M. Alam, K.M. Abdullah, B.R. Singh, A.H. Naqvi, I. Naseem, Ameliorative effect of quercetin nanorods on diabetic mice: mechanistic and therapeutic strategies, RSC Adv. 6 (60) (2016) 55092–55103.

[73] S.N. Abd El-Rahman, S.S. Al-Jameel, Synergistic effect of quercetin nanoparticles on liver and pancreas tissues and oxidative stress of streptozotocin-induced diabetic rats, Asian J. Chem. 29 (5) (2017) 1003–1010.

[74] F. Tong, S. Liu, B. Yan, X. Li, S. Ruan, S. Yang, Quercetin nanoparticle complex attenuated diabetic nephropathy via regulating the expression level of ICAM-1 on endothelium, Int. J. Nanomedicine 12 (2017) 7799–7813.
[75] S. Ebrahimpour, A. Esmaeili, S. Beheshti, Effect of quercetin-conjugated superparamagnetic iron oxide nanoparticles on diabetes-induced learning and memory impairment in rats, Int. J. Nanomedicine 13 (2018) 6311–6324.
[76] S. Ebrahimpour, A. Esmaeili, F. Dehghanian, S. Beheshti, Effects of quercetin-conjugated with superparamagnetic iron oxide nanoparticles on learning and memory improvement through targeting microRNAs/NF-κB pathway, Sci. Rep. 10 (2020), 15070.
[77] S. Ebrahimpour, S.B. Shahidi, M. Abbasi, Z. Tavakoli, A. Esmaeili, Quercetin-conjugated superparamagnetic iron oxide nanoparticles (QCSPIONs) increases Nrf2 expression via miR-27a mediation to prevent memory dysfunction in diabetic rats, Sci. Rep. 10 (2020), 15957.
[78] J. Singh, P. Mittal, G. Vasant Bonde, G. Ajmal, B. Mishra, Design, optimization, characterization and in vivo evaluation of Quercetin enveloped Soluplus/P407 micelles in diabetes treatment, Artif. Cells Nanomed. Biotechnol. 46 (3) (2018) S546–S555.
[79] P. Mukhopadhyay, S. Maity, S. Mandal, A.S. Chakraborti, A.K. Prajapati, P.P. Kundu, Preparation, characterization and in vivo evaluation of pH sensitive, safe quercetin-succinylated chitosan-alginate core-shell-corona nanoparticle for diabetes treatment, Carbohydr. Polym. 182 (2018) 42–51.
[80] K. Posokhova, I. Stechyshyn, I. Krynytska, M. Marushchak, I. Birchenko, I. Klishch, Comparative study of the effect of various forms of quercetin on experimental diabetes, Roman. J. Diabet. Nutr. Metabol. Dis. 25 (4) (2018) 383–388.
[81] S. Singh, V. Kushwah, A.K. Agrawal, S. Jain, Insulin- and quercetin-loaded liquid crystalline nanoparticles: implications on oral bioavailability, antidiabetic and antioxidant efficacy, Nanomedicine (London, England) 13 (5) (2018) 521–537.
[82] S. Pathak, S. Regmi, T.T. Nguyen, B. Gupta, M. Gautam, C.S. Yong, J.O. Kim, Y. Son, J.R. Kim, M.H. Park, Y.K. Bae, S.Y. Park, D. Jeong, S. Yook, J.H. Jeong, Polymeric microsphere-facilitated site-specific delivery of quercetin prevents senescence of pancreatic islets in vivo and improves transplantation outcomes in mouse model of diabetes, Acta Biomater. 75 (2018) 287–299.
[83] L. Tang, K. Li, Y. Zhang, H. Li, A. Li, Y. Xu, B. Wei, Quercetin liposomes ameliorate streptozotocin-induced diabetic nephropathy in diabetic rats, Sci. Rep. 10 (2020), 2440.
[84] M.X. Xu, M. Wang, W.W. Yang, Gold-quercetin nanoparticles prevent metabolic endotoxemia-induced kidney injury by regulating TLR4/NF-kB signaling and Nrf2 pathway in high fat diet fed mice, Int. J. Nanomedicine 12 (2017) 327–345.
[85] A. Ghosh, S. Sarkar, A.K. Mandal, N. Das, Neuroprotective role of nanoencapsulated quercetin in combating ischemia-reperfusion induced neuronal damage in young and aged rats, PLoS One 8 (4) (2013), e57735.
[86] G. Wang, Q. Li, D. Chen, B. Wu, Y. Wu, W. Tong, P. Huang, Kidney-targeted rhein-loaded liponanoparticles for diabetic nephropathy therapy via size control and enhancement of renal cellular uptake, Theranostics 9 (21) (2019) 6191–6208.
[87] L. Wang, M. Feng, Y. Li, Y. Du, H. Wang, Y. Chen, L. Li, Fabrication of superparamagnetic nano-silica@ quercetin-encapsulated PLGA nanocomposite: potential application for cardiovascular diseases, J. Photochem. Photobiol. B Biol. 196 (2019), 111508.
[88] M. Giannouli, V. Karagkiozaki, F. Pappa, I. Moutsios, C. Gravalidis, S. Logothetidis, Fabrication of quercetin-loaded PLGA nanoparticles via electrohydrodynamic atomization for cardiovascular disease, Mater. Today: Proc. 5 (8) (2018) 15998–16005.
[89] Y.D. Taghipour, M. Hajialyani, R. Naseri, M. Hesari, P. Mohammadi, A. Stefanucci, A. Mollica, M.H. Farzaei, M. Abdollahi, Nanoformulations of natural products for management of metabolic syndrome, Int. J. Nanomedicine 14 (2019) 5303–5321.

[90] S. Maity, P. Mukhopadhyay, P.P. Kundu, A.S. Chakraborti, Alginate coated chitosan core-shell nanoparticles for efficient oral delivery of naringenin in diabetic animals—an in vitro and in vivo approach, Carbohydr. Polym. 170 (2017) 124–132.

[91] S. Maity, A.S. Chakraborti, Formulation, physico-chemical characterization and antidiabetic potential of naringenin-loaded poly D, L lactide-co-glycolide (N-PLGA) nanoparticles, Eur. Polym. J. 134 (2020), 109818.

[92] Y. Zhang, Effect of apigenin-loaded nanoliposomes on myocardial cells apoptosis induced by diabetic cardiomyopathy, Herald Med. 38 (5) (2019) 555–559.

[93] P. Li, S.N.A. Bukhari, T. Khan, R. Chitti, D.B. Bevoor, A.R. Hiremath, N. SreeHarsha, Y. Singh, K.S. Gubbiyappa, Apigenin-loaded solid lipid nanoparticle attenuates diabetic nephropathy induced by streptozotocin nicotinamide through Nrf2/HO-1/NF-kB signalling pathway, Int. J. Nanomedicine 15 (2020) 9115–9124.

[94] X. Yang, Design and optimization of crocetin loaded PLGA nanoparticles against diabetic nephropathy via suppression of inflammatory biomarkers: a formulation approach to preclinical study, Drug Deliv. 26 (1) (2019) 849–859.

[95] R. Ravichandran, Studies on gymnemic acids nanoparticulate formulations against diabetes mellitus, Int. J. Biomed. Clin. Eng. 1 (2) (2012) 1–12.

[96] D. Chen, S. Han, Y. Zhu, F. Hu, Y. Wei, G. Wang, Kidney-targeted drug delivery via rhein-loaded polyethyleneglycol-co-polycaprolactone-co-polyethylenimine nanoparticles for diabetic nephropathy therapy, Int. J. Nanomedicine 13 (2018) 3507–3527.

[97] F. Shi, Z. Wei, Y. Zhao, X. Xu, Nanostructured lipid carriers loaded with baicalin: an efficient carrier for enhanced antidiabetic effects, Pharmacogn. Mag. 12 (47) (2016) 198–202.

[98] J. Wang, J. Tan, J. Luo, P. Huang, W. Zhou, L. Chen, L. Long, L. Zhang, B. Zhu, L. Yang, D.Y.B. Yeng, Enhancement of scutellarin oral delivery efficacy by vitamin B12-modified amphiphilic chitosan derivatives to treat type II diabetes induced-retinopathy, J. Nanobiotechnol. 15 (2017), 18.

[99] Purbowatiningrum, Ngadiwiyana, Ismiyarto, E. Fachriyah, I. Eviana, O. Eldiana, N. Amaliyah, A.N. Sektianingrum, Antidiabetic activity from gallic acid encapsulated nanochitosan, IOP Conf. Ser. Materi. Sci. Eng. 172 (1) (2017), 012042.

[100] Y. Zhang, L. Zhang, Q. Ban, J. Li, C.-H. Li, Y.-Q. Guan, Preparation and characterization of hydroxyapatite nanoparticles carrying insulin and gallic acid for insulin oral delivery, Nanomedicine 14 (2) (2018) 353–364.

[101] S. Das, P. Roy, R. Pal, R.G. Auddy, A.S. Chakraborti, A. Mukherjee, Engineered silybin nanoparticles educe efficient control in experimental diabetes, PLoS One 9 (7) (2014), e101818.

[102] I. Barwal, A. Sood, M. Sharma, B. Singh, S.C. Yadav, Development of stevioside pluronic-F-68 copolymer based PLA-nanoparticles as an antidiabetic nanomedicine, Colloids Surf. B: Biointerfaces 101 (2013) 510–516.

[103] A. Ahangarpour, A.A. Oroojan, L. Khorsandi, M. Kouchak, M. Badavi, Solid lipid nanoparticles of myricitrin have antioxidant and antidiabetic effects on streptozotocin-nicotinamide-induced diabetic model and myotube cell of male mouse, Oxidative Med. Cell. Longev. 2018 (2018), 7496936.

[104] D. Paul, T.K. Dey, S. Mukherjee, M. Ghosh, P. Dhar, Comparative prophylactic effects of α-eleostearic acid rich nano and conventional emulsions in induced diabetic rats, J. Food Sci. Technol. 51 (9) (2014) 1724–1736.

[105] M.S. Lee, S. Jung, Y. Shin, S. Lee, C.T. Kim, Y. Kim, Lipolytic efficacy of alginate double-layer nanoemulsion containing oleoresin capsicum in differentiated 3T3-L1 adipocytes, Food Nutr. Res. 61 (1) (2017) 1339553.

[106] J.Y. Kim, M.S. Lee, S. Jung, H. Joo, C.T. Kim, I.H. Kim, S. Seo, S. Oh, Y. Kim, Anti-obesity efficacy of nanoemulsion oleoresin capsicum in obese rats fed a high-fat diet, Int. J. Nanomedicine 9 (1) (2014) 301–310.

[107] S. Tan, B. Gao, Y. Tao, J. Guo, Z.Q. Su, Antiobese effects of capsaicin-chitosan microsphere (CCMS) in obese rats induced by high fat diet, J. Agric. Food Chem. 62 (8) (2014) 1866–1874.
[108] M. Roy, S. Sen, A.S. Chakraborti, Pelargonidin-PLGA nanoparticles: fabrication, characterization, and their effect on streptozotocin induced diabetic rats, Indian J. Exp. Biol. 55 (12) (2017) 819–830.
[109] A. Samadder, S.K. Abraham, A.R. Khuda-Bukhsh, Nanopharmaceutical approach using pelargonidin towards enhancement of efficacy for prevention of alloxan-induced DNA damage in L6 cells via activation of PARP and p53, Environ. Toxicol. Pharmacol. 43 (2016) 27–37.
[110] J.A. Daunde, S.S. Desai, P.J. Desai, P.S. Kamble, A.V. Bhoi, P.R. Gaiwad, M.V. Walvekar, Nano-scaling of trigonelline improves antioxidative status of HFD-STZ induced diabetic mice, Int. J. Res. Appl. Sci. Eng. Technol. 6 (2) (2018) 2547–2552.
[111] M. Sechi, D.N. Syed, N. Pala, A. Mariani, S. Marceddu, A. Brunetti, H. Mukhtar, V. Sanna, Nanoencapsulation of dietary flavonoid fisetin: formulation and in vitro antioxidant and α-glucosidase inhibition activities, Mater. Sci. Eng. C Mater. Biol. Appl. 68 (2016) 594–602.
[112] P.K. Sharma, P. Saxena, A. Jaswanth, M. Chalamaiah, A. Balasubramaniam, Anti-diabetic activity of lycopene niosomes. Experimental observation, J. Pharm. Drug Dev. 4 (1) (2017) 103.
[113] Z. Goktas, Y. Zu, M. Abbasi, S. Galyean, D. Wu, Z. Fan, S. Wang, Recent advances in nanoencapsulation of phytochemicals to combat obesity and its comorbidities, J. Agric. Food Chem. 68 (31) (2020) 8119–8131.

SECTION B

CHAPTER 4

Genetic effects of phytonutrients in metabolic disorders

Shabana Bibi[a,b], Mohammad Mehedi Hasan[c], Anastasiia Shkodina[d], Muhammad Ajmal Shah[e], Ghulam Mujtaba Shah[e,f], Ajmal Khan[g], and Ahmed Al-Harrasi[g]

[a]Department of Biosciences, Shifa Tameer-e-Millat University, Islamabad, Pakistan
[b]Yunnan Herbal Laboratory, School of Ecology and Environmental Sciences, Yunnan University, Kunming, China
[c]Department of Biochemistry and Molecular Biology, Mawlana Bhashani Science and Technology University, Tangail, Bangladesh
[d]Poltava State Medical University, Poltava, Ukraine
[e]Department of Pharmacy, Hazara University, Mansehra, Pakistan
[f]Department of Botany, Hazara University, Mansehra, Pakistan
[g]Natural and Medical Sciences Research Centre, University of Nizwa, Nizwa, Oman

1. Introduction

Phytonutrients could involve in the pathogenesis of fatal diseases directly or indirectly. Micronutrients present in the daily food intake usually interact with the genes in a pattern. Still, this kind of interaction occasionally could produce adverse results [1,2]. Individuals could be affected by genetic and environmental factors, so it is highly suggested to consider both factors to understand health-related circumstances [3]. Literature highlights that the individual could be affected solely by one factor, and it could be either environmental or genetic only. Scientists have clarified the phenomenon of genes and micronutrient interactions in developing and preventing disease [3,4].

Metabolic diseases (MDs) represent a growing interest in the research to gain more insight into public health issues. MD results from the interaction of heritable factors with weak linkage with environmental influences [5]. To explore the extent of human molecular genetics of an MD, an understanding of the ongoing pathophysiological phenomenon is needed [6]. As DNA methylation is the paradigm of epigenetic alteration associated with the gene's expression physiologically and pathologically and abruptly move toward the development of MD [7]. Many phyto- and micronutrients and vitamins are essential for modulating mechanisms of DNA metabolism. Indeed, it is necessary to understand that folate has a unique function as a

The Role of Phytonutrients in Metabolic Disorders
https://doi.org/10.1016/B978-0-12-824356-5.00006-0

facilitator aimed at one-carbon transfer elements for nucleotide synthesis. Current studies have presented that folate deficiency can promote the disruption of DNA synthesis/repair-related mechanism and influence the DNA methylation. While there is an evidence of gene-phytonutrient (folate), interaction suggested polymorphism in the methylenetetrahydrofolate reductase gene and promoted the mechanism of DNA methylation [8]. With dietary components (DCs) rich natural and eating food with significant oils such as olive oil and fish oils twice a week, it could improve the lifestyle of hypertriglyceridemia and hyperchylomicronemia patients to maintain their cholesterol levels with ideal body weight [9].

Genetic alteration proceeds toward the development of MD. It is investigated gender and concluded that insulin productions, glucose levels, triglycerides (TG), and cholesterols levels were the same in both genders [10]. DC as food interventions may eventually be a supportable technique to avoid MD because specific bioactive components can significantly improve individuals' health in the era of infectious pathogens [11]. Plants, vegetables, and fruits are rich sources of phytonutrients that could improve the MD frequently and improve the immune system of individuals [12,13]. Serum cholesterol management is critical to manage MD, plants sterols esters-rich DC lower the cholesterol level in children having familial hypercholesterolemia [14]. Due to abnormal lipid profiles in our body, various metabolic difficulties such as obesity, hypertension, cardiovascular diseases (CVDs), insulin resistance (IR)-related disorders, atherogenic dyslipidemia, and cancer threats have increased [15,16]. Phytonutrient-rich food components play an essential role in preventing and developing several diseases; dietary fats (DFs) are the leading cause of any MD [17]. High-fat diets (HFDs), such as saturated fatty acid (FA) contents when present in high concentration in the diet plans might process lead to the development of fatal MD, such as diabetes mellitus (DM), adiposity, obesity, IR-related disorders and inflammatory disorders [18]. In fact foods with high contents of monounsaturated fatty acids (MUFAs) have been associated with insulin sensitivity and IR-related health issues [19]. Another study reported that if obese patients are treated with MUFA-rich foods, it could have significant effects on the production of insulin and management of glucose levels and can be linked with the reduction of fats in the body [20]. Treatment with polyunsaturated fatty acids (PUFAs) in animal models, when $n-3$, has presented that it could improve the insulin sensitivity and manage the inflammatory events in anti-DM patients; although, in the case of trials in humans, results correlated and found difficulties in terms of the epidemiology of DM patients and their response toward the IR [20,21].

2. Phytonutrient-rich dietary components and genetic interactions

Nutritional factors have been studied with respect to gene expressions in MD research by genomics and transcriptomics analysis proceed to protein studies known as proteomics [22–24]. More advance study of secondary metabolites extended to metabolomics explaining the different pathways and expression of important chemicals in the body important in the management of MD [25]. Nutraceutical companies are working to understand the changes of gene expression profiles with respect to proteins that influence the regulation and transportation of certain nutrients and secondary metabolites in body, and helpful in the treatment of MD. Therefore, a novel approach has been designed known as patient-centered health care that helps to achieve more significant nutrition and healthy lifestyle-related results with respect to gene expressions that modulate the signaling pathways [26] (Fig. 1).

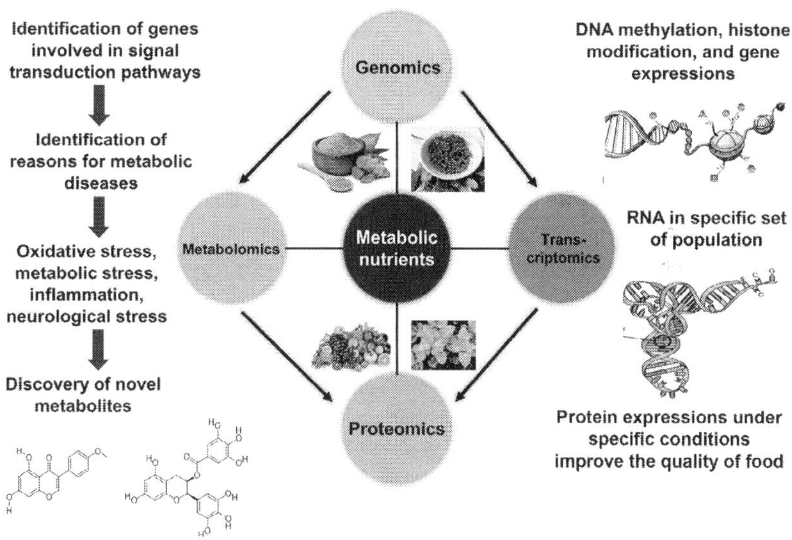

Fig. 1 Nutrigenetic/nutrigenomic research pipelines lead to the gene expression and assist in the biochemical functions in body, regulate the signal transduction pathways, and improve the physiological health effects or promote the fundamental metabolic disturbances, such as diabetes, obesity, cancers, inflammatory, oxidative, metabolic, and neurological stress. Genetics deals with the changes promoted to the next generations, transcriptomics deals with the study of RNA and gene expressions, proteomic study helps to improve the quality of phytonutrients and natural food contents in different environmental and stress conditions, and metabolomics assist the study of small molecules significant for the promotion or suppression of metabolic diseases.

The Human Genome Project supports the researchers to understand the relationship of DC making interactions with different genes and could affect the signaling pathways and results in the development of diseases [27] such as cancer, diabetes, obesity, neurodegenerative, and CVD [3,17]. Specific DCs have potential to change the gene expressions due to different reasons, might act as ligand and perform activity with transcription factor receptor, may interact with any protein and affect the signal transduction pathway, and also may be having ability to metabolize the MD-related signaling pathway and affect the concentrations of substrates [22] (Fig. 1). Specific DCs such as plant sterols manage cholesterol-related disease by predicting the interaction with individuals' genetic modifications and proceed to decrease or increase the regulatory events of specific MD pathways [28].

Sequence information assists the significance of genetic heterogeneity linkage between human populations. A large number of single-nucleotide polymorphism (SNP) investigations have presented a clear relationship of genes with food components [29]. SNPs explained the phenomenon of involved genes in the metabolism of drugs, environmental agents, or DC that might significantly influence the individual reactions toward intake of specific diet plans [12]. The effect of DC on the genetics of an individual revealed the link among SNPs and dietary nutrients, e.g., it is investigated that high-density lipoproteins (HDL) when are in high concentration in the carriers of A allele for an SNP positioned in the promoter site of apolipoprotein (APO) A1 subsequently due to polyunsaturated fatty acids (PUFAs) rich components diet. While in the case of APO E polymorphism, specifically, the carriers of APO E4 isoforms were linked with a high chance of developing CVD compared with the carriers of the APO E3 isoforms [3,30].

The interaction between DC, metabolism, and gene expression must be valuable to keep the balanced homeostasis in the body. The phytonutrient combination, not a single one, has been described as the cause of the disease-causing food components [31,32]. Genetic variation is the primary cause of individual differences in response to particular diet programs. Studies in nutrigenetics are focused on gaining an understanding of genetic variation that relates to different gene expressions and identifying genetic modifications as risk factors linked to dietary nutrients-associated diseases such as psychiatric, cancer, heart disease, neurodegenerative, and mitochondrial diseases [3,33,34].

To counteract the growing threat of cancer, the phytonutrient-rich DC group may be able to do so; they can be classified based on their interaction with specific genetic polymorphisms, studied for their influence on one another, and determined to be either carcinogens or anticarcinogens in dietary foods [35]. Interactions amongst diverse types of dietary foods might influence the overall response [1,36]. An important phenomenon of polymorphisms of genetic variants associated with tumorigenesis is frequently investigated for those adaptations of drug-like bioavailability, absorption, and the efficacy of several dietary phytonutrients. Furthermore, genes that can affect the other regulatory process of tumorigenesis, e.g., DNA methylation and replication and repair-related events, are also studied in detail [37].

Several alcohol-associated bioactive DC could regulate several intracellular pathways, prompting cancer development or protection [38,39]. Heavy consumption of food available in combination with alcohol components affects the body badly and may proceed toward the development of MD and act as metabolic sensors [38,40,41]. It is known that alcohol metabolites, enzymatically activated by liver cytochromes to become early cancer inductors, are managed by glutathione-S-transferase mu 1 (GSTM1) enzymes with the function of detoxification. It was recently indicated that GSTM1 null genotype had defensive properties against esophageal carcinoma [42]. There is a correlation between phytonutrients from the flavonol class and the wine-related compounds in esophageal carcinoma, and another study found that healthy women with the GSTM1 null genotype excrete more flavonols and epigallocatechin in their urine, which was associated with a lower risk for breast cancer. Genes and AABDCs may be responsible for this strategy's success. A cancer-protective phenotype shows that interactions between genes have a greater impact on cancer susceptibility than the single-gene phenomena [42]. The mutation develops phenylketonuria disease in a single gene, and the affected patients of this disease should avoid the food rich in phenylalanine. However, in Asia, people have this disease due to a lack of an important enzyme known as aldehyde dehydrogenase that accounts for ethanol metabolism in the body. It could not be adequately managed in patients due to ingestion of diet-containing alcohol [43].

3. Phytonutrients/natural biomolecules targeting metabolic cell signaling pathways

According to the history of medical science, natural products are the backbone of pharmaceutical industry because selected drugs identified by the results of molecular or combinatorial chemistry are very costly and have unbearable side effects [44]. Cancer is the consequence of chronic inflammatory events and moves toward the rapid growth of intrinsic origin; typical characteristics of cancers include carcinogen invasion and metastasis, inducing angiogenesis, production, and replicating carcinogens without any limit [17,45]. This contributes to why traditional Chinese medicines (TCM) have been popular and extensively utilized for anticancer treatment among various regions in China even before. Now, these herbal treatments are more acceptable worldwide because the human body was observed to be more tolerable toward TCM [46].

Recent studies have now explored the mechanism of PI3K/Akt/mTOR intracellular cascade for cancer inhibition by TCM [47]. Numerous natural food's bioactive molecules have presented significant properties against MD [17] (Table 1). The literature highlighted that multiple dietary food constituents might adapt the neoplastic progression in addition to the programmed cell death of cancer cells. Protein kinase complexes belonging to the cyclin and cyclin-dependent kinase (CDK) families are involved in the regulation of cell cycle (CC) sites [48]. In the same way, the importance of these CC sites is determined by DC. Consumption of necessary and nonessential nutrients has been shown to alter the CC checkpoints in order to reduce cancer progression and proliferation [49,50].

Colorectal neoplasia has abnormalities linked to DNA methylation accumulation. DC could have an impact on the health, such as encouraging these patients to eat more fruits and vegetables rich in folates, methionine, and alcohol in moderation [39]. Many plants' seeds include methionine, which is a highly active DC and biologically active to prevent cancer cell progression; a lack of folate and methionine in the diet, as well as the consumption of alcohol, may raise the risk of breast cancer [51]. Mechanism of action of phytonutrients in breast cancer disease has been explained in Fig. 2. Methionine-rich food is essential, as it is prevalent in the average diet and can help slow the proliferation of cancer cells [39]. A wide range of cancer types and phases of oncogenesis have been linked to DNA methylation, which is involved in a wide range of cellular and genetic processes [52]. In cancers that are dependent on methionine for their survival and proliferation, suppression of the enzyme MTHFR may be a novel approach to cancer development control. Methionine dependency in cancer may be due to a single or a group of deletions, polymorphisms, or modifications in the expression of genes involved in the methionine recovery process. Cancer cells with these defects are therefore unable to replenish methionine through these pathways [53].

Table 1 Chemical structures of phytochemicals that have a direct impact on metabolic diseases.

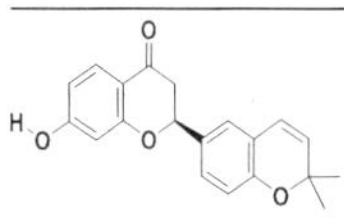 Abyssinones I	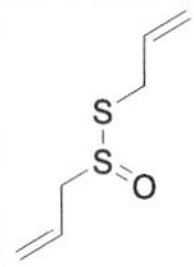 Allicin	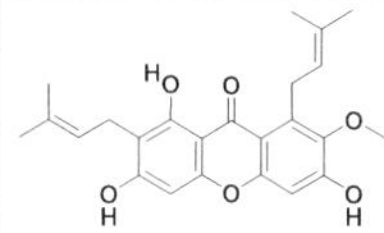 Alpha-mangostin
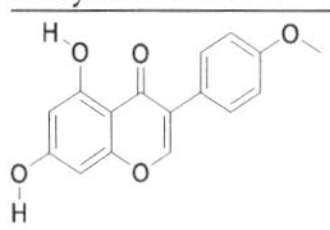 Biochanin A	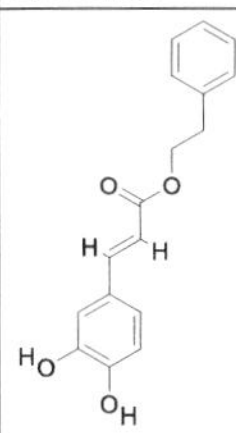 Caffeic acid phenethyl ester	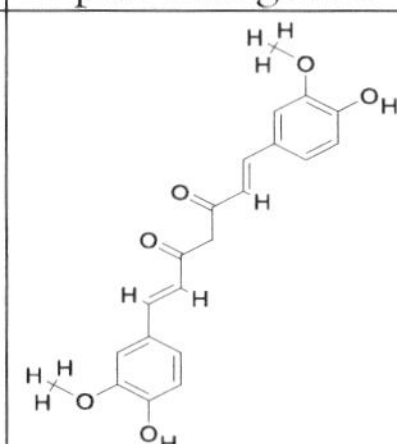 Curcumin
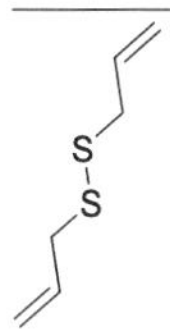 Diallyl disulfide	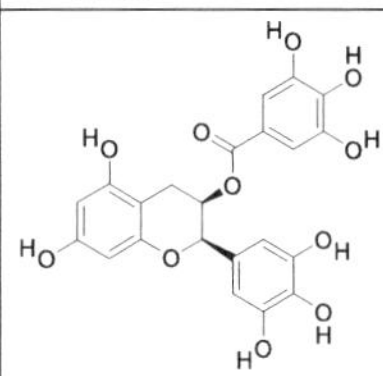 Epigallocatechin-3-gallate	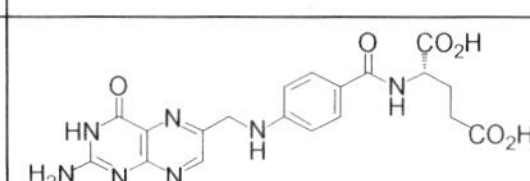 Folic acid
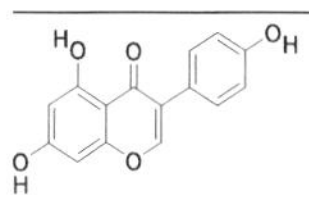 Genistein	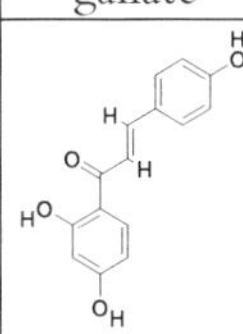 Isoliquiritigenin	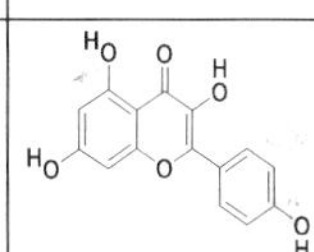 Kaempferol
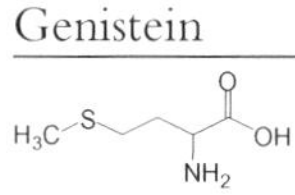 methionine	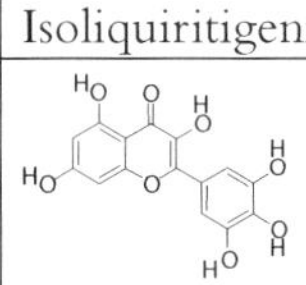 Myricetin	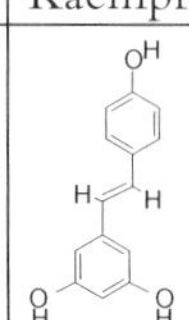 Resveratrol
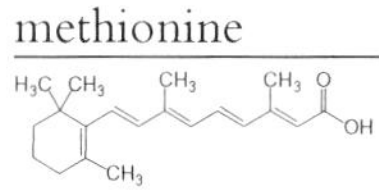 Retinoic acid	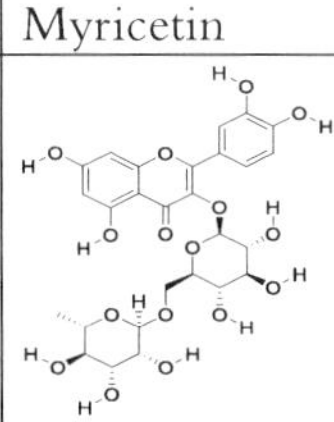 Rutin	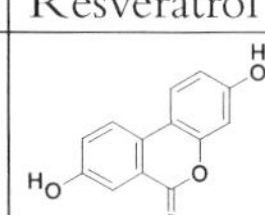 Urolithin A

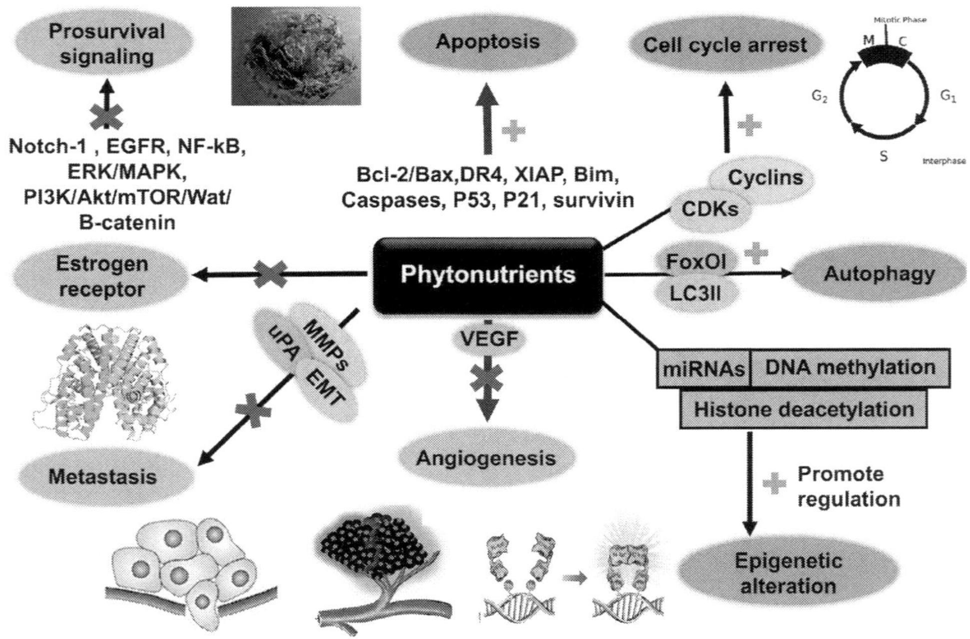

Fig. 2 Phytonutrients influence the metabolic cell signaling pathways in cancer disease.

Folates are another important bioactive molecule present in natural products also known as vitamins B9 and found abundantly in vegetables such as spinach; folates in the form of folic acid are used as supplementary contents for the treatment of several diseases caused due to folates deficiency, folates play a role in neural tube abnormalities, and several insulin's and lipid profile-related issues in CVD [54], neurodegenerative [55], and cancer disease [39,56]. Fresh green vegetables, beans, grains, and fruits are all renowned sources of folates [57]. The genome's stability can be affected by both a lack of micronutrients and an abundance of micronutrients, which have an effect on interactions between phytonutrients and genes and vice versa [58].

SNPs can impact how prominent micronutrients interactions are in choric syndrome, and hence how likely it is that these interactions will enhance or decrease the likelihood of disease onset [3]. An interaction between a gene and a phytonutrient known as the MTHFR gene is unique. Folic acid metabolism and homocysteine (Hcy) levels in the blood are closely linked via the MTHFR gene. When folic acid shortage is present in the diet, carriers of a certain MTHFR gene SNP have elevated Hcy levels in their blood [59]. Hcy levels above the recommended daily intake of folic acid are linked to cardiovascular disease (CVD) and an increased risk of colon cancer [12]. A real-life example is how folate intake can change the level of Hcy in the body. Plasma Hcy is a good indicator of how much folate, vitamin B6, and vitamin B12 you eat, but it also correlates with how much alcohol you drink [60]. The storage of Hcy is a commentator of CVD risk [61,62]. Numerous mechanisms have been hypothesized to encourage CVD onset and upgrade inflammatory events [63]. Plasma Hcy has a heredity evaluation of between 8% and 57% [64,65]. The C677T polymorphism (rs1801133) in the 5, 10 MTHFR gene has been associated to an increase in plasma Hcy. The T allele transporters are less able to convert methylenetetrahydrofolate to methyltetrahydrofolate, causing OCCP dysregulation [66]. For people with the TT genotypes, greater plasma Hcy levels, lower serum folate levels, and poor responsiveness to short-term folate supplementation have all been found in a recent meta-analysis [67]. These findings indicate the need to identify MTHFR TT carriers to minimize genetic consequences. The success of hyperhomocysteinemia treatment with folate relies on the MTHFR genotype [68].

Retinoids, generally known as vitamin A, are micronutrients present in phytochemicals such as beta-carotenoids extracted from plants. Retinoic acid is the active metabolite found in many foods and is linked to homeostasis [69]. For example, in fruits and vegetables, retinoids are provitamin beta-carotenes that can be cleaved by an enzyme in the small intestine and transformed to retinol. Several studies have been conducted to understand elevated circulation vitamin A or RBP4 levels in type 2 diabetes. In vivo, RBP4 expression was increased in adipose tissue of mice with decreased insulin action [70]. Several studies have shown that serum RBP regulates the liver's phosphoenolpyruvate carboxykinase, an important gluconeogenic enzyme, allowing for better blood glucose levels as a result of lower liver glucose levels [70]. Deficit in vitamin A or genetic intervention to lower endogenous retinoic acid synthesis and consequently retinoic acid signaling reduces fasting blood glucose and gluconeogenesis in the liver of mice [71,72]. Supplementing with high concentrations of carotenoids and flavonoids may not lessen the risk of cancer development [73].

Phyto-polyphenolic substances found in fruits and vegetables may have antioxidant and antiinflammatory qualities, which may lessen the chance of developing MD [74]. Garcinia mangostana (mangosteen fruit) has a bioactive component, alpha-mangostin, that can inhibit, reverse, or halt several breast cancer cell lines [75]. There is evidence that the protein alpha-mangostin manages the PI3K, Akt, and mTOR cascade to prevent the growth of skin cancer in mice, which has been stimulated by DMBA or TPA [76]. Healthy food and medicine have been made with pomegranates for a long time. It is an important part of many remedies because it is an antioxidant, an antiinflammatory, and an anticancer agent. Cancer cell lines from skin, lung, colorectal, breast, and prostate have been shown to be resistant to pomegranate-derived metabolites [77]. Urolithin A is an important bioactive component of pomegranate fruit, has been shown to reduce cell growth and increase cell death by blocking the PI3K/AKT/mTOR signaling cascade, which suggests a possible pancreatic cancer treatment from a healthy food source [78].

Few important phytonutrients, such as Apigenin found in celery and parsley, are significant bioactive compounds that play a role as anticarcinogen [1,48]. Plant-derived food and herbal medicine are said to control different forms of liver cancers. Antioxidant, antiinflammatory, and antiproliferative characteristics have been demonstrated for apigenin, an abundant phytonutrient found in fruits and vegetables. The inhibition of PI3K/Akt/mTOR signaling also increases autophagy in liver cell carcinoma, which offers an effective treatment for liver cancer [79].

Abyssinones I induced programmed cell death by downregulating Bcl-2 and upregulating p53 and Bax. The mitochondrial route producing cytochrome c and Apaf-1 into cytosol related to caspase-3 activation may help initiate apoptosis and also about to lower the antiproliferative markers PCNA and cyclin D1 [80]. Allicin is an important DC found in garlic and as an anticarcinogen in several animal models experiments. It could significantly promote apoptotic cell death via the regulatory mechanism of p53 gene modulatory effects in human hepatic carcinoma and is involved in developing autophagy and apoptotic procedures [81]. Biochanin A is an active natural bioactive component of red clover and has presented an excellent proliferative mechanism in lung cancer studies; it also added knowledge of CC arrest and apoptotic activity by regulating CC-associated proteins expressions and activated Bcl-2 and caspase three signaling pathways [82]. Caffeic acid phenethyl ester is an excellent phytonutrient found in most plants, intake of it can help inactivation of mitogen-activated protein kinase (MAPK) signaling pathway by increasing the NDRG1 gene expression by the phosphorylated mechanism of ERK1/2 gene expression to suppress the human oral carcinoma [83]. It is also widely investigated for the A431 skin cancer cell line and promoted apoptosis, cell cycle arrest, improvement of the ROS-mediated alteration in MMP, and blockage of the PI3K/Akt/mTOR signaling cascade [84].

Curcumin found in turmeric and other medicinal plants mediate anticancer effects by the regulatory mechanism of multiple signaling pathways [85,86] among 61 reported curcumin metabolites, four compounds (E10, F10, FN1, and FN2) were reported to inhibit colon, prostate, and pancreas cancers with significant efficacy [87]. Diallyl disulfide is a vital phytonutrient that could induce single-regulated kinases phosphorylation and display alteration in the genetic profile in the case of colon cancer cell lines [48].

Epigallocatechin-3-gallate is found in tea leaves, and intake of it as a supplementary mixture have presented that in mouse liver, it improves the expression of genes responsible for the treatment of cancer-related activities such as cell growth, apoptosis, and cell adhesion, regulates the detoxification, transportation, and phosphorylation of kinases along with transcription factors, plays a role in the Nrf2 signaling pathway and involves in chemoprevention [88]. Epigallocatechin-3-gallate has been studied in PANC-1 pancreatic cancer cell line [89]. It has been discovered that the PI3K/Akt/mTOR signaling pathway is significantly modulated by the upregulation of PTEN mRNA and protein expression levels as well as the downregulation of P-Akt and p-mTOR [90]. Genistein found abundantly in soybeans and allyl sulfur found in garlic have been sufficiently studied for their behavior as a protector of cancer-related mechanisms and are involved in the CC by numerous routes and changes the posttranslational activities, and bring changes to phosphorylation events of the chief regulatory factors associated with cell division [1,48].

A natural phenolic compound called isoliquiritigenin, isolated from Medicago spp., can inhibit the GES-1 MKN28 gastric cancer cell proliferation and metastasis by the deregulation of PI3K/Akt pathway [91]. Isoliquiritigenin is significant for the management of oxidative stress, inflammatory parameters, and mechanism of cell apoptosis in cancer cells, also upregulates antioxidant and enhanced Nrf2 along with the inhibition of the NF-kB pathway and proceed the activation of SIRT1 [92]. Kaempferol is found in several vegetables and fruits and can induce CC arrest and inhibit the activity of CDKs and exhibit anticarcinogenic activity in colon cancer [93]. As an anticarcinogen and major chemoprotective agent in the fight against malignancies of the breast, the colon, the liver, and the ovary, myricetin is found in a variety of foods [17,94].

Grapes, peanuts, and all kind of berries contain resveratrol. Antiproliferation and related mechanisms are enhanced by the use of DCs, such as resveratrol, which has been shown to regulate the MAPK signaling pathway and reduce the activated p38, JNK1, and ERK2 gene expressions and improve antiproliferation mechanisms [95,96].

Rutin is involved in modulating several intracellular signaling pathways such as the Wnt signaling pathway, cytokine-receptor-associated Janus-family kinases signaling pathway, and epidermal growth factors induced signaling pathway the progression of different types of cancer [97]. Kim et al. have presented an alternative mechanism by which other DC can modify the cancer cell behavior through fast-tracking cell death and increasing apoptosis. Programmed cell death of cancer cells occurs by the two well-known processes: the fundamental, mitochondrial-arbitrated process and the other death receptor-mediated process [98]. Apoptosis can be influenced by dietary anticarcinogen strategies that impact mRNA transcription, protein expression, and function. Free radical creation and synthesis in the cell were stimulated by these phytochemicals and anticarcinogens, which boosted the mechanism of apoptosis (Fig. 1) [98].

4. Dietary fats involved with gene interactions in metabolic disorders

Obesity and CVD are essential research topics due to their high prevalence worldwide; expanding the information of fat intake and cardiometabolic disorder, it is necessary to know the abuse among low-fat (LF) and low-carb diets. LF diets have been intensely encouraged as antiatherogenic throughout the last decades and may not lead to adverse lipid metabolism-related disorders [99]. Single or multiple mutations in genes are also a significant cause of obesity, such as leptin, leptin receptor, pro-opiomelanocortin, and melanocortin-4 receptor [100].

Dyslipidemia is prolonged and proceeds toward obesity and other MDs and other instabilities of IR and glucose levels. Both fasting and postprandial lipid metabolism (LM) are affected by associated MD, such as in type 2 diabetic patients having low immunity and impaired metabolic homeostasis [20,101]. Several studies explained the linking of candidate genes with the regulatory mechanism of postprandial LM, genetic interactions of apolipoproteins, APOB, APOE, cholesterol ester transfer receptor, liver and lipoprotein enzymes, glucokinases, FA-binding proteins, microsomal TG transfer protein, and peroxisome proliferator-activated receptor-gamma (PPAR-gamma) had been studied extensively [102]. Lipid sensitivity and transcription factor PPAR-gamma Pro12Ala polymorphism are the utmost broadly mimicked genetic variants for type 2 DM threat in individuals [20]. The PPAR-gamma Pro12Ala polymorphism offers remarkable results in gene-phytonutrient interactions for MD. A forthcoming population-based cohort analysis guided that an imperative interaction between daily DF composition and relationship with PPAR-gamma locus [103,104].

Numerous phytonutrigenetic analyses by adding the information of different genetic alleles, it is debated that the intake of HFD or LF diets for 12 months in personalized nutritional strategies aimed to decrease weight loss and improve the insulin secretions, lipid profile, and glycemic control [105]. Numerous studies highlight that genotype variation could predispose individuals to different weight loss by management of lipid profile and that fluctuates by diet plan types [106–108]. Furthermost, numerous investigated genes were identified to associate with food intake closely plans to control and regulate the energy homeostatic events in the body, such as genetic variants FTO and MC3R and glucose-related and LM as genetic variants ADIPOQ and CETP [108,109].

STAT3 is essential for leptin signaling, and hypothalamic FTO overexpression leads to fourfold increase in STAT3 expression [110]. Sustainable cancer progression has been found to be dependent on the metabolism of FA, aberrant STAT3 has been seen in numerous cancer types, and it is a critical mechanism of STAT3-regulated lipid metabolism for cancer stem cell regeneration. Treatment confrontation phytonutrients are a potential basis for novel cancer therapeutic options. DC is recognized as a modulator of the signaling cascade involved in LM, including the STAT3 signaling for cancer [111]. Remarkably, the gene variants in the FTO and MC4R are linked with food craving desire and have explored the discrepancy in the state of being fed in response to the intake of dietary proteins [112,113]. After eating low-energy DCs, different people had different reactions. This was also observed, how the FTO, PPAR, and NPY gene expressions could predict that how much weight and inflammation would be reduced [114,115].

Grapes are the rich source of phytonutrients; studies conducted on the grapes extracted polyphonic compounds results concluded that the intake of supplementation containing polyphenols considerably decrease the TMAO serum levels, which are a high threat for the development of MD such as obesity and CVD [116,117].

It is evident from the literature that single-nucleotide polymorphism in the PON1 gene is closely linked with probability to development of MD such as CVD and atherosclerosis, and phytonutrigenetic linkage for the individual response toward intake of polyphenols has been formulated with the gene encoding for PON1 enzyme [118].

It is investigated that coffee contains caffeine components and extensive intake of coffee as DC is associated with the development of MD that depends on the high blood pressure cholesterol levels such as HDL, LDL, and TG in patients with psoriatic arthritis [119]. Knowledge of photonutrigenetic interactions is preliminary information to suggest that MD such as CVD is associated with drinking coffee. Numerous polymorphic genes information is linked with the metabolism of caffeine, such as CYP1A2, have been studied and concluded that it could be a treat for CVD development due to intake of coffee [120].

5. Conclusions

DCs are projected to be helpful as an adjuvant for their prospective antiinflammatory effect by consuming polyphenols food. There is a considerable significance in the patients with MD when regularly intake DC, especially in CVD, obesity, DM, and cancer. It could be clarified to understand their conditions by the difference in their genetic polymorphisms. Mother Nature provided us plants with excellent therapeutic options, so genetic differences by the intake of DC led to the emergence of the new field of phytonutrigenetics, which explain the healthy and unhealthy aspects of specific nutrient intake with genetic variations such as in cancer pathogenesis. These days more researchers focused the phytonutrigenetics on understanding the phenomenon of personalized DC for treating LM-related disorders and MD. Regarding the effective management of carcinogens, individualized natural

DCs are appropriate and have been studied concerning individuals' genetic profiles that seem highly competent to manage MD.

Other adaptable environmental influences that could interact with the DC should be deliberated in gene-environment studies, such as physical movement, alcohol, and tobacco intake, and smoking habits diagonally relating to various MD conditions. However, this chapter provided clear evidence of the concept of phytonutrients and genetic interaction in MD and explained the influence of alcohol and aflatoxin in MD. There is a need to shift toward personalized DC, which is an attractive proposition for the management of MD. Phytonutrigenetics presents a clear perspective to alter DC-related disorders expectation and treatment options because the natural bioactive therapeutic agents are gaining extensive attention for the management of lipid profile in MD patients. Such as phytochemicals discussed and presented in Table 1 are studied extensively through animal-based studies to validate chemical properties against MD. It is highly recommended to add fresh fruits, vegetables, and fiber food in diet plans to reduce the chance of development of MD such as cancer, obesity, DM, and CVD.

References

[1] A.Z. Elsamanoudy, M.A.M. Neamat-Allah, F.A.H. Mohammad, M. Hassanien, H.A. Nada, The role of nutrition related genes and nutrigenetics in understanding the pathogenesis of cancer, J. Microsc. Ultrastruct. 4 (2016) 115–122.

[2] C. Henrich, The role of nutrition in integrative oncology, in: Integrative and Functional Medical Nutrition Therapy, Springer, 2020, pp. 407–436.

[3] L. Barrea, G. Annunziata, L. Bordoni, G. Muscogiuri, A. Colao, S. Savastano, Nutrigenetics—personalized nutrition in obesity and cardiovascular diseases, Int. J. Obes. Suppl. 10 (2020) 1–13.

[4] A. Nasir, M.M.H. Bullo, Z. Ahmed, A. Imtiaz, E. Yaqoob, M. Jadoon, H. Ahmed, A. Afreen, S. Yaqoob, Nutrigenomics: epigenetics and cancer prevention: a comprehensive review, Crit. Rev. Food Sci. Nutr. 60 (2020) 1375–1387.

[5] J. Parker, C. O'Brien, J. Hawrelak, F.L. Gersh, Polycystic ovary syndrome: an evolutionary adaptation to lifestyle and the environment, Int. J. Environ. Res. Public Health 19 (2022) 1336.

[6] P.-Y. Robillard, G. Dekker, M. Scioscia, S. Saito, Progress in the understanding of the pathophysiology of immunologic maladaptation related to early-onset preeclampsia and metabolic syndrome related to late-onset preeclampsia, Am. J. Obstet. Gynecol. 226 (2022).

[7] R. Barres, J.R. Zierath, DNA methylation in metabolic disorders, Am. J. Clin. Nutr. 93 (2011) 897S–900S.

[8] L. Donnellan, B.S. Simpson, V.S. Dhillon, M. Costabile, M. Fenech, P. Deo, Folic acid deficiency increases sensitivity to DNA damage by glucose and methylglyoxal, Mutagenesis (2022).

[9] L.H. Kushi, C. Doyle, M. McCullough, C.L. Rock, W. Demark-Wahnefried, E.V. Bandera, S. Gapstur, A.V. Patel, K. Andrews, T. Gansler, et al., American Cancer Society Guidelines on nutrition and physical activity for cancer prevention: reducing the

risk of cancer with healthy food choices and physical activity, CA, Cancer J. Clin. 62 (2012) 30–67.
[10] O. Tabatabaei-Malazy, S. Saeedi Moghaddam, M. Masinaei, N. Rezaei, S. Mohammadi Fateh, A. Dilmaghani-Marand, E. Abdolhamidi, F. Razi, P. Khashayar, A. Mahdaviheza-veh, et al., Association between being metabolically healthy/unhealthy and metabolic syndrome in Iranian adults, PLoS One 17 (2022), e0262246.
[11] A.R. Williams, A.I.S. Andersen-Civil, L. Zhu, A. Blanchard, Dietary phytonutrients and animal health: regulation of immune function during gastrointestinal infections, J. Anim. Sci. 98 (2020) skaa030.
[12] M. Fenech, Genome health nutrigenomics and nutrigenetics—diagnosis and nutritional treatment of genome damage on an individual basis, Food Chem. Toxicol. 46 (2008) 1365–1370.
[13] A. Salter, H. Wiseman, G. Tucker, Phytonutrients, John Wiley & Sons, 2012.
[14] Å.L. Amundsen, L. Ose, M.S. Nenseter, F.Y. Ntanios, Plant sterol ester-enriched spread lowers plasma total and LDL cholesterol in children with familial hypercholesterolemia, Am. J. Clin. Nutr. 76 (2002) 338–344.
[15] G.R. Caponio, D.Q.-H. Wang, A. Di Ciaula, M. De Angelis, P. Portincasa, Regulation of cholesterol metabolism by bioactive components of soy proteins: novel translational evidence, Int. J. Mol. Sci. 22 (2021) 227.
[16] J. Swierczynski, A. Hebanowska, T. Sledzinski, Role of abnormal lipid metabolism in development, progression, diagnosis and therapy of pancreatic cancer, World J Gastroenterol: WJG 20 (2014) 2279.
[17] S. Subramaniam, K.R. Selvaduray, A.K. Radhakrishnan, Bioactive compounds: natural defense against cancer? Biomolecules. 9 (2019) 758.
[18] P. Sharma, S. Dwivedi, Nutrigenomics and nutrigenetics: new insight in disease prevention and cure, Indian J. Clin. Biochem. 32 (2017).
[19] A. Due, T.M. Larsen, K. Hermansen, S. Stender, J.J. Holst, S. Toubro, T. Martinussen, A. Astrup, Comparison of the effects on insulin resistance and glucose tolerance of 6-mo high-monounsaturated-fat, low-fat, and control diets, Am. J. Clin. Nutr. 87 (2008) 855–862.
[20] C.M. Phillips, Nutrigenetics and metabolic disease: current status and implications for personalised nutrition, Nutrients 5 (2013) 32–57.
[21] A.C. Tierney, J. McMonagle, D.I. Shaw, H.L. Gulseth, O. Helal, W.H.M. Saris, J.A. Paniagua, I. Gołkabek-Leszczyñska, C. Defoort, C.M. Williams, et al., Effects of dietary fat modification on insulin sensitivity and on other risk factors of the metabolic syndrome—LIPGENE: a European randomized dietary intervention study, Int. J. Obes. 35 (2011) 800–809.
[22] M.J. Gonzalez, J.R. Miranda-Massari, J. Duconge, J.R. Rodriguez, K. Cintron, M.J. Berdiel, J.W. Rodriguez, et al., Nutrigenomics, metabolic correction and disease, J. Restor. Med. 4 (2015) 74–82.
[23] S. Vakili, M.A. Caudill, Personalized nutrition: nutritional genomics as a potential tool for targeted medical nutrition therapy, Nutr. Rev. 65 (2007) 301–315.
[24] P. Wang, A.M. Schumacher, S.-H. Shiu, Computational prediction of plant metabolic pathways, Curr. Opin. Plant Biol. 66 (2022), 102171.
[25] A.K. Pathak, K. Sukhavasi, D. Marnetto, G. Chaubey, A.K. Pandey, Human population genomics approach in food metabolism, in: Future Foods, Elsevier, 2022, pp. 433–449.
[26] J.R. Keathley, A. Arbour, M.-C. Vohl, Towards a standardized definition of medical nutrition therapy and regulatory reform in Canada, Can. J. Diet. Pract. Res. (2022) 1–6.
[27] A. El-Sohemy, Nutrigenetics, Nutr. Asia 60 (2007) 25–30.
[28] I. Vazquez-Vidal, P.J.H. Jones, Nutrigenetics and blood cholesterol levels in response to plant sterols, in: Principles of Nutrigenetics and Nutrigenomics, Elsevier, 2020, pp. 227–230.

[29] C.M. Williams, J.M. Ordovas, D. Lairon, J. Hesketh, G. Lietz, M. Gibney, B. Van Ommen, The challenges for molecular nutrition research 1: linking genotype to healthy nutrition, Genes Nutr. 3 (2008) 41–49.
[30] J. Hou, Q. Deng, X. Guo, X. Deng, W. Zhong, Z. Zhong, Association between apolipoprotein E gene polymorphism and the risk of coronary artery disease in Hakka postmenopausal women in southern China, Lipids Health Dis. 19 (2020) 1–7.
[31] K.R. Martin, Using nutrigenomics to evaluate apoptosis as a preemptive target in cancer prevention, Curr. Cancer Drug Targets 7 (2007) 438–446.
[32] C.D. Davis, J.A. Milner, Nutrigenomics, vitamin D and cancer prevention, Lifestyle Genom. 4 (2011) 1–11.
[33] C.B. Williamson, J.M. Pizano, A nutritional genomics approach to epigenetic influences on chronic disease, in: Integrative and Functional Medical Nutrition Therapy, Springer, 2020, pp. 235–268.
[34] A.P. Simopoulos, Genetic variants in the metabolism of omega-6 and omega-3 fatty acids: their role in the determination of nutritional requirements and chronic disease risk, Exp. Biol. Med. 235 (2010) 785–795.
[35] D. Panagiotakos, M. Sitara, C. Pitsavos, C. Stefanadis, Estimating the 10-year risk of cardiovascular disease and its economic consequences, by the level of adherence to the Mediterranean diet: the ATTICA study, J. Med. Food 10 (2007) 239–243.
[36] A.V. Krishnan, S. Swami, J. Moreno, R.B. Bhattacharyya, D.M. Peehl, D. Feldman, Potentiation of the growth-inhibitory effects of vitamin D in prostate cancer by genistein, Nutr. Rev. 65 (2007) S121–S123.
[37] J.W. Lampe, J.-L. Chang, Interindividual differences in phytochemical metabolism and disposition, Semin. Cancer Biol. (2007) 347–353.
[38] F. Caradonna, I. Cruciata, C. Luparello, Nutrigenetics, nutrigenomics and phenotypic outcomes of dietary low-dose alcohol consumption in the suppression and induction of cancer development: evidence from in vitro studies, Crit. Rev. Food Sci. Nutr. (2020) 1–32.
[39] E. Giovannucci, M.J. Stampfer, G.A. Colditz, E.B. Rimm, D. Trichopoulos, B.A. Rosner, F.E. Speizer, W.C. Willett, Folate, methionine, and alcohol intake and risk of colorectal adenoma, J. Natl. Cancer Inst. 85 (1993) 875–883.
[40] P. Gut, E. Verdin, The nexus of chromatin regulation and intermediary metabolism, Nature 502 (2013) 489–498.
[41] L.I. Gavrilas, C. Ionescu, O. Tudoran, C. Lisencu, O. Balacescu, D. Miere, The role of bioactive dietary components in modulating miRNA expression in colorectal cancer, Nutrients 8 (2016) 590.
[42] F. Zhao, J.-F. Su, S.-M. Lun, Y.-J. Hou, L.-J. Duan, N.-C. Wang, F.-F. Shen, Y.-W. Zhang, Z.-W. Gao, J. Li, et al., Association between polymorphisms in the CYP1A1, CYP2E1 and GSTM1 genes, and smoking, alcohol and upper digestive tract carcinomas in a high-incidence area of northern China, Oncol. Lett. 18 (2019) 1267–1277.
[43] D. Farhud, M. Shalileh, Phenylketonuria and its dietary therapy in children, Iran. J. Pediatr. 18 (2008).
[44] S. Bibi, K. Sakata, An integrated computational approach for plant-based protein tyrosine phosphatase non-receptor type 1 inhibitors, Curr. Comput. Aided Drug Des. 13 (2017) 319–335.
[45] D. Hanahan, R.A. Weinberg, Hallmarks of cancer: the next generation, Cell 144 (2011) 646–674.
[46] Y.-T. Liu, B.-S. Tzang, J. Yow, Y.-H. Chiang, C.-Y. Huang, T.-C. Hsu, Traditional Chinese medicine formula T33 inhibits the proliferation of human colorectal cancer cells by inducing autophagy, Environ. Toxicol. (2022).
[47] D. Tewari, P. Patni, A. Bishayee, A.N. Sah, A. Bishayee, Natural products targeting the PI3K-Akt-mTOR signalling pathway in cancer: a novel therapeutic strategy, Semin. Cancer Biol. 80 (2019).

[48] L.M. Knowles, J.A. Milner, Diallyl disulfide induces ERK phosphorylation and alters gene expression profiles in human colon tumor cells, J. Nutr. 133 (2003) 2901–2906.
[49] M. Rayner, P. Scarborough, C. Williams, The origin of guideline daily amounts and the food standards agency's guidance on what counts as 'a lot' and 'a little', Public Health Nutr. 7 (2004) 549–556.
[50] S.M. Meeran, S.K. Katiyar, Cell cycle control as a basis for cancer chemoprevention through dietary agents, Front. Biosci. J. Virtual Libr. 13 (2008) 2191.
[51] H.S. Feigelson, C.R. Jonas, A.S. Robertson, M.L. McCullough, M.J. Thun, E.E. Calle, Alcohol, folate, methionine, and risk of incident breast cancer in the American Cancer Society Cancer Prevention Study II Nutrition Cohort, Cancer Epidemiol. Biomarkers Prev. 12 (2003) 161–164.
[52] P.W. Laird, R. Jaenisch, The role of DNA methylation in cancer genetics and epigenetics, Annu. Rev. Genet. 30 (1996) 441–464.
[53] P. Cavuoto, M.F. Fenech, A review of methionine dependency and the role of methionine restriction in cancer growth control and life-span extension, Cancer Treat. Rev. 38 (2012) 726–736.
[54] M.J. Akhtar, M.A. Khan, I. Ahmad, High performance liquid chromatographic determination of folic acid and its photodegradation products in the presence of riboflavin, J. Pharm. Biomed. Anal. 16 (1997) 95–99.
[55] D.A. Snowdon, C.L. Tully, C.D. Smith, K.P. Riley, W.R. Markesbery, Serum folate and the severity of atrophy of the neocortex in Alzheimer disease: findings from the Nun study, Am. J. Clin. Nutr. 71 (2000) 993–998.
[56] B.A. Jennings, G. Willis, How folate metabolism affects colorectal cancer development and treatment; a story of heterogeneity and pleiotropy, Cancer Lett. 356 (2015) 224–230.
[57] N. Delchier, A.-L. Herbig, M. Rychlik, C.M.G.C. Renard, Folates in fruits and vegetables: contents, processing, and stability, Compr. Rev. Food Sci. Food Saf. 15 (2016) 506–528.
[58] V.S. Reddy, R. Palika, A. Ismail, R. Pullakhandam, G.B. Reddy, Nutrigenomics: opportunities & challenges for public health nutrition, Indian J. Med. Res. 148 (2018) 632.
[59] K.S. Crider, J.-H. Zhu, L. Hao, Q.-H. Yang, T.P. Yang, J. Gindler, D.R. Maneval, E.P. Quinlivan, Z. Li, L.B. Bailey, et al., MTHFR 677C→T genotype is associated with folate and homocysteine concentrations in a large, population-based, double-blind trial of folic acid supplementation, Am. J. Clin. Nutr. 93 (2011) 1365–1372.
[60] J. Selhub, Folate, vitamin B12 and vitamin B6 and one carbon metabolism, J. Nutr. Health Aging 6 (2002) 39–42.
[61] P.M. Ridker, J. Shih, T.J. Cook, M. Clearfield, J.R. Downs, A.D. Pradhan, S.E. Weis, A.M. Gotto Jr., Plasma homocysteine concentration, statin therapy, and the risk of first acute coronary events, Circulation 105 (2002) 1776–1779.
[62] J. Selhub, The many facets of hyperhomocysteinemia: studies from the Framingham cohorts, J. Nutr. 136 (2006) 1726S–1730S.
[63] D. Djuric, V. Jakovljevic, V. Zivkovic, I. Srejovic, Homocysteine and homocysteine-related compounds: an overview of the roles in the pathology of the cardiovascular and nervous systems, Can. J. Physiol. Pharmacol. 96 (2018) 991–1003.
[64] M. Cesari, A.B. Burlina, K. Narkiewicz, M.T. Sartori, A. Sacchetto, G.P. Rossi, Are fasting plasma homocyst(e)ine levels heritable? A study of normotensive twins, J. Investig. Med. 48 (2000) 351–358.
[65] S. Vermeulen, G.M. Van Der Vleuten, J. De Graaf, A.R. Hermus, H.J. Blom, A.F.H. Stalenhoef, M. Den Heijer, A genome-wide linkage scan for homocysteine levels suggests three regions of interest, J. Thromb. Haemost. 4 (2006) 1303–1307.
[66] A. Hazra, P. Kraft, R. Lazarus, C. Chen, S.J. Chanock, P. Jacques, J. Selhub, D.J. Hunter, Genome-wide significant predictors of metabolites in the one-carbon metabolism pathway, Hum. Mol. Genet. 18 (2009) 4677–4687.

[67] N.J. Colson, H.L. Naug, E. Nikbakht, P. Zhang, J. McCormack, The impact of MTHFR 677 C/T genotypes on folate status markers: a meta-analysis of folic acid intervention studies, Eur. J. Nutr. 56 (2017) 247–260.

[68] B. Du, H. Tian, D. Tian, C. Zhang, W. Wang, L. Wang, M. Ge, Q. Hou, W. Zhang, Genetic polymorphisms of key enzymes in folate metabolism affect the efficacy of folate therapy in patients with hyperhomocysteinaemia, Br. J. Nutr. 119 (2018) 887–895.

[69] Y. Shirakami, S.-A. Lee, R.D. Clugston, W.S. Blaner, Hepatic metabolism of retinoids and disease associations, Biochim. Biophys. Acta (BBA)-Mol. Cell Biol. Lipids 1821 (2012) 124–136.

[70] Q. Yang, T.E. Graham, N. Mody, F. Preitner, O.D. Peroni, J.M. Zabolotny, K. Kotani, L. Quadro, B.B. Kahn, Serum retinol binding protein 4 contributes to insulin resistance in obesity and type 2 diabetes, Nature 436 (2005) 356–362.

[71] D.-J. Shin, D.P. Odom, K.B. Scribner, S. Ghoshal, M.M. McGrane, Retinoid regulation of the phosphoenolpyruvate carboxykinase gene in liver, Mol. Cell. Endocrinol. 195 (2002) 39–54.

[72] F.W. Kiefer, G. Orasanu, S. Nallamshetty, J.D. Brown, H. Wang, P. Luger, N.R. Qi, C.F. Burant, G. Duester, J. Plutzky, Retinaldehyde dehydrogenase 1 coordinates hepatic gluconeogenesis and lipid metabolism, Endocrinology 153 (2012) 3089–3099.

[73] R. Garcia, C.A. Gonzalez, A. Agudo, E. Riboli, High intake of specific carotenoids and flavonoids does not reduce the risk of bladder cancer, Nutr. Cancer 35 (1999) 212–214.

[74] M. Rahman, M. Rahaman, M. Islam, F. Rahman, F.M. Mithi, T. Alqahtani, M.A. Almikhlafi, S.Q. Alghamdi, A.S. Alruwaili, M. Hossain, et al., Role of phenolic compounds in human disease: current knowledge and future prospects, Molecules 27 (2022) 233.

[75] S.E. Simon, H.S. Lim, F.A. Jayakumar, E.W. Tan, K.O. Tan, Alpha-mangostin activates MOAP-1 tumor suppressor and mitochondrial signalling in MCF-7 human breast cancer cells, Evidence-Based Complement. Altern. Med. 2022 (2022).

[76] F. Wang, H. Ma, Z. Liu, W. Huang, X. Xu, X. Zhang, α-Mangostin inhibits DMBA/TPA-induced skin cancer through inhibiting inflammation and promoting autophagy and apoptosis by regulating PI3K/Akt/mTOR signalling pathway in mice, Biomed. Pharmacother. 92 (2017) 672–680.

[77] P. Sharma, S.F. McClees, F. Afaq, Pomegranate for prevention and treatment of cancer: an update, Molecules 22 (2017) 177.

[78] T.M. Totiger, S. Srinivasan, V.R. Jala, P. Lamichhane, A.R. Dosch, A.A. Gaidarski, C. Joshi, S. Rangappa, J. Castellanos, P.K. Vemula, et al., Urolithin A, a novel natural compound to target PI3K/AKT/mTOR pathway in pancreatic cancer, Mol. Cancer Ther. 18 (2019) 301–311.

[79] J. Yang, C. Pi, G. Wang, Inhibition of PI3K/Akt/mTOR pathway by apigenin induces apoptosis and autophagy in hepatocellular carcinoma cells, Biomed. Pharmacother. 103 (2018) 699–707.

[80] K.K.L. Samaga, G.V. Rao, G.C. Reddy, A.K. Kush, L. Diwakar, Synthetic racemates of abyssinone I and II induces apoptosis through mitochondrial pathway in human cervix carcinoma cells, Bioorg. Chem. 56 (2014) 54–61.

[81] Y.-L. Chu, C.-T. Ho, J.-G. Chung, R. Raghu, Y.-C. Lo, L.-Y. Sheen, Allicin induces anti-human liver cancer cells through the p53 gene modulating apoptosis and autophagy, J. Agric. Food Chem. 61 (2013) 9839–9848.

[82] Y. Li, H. Yu, F. Han, M. Wang, Y. Luo, X. Guo, Biochanin A induces S phase arrest and apoptosis in lung cancer cells, Biomed. Res. Int. 2018 (2018).

[83] L.-C. Chung, K.-C. Chiang, T.-H. Feng, K.-S. Chang, S.-T. Chuang, Y.-J. Chen, K.-H. Tsui, J.-C. Lee, H.-H. Juang, Caffeic acid phenethyl ester upregulates N-myc downstream regulated gene 1 via ERK pathway to inhibit human oral cancer cell growth in vitro and in vivo, Mol. Nutr. Food Res. 61 (2017) 1600842.

[84] N. Zeng, T. Hongbo, Y. Xu, M. Wu, Y. Wu, Anticancer activity of caffeic acid n-butyl ester against A431 skin carcinoma cell line occurs via induction of apoptosis and inhibition of the mTOR/PI3K/AKT signalling pathway, Mol. Med. Rep. 23 (2021).
[85] A.B. Kunnumakkara, D. Bordoloi, C. Harsha, K. Banik, S.C. Gupta, B.B. Aggarwal, Curcumin mediates anticancer effects by modulating multiple cell signalling pathways, Clin. Sci. 131 (2017) 1781–1799.
[86] M.N. Khan, Y.A. Haggag, M.E. Lane, P.A. McCarron, M.M. Tambuwala, Polymeric nano-encapsulation of curcumin enhances its anti-cancer activity in breast (MDA-MB231) and lung (A549) cancer cells through reduction in expression of HIF-1α and nuclear p65 (REL A), Curr. Drug Deliv. 15 (2018) 286–295.
[87] X. Wei, Z.-Y. Du, X. Zheng, X.-X. Cui, A.H. Conney, K. Zhang, Synthesis and evaluation of curcumin-related compounds for anticancer activity, Eur. J. Med. Chem. 53 (2012) 235–245.
[88] G. Shen, C. Xu, R. Hu, M.R. Jain, S. Nair, W. Lin, C.S. Yang, J.Y. Chan, A.-N.T. Kong, Comparison of (-)-epigallocatechin-3-gallate elicited liver and small intestine gene expression profiles between C57BL/6J mice and C57BL/6J/Nrf2 (-/-) mice, Pharm. Res. 22 (2005) 1805–1820.
[89] S. Liu, X.-J. Wang, Y. Liu, Y.-F. Cui, PI3K/AKT/mTOR signalling is involved in (-)-epigallocatechin-3-gallate-induced apoptosis of human pancreatic carcinoma cells, Am. J. Chin. Med. 41 (2013) 629–642.
[90] J. Yi, S. Li, C. Wang, N. Cao, H. Qu, C. Cheng, Z. Wang, L. Wang, L. Zhou, Potential applications of polyphenols on main ncRNAs regulations as novel therapeutic strategy for cancer, Biomed. Pharmacother. 113 (2019), 108703.
[91] L. Jia, B. Lei, H. Gao, L. Jia, D. Luo, J. Han, B. Jia, miR-130b suppresses the invasion and migration of prostate cancer via inhibiting DLL1 and regulating the PI3K/Akt pathways, Exp. Ther. Med. 23 (2022) 1–9.
[92] W.H. Al-Qahtani, G.M. Alshammari, J.S. Ajarem, A.Y. Al-Zahrani, A. Alzuwaydi, R. Eid, M.A. Yahya, Isoliquiritigenin prevents Doxorubicin-induced hepatic damage in rats by upregulating and activating SIRT1, Biomed. Pharmacother. 146 (2022), 112594.
[93] H.J. Cho, J.H.Y. Park, Kaempferol induces cell cycle arrest in HT-29 human colon cancer cells, J. Cancer Prev. 18 (2013) 257.
[94] J.K. Jayakumar, P. Nirmala, B.A.P. Kumar, A.P. Kumar, Evaluation of protective effect of myricetin, a bioflavonoid in dimethyl benzanthracene-induced breast cancer in female Wistar rats, South Asian J. Cancer 3 (2014) 107.
[95] R. Yu, V. Hebbar, D.W. Kim, S. Mandlekar, J.M. Pezzuto, A.-N.T. Kong, Resveratrol inhibits phorbol ester and UV-induced activator protein 1 activation by interfering with mitogen-activated protein kinase pathways, Mol. Pharmacol. 60 (2001) 217–224.
[96] J.-H. Ko, G. Sethi, J.-Y. Um, M.K. Shanmugam, F. Arfuso, A.P. Kumar, A. Bishayee, K.S. Ahn, The role of resveratrol in cancer therapy, Int. J. Mol. Sci. 18 (2017) 2589.
[97] A.A. Perk, I. Shatynska-Mytsyk, Y.C. Gerçek, K. Boztacs, M. Yazgan, S. Fayyaz, A.A. Farooqi, Rutin mediated targeting of signalling machinery in cancer cells, Cancer Cell Int. 14 (2014) 1–5.
[98] T.-M. Kim, S.-H. Yim, Y.-J. Chung, Copy number variations in the human genome: potential source for individual diversity and disease association studies, Genom. Inform. 6 (2008) 1–7.
[99] T. Hu, L.A. Bazzano, The low-carbohydrate diet and cardiovascular risk factors: evidence from epidemiologic studies, Nutr. Metab. Cardiovasc. Dis. 24 (2014) 337–343.
[100] C.H. Andreasen, G. Andersen, Gene-environment interactions and obesity—further aspects of genomewide association studies, Nutrition 25 (2009) 998–1003.
[101] A.I. Perez-Caballero, J.F. Alcala-Diaz, P. Perez-Martinez, A. Garcia-Rios, N. Delgado-Casado, C. Marin, E. Yubero-Serrano, A. Camargo, J. Caballero, M.M.

Malagon, et al., Lipid metabolism after an oral fat test meal is affected by age-associated features of metabolic syndrome, but not by age, Atherosclerosis 226 (2013) 258–262.
[102] C. Phillips, G. Murugasu, D. Owens, P. Collins, A. Johnson, G.H. Tomkin, Improved metabolic control reduces the number of postprandial apolipoprotein B-48-containing particles in type 2 diabetes, Atherosclerosis 148 (2000) 283–291.
[103] J. Luan, P.O. Browne, A.-H. Harding, D.J. Halsall, S. O'Rahilly, V.K.K. Chatterjee, N.J. Wareham, Evidence for gene-nutrient interaction at the PPARγ locus, Diabetes 50 (2001) 686–689.
[104] M. Ghoussaini, D. Meyre, S. Lobbens, G. Charpentier, K. Clément, M.-A. Charles, M. Tauber, J. Weill, P. Froguel, Implication of the Pro12Ala polymorphism of the PPAR-gamma 2 gene in type 2 diabetes and obesity in the French population, BMC Med. Genet. 6 (2005) 1–8.
[105] C.D. Gardner, J.F. Trepanowski, L.C. Del Gobbo, M.E. Hauser, J. Rigdon, J.P.A. Ioannidis, M. Desai, A.C. King, Effect of low-fat vs low-carbohydrate diet on 12-month weight loss in overweight adults and the association with genotype pattern or insulin secretion: the DIETFITS randomized clinical trial, JAMA 319 (2018) 667–679.
[106] Q. Qi, G.A. Bray, S.R. Smith, F.B. Hu, F.M. Sacks, L. Qi, Insulin receptor substrate 1 gene variation modifies insulin resistance response to weight-loss diets in a 2-year randomized trial: the Preventing Overweight Using Novel Dietary Strategies (POUNDS LOST) trial, Circulation 124 (2011) 563–571.
[107] D. Sun, Y. Heianza, X. Li, X. Shang, S.R. Smith, G.A. Bray, F.M. Sacks, L. Qi, Genetic, epigenetic and transcriptional variations at NFATC2IP locus with weight loss in response to diet interventions: the POUNDS Lost Trial, Diabetes, Obes. Metab. 20 (2018) 2298–2303.
[108] Q. Qi, R. Durst, D. Schwarzfuchs, E. Leitersdorf, S. Shpitzen, Y. Li, H. Wu, C.M. Champagne, F.B. Hu, M.J. Stampfer, et al., CETP genotype and changes in lipid levels in response to weight-loss diet intervention in the POUNDS LOST and DIRECT randomized trials, J. Lipid Res. 56 (2015) 713–721.
[109] D.A. de Luis, O. Izaola, D. Primo, R. Aller, A. Ortola, E. Gómez, J.J. Lopez, The association of SNP276G>T at adiponectin gene with insulin resistance and circulating adiponectin in response to two different hypocaloric diets, Diabetes Res. Clin. Pract. 137 (2018) 93–99.
[110] R.A. Coleman, T.M. Lewin, D.M. Muoio, Physiological and nutritional regulation of enzymes of triacylglycerol synthesis, Annu. Rev. Nutr. 20 (2000) 77–103.
[111] C. Tse, A. Warner, R. Farook, J.G. Cronin, Phytochemical targeting of STAT3 orchestrated lipid metabolism in therapy-resistant cancers, Biomolecules 10 (2020) 1118.
[112] T. Huang, Y. Zheng, A. Hruby, D.A. Williamson, G.A. Bray, Y. Shen, F.M. Sacks, L. Qi, Dietary protein modifies the effect of the MC4R genotype on 2-year changes in appetite and food craving: the POUNDS Lost Trial, J. Nutr. 147 (2017) 439–444.
[113] T. Huang, Q. Qi, Y. Li, F.B. Hu, G.A. Bray, F.M. Sacks, D.A. Williamson, L. Qi, FTO genotype, dietary protein, and change in appetite: the Preventing Overweight Using Novel Dietary Strategies trial, Am. J. Clin. Nutr. 99 (2014) 1126–1130.
[114] M.L.R. Curti, M.M. Rogero, V.T. Baltar, C.R. Barros, A. Siqueira-Catania, S.R.G. Ferreira, FTO T/A and peroxisome proliferator-activated receptor-γ Pro12Ala polymorphisms but not ApoA1-75 are associated with better response to lifestyle intervention in Brazilians at high cardiometabolic risk, Metab. Syndr. Relat. Disord. 11 (2013) 169–176.
[115] D.A. de Luis, O. Izaola, B. de la Fuente, D. Primo, R. Aller, Polymorphism of neuropeptide Y gene rs16147 modifies the response to a hypocaloric diet on cardiovascular risk biomarkers and adipokines, J. Hum. Nutr. Diet. 30 (2017) 159–165.

[116] G. Annunziata, M. Maisto, C. Schisano, R. Ciampaglia, V. Narciso, S.T.S. Hassan, G.C. Tenore, E. Novellino, Effect of grape pomace polyphenols with or without pectin on TMAO serum levels assessed by LC/MS-based assay: a preliminary clinical study on overweight/obese subjects, Front. Pharmacol. 10 (2019) 575.

[117] G. Annunziata, M. Maisto, C. Schisano, R. Ciampaglia, V. Narciso, G.C. Tenore, E. Novellino, Effects of grape pomace polyphenolic extract (Taurisolo) in reducing TMAO serum levels in humans: preliminary results from a randomized, placebo-controlled, cross-over study, Nutrients 11 (2019) 139.

[118] N. Shunmoogam, P. Naidoo, R. Chilton, Paraoxonase (PON)-1: a brief overview on genetics, structure, polymorphisms and clinical relevance, Vasc. Health Risk Manag. 14 (2018) 137.

[119] L. Barrea, G. Muscogiuri, C. Di Somma, G. Annunziata, M. Megna, A. Falco, A. Balato, A. Colao, S. Savastano, Coffee consumption, metabolic syndrome and clinical severity of psoriasis: good or bad stuff? Arch. Toxicol. 92 (2018) 1831–1845.

[120] P. Palatini, G. Ceolotto, F. Ragazzo, F. Dorigatti, F. Saladini, I. Papparella, L. Mos, G. Zanata, M. Santonastaso, CYP1A2 genotype modifies the association between coffee intake and the risk of hypertension, J. Hypertens. 27 (2009) 1594–1601.

CHAPTER 5

Therapeutic role of nutraceuticals in the management of brain disorders

Amira Yasmine Benmelouka[a], Muhammad Ajmal Shah[b], Uzma Saleem[c], Alaa Ahmed Elshanbary[d], Mostafa Meshref[e], Ghulam Mujtaba Shah[b,f], Ifat Alsharif[g], Norah A. Althobaiti[h], and Reem Hasaballah Alhasani[i]

[a]Faculty of Medicine, University of Algiers, Algiers, Algeria
[b]Department of Pharmacy, Hazara University, Mansehra, Pakistan
[c]Department of Pharmacology, Faculty of Pharmaceutical Sciences, Government College University, Faisalabad, Pakistan
[d]Faculty of Medicine, Alexandria University, Alexandria, Egypt
[e]Department of Neurology, Al-Azhar University, Cairo, Egypt
[f]Department of Botany, Hazara University, Mansehra, Pakistan
[g]Department of Biology, Jamoum University College, Umm Al-Qura University, Makkah, Saudi Arabia
[h]Department of Biology, College of Science and Humanities, Shaqra University, Al-Quwaiiyah, Saudi Arabia
[i]Department of Biology, Faculty of Applied Science, Umm Al-Qura University, Makkah, Saudi Arabia

1. Introduction

In the last few years, the advancements in understanding of world properties and the extension of industrialization have impacted humans' lifestyle and their dietary habits leading to the adoption of a more sedentary lifestyle. These modifications have consequently influenced individuals' health and led to the appearance of various metabolic dysfunctions that can affect the brain [1]. Dietary factors may affect many brain processes through the modification of the metabolism of gut and brain hormones. For instance, they can influence some synaptic plasticity regulators leading to a considerable impact on cognitive capacities [2]. Furthermore, diet can have various effects on the epigenomic mechanisms in human cells, and consequently on the internal cellular metabolism [3]. Lifestyle, physical activity, and environment can also modulate the functional processes in the brain tissue [4]. They may directly influence the progeny of neural stem cells and can modify the metabolism of microglia, which can indirectly mediate neurogenesis [4].

Moreover, blood-brain barrier (BBB) is composed of highly differentiated endothelial cells that serve as a separator between the blood and the nervous

The Role of Phytonutrients in Metabolic Disorders
https://doi.org/10.1016/B978-0-12-824356-5.00012-6

tissue [5]. BBB dysfunctions are associated with various pathologies including Alzheimer's disease (AD) [6], Parkinson's disease [7], Huntington's disease [8], depression [9], anxiety [10], bipolar disorders [11], autism spectrum disorders (ASDs) [12], and schizophrenia [13]. Some nutrients such as phytochemicals and vitamins seem to exert a protective effect on BBB [14–16]. The modifications of BBB can be triggered by multiple mechanisms such as the secretion of metabolites by gut microbiome. The dysfunctions of the normal gut microbiota affect human BBB permeability [17]. The alteration of metabolic pathways in some clinical conditions like diabetes may also increase the BBB permeability and enhance β-amyloid deposition in the brain, which can engender the progression to nerve degeneration [18]. Some food components are able to control the integrity of this barrier and reverse brain injury [19–21].

Furthermore, it is known that inflammatory processes that can occur in the central nervous system (CNS) ensure protection against many aggressive phenomena and reverse glial and neuronal damages. Yet, excessive and prolonged neuroinflammation after nerve injury may negatively impact the regeneration of the nervous system [22]. This neuroinflammation may be caused by various conditions that accompany the release of inflammatory mediators including malignant proliferations, traumatic accidents, pathologic metabolic changes in diabetes and dyslipidemia, and the exposure to some toxins and drugs [23]. Many nutraceuticals have antiinflammatory properties and can attenuate this inflammation and lead to the promotion of brain health [24]. Also, some dietary patterns and supplementation with probiotics and prebiotics may play a crucial role in the determination of gut microbiota composition affecting cerebral metabolism via the gut-brain axis. Nutraceuticals can therefore indirectly modulate the progression of psychiatric and neurodegenerative troubles namely depression, anxiety, and AD (Fig. 1) [25,26].

The aim of this chapter is to review the findings of previously published scientific articles on the possible effects of nutraceutical products in the major human neurologic disorders that are associated with the existence of metabolic dysfunctions in the brain.

2. Classes of neutraceuticals and their mechanisms of action

There are many categories of nutraceuticals (Fig. 2) that can be applied in different brain disorders due to their potential roles and their involvement in various human pathways and processes (see Table 1).

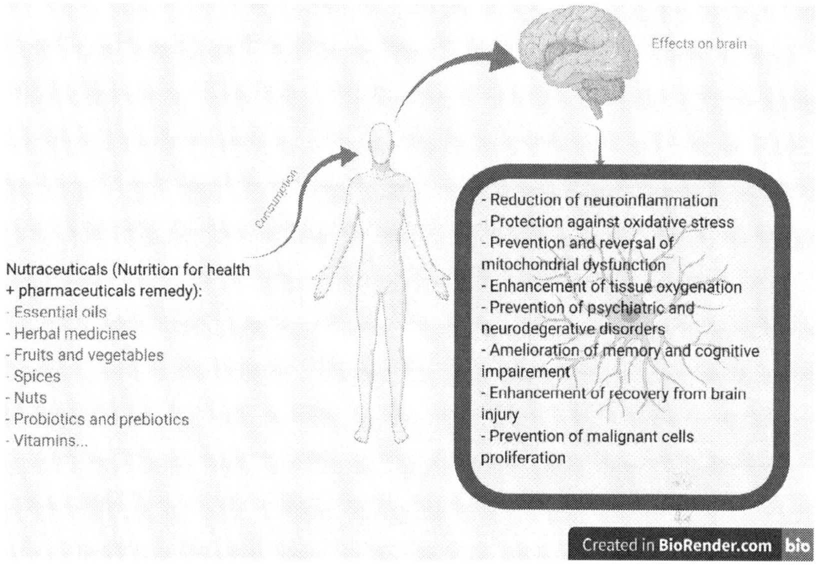

Fig. 1 Effects of the consumption of nutraceuticals on human brain.

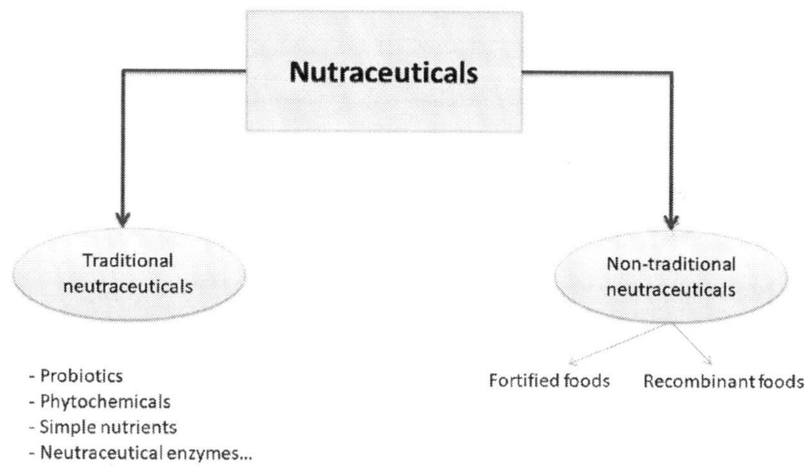

Fig. 2 The different categories of neutraceuticals.

2.1 Traditional nutraceuticals

Traditional nutraceuticals or food nutraceuticals are represented by compounds that can be obtained directly from natural products without additional changes [27]. They include many classes such as nutrients that mainly include fatty acids, minerals, amino acids, and other active element like

Table 1 Mechanisms of action of some nutraceuticals classes in neurologic and neuropsychiatric disorders.

Disease	Categories	Class	Example	Mechanism of action	Reference
Alzheimer's Disease	Herbals or Extracts	Flavonoids	Catechin, epigallocatechin, and epicatechin	(1) Alter cerebral blood flow (2) Activate antioxidant enzymes and proteins engaged in neuronal repair synaptic plasticity (3) Prevent neuropathological activities in brain	[74,75,208]
		Diterpenoid	Crocin	(1) Enhance cognition through ADAS-Cog and CDR-SD-mediated enzymes (2) Change the levels of oxidative markers in the hippocampus (3) Eliminate the deleterious impacts on learning and memory due to chronic stress	
		7-Hydroxyflavonoid	Cyanidin	(1) Inhibition of phospholipase A2 engaged in the signaling of proinflammatory cytokines and oxidative stress factors which conducts neuroprotection	
		Flavone	Luteolin	(1) Keeps DNA against hydrogen peroxide-mediated toxicity (2) Blocks inflammation and cell damage	

MS	Herbals or Extracts	Curcuminoids	Curcumin	(1) Control expression of some genes which control programmed cell death 1, micro-rnas32 and 45, interferon gamma, chemokine ligand 2 and 5 and NFKB	[88–90]
	Herbals or Extracts	Organosulfur compound	Alpha Lipoic acid	(1) Inhibit the enhancement of secretion of some inflammatory markers such as interleukin 6, tumor necrosis factor alpha and matrix metallopeptide 9	
	Herbals or Extracts	Flavonoids	Ginkgo biloba	(1) Alter the action of acetylcholine release, glycine and GABA receptors and platelet-activating factor	
Parkinson's Disease	Nutrients	Vitamines	Vitamine-B12	(1) Increases endogenous H2S production	[78,122,136,208]
	Herbals or Extracts	Polyphenols	Epigallocatechi$n-3$ gallate	(1) Skip the blood-brain barrier (BBB) (2) Extreme scavenging activity and iron chelation property of the phytoconstituent (3) Xecrease neurotoxicity by improving DA levels in the brain striatal region	
		Flavonoids	Bicalein	(1) Inhibits fibrillation and neurotoxicity by stopping the synthesis of oligomer of α-syn (2) Stimulate autophagy, reduce inflammation and inflammatory cytokines, and hinder apoptosis, so repairing the levels of DA in an MPP-induced model	

Continued

Table 1 Mechanisms of action of some nutraceuticals classes in neurologic and neuropsychiatric disorders—cont'd

Disease	Categories	Class	Example	Mechanism of action	Reference
	Herbals or Extracts	Curcuminoids	Curcumin	(1) Antioxidant activity and anti-inflammatory	
	Herbals or Extracts	Vinca alkaloid	Vibcamine	(1) Anti-PD action via various mechanisms; vasodilation, muscle relaxation of the neuronal capillaries, enhanced flow of nutrients and glucose to the brain which increase in ATP production via the Krebs cycle	
Depression	Nutrients	Fatty acids	Omega-3 fatty acids (eicosapentaenoic and docosahexaenoic acids)	(1) Preventing reuptake of monoamines during neurological transmission and encourages neurotransmission by improving the fluidity in membranes of cell (2) Decline inflammatory mediators and their production (3) Enhancing neurogenesis and prevents depressive attacks	[167,170]
		Amino adecids	N-acetyl Cystein	(1) Antiinflammatory and antioxidant effects which lead to refill glutathione levels and improves neurogenesis (2) Defend against mitochondrial toxicity and regulate glutamate pathway thus inhibiting depression	

		Vitamines	L-Tryptophan/5-HTP	(1) Conversion into serotonin in the presence of B6 and Mg to actively form 5-HTP via an intermediate process	
			Vitamin D	(1) Ligand for receptors in the hypothalamus, prefrontal cortex, and substantia nigra (2) Controls the genetic expression leading to coding of protein tyrosine hydroxylase	
		Minerals	Zinc	(1) Increasing BNDF so improving neurogenesis in hippocampal (2) Modify the action of NMDA and glutamate receptors	
Huntington's disease	Nutrients	Fatty acids	Triheptanoin	(1) Increase krebs cycle intermediates as their reduction leads to reduce bcaas (2) Provide keton bodies which cross BBB and increase levels of ATP and pcr	[143]
			Eicosapentaenoic acid	(1) Reduce phospholipase A2 (2) Lower neuronal membrane phospholipid turnover and a reverse of the cerebral atrophic procedure in primary period of schizophrenia	[148,149]
	Phytochemicals	Phenolic acids	Curcumin	(1) Antioxidant, antiinflammatory and antiprotein cluster	[193,195]

Continued

Table 1 Mechanisms of action of some nutraceuticals classes in neurologic and neuropsychiatric disorders—cont'd

Disease	Categories	Class	Example	Mechanism of action	Reference
Brain ataxia	Nutrients/ Vitamins	Vitamine E	Tocotrienols	(1) Enhance FXN-3 expression (2) Augment transcription of IKBKAP gene, thus increase normal protein (3) Antifibrosis (4) Decrease inflammation by inhibition of TNF-a and NF-jb and the LPS stimulated IL-630 expression	[158]
	Nutraceutical Enzymes	Coenzyme	Coq10	(1) Acts as electron carrier in MRC, transporting electrons from complex I and II to complex III [1] and participate in ATP synthesis (2) Inhibit the development of lipid peroxidation in membranes or the reprocessing of other antioxidants, e.g., vitamin E	[160]
	Nutrients	Minerals	Zinc	(1) Control GABA, NMDA, and glycine receptors expressed in neurons	[159]
Psychotic and mood disorders	Nutrients	Fatty acids	Omega-3 fatty acids (eicosapentaenoic and docosahexaenoic acids)	(1) Enhance dopamine and serotonin neurotransmission (2) Reduce microinflammation and oxidative stress (3) Regulate the function of mitochondria (4) Inhibits apoptosis induced toxicity (5) Modulated expression of brain-derived neurotrophic factor (BDNF) gene	[170]

Brain neoplasms	Nutrients	Essential oils	Ocimum basilicum	(1) Antiinflammatory and antiproliferative	[181,182]
			Hypericum hircinum	(1) Antiproliferative	
	Herbals or Extracts	Flavonoids	Hispidulin	(1) Enhance AMPK (2) Control mTOR signaling	[185]
			Luteolin	(1) Inhibits cellular invasion (2) Reduce MMP and FAK (3) Inhibit PI3K/Akt signaling	[203]
	Herbals or Extracts	Terpens, Monoterpens	Carvacrol	(1) Apoptosis induced by ROS (2) Reduce TRPM7 correlated to invasion of tumor cells (3) Stop Ras/MEK/MAPK and PI3K/Akt signaling pathways (4) Decreasing the migration of U87MG cells	[191,192]
	Herbals or Extracts	Cannabinoid	Tetrahydrocannabinol	(1) Reduce synthesis of VEGF and enhance VEGFR-2 (2) Inhibit action of angiopoietin-2 in endothelial cells	[197–199,205]
			Cannabidiol	(1) Enhance sphingolipid ceramide which leads to apoptosis (2) Inhibit GBM tumor through 5-lipoxygenase enzyme and FAAH (3) Inhibit Erk/Akt signaling and VEGF expression (4) Decline transcriptional action of Id-1 in glioma	

vitamins. These nutrients can modulate cholesterol metabolism and other pathways leading to the enhancement of nervous system health and to the amelioration of neuronal transmission [28]. The second type of traditional nutraceuticals includes nutraceutical enzymes, which have less benefits in treating brain alterations [28]. The third class is represented by herbals and herbal extracts. They are considered as potential therapeutics that can be used in mental health and neurologic sicknesses management due to their multiple actions. For instance, curcumin can enhance the levels of some neurotransmitters and improve noradrenaline concentrations in the frontal cortex and striatum regions and in their frontal cortex [29,30]. It can also lead to pathways impairment including the nuclear factor kappa-light-chain-enhancer of activated B cells (NFκB) pathway, and some interleukins production and releasing [31]. Furthermore, curcumin, garlic, ginger, ginkgo biloba, and flavonoids may exhibit antiinflammatory, neuroprotective, and antioxidative properties that can be exploited in degenerative neurologic disorders and other brain alterations [32,33]. Despite the lack of strong evidence and the existence of some controversial data, probiotics are also modern natural nutraceutical compounds that may be helpful in treating many human diseases that are associated with the occurrence of gastrointestinal dysbiosis [34].

2.2 Nontraditional nutraceuticals

This category is mainly represented by fortified foods, which may be obtained via improvement of nutritional quality of the products using technological methods, and recombinant nutraceuticals [35,36]. The development of the latter class results from advances in biotechnology [35].

2.2.1 Phytonutrients or phytochemicals

Phytonutrients are chemical substances that are manufactured and generated by various types of plants. They are known as phytochemicals too [37,38]. They are produced by plants via either primary or secondary metabolism, which help the plants to resist various infections and promotes plant growth [39]. They are found in different plants including red, orange, and yellow vegetables and fruit and in gloomy green leafy vegetables such as spinach, kale, broccoli, and Swiss chard. Moreover, whole grain products and grain breads and cereals (such as different rice types, quinoa, and barley). Nuts and seeds are also sources including walnuts, sunflower, almonds, sesame, and flax seeds. Dark chocolate, tea, and coffee with their different subtypes are known sources too [39–43]. The phytonutrients consist of varying substances such as flavonoids and its alternatives including (catechin, epigallocatechin, epicatechin, bicalein, ginkgo biloba, and 7-hydroxyflavonoid). Also, curcumin, polyphenols, alpha lipoic acid, and cannabinoid (tetrahydrocannabinol and cannabidiol) [41–43]. The phytonutrients can affect brain health via different mechanisms as they act as an important functioning role in preserving the balance of brain chemical substances through affecting the receptors functions for the major inhibitory neurotransmitters. In conventional medicine, many plants have beneficial effects on cognitive disorders treatment [44]. Also, they contain multiple antioxidants, which hinder aging processes [45]. In addition to that, they also promote autophagy, improve cognitive performance, and eliminate free radicals from the body [46]. Moreover, they play a major protection against neuroinflammation [47]. Also, they mediate the activation of signaling pathways, leading to the expression of cytoprotective and restorative proteins [48,49].

2.2.2 Consumption and safety of nutraceuticals

Nutraceuticals are widely consumed in many regions; about 50% of adult subjects from the United States reported that they have applied at least one dietary supplement during the previous 30 days [50]. The consumption of nutraceuticals is also common and valuated in many populations from Malaysia, China, Taiwan, United Arab Emirates, Bangladesh, Jordan, and other areas [51–57]. They are thought to be generally safe and their administration usually does not engender harmful major adverse action in many reports [54]. However, the health benefits and outcomes of these dietary supplements are still unclear and questionable and some of them can cause harmful drug interactions and produce significant toxicity [58]. Botanicals are associated with rare direct adverse events of a mild intensity such as nausea, headache, and sensation of fatigue but their administration with concomitant substances may cause potential toxic effects [58,59]. Although rare, compounds such as garlic and ginkgo biloba may be linked to the onset of spontaneous hemorrhage [60,61]. Also, herbals and their extracts may cause the induction of cytochrome P450 resulting in some cases of herb-drug interactions [62,63]. Therefore, medical care providers should consider these risks in the implementation of management strategies including herbals and some dietary supplements.

2.2.3 Nutraceuticals in Alzheimer's disease

Alzheimer's disease is one of the progressive debilitating illnesses that can have great impacts on the life of patients, their families, and their caregivers. This neurodegenerative disease is therefore considered as one of the major global public health issues [64]. One of the major neurologic characteristics of AD is the decrease of acetylcholine, which is an important neurotransmitter involved in synaptogenesis and in the development cognitive processes. This decline in acetylcholine levels is due to the damage of cholinergic neurons [65]. Alterations in the process of forming neuronal synapsis in neuronal cells, and the increase of oxidative stress are, in addition to the accumulation of beta-amyloid plaques in brain and the production of neurofibrillary tangles, the major hallmarks of this disease [66,67]. Dysfunction of mitochondrial metabolism, loss of lipids and proteins homeostasis, alterations in biometal distribution, neuronal senescence, and decline of nutrient sensing are also linked to the pathogenesis of AD [68,69].

Diets which are rich in antioxidants and polyunsaturated fatty acids and antioxidant molecules vegetables, fruits, and fish may contribute in lowering the incidence of AD [70]. For instance, piperine, which is an alkaloid found in fruits called *Piper nigrum*, can enhance memory and improve neurodegeneration [71]. Various polyphenolic substances have shown a potential effect in modifying the course of AD and other similar conditions. These compounds are classified into different categories according to their structural properties [72]. They mainly exert their action via the upregulation of a key regulator called SIRT1, which is responsible of the control of multiple human cellular pathways [73]. Polyphenols can also serve as antiamyloid molecules since they can modulate the enzymatic activity of brain secretases [74,75].

In addition, ascorbic acid and carotenes can lead to the depression of the process lipid peroxidation and can decease AD [76]. Caffeine, which is a widely consumed phytochemical, can provide a certain protection against oxidative stress in patients with AD [77]. Finally, supplementation with other compounds including taurins, cysteine, and molecules that can enhance the availability of methyl groups in human cells such as folate, betaine, vitamin B12, and S-adenosylmethionine (also known as SAM) can help in preventing the onset of AD through the increase of H_2S production [78].

3. Current evidence on the use of neutraceuticals in multiple sclerosis

Multiple sclerosis (MS) represents a long-term inflammatory demyelination of the nervous tissue resulting in the loss of various neuronal functions [79]. It is characterized by the development of reversible episodes of total or partial neurological disabilities such as limb weakness, ataxia, and visual problems like diplopia and mononuclear visual loss [80].

Unfortunately, the deterioration of the neurologic functions among MS patients cannot be prevented by the presently applied pharmacotherapies and the evidence on the effects of the current disease-modifying medications is still controversial [79]. The direct implication of nutritional factors in this disease is not clear yet, but it was recently admitted that a high dietary consumption of some foods during adolescence may reduce the risk of developing MS [81]. These foods include fruits, vegetables yogurt, cheese, butter fresh fish, and canned tuna. But not red meat, margarine and shrimp [81]. Nutraceutical interventions have been used in different trials involving individuals with MS and were reported to ameliorate both biological and clinical characteristics in MS patients [82]. These nutraceuticals include various categories such as vitamins, gingko biloba, green tea, lemon verbena, coenzyme Q10, and probiotics. Many of the used molecules and plants extracts did not show any efficacy in treating various MS symptoms in clinical trials such as gamma-tocopherol [83], Cranberry extract [84], creatine monohydrate [85], melatonin [86], and retinyl-palmitate [87].

The administration of some nutraceuticals in MS patients may affect the inflammatory processes that characterize this disease, for example, curcumin can modulate the expression of different genes that are responsible of many immune inflammatory and immune molecules including programmed cell death 1 (PDCD1), micro-RNAs 32 and 45, interferon gamma (IFN-γ), chemokine ligand (CCL) 2 and 5, forkhead box P3 (FOXP3), SIRT1, sex-determining region Y box-2 (Sox2), activator protein 1 (AP-1), signal transducer and activator of transcription (STAT) types 1 and 5, and NFκB [88]. Some human trials showed that alpha lipoic acid significantly impacted the change in brain volume but there was no effect on quality of life, mobility, cognition, fatigue, and on the scores of the expanded disability status scale (EDSS) [89,90]. However, in Khallli et al. report, alpha lipoic acid significantly improved EDSS in people with a baseline EDSS of more than zero ($p = 0.036$) [89]. Lipoic acid did not ameliorate the secretion of some crucial inflammatory markers that intervene in the pathogenesis of MS including interleukin 6 (IL-6), tumor necrosis factor-alpha (TNF-α) [91,92], and matrix metallopeptidase-9 (MMP-9) [93]. Lemon verbena, in its turn, may decrease the serum concentrations of C-reactive protein (or CRP), IL-10, and IL-4 in individuals having secondary progressive MS. However, it does not modify the levels of IL-12, IL-6, IL-23, or TNF-α [94]. Probiotics may also have a positive influence on the regulation of metabolic, inflammatory, immune, and oxidative stress parameters in this neurodegenerative illness [95]. An interesting investigation assessed the effects of multistrain probiotic formulation composed of *Lactobacillus casei*, *Lactobacillus acidophilus*, and *Lactobacillus fermentum* and *Bifidobacterium bifidum*. This supplementation was associated with an improvement in the function of beta cells, insulin markers, and in total/HDL cholesterol levels [96]. MS patients had also improved concentrations of nitric oxide metabolites, malondialdehyde, and CRP. Regarding clinical results, there was an amelioration in EDSS, depression levels, and quality of life [96]. Moreover, ginkgo biloba, as well as biotin may improve some MS outcomes such as retrospective memory and concentration for ginkgo biloba [97] and disability reversal [98] for biotin. However, biotin is not linked to any significant effects in measures of quality of life, visual acuity, and subject or clinician assessed Clinical Global Impression Scale scores [99]. Furthermore, the real effect of both and biotin ginko biloba on many MS symptoms is still not understood and more investigations are required to determine whether it can be used in MS management. Regarding caffeine and coffee, it is thought that they have a great impact on MS course due to their neuroprotective actions [77,100]. Other phytochemicals may be also used like andrographolide, which may be associated with a potential role in preventing MS-related disabilities and brain atrophy [101].

Finally, many vitamins may help patients living with MS including vitamin D, which is thought to enhance brain blood perfusion and cellular tissue oxygenation [102]. Yet, the improvements associated with vitamin D supplementation may be more apparent in patients with a low baseline concentration of vitamin D [103] and the existing evidence does not allow to use this vitamin as a disease-modifying medication and it is only recommended that the serum levels should be kept between 50 and 125 nmol/L, meaning that the intake should be of 600–4000 IU/day [104].

4. Amyotrophic lateral sclerosis and nutritional supplementations

Amyotrophic lateral sclerosis, or ALS or Lou Gehrig's disease, is an intractable degenerative neurologic illness that develops from the progressive loss of both lower and upper motor neurons in patients' nervous system. Its typical symptoms are represented by the progressive installation of weakness, muscle fasciculation and atrophy, pain, and spasticity [105]. There is an inverse relation between ALS and overall consumption of fish [106]. Also, the consumption of foods with high mega 3 fatty acids may help prevent or delay or even prevent the onset of this motor nerve degeneration [107]. But, the risk associated with the intake of some dietary components, particularly those that contain amino acids, in addition to some vitamins and minerals like selenium, is still undetermined [106]. A report suggested that there is no statistically significant association between exposures to coffee or tea and mortality due to ALS [108]. Furthermore, after comparing the composition of the intestinal microbiota of patients suffering from ALS and healthy individuals, scientists could reveal a difference between these two populations with a low abundance of yeasts and a higher proportion of enterobacteria and Escherichia coli in ALS patients microbiota [109]. In addition, ALS patients tend to have higher levels of vitamins A and E and diminished levels of vitamins B2, B9, and C in comparison to healthy controls. Serum concentration of vitamin C may be lower in early-onset ALS patients compared to those in late-onset ALS patients [110]. Several large investigations demonstrated that regular administration of vitamin E was associated with a reduced risk of the ALS occurrence [111]. It was also found that vitamin D levels can be correlated to poor mobility in ALS patients, but it cannot predict the degree of the progression of the disease [112]. The administration of vitamin D can reduce brain damage caused by hypoxia, and consequently decreases the death of nervous cells due to the exposition to glutamate insult [113]. G93A mouse model of ALS having high doses of vitamin D has a better functional capacity. In fact, various aspects of the disease can be targeted by vitamin D leading to a cumulative effect that can be greater than antiglutaminergic medications [114]. Moreover, a pilot study showed that biotin is tolerated in this disease but its efficacy needs to be assessed [115].

Many phytochemicals have been exploited to identify potential management tools for ALS. The use of curcumin showed some encouraging effects with an improvement of some patterns of the disease such as oxidative damage leading to a slight decrease in ALS [116]. Cannabis derivatives may be used as symptomatic therapy for ALS spasticity [117].

Lastly, not all nutraceuticals showed conclusive results in ALS investigations. A recent long-term randomized study using B12 concluded that high doses of this vitamin may promote the survival of ALS subjects but investigators did not record a significant efficacy in the whole study sample [118]. Also, β-carotene supplementation was not associated with ALS [111]. Although the evidence is scarce, the different works done on the effect of supplying ALS subjects with nutritional compounds may help not only in establishing new management approaches but also in understanding the factors and the phenomena that potentially trigger this disease such as neuroinflammation and some pathways related to oxidative stress.

5. Effects of neutraceuticals supplementation in Parkinson's disease

Parkinson's disease (PD) arises from the lethality of dopamine neurons in the substantia nigra greatly impacting the process of controlling body movements [119]. Recently, this neurodegenerative condition was considered as multisystem disorder characterized by neuroinflammation leading to impaired nonmotor and motor human functions [120].

The risk of PD is majored in some circumstances such as increased exposure to pesticides and to some dairy products, in addition to the presence of medical history of brain injury and melanoma [121]. It is, however, reduced by some other factors such as caffeine, smoking, physical activity, elevated concentrations of serum urate, and the consumption of some drugs such as ibuprofen [121]. Furthermore, some dietary panels have been suggested as adjunctives to PD therapy including ketogenetic diet, muscular exercise, and supplementation with nutraceutical and antioxidative products including niacin, nicotine, melatonin, caffeine, butyrate, and glutathione [122]. But some results did not support the administration of vitamins with antioxidant potentials to reduce PD risk [123].

Actually, the rate of using dietary supplements is high among PD subjects. In a cross-sectional study, 83.4% of the participants reported taking at least one dietary compound and more than half of patients have had multivitamins, vitamins B12 and vitamin D as supplements [124]. Regarding PD progression nuts, fresh fruits and vegetables, nonfried fish, olive and coconut oils, spices, seeds, and nuts are correlated to low rate of progression [125], while canned fruits and vegetables, fried foods, soda and other compound may be implicated in the acceleration of PD [125]. Supplementation with iron may also be associated with rapid PD progression [125].

Caffeine exerts its actions by blocking A_{2A}Rs and by reducing the depletion of dopamine leading to some improvements in the locomotor functions [126]. The consumption of caffeine may stabilize the BBB during PD via attenuating neuroinflammation [127]. It can also affect oxidative stress processes through inhibiting lipid peroxidation and decreasing the release of reactive oxygen species (ROS) such as singlet oxygen and hydroxyl radicals [128]. Probiotics supplementation for 12 weeks in PD patients may also affect the neuroinflammatory disorder since it significantly improved gene expression of interleukins 1 and 8, TNF-α, PPAR-γ, and TGF-β but did not modify the expression ofVEGF and LDLR genes [129]. Compared to placebo, the consumption of probiotic decreased MDS-UPDRS and positively modified lab test results showing amelioration in inflammatory and oxidative stress markers such as CRP, malondialdehyde, and glutathione [130]. In addition, they are associated with reduced insulin and diminished insulin resistance with a statistically significant increase of sensitivity to insulin effects [130]. However, the available clinical evidence on probiotics in PD treatment is not solid and their effects on motor symptoms or progression of PD are not well characterized [131]. Besides, prebiotics and fermented milk which contains various strains of probiotics may improve constipation in PD patients [132]. Cosupplementation with vitamin E and omega-3 fatty acids can also have positive effects on UPDRS and on inflammatory and metabolic markers [133]. Macrophage polarization during PD can be triggered by the effects of nutritional elements such as niacin, which modifies the polarization from the pro-inflammatory phenotype (M1) to the antiinflammatory form (M2) [134]. It also causes a declined NF-κB translocation and may lead to a drop in pro-inflammatory cytokines [135].

Finally, nutraceuticals that target the production of peroxynitrite and its actions can play a role in preventing and controlling the course of PD. These elements include omega-3 fatty acids, ferulic acid, vitamins, taurine, butyrogenic dietary fibers, N-acetylcysteine, *epigallocatechin-gallate*, probiotics, caffeine, and phycocyanobilin of *spirulina* [136].

6. Effects of nutraceuticals in Huntington's disease

Huntington's disease (HD) is a clinical condition characterized by a neurodegeneration induced by an unstable expansion of the CAG trinucleotide repeat in a specific gene called the *Huntingtin (HTT)* gene [137]. Currently, no disease-modifying therapy has been approved for HD despite its debilitating character [137]. It is also characterized by the existence of an energy-deficient state; meaning that individuals affected by this condition need to be supplemented by a high-calorie nutritional diet [138]. Unfortunately, until now, the investigations did not find any nutraceuticals that can provide a disease modification for HD patients [139]. As it is well known, decreased energy production induced by mitochondrial dysfunction and oxidative stress are related to HD and many other degenerative diseases [140]. A variety of nutraceuticals and multiple diets can impact the oxidative stress and mitochondrial impairment [141]. For instance models of HD in which quercetin was used, showed an attenuated mitochondrial oxidative stress and a significant reduction in pyknotic nuclei and astrogliosis that were engendered by 3-nitropropionic acid in striatum [142]. Triheptanoin, which is an important source of heptanoate fatty acids, is capable of the amelioration of the bioenergetic profile in the nervous tissue of individuals having HD [143]. Moreover, CoQ10 is a well-known antioxidant that is involved in electron transfer in mitochondria [144]. Its use in HD patients was generally safe but did not impact the outcomes of the illness [145]. Similarly, the results of a recent study did not support creatine, which is also involved in many mitochondrial processes, for the treatment of HD [146]. Furthermore, curcumin can also target oxidative stress processes and neuroinflammation in HD. It can additionally modulate transcriptional alterations and enhance the functions of molecular chaperons [147]. Eicosapentaenoic acid, which is one of the well-characterized fatty acids, may positively influence motor functioning in HD patients. This effect was not consistent among all the reported trials [148]. Yet, eicosapentaenoic acid could reverse the progression of brain atrophy [149]. Actually, there is a paucity of studies investigating the effects of neutraceutical compounds in HD patients, however, it is established that patients with determined deficiencies. This is, for example, the case of patients having decreased carnitinemia who may be supplied with levocarnitine [150] and of patients with pantothenate deficiency who can be treated with B5 [151].

7. The role of nutraceuticals supplementation in brain ataxia

Different causes of brain ataxia have been associated with metabolic dysfunctions in the nervous system [152–155]. Oxidative stress has been incriminated in the pathological processes of such disorders including Friedreich's ataxia, which is an orphan genetic disease with reduced expression of frataxin (FXN) engendering neuronal loss [155]. Tocotrienols may be beneficial since they are associated with a decline in inflammatory disorders in Friedreich's ataxia and with decreased oxidative stress [156]. Low doses of tocotrienol can significantly enhance the production of the FXN isoform FXN-3 but not FXN-1, FXN-2 in patients [157]. Furthermore, it is well established that, in Ataxia with vitamin E deficiency (AVED), the supplementation protects from the progress of the degeneration and influences the clinical symptoms [158].

In a randomized trial involving individuals with spinocerebellar ataxia (SCA) type 2, 6 months oral zinc sulfate supplementation increased Zn amounts in the cerebrospinal fluid, ameliorated lipids induced oxidative stress and positively impacted the clinical outcomes in the SCA2 group including posture and dysdiadochocinesia [159]. Also, the use of the antioxidant compound CoQ 10 can lead to a significant amelioration in clinical outcome of patients with SCA1 and SCA 3 [160]. Finally, cerebellar ataxia associated with deficiency in CoQ 10 can be improved by supplementation with this important cofactor [161].

7.1 Psychiatric disorders

Psychiatric disorders share some common pathologic features including the upregulation of neuroinflammatory cytokines [162], the disruption of cerebral blood flow [163], and the alteration of the cerebral white matter [164] and of the BBB [12]. There is some evidence of efficacy of the use of nutritional supplements in many psychiatric troubles [165]. A recent systematic review on the application of nutraceuticals in the treatment of psychotic and mood disorders found that 10 out of 11 studies investigating the role of omega-3 demonstrated a significant effect of this category of nutraceuticals [166]. However, no evidence was found after reviewing the published reports on some other nutrients such as vitamins B9 and B12, carnitine, and vitamin D [166]. For instance, supplementing diabetes patients with vitamin D may provide a sort of protection against the occurrence of major depressive disorder [167]. Actually, the use of certain compounds can be very prevalent among individuals with psychiatric diseases. In a cross-sectional study evaluating young patients suffering from autism spectrum disorder (ASD), 75% of the involved population reported the use of a wide range of nutraceuticals supplements including multivitamins, magnesium, probiotics, and omega 3 [168]. Some patients reported that they were consuming the supplements without any prescription. Although there is some evidence on the efficacy of the different supplementations in improving functional domains in patients with ASD, the current knowledge is still limited and their use should be restricted to patients who already have some nutritional deficiencies [169].

In terms of depression, many neutraceuticals categories including folate, vitamin D, omega-3 fatty acids, and S-adenosylmethionine have shown considerable effects on depressive symptoms supporting the possibility of their clinical use [170]. Furthermore, CoQ10 can be used safely in the management of the depressive phase of bipolar disorder [171]. It is associated with an amelioration of symptoms in the patients with bipolar depression [172] and with an improvement of levels of some inflammatory cytokines such as IL-10 and TNF-α but not IL-6 [171]. Moreover, the application of probiotics and prebiotics as nutritional supplements has shown some beneficial effects not only in depression [173] but also in managing stress in healthy people [174].

The supplementation with nutraceuticals has been also investigated to treat schizophrenia, yet, scientists do not recommend their prescription in clinical practice except for individuals with mineral and vitamin deficiencies [175]. In general, nutrient supplements can be very safe in patients with mood and psychiatric issues and can be used along with the specific psychiatric drugs without counter indications but it is still early to incorporate them in the treatment recommendations according to the existent evidence [176].

7.2 Effects of nutraceuticals in brain neoplasms

Interest in nutraceuticals role in cancer treatment has expanded in recent years [177,178]. Medical plant components such as essential oils (EO) demonstrated their anticancer effect [179,180]. Regarding glioblastoma, EOs of *Hypericum hircinum* had an antiproliferative effect on T98G cells. Also, *Zanthoxylum tinguassuiba* contains α-bisabolol, which is an antiglioma sesquiterpene so they could be an effective alternative therapy [181,182]. C6-ceramide (CER) showed an effective combination with paclitaxel (PTX) in novel oil-in-water nanoemulsions, which enhanced its therapeutic activity in glioblastoma [183]. *Ocimum basilicum* and *Lippia multiflora* EOS had an aggressive effect on SF-767 glioblastoma cell line proliferation, whereas essential oil of *Ageratum conyzoides* revealed the maximum activity on SF-763 cells [180]. EOS of croton Regelianus and its component Ascaridole can exert an antitumor effect in brain (SF-295) human cancer cells [184]. Flavonoids such as hispidulin caused a dose-dependent inhibition of the proliferation of GBM cells through stimulation of AMP-activated protein kinase (AMPK) [185].

Furthermore, monoterpenes such as perillyl alcohol (POH) is an active chemotherapeutic agent for recurrent glioblastoma multiforme cell lines (U87 and A172) with morphological modifications [186]. Intranasal administration of POH improved the overall survival of patients with recurrent GBM compared to supportive treatment [187]. POH also demonstrated an antimetastatic effect in C6 cell line of chick embryo model [188]. An experiment by Fonseca et al. showed that POH can exert antiproliferative effects, can decrease protein synthesis, also can result in cell morphology modifications, and causes an alteration in membrane permeability with extra changes in the architecture of C6, U87MG, and A172 cell [189]. POH decreased the angiogenesis process through inhibition of the cytokine IL-8 and VEGF [190]. In addition, Chen et al. reported that carvacrol reduced the activity and expression of transient receptor potential cation channel subfamily M member 7 (TRPM7) at the transcript and protein stages in U87MG cells, which lead to antiproliferative effect and activation of caspase-3 [191]. Moreover, carvacrol decreased the expression of MMP2, which is critical in the invasive capabilities of U87MG cells [192].

Curcumin had also an antiproliferative effect in GBM cells, activated caspase-3, and suppressed antiapoptotic genes such as NF-κβ, AP-1, and Bcl-2 [193]. Demethoxycurcumin causes Bcl-2 facilitated G2/M arrest and apoptosis in U87 human glioma cells [194]. Curcumin deactivated gliomas progression in xenograft models through inhibition of angiogenesis by the reduction synthesis of blood vessels from endothelial cell markers [195]. Langone et al. showed that curcumin inhibited Akt-1, BCl XL, and cyclin D1 and could be a promising therapy for glioblastoma [196].

Tetrahydrocannabinol (THC) and cannabidiol (CBD) are of the major phytocannabinoids existing in marijuana, with a useful anticancer effect in a variety of cancer animal models, involving GBM [197]. Cannabinoids release sphingolipid ceramide and regulate cell proliferation and differentiation and mediate apoptosis [197]. THC in combination with temozolomide (TMZ) significantly decreased the viability of a HG19 primary culture and U87MG and T98G cell lines [198]. This combination also elevated the activity of caspase-3 up to 5 times more than TMZ alone [198]. Furthermore, Solinas et al. reported that CBD treatment had an antitumor effect through a dose-related downregulation of ERK and Akt signaling pathways in T98G and U87-MG cells and reduces hypoxia-inducible factor HIF-1a expression in U87-MG cells [199].

Finally, polyphenols as resveratrol can reduce glioma proliferation, stop S phase of the cell cycle, stimulate apoptosis in vitro, and inhibit intracranial C6 tumor growth in vivo and extend survival in rats [200]. Furthermore, it regulates the PI3K/Akt signaling pathway, which is implicated in controlling angiogenesis control in glioma [201,202]. In vivo studies proved that miR-7-1-3p high expression improved antitumor effects of luteolin and silibinin flavonoids, which prevent autophagy and provoke apoptosis in U87MG and T98G tumors after rapamycin treatment [203]. Resveratrol ($40\,\mathrm{mg\,kg^{-1}\,day^{-1}}$) showed an antiangiogenic effect in a glioma rat model by decreasing CD31 expression [204]. Cannabidiol (CBD) decreased GBM growth through mediating enzyme 5-lipoxygenase and fatty acid amide hydrolase [205]. Many of these nutraceuticals have moved to human clinical trials and some showed some efficacy.

8. Proposed neuroprotective mechanisms of some popular nutraceuticals

8.1 Curcumin

Curcumin contribute to the amelioration of antioxidant status and to the prevention of neuronal damage via the Nrf2 and NF-κB signaling pathways [206]. It modulates the activity of Aβ amyloid/β secretase and participates in the restoration of autophagy machinery and in decreasing neuroinflammation [207]. Decrease of cortisol levels and inhibition of acetyl/butyryl choline esterase and monoamine oxidase A and B activity is also observed after curcumin use [208]. This nutraceutical also helps ameliorate mitochondrial dynamics and enhances neurotropic growth factors [209].

8.2 Coenzyme Q10 (CoQ10)

CoQ10 is a ubiquitous molecule that participates in energy metabolism providing various neuroprotective effects. It attenuates inflammation and decreases cytokines by downregulating NF-κB and helps protect dopaminergic cells [210]. It can suppress AChE activity and decrease α-syn aggregation leading to protection against neurodegeneration observed in AD and PD [172]. Also, supplementation with CoQ10 enhances mitochondrial and neuronal and locomotory functions via the modulation of PPAR-γ and Akt metabolism [211].

8.3 Polyphenols

They can help in maintaining BBB integrity and decreasing neuroinflammation via different pathways including NF-κB, JNK/MAPK Nrf2/HO-1 and PI3K/Akt pathways [212]. Resveratrol may improve autophagy and improve mitochondrial function through the modulation of SIRT1, PPAR, and ERK [213,214]. It also has antiamyloidogenic properties [214].

8.4 Polyunsaturated fatty acids

Polyunsaturated fatty acids promote neurogenesis pathways and inactivate microglia/astrocytes through PPAR-γ and JNK signaling pathway and reduce brain inflammation [215,216]. They can exert antiamyloidogenic properties and help reduce aggregation of tau protein and amyloid β plaque by improving phagocytosis processes and by inhibiting β/γ secretase enzyme [215].

9. Conclusions

Emerging evidence on the use of nutrient components in managing multiple brain disorders is very promising since these methods are associated with potential benefits along with the possibility of having low incidence of undesirable events. Unfortunately, many limitations prevented the release of full recommendations, which may be applicable in clinical management. These limitations are mainly represented by the small sample sizes of the studies that have been accomplished, the great variability in measured outcomes, and the heterogeneity among the existent studies. Large randomized trials are needed to expand our current knowledge and to assess the potential effects of the unexplored molecules.

Authors' contribution

All authors contributed in data collection, and in the process of writing and revising the manuscript.

References

[1] F. Gomez-Pinilla, X. Yang, System biology approach intersecting diet and cell metabolism with pathogenesis of brain disorders, Prog. Neurobiol. 169 (2018) 76–90.
[2] F. Gómez-Pinilla, Brain foods: the effects of nutrients on brain function, Nat. Rev. Neurosci. 9 (7) (2008) 568–578.
[3] D. Albuquerque, E. Stice, R. Rodríguez-López, L. Manco, C. Nóbrega, Current review of genetics of human obesity: from molecular mechanisms to an evolutionary perspective, Mol. Gen. Genomics. 290 (4) (2015) 1191–1221.
[4] J. Valero, I. Paris, A. Sierra, Lifestyle shapes the dialogue between environment, microglia, and adult neurogenesis, ACS Chem. Neurosci. 7 (4) (2016) 442–453.
[5] R. Daneman, A. Prat, The blood-brain barrier, Cold Spring Harb. Perspect. Biol. 7 (1) (2015), a020412.
[6] R.D. Bell, B.V. Zlokovic, Neurovascular mechanisms and blood-brain barrier disorder in Alzheimer's disease, Acta Neuropathol. 118 (1) (2009) 103–113.
[7] B.S. Desai, A.J. Monahan, P.M. Carvey, B. Hendey, Blood-brain barrier pathology in alzheimer's and parkinson's disease: implications for drug therapy, Cell Transplant. 16 (3) (2007) 285–299. [Internet]. Available from https://doi.org/10.3727/000000007783464731.
[8] J. Drouin-Ouellet, S.J. Sawiak, G. Cisbani, M. Lagacé, W.-L. Kuan, M. Saint-Pierre, et al., Cerebrovascular and blood-brain barrier impairments in Huntington's disease: potential implications for its pathophysiology, Ann. Neurol. 78 (2) (2015) 160–177. Available from: https://doi.org/10.1002/ana.24406.
[9] S. Najjar, D.M. Pearlman, O. Devinsky, A. Najjar, D. Zagzag, Neurovascular unit dysfunction with blood-brain barrier hyperpermeability contributes to major depressive disorder: a review of clinical and experimental evidence, J. Neuroinflammation 10 (1) (2013) 906. Available from: https://doi.org/10.1186/1742-2094-10-142.
[10] Z. Gal, R.J. Huse, X. Gonda, S. Kumar, G. Juhasz, G. Bagdy, et al., Anxiety and depression—the role of blood-brain barrier integrity, Neuropsychopharmacol. Hung. 21 (1) (2019) 19–25. Available from: http://europepmc.org/abstract/MED/30962406.

[11] L. Kamintsky, K.A. Cairns, R. Veksler, C. Bowen, S.D. Beyea, A. Friedman, et al., Blood-brain barrier imaging as a potential biomarker for bipolar disorder progression, NeuroImage Clin. 26 (2020), 102049. Available from: http://www.sciencedirect.com/science/article/pii/S2213158219303961.

[12] J. Kealy, C. Greene, M. Campbell, Blood-brain barrier regulation in psychiatric disorders, Neurosci. Lett. 726 (2020), 133664. Available from: http://www.sciencedirect.com/science/article/pii/S0304394018304361.

[13] S. Pong, Brain Microvascular Endothelial Cell Dysfunction in Schizophrenia: A Preliminary Report, 2020, Available from: https://hdl.handle.net/2144/41156.

[14] X. Chen, O. Ghribi, J.D. Geiger, Caffeine protects against disruptions of the blood-brain barrier in animal models of Alzheimer's and Parkinson's diseases, J. Alzheimers Dis. 20 (2010) S127–S141.

[15] C.-Y. Chang, J.-Y. Chen, M.-H. Wu, M.-L. Hu, Therapeutic treatment with vitamin C reduces focal cerebral ischemia-induced brain infarction in rats by attenuating disruptions of blood brain barrier and cerebral neuronal apoptosis, Free Radic. Biol. Med. 155 (2020) 29–36. Available from: http://www.sciencedirect.com/science/article/pii/S0891584919324529.

[16] M.O. Welcome, Blood brain barrier inflammation and potential therapeutic role of phytochemicals, PharmaNutrition 11 (2020), 100177. Available from: http://www.sciencedirect.com/science/article/pii/S2213434420300025.

[17] V. Braniste, M. Al-Asmakh, C. Kowal, F. Anuar, A. Abbaspour, M. Tóth, et al., The gut microbiota influences blood-brain barrier permeability in mice, Sci. Transl. Med. 6 (263) (2014), 263ra158.

[18] N.K. Acharya, E.C. Levin, P.M. Clifford, M. Han, R. Tourtellotte, D. Chamberlain, et al., Diabetes and hypercholesterolemia increase blood-brain barrier permeability and brain amyloid deposition: beneficial effects of the LpPLA2 inhibitor darapladib, J. Alzheimers Dis. 35 (1) (2013) 179–198.

[19] M. Lehmann, B. Regland, K. Blennow, C.G. Gottfries, Vitamin B_{12}-B_6-Folate treatment improves blood-brain barrier function in patients with hyperhomocysteinaemia and mild cognitive impairment, Dement. Geriatr. Cogn. Disord. 16 (3) (2003) 145–150. Available from: https://www.karger.com/DOI/10.1159/000071002.

[20] F. Mohagheghi, M.R. Bigdeli, B. Rasoulian, A.A. Zeinanloo, A. Khoshbaten, Dietary virgin olive oil reduces blood brain barrier permeability, brain edema, and brain injury in rats subjected to ischemia-reperfusion, ScientificWorldJournal 10 (2010), 246470. Available from: https://doi.org/10.1100/tsw.2010.128.

[21] S. Won, I. Sayeed, B.L. Peterson, B. Wali, J.S. Kahn, D.G. Stein, Vitamin D prevents hypoxia/reoxygenation-induced blood-brain barrier disruption via vitamin D receptor-mediated NF-kB signaling pathways, PLoS One 10 (3) (2015), e0122821. Available from: https://doi.org/10.1371/journal.pone.0122821.

[22] D. Kempuraj, R. Thangavel, P.A. Natteru, G.P. Selvakumar, D. Saeed, H. Zahoor, et al., Neuroinflammation induces neurodegeneration, J. Neurol. Neurosurg. Spine 1 (1) (2016).

[23] R.M. Barrientos, M.M. Kitt, L.R. Watkins, S.F. Maier, Neuroinflammation in the normal aging hippocampus, Neuroscience 309 (2015) 84–99.

[24] M.N. Catorce, G. Gevorkian, Evaluation of anti-inflammatory nutraceuticals in LPS-induced mouse neuroinflammation model: an update, Curr. Neuropharmacol. 18 (2020).

[25] R.A. Luna, J.A. Foster, Gut brain axis: diet microbiota interactions and implications for modulation of anxiety and depression, Curr. Opin. Biotechnol. 32 (2015) 35–41.

[26] A. Benmelouka, A.M. Sherif, M.A. Ebada, A review of the relationship between gut microbiota and memory, in: Biological, Diagnostic and Therapeutic Advances in Alzheimer's Disease, Springer, Singapore, 2019, pp. 151–165.

[27] K. Bhaskarachary, Traditional foods, functional foods and nutraceuticals, Proc. Indian Natl. Sci. Acad. 82 (5) (2016) 1565–1577.
[28] R. Makkar, T. Behl, S. Bungau, G. Zengin, V. Mehta, A. Kumar, et al., Nutraceuticals in neurological disorders, Int. J. Mol. Sci. 21 (12) (2020) 4424.
[29] Y. Xu, B.-S. Ku, H.-Y. Yao, Y.-H. Lin, X. Ma, Y.-H. Zhang, et al., The effects of curcumin on depressive-like behaviors in mice, Eur. J. Pharmacol. 518 (1) (2005) 40–46.
[30] S.K. Kulkarni, M.K. Bhutani, M. Bishnoi, Antidepressant activity of curcumin: involvement of serotonin and dopamine system, Psychopharmacology 201 (3) (2008) 435–442.
[31] I. Morales, C. Cerda-Troncoso, V. Andrade, R.B. Maccioni, The natural product curcumin as a potential coadjuvant in Alzheimer's treatment, J. Alzheimers Dis. 60 (2) (2017) 451–460.
[32] S.K. Kulkarni, A. Dhir, An overview of curcumin in neurological disorders, Indian J. Pharm. Sci. 72 (2) (2010) 149–154. Available from: https://pubmed.ncbi.nlm.nih.gov/20838516.
[33] C. Calfio, A. Gonzalez, S.K. Singh, L.E. Rojo, R.B. Maccioni, The emerging role of nutraceuticals and phytochemicals in the prevention and treatment of Alzheimer's disease, J. Alzheimers Dis. (2020) 1–19.
[34] J. Zucko, A. Starcevic, J. Diminic, D. Oros, A.M. Mortazavian, P. Putnik, Probiotic—friend or foe? Curr. Opin. Food Sci. 32 (2020) 45–49.
[35] W. Andlauer, P. Fürst, Nutraceuticals: a piece of history, present status and outlook, Food Res. Int. 35 (2–3) (2002) 171–176.
[36] P.B. Ottaway, Food Fortification and Supplementation: Technological, Safety and Regulatory Aspects, Elsevier, 2008.
[37] J. Szalay, What Are Phytonutrients?, Live Science, 2015.
[38] S. Yoo, K. Kim, H. Nam, D. Lee, Discovering health benefits of phytochemicals with integrated analysis of the molecular network, chemical properties and ethnopharmacological evidence, Nutrients 10 (8) (2018) 1042.
[39] R.J. Molyneux, S.T. Lee, D.R. Gardner, K.E. Panter, L.F. James, Phytochemicals: the good, the bad and the ugly? Phytochemistry 68 (22–24) (2007) 2973–2985.
[40] webmd. Phytonutrients.
[41] D.M. Minich, A review of the science of colorful, plant-based food and practical strategies for "eating the rainbow", J. Nutr. Metab. 2019 (2019) 1–19.
[42] C. Gupta, D. Prakash, Phytonutrients as therapeutic agents, J. Complement. Integr. Med. 11 (3) (2014).
[43] C. Leitzmann, Characteristics and health benefits of phytochemicals, Complement. Med. Res. 23 (2) (2016) 69–74.
[44] G.P. Kumar, F. Khanum, Neuroprotective potential of phytochemicals, Pharmacogn. Rev. 6 (12) (2012) 81.
[45] R.F.M. Silva, L. Pogačnik, Polyphenols from food and natural products: neuroprotection and safety, Antioxidants 9 (1) (2020) 61.
[46] J. Bensalem, S. Dudonné, N. Etchamendy, H. Pellay, C. Amadieu, D. Gaudout, et al., Polyphenols from grape and blueberry improve episodic memory in healthy elderly with lower level of memory performance: a bicentric double-blind, randomized, placebo-controlled clinical study, J. Gerontol. Ser. A 74 (7) (2019) 996–1007.
[47] R. Hornedo-Ortega, A.B. Cerezo, R.M. de Pablos, S. Krisa, T. Richard, M.C. García-Parrilla, et al., Phenolic compounds characteristic of the mediterranean diet in mitigating microglia-mediated neuroinflammation, Front. Cell. Neurosci. 12 (2018).
[48] S. Davinelli, N. Sapere, D. Zella, R. Bracale, M. Intrieri, G. Scapagnini, Pleiotropic protective effects of phytochemicals in Alzheimer's disease, Oxidative Med. Cell. Longev. 2012 (2012) 1–11.

[49] S. Davinelli, M. Maes, G. Corbi, A. Zarrelli, D.C. Willcox, G. Scapagnini, Dietary phytochemicals and neuro-inflammaging: from mechanistic insights to translational challenges, Immun. Ageing 13 (1) (2016) 16.

[50] R.L. Bailey, J.J. Gahche, P.E. Miller, P.R. Thomas, J.T. Dwyer, Why US adults use dietary supplements, JAMA Intern. Med. 173 (5) (2013) 355–361.

[51] S. Rautiainen, J.E. Manson, A.H. Lichtenstein, H.D. Sesso, Dietary supplements and disease prevention - a global overview, Nat. Rev. Endocrinol. 12 (7) (2016) 407–420.

[52] C.-H. Chuang, S.-H. Yang, P.-J. Chang, P.-C. Chen, Y.C. Chen, Dietary supplement intake by 6-month-old Taiwanese infants, J. Pediatr. Gastroenterol. Nutr. 54 (1) (2012). Available from: https://journals.lww.com/jpgn/Fulltext/2012/01000/Dietary_Supplement_Intake_by_6_month_old_Taiwanese.14.aspx.

[53] P.B. James, A.I. Kaikai, A.J. Bah, A. Steel, J. Wardle, Herbal medicine use during breastfeeding: a cross-sectional study among mothers visiting public health facilities in the Western area of Sierra Leone, BMC Complement. Altern. Med. 19 (1) (2019) 66. Available from: https://doi.org/10.1186/s12906-019-2479-7.

[54] N.M. Abdulla, F. Aziz, I. Blair, M. Grivna, B. Adam, T. Loney, Prevalence of, and factors associated with health supplement use in Dubai, United Arab Emirates: a population-based cross-sectional study, BMC Complement. Altern. Med. 19 (1) (2019) 172. Available from: https://doi.org/10.1186/s12906-019-2593-6.

[55] M. Ahmed, J.H. Hwang, M.A. Hasan, D. Han, Herbal medicine use by pregnant women in Bangladesh: a cross-sectional study, BMC Complement. Altern. Med. 18 (1) (2018) 333. Available from: https://doi.org/10.1186/s12906-018-2399-y.

[56] T.M. Khan, M.A. Hassali, M.S.M. Al-Haddad, Nutraceuticals use among the inhabitants of Penang, Malaysia, Int. J. Collab. Res. Intern. Med. Public Heal. 3 (5) (2011).

[57] D.H. Abdel-Qader, A. Albassam, N.S. Ismael, M.S. Aljamal, L.-C. Chen, K. Mansoor, et al., Herbal medicine use in the Jordanian population: a nationally representative cross-sectional survey, J. Pharm. Pharmacogn. Res. 8 (6) (2020) 525–536.

[58] M.J.J. Ronis, K.B. Pedersen, J. Watt, Adverse effects of nutraceuticals and dietary supplements, Annu. Rev. Pharmacol. Toxicol. 58 (2018) 583–601. Available from: https://pubmed.ncbi.nlm.nih.gov/28992429.

[59] C. Di Lorenzo, A. Ceschi, H. Kupferschmidt, S. Lüde, N.E. De Souza, A. Dos Santos, et al., Adverse effects of plant food supplements and botanical preparations: a systematic review with critical evaluation of causality, Br. J. Clin. Pharmacol. 79 (4) (2015) 578–592.

[60] S. Bent, H. Goldberg, A. Padula, A.L. Avins, Spontaneous bleeding associated with ginkgo biloba: a case report and systematic review of the literature: a case report and systematic review of the literature, J. Gen. Intern. Med. 20 (7) (2005) 657–661.

[61] A. Woodbury, R. Sniecinski, Garlic-induced surgical bleeding: how much is too much? A A Case Rep. 7 (12) (2016) 266–269.

[62] R.G. Tirona, D.G. Bailey, Herbal product-drug interactions mediated by induction, Br. J. Clin. Pharmacol. 61 (6) (2006) 677–681.

[63] T.K.H. Chang, Activation of pregnane X receptor (PXR) and constitutive androstane receptor (CAR) by herbal medicines, AAPS J. 11 (3) (2009) 590–601.

[64] World Health Organization, Dementia Cases Set to Triple by 2050 But Still Largely Ignored, Geneva, Switz, 2012.

[65] V.N. Talesa, Acetylcholinesterase in Alzheimer's disease, Mech. Ageing Dev. 122 (16) (2001) 1961–1969.

[66] D. Praticò, Oxidative stress hypothesis in Alzheimer's disease: a reappraisal, Trends Pharmacol. Sci. 29 (12) (2008) 609–615.

[67] P. Sharma, P. Srivastava, A. Seth, P.N. Tripathi, A.G. Banerjee, S.K. Shrivastava, Comprehensive review of mechanisms of pathogenesis involved in Alzheimer's disease and potential therapeutic strategies, Prog. Neurobiol. 174 (2019) 53–89.

[68] A.C. Kim, S. Lim, Y.K. Kim, Metal ion effects on Aβ and Tau aggregation, Int. J. Mol. Sci. 19 (1) (2018).

[69] A.M. Elmatboly, A.M. Sherif, D.A. Deeb, A. Benmelouka, M.N. Bin-Jumah, L. Aleya, et al., The impact of proteostasis dysfunction secondary to environmental and genetic causes on neurodegenerative diseases progression and potential therapeutic intervention, Environ. Sci. Pollut. Res. (2020). Available from: https://doi.org/10.1007/s11356-020-07914-1.

[70] G.C. Román, R.E. Jackson, R. Gadhia, A.N. Román, J. Reis, Mediterranean diet: the role of long-chain ω-3 fatty acids in fish; polyphenols in fruits, vegetables, cereals, coffee, tea, cacao and wine; probiotics and vitamins in prevention of stroke, age-related cognitive decline, and Alzheimer disease, Rev. Neurol. (Paris) 175 (10) (2019) 724–741.

[71] M.H. Farzaei, Z. Shahpiri, M.R. Mehri, R. Bahramsoltani, M. Rezaei, A. Raeesdana, et al., Medicinal plants in neurodegenerative diseases: perspective of traditional Persian medicine, Curr. Drug Metab. 19 (5) (2018) 429–442.

[72] C. Manach, A. Scalbert, C. Morand, C. Rémésy, L. Jiménez, Polyphenols: food sources and bioavailability, Am. J. Clin. Nutr. 79 (5) (2004) 727–747.

[73] S. Chung, H. Yao, S. Caito, J.-W. Hwang, G. Arunachalam, I. Rahman, Regulation of SIRT1 in cellular functions: role of polyphenols, Arch. Biochem. Biophys. 501 (1) (2010) 79–90.

[74] K. Jiménez-Aliaga, P. Bermejo-Bescós, J. Benedí, S. Martín-Aragón, Quercetin and rutin exhibit antiamyloidogenic and fibril-disaggregating effects in vitro and potent antioxidant activity in APPswe cells, Life Sci. 89 (25–26) (2011) 939–945.

[75] M. Kostomoiri, A. Fragkouli, M. Sagnou, L.A. Skaltsounis, M. Pelecanou, E.C. Tsilibary, et al., Oleuropein, an anti-oxidant polyphenol constituent of olive promotes α-secretase cleavage of the amyloid precursor protein (AβPP), Cell. Mol. Neurobiol. 33 (1) (2013) 147–154.

[76] L.I. da Hage-Melim, J.V. Ferreira, N.K.S. de Oliveira, L.C. Correia, M.R.S. Almeida, J.G.C. Poiani, et al., The impact of natural compounds on the treatment of neurodegenerative diseases, Curr. Org. Chem. 23 (3) (2019) 335–360.

[77] M. Kolahdouzan, M.J. Hamadeh, The neuroprotective effects of caffeine in neurodegenerative diseases, CNS Neurosci. Ther. 23 (4) (2017) 272–290.

[78] M.F. McCarty, J.H. O'Keefe, J.J. DiNicolantonio, A diet rich in taurine, cysteine, folate, B(12) and betaine may lessen risk for Alzheimer's disease by boosting brain synthesis of hydrogen sulfide, Med. Hypotheses 132 (2019), 109356.

[79] D.S. Reich, C.F. Lucchinetti, P.A. Calabresi, Multiple sclerosis, N. Engl. J. Med. 378 (2) (2018) 169–180.

[80] W.J. Brownlee, T.A. Hardy, F. Fazekas, D.H. Miller, Diagnosis of multiple sclerosis: progress and challenges, Lancet (London, England) 389 (10076) (2017) 1336–1346.

[81] I. Abdollahpour, M.P. Sormani, S. Nedjat, M.A. Mansournia, I. van der Mei, The role of nutritional factors during adolescence in multiple sclerosis onset: a population-based incident case-control study, Nutr. Neurosci. 1–8 (2019).

[82] W. Marx, M. Hockey, A.J. McGuinness, M. Lane, J. Christodoulou, I. van der Mei, et al., The effect of emerging nutraceutical interventions for clinical and biological outcomes in multiple sclerosis: a systematic review, Mult. Scler. Relat. Disord. 37 (2020), 101486.

[83] M.C. Pantzaris, G.N. Loukaides, E.E. Ntzani, I.S. Patrikios, A novel oral nutraceutical formula of omega-3 and omega-6 fatty acids with vitamins (PLP10) in relapsing remitting multiple sclerosis: a randomised, double-blind, placebo-controlled proof-of-concept clinical trial, BMJ Open 3 (4) (2013).

[84] P. Gallien, G. Amarenco, N. Benoit, V. Bonniaud, C. Donzé, J. Kerdraon, et al., Cranberry versus placebo in the prevention of urinary infections in multiple sclerosis: a multicenter, randomized, placebo-controlled, double-blind trial, Mult. Scler. J. 20 (9) (2014) 1252–1259.

[85] S.K. Malin, N. Cotugna, C.-S. Fang, Effect of creatine supplementation on muscle capacity in individuals with multiple sclerosis, J. Diet Suppl. 5 (1) (2008) 20–32.
[86] M.J. Drake, L. Canham, N. Cotterill, D. Delgado, J. Homewood, K. Inglis, et al., Results of a randomized, double blind, placebo controlled, crossover trial of melatonin for treatment of Nocturia in adults with multiple sclerosis (MeNiMS), BMC Neurol. 18 (1) (2018) 107.
[87] S. Bitarafan, Z. Mohammadpour, S. Jafarirad, M.-H. Harirchian, M.S. Yekaninejad, A.A. Saboor-Yaraghi, The effect of retinyl-palmitate on the level of pro and anti-inflammatory cytokines in multiple sclerosis patients: a randomized double blind clinical trial, Clin. Neurol. Neurosurg. 177 (2019) 101–105.
[88] S. Dolati, M. Ahmadi, L. Aghebti-Maleki, A. Nikmaram, F. Marofi, R. Rikhtegar, et al., Nanocurcumin is a potential novel therapy for multiple sclerosis by influencing inflammatory mediators, Pharmacol. Rep. 70 (6) (2018) 1158–1167.
[89] M. Khallli, G. Eskandari, M. Ghajarzadeh, A. Azimi, S. Eghtesadi, M. Sahraian, et al., Lipoic acid and multiple sclerosis: a randomized controlled conical trial, Curr. Top Nutraceutical Res. 10 (2012) 95–100.
[90] R. Spain, K. Powers, C. Murchison, E. Heriza, K. Winges, V. Yadav, et al., Lipoic acid in secondary progressive MS: a randomized controlled pilot trial, Neurol. Neuroinflam. 4 (5) (2017).
[91] M. Khalili, S. Eghtesadi, A. Mirshafiey, G. Eskandari, M. Sanoobar, M.A. Sahraian, et al., Effect of lipoic acid consumption on oxidative stress among multiple sclerosis patients: a randomized controlled clinical trial, Nutr. Neurosci. 17 (1) (2014) 16–20.
[92] M. Khalili, A. Azimi, V. Izadi, S. Eghtesadi, A. Mirshafiey, M.A. Sahraian, et al., Does lipoic acid consumption affect the cytokine profile in multiple sclerosis patients: a double-blind, placebo-controlled, randomized clinical trial, Neuroimmunomodulation 21 (6) (2014) 291–296.
[93] V. Yadav, G. Marracci, J. Lovera, W. Woodward, K. Bogardus, W. Marquardt, et al., Lipoic acid in multiple sclerosis: a pilot study, Mult. Scler. J. 11 (2) (2005) 159–165.
[94] E. Mauriz, D. Vallejo, M.J. Tuñón, J.M. Rodriguez-López, R. Rodríguez-Pérez, J. Sanz-Gómez, et al., Effects of dietary supplementation with lemon verbena extracts on serum inflammatory markers of multiple sclerosis patients, Nutr. Hosp. 31 (2) (2015) 764–771.
[95] M. Morshedi, R. Hashemi, S. Moazzen, A. Sahebkar, E.-S. Hosseinifard, Immunomodulatory and anti-inflammatory effects of probiotics in multiple sclerosis: a systematic review, J. Neuroinflammation 16 (1) (2019) 231.
[96] E. Kouchaki, O.R. Tamtaji, M. Salami, F. Bahmani, R.D. Kakhaki, E. Akbari, et al., Clinical and metabolic response to probiotic supplementation in patients with multiple sclerosis: a randomized, double-blind, placebo-controlled trial, Clin. Nutr. 36 (5) (2017) 1245–1249.
[97] J. Lovera, B. Bagert, K. Smoot, C.D. Morris, R. Frank, K. Bogardus, et al., Ginkgo biloba for the improvement of cognitive performance in multiple sclerosis: a randomized, placebo-controlled trial, Mult. Scler. J. 13 (3) (2007) 376–385.
[98] A. Tourbah, C. Lebrun-Frenay, G. Edan, M. Clanet, C. Papeix, S. Vukusic, et al., MD1003 (high-dose biotin) for the treatment of progressive multiple sclerosis: a randomised, double-blind, placebo-controlled study, Mult. Scler. J. 22 (13) (2016) 1719–1731.
[99] A. Tourbah, O. Gout, A. Vighetto, V. Deburghgraeve, J. Pelletier, C. Papeix, et al., MD1003 (high-dose pharmaceutical-grade biotin) for the treatment of chronic visual loss related to optic neuritis in multiple sclerosis: a randomized, double-blind, placebo-controlled study, CNS Drugs 32 (7) (2018) 661–672.
[100] L. Herden, R. Weissert, The Impact of coffee and caffeine on multiple sclerosis compared to other neurodegenerative diseases, Front. Nutr. 5 (2018) 133. Available from: https://pubmed.ncbi.nlm.nih.gov/30622948.

[101] E. Ciampi, R. Uribe-San-Martin, C. Cárcamo, J.P. Cruz, A. Reyes, D. Reyes, et al., Efficacy of andrographolide in not active progressive multiple sclerosis: a prospective exploratory double-blind, parallel-group, randomized, placebo-controlled trial, BMC Neurol. 20 (2020) 1–10.

[102] T. Müller, L. Lohse, A. Blodau, K. Frommholz, Vitamin D rise enhances blood perfusion in patients with multiple sclerosis, J. Neural Transm. 126 (12) (2019) 1631–1636.

[103] M. Berezowska, S. Coe, H. Dawes, Effectiveness of vitamin D supplementation in the management of multiple sclerosis: a systematic review, Int. J. Mol. Sci. 20 (6) (2019).

[104] S.A. Atkinson, J.C. Fleet, Canadian recommendations for vitamin D intake for persons affected by multiple sclerosis, J. Steroid Biochem. Mol. Biol. 199 (2020), 105606.

[105] M.C. Kiernan, S. Vucic, B.C. Cheah, M.R. Turner, A. Eisen, O. Hardiman, et al., Amyotrophic lateral sclerosis, Lancet (London, England) 377 (9769) (2011) 942–955.

[106] T. Filippini, M. Fiore, M. Tesauro, C. Malagoli, M. Consonni, F. Violi, et al., Clinical and lifestyle factors and risk of amyotrophic lateral sclerosis: a population-based case-control study, Int. J. Environ. Res. Public Health 17 (3) (2020).

[107] K.C. Fitzgerald, É.J. O'Reilly, G.J. Falcone, M.L. McCullough, Y. Park, L.N. Kolonel, et al., Dietary ω-3 polyunsaturated fatty acid intake and risk for amyotrophic lateral sclerosis, JAMA Neurol. 71 (9) (2014) 1102–1110.

[108] J. Petimar, É. O'Reilly, H.-O. Adami, P.A. van den Brandt, J. Buring, D.R. English, et al., Coffee, tea, and caffeine intake and amyotrophic lateral sclerosis mortality in a pooled analysis of eight prospective cohort studies, Eur. J. Neurol. 26 (3) (2019) 468–475. Available from: https://doi.org/10.1111/ene.13840.

[109] L. Mazzini, L. Mogna, F. De Marchi, A. Amoruso, M. Pane, I. Aloisio, et al., Potential role of gut microbiota in ALS pathogenesis and possible novel therapeutic strategies, J. Clin. Gastroenterol. 52 (Suppl 1) (2018) S68–S70.

[110] M. Wang, Z. Liu, W. Sun, Y. Yuan, B. Jiao, X. Zhang, et al., Association between vitamins and amyotrophic lateral sclerosis: a center-based survey in mainland china, Front. Neurol. 11 (2020) 488. Available from: https://pubmed.ncbi.nlm.nih.gov/32625160.

[111] D. Michal Freedman, R.W. Kuncl, S.J. Weinstein, N. Malila, J. Virtamo, D. Albanes, Vitamin E serum levels and controlled supplementation and risk of amyotrophic lateral sclerosis, Amyotroph. Lateral Scler. Frontotemporal Degener. 14 (4) (2013) 246–251.

[112] S. Paganoni, E.A. Macklin, C. Karam, H. Yu, F. Gonterman, K.A. Fetterman, et al., Vitamin D levels are associated with gross motor function in amyotrophic lateral sclerosis, Muscle Nerve 56 (4) (2017) 726–731.

[113] K.v.q. Long, N. LTH, Roles of vitamin D in amyotrophic lateral sclerosis: possible genetic and cellular signaling mechanisms, Mol. Brain 6 (2013) 16. Available from: https://pubmed.ncbi.nlm.nih.gov/23570271.

[114] A. Gianforcaro, M.J. Hamadeh, Vitamin D as a potential therapy in amyotrophic lateral sclerosis, CNS Neurosci. Ther. 20 (2) (2014) 101–111.

[115] R. Juntas-Morales, N. Pageot, A. Bendarraz, S. Alphandéry, F. Sedel, S. Seigle, et al., High-dose pharmaceutical grade biotin (MD1003) in amyotrophic lateral sclerosis: a pilot study, EClinicalMedicine 19 (2020), 100254. Available from: https://pubmed.ncbi.nlm.nih.gov/32140672.

[116] L. Chico, E.C. Ienco, C. Bisordi, A. Lo Gerfo, L. Petrozzi, A. Petrucci, et al., Amyotrophic lateral sclerosis and oxidative stress: a double-blind therapeutic trial after curcumin supplementation, CNS Neurol. Disord. Drug Targets 17 (10) (2018) 767–779.

[117] T. Meyer, A. Funke, C. Münch, D. Kettemann, A. Maier, B. Walter, et al., Real world experience of patients with amyotrophic lateral sclerosis (ALS) in the treatment of spasticity using tetrahydrocannabinol:cannabidiol (THC:CBD), BMC Neurol. 19 (1) (2019) 222. Available from: https://pubmed.ncbi.nlm.nih.gov/31493784.

[118] R. Kaji, T. Imai, Y. Iwasaki, K. Okamoto, M. Nakagawa, Y. Ohashi, et al., Ultra-high-dose methylcobalamin in amyotrophic lateral sclerosis: a long-term phase II/III randomised controlled study, J. Neurol. Neurosurg. Psychiatry 90 (4) (2019) 451–457.

[119] M.A. Qamar, A. Sauerbier, M. Politis, H. Carr, P. Loehrer, K.R. Chaudhuri, Presynaptic dopaminergic terminal imaging and non-motor symptoms assessment of Parkinson's disease: evidence for dopaminergic basis? npj Park Dis. 3 (1) (2017) 1–20.
[120] F. Magrinelli, A. Picelli, P. Tocco, A. Federico, L. Roncari, N. Smania, et al., Pathophysiology of motor dysfunction in Parkinson's disease as the rationale for drug treatment and rehabilitation, Parkinsons Dis. 2016 (2016).
[121] A. Ascherio, M.A. Schwarzschild, The epidemiology of Parkinson's disease: risk factors and prevention, Lancet Neurol. 15 (12) (2016) 1257–1272.
[122] G. Bjørklund, M. Dadar, G. Anderson, S. Chirumbolo, M. Maes, Preventive treatments to slow substantia nigra damage and Parkinson's disease progression: a critical perspective review, Pharmacol. Res. 161 (2020), 105065.
[123] K.C. Hughes, X. Gao, I.Y. Kim, E.B. Rimm, M. Wang, M.G. Weisskopf, et al., Intake of antioxidant vitamins and risk of Parkinson's disease, Mov. Disord. 31 (12) (2016) 1909–1914.
[124] C.C. Ferguson, L.L. Knol, A. Halli-Tierney, A.C. Ellis, Dietary supplement use is high among individuals with Parkinson disease, South. Med. J. 112 (12) (2019) 621–625.
[125] L.K. Mischley, R.C. Lau, R.D. Bennett, Role of diet and nutritional supplements in Parkinson's disease progression, Oxidative Med. Cell. Longev. 2017 (2017), 6405278.
[126] J.F. Chen, K. Xu, J.P. Petzer, R. Staal, Y.H. Xu, M. Beilstein, et al., Neuroprotection by caffeine and A(2A) adenosine receptor inactivation in a model of Parkinson's disease, J. Neurosci. 21 (10) (2001) RC143.
[127] X. Chen, X. Lan, I. Roche, R. Liu, J.D. Geiger, Caffeine protects against MPTP-induced blood-brain barrier dysfunction in mouse striatum, J. Neurochem. 107 (4) (2008) 1147–1157.
[128] K.C. Teo, S.-L. Ho, Monoamine oxidase-B (MAO-B) inhibitors: implications for disease-modification in Parkinson's disease, Transl. Neurodegener. 2 (1) (2013) 19.
[129] S. Borzabadi, S. Oryan, A. Eidi, E. Aghadavod, R. Daneshvar Kakhaki, O.R. Tamtaji, et al., The Effects of probiotic supplementation on gene expression related to inflammation, insulin and lipid in patients with Parkinson's disease: a randomized, double-blind, Arch. Iran. Med. 21 (7) (2018) 289–295.
[130] O.R. Tamtaji, M. Taghizadeh, R. Daneshvar Kakhaki, E. Kouchaki, F. Bahmani, S. Borzabadi, et al., Clinical and metabolic response to probiotic administration in people with Parkinson's disease: a randomized, double-blind, placebo-controlled trial, Clin. Nutr. 38 (3) (2019) 1031–1035.
[131] T. Van Laar, J.M. Boertien, A.H. Herranz, Faecal transplantation, pro- and prebiotics in Parkinson's disease; hope or hype? J. Parkinsons Dis. 9 (s2) (2019) S371–S379.
[132] M. Barichella, C. Pacchetti, C. Bolliri, E. Cassani, L. Iorio, C. Pusani, et al., Probiotics and prebiotic fiber for constipation associated with Parkinson disease: an RCT, Neurology 87 (12) (2016) 1274–1280.
[133] M. Taghizadeh, O.R. Tamtaji, E. Dadgostar, R. Daneshvar Kakhaki, F. Bahmani, J. Abolhassani, et al., The effects of omega-3 fatty acids and vitamin E co-supplementation on clinical and metabolic status in patients with Parkinson's disease: a randomized, double-blind, placebo-controlled trial, Neurochem. Int. 108 (2017) 183–189.
[134] C. Wakade, B. Giri, A. Malik, H. Khodadadi, J.C. Morgan, R.K. Chong, et al., Niacin modulates macrophage polarization in Parkinson's disease, J. Neuroimmunol. 320 (2018) 76–79.
[135] B. Giri, K. Belanger, M. Seamon, E. Bradley, S. Purohit, R. Chong, et al., Niacin ameliorates neuro-inflammation in Parkinson's disease via GPR109A, Int. J. Mol. Sci. 20 (18) (2019).
[136] M.F. McCarty, A. Lerner, Nutraceuticals targeting generation and oxidant activity of peroxynitrite may aid prevention and control of Parkinson's disease, Int. J. Mol. Sci. 21 (10) (2020).

[137] L.A. Barboza, N.C. Ghisi, Evaluating the current state of the art of Huntington disease research: a scientometric analysis, Braz. J. Med. Biol. Res. 51 (3) (2018) e6299.

[138] R.R. Handley, S.J. Reid, S. Patassini, S.R. Rudiger, V. Obolonkin, C.J. McLaughlan, et al., Metabolic disruption identified in the Huntington's disease transgenic sheep model, Sci. Rep. 6 (2016) 20681.

[139] M. Yu, D. Bega, A review of the clinical evidence for complementary and alternative medicine in Huntington's disease, Tremor Other Hyperkinet. Mov. (N Y) 9 (2019), https://doi.org/10.7916/tohm.v0.678. Available from: https://pubmed.ncbi.nlm.nih.gov/31523487.

[140] A. Agnihotri, O.I. Aruoma, Alzheimer's disease and Parkinson's disease: a nutritional toxicology perspective of the impact of oxidative stress, mitochondrial dysfunction, nutrigenomics and environmental chemicals, J. Am. Coll. Nutr. 39 (1) (2020) 16–27.

[141] V.P. Dadhania, P.P. Trivedi, A. Vikram, D.N. Tripathi, Nutraceuticals against neurodegeneration: a mechanistic insight, Curr. Neuropharmacol. 14 (6) (2016) 627–640.

[142] R. Sandhir, A. Mehrotra, Quercetin supplementation is effective in improving mitochondrial dysfunctions induced by 3-nitropropionic acid: implications in Huntington's disease, Biochim. Biophys. Acta 1832 (3) (2013) 421–430.

[143] I.M. Adanyeguh, D. Rinaldi, P.-G. Henry, S. Caillet, R. Valabregue, A. Durr, et al., Triheptanoin improves brain energy metabolism in patients with Huntington disease, Neurology 84 (5) (2015) 490–495.

[144] G.P. Littarru, L. Tiano, Bioenergetic and antioxidant properties of coenzyme Q 10: recent developments, Mol. Biotechnol. 37 (1) (2007) 31–37.

[145] A. McGarry, M. McDermott, K. Kieburtz, E.A. de Blieck, F. Beal, K. Marder, et al., A randomized, double-blind, placebo-controlled trial of coenzyme Q10 in Huntington disease, Neurology 88 (2) (2017) 152–159.

[146] S.M. Hersch, G. Schifitto, D. Oakes, A.-L. Bredlau, C.M. Meyers, R. Nahin, et al., The CREST-E study of creatine for Huntington disease: a randomized controlled trial, Neurology 89 (6) (2017) 594–601.

[147] F. Labanca, H. Ullah, H. Khan, L. Milella, J. Xiao, Z. Dajic-Stevanovic, et al., Therapeutic and mechanistic effects of curcumin in Huntington's disease, Curr. Neuropharmacol. 19 (2020).

[148] J.J. Ferreira, A. Rosser, D. Craufurd, F. Squitieri, B.L. Nicholas Mallard, Randomized controlled trial of ethyl-eicosapentaenoic acid in Huntington disease: the TREND-HD study, Arch. Neurol. 65 (12) (2008) 1582–1589.

[149] B.K. Puri, G.M. Bydder, S.J. Counsell, B.J. Corridan, A.J. Richardson, J.V. Hajnal, et al., MRI and neuropsychological improvement in Huntington disease following ethyl-EPA treatment, Neuroreport 13 (1) (2002) 123–126.

[150] M. Cuturic, R.K. Abramson, R.R. Moran, J.W. Hardin, E.M. Frank, A.A. Sellers, Serum carnitine levels and levocarnitine supplementation in institutionalized Huntington's disease patients, Neurol. Sci. 34 (1) (2013) 93–98.

[151] S. Patassini, P. Begley, J. Xu, S.J. Church, N. Kureishy, S.J. Reid, et al., Cerebral vitamin B5 (D-pantothenic acid) deficiency as a potential cause of metabolic perturbation and neurodegeneration in Huntington's disease, Metabolites 9 (6) (2019).

[152] B. Soong, R. Liu, L. Wu, Y. Lu, H. Lee, Metabolic characterization of spinocerebellar ataxia type 6, Arch. Neurol. 58 (2) (2001) 300–304.

[153] J.L. Griffin, C.K. Cemal, M.A. Pook, Defining a metabolic phenotype in the brain of a transgenic mouse model of spinocerebellar ataxia 3, Physiol. Genomics 16 (3) (2004) 334–340.

[154] F. Palau, C. Espinós, Autosomal recessive cerebellar ataxias, Orphanet. J. Rare Dis. 1 (2006) 47.

[155] M. Pandolfo, Friedreich ataxia, in: Rosenberg's Molecular and Genetic Basis of Neurological and Psychiatric Disease, Elsevier, 2020, pp. 99–112.

[156] A. Bolotta, A. Pini, P.M. Abruzzo, A. Ghezzo, A. Modesti, T. Gamberi, et al., Effects of tocotrienol supplementation in Friedreich's ataxia: a model of oxidative stress pathology, Exp. Biol. Med. (Maywood) 245 (3) (2020) 201–212.

[157] P.M. Abruzzo, M. Marini, A. Bolotta, G. Malisardi, S. Manfredini, A. Ghezzo, et al., Frataxin mRNA isoforms in FRDA patients and normal subjects: effect of tocotrienol supplementation, Biomed. Res. Int. 2013 (2013), 276808.

[158] I. Di Donato, S. Bianchi, A. Federico, Ataxia with vitamin E deficiency: update of molecular diagnosis, Neurol. Sci. 31 (4) (2010) 511–515.

[159] L. Velázquez-Pérez, J. Rodríguez-Chanfrau, J.C. García-Rodríguez, G. Sánchez-Cruz, R. Aguilera-Rodríguez, R. Rodríguez-Labrada, et al., Oral zinc sulphate supplementation for six months in SCA2 patients: a randomized, double-blind, placebo-controlled trial, Neurochem. Res. 36 (10) (2011) 1793–1800.

[160] R.Y. Lo, K.P. Figueroa, S.M. Pulst, C.-Y. Lin, S. Perlman, G. Wilmot, et al., Coenzyme Q10 and spinocerebellar ataxias, Mov. Disord. 30 (2) (2015) 214–220.

[161] R. Artuch, G. Brea-Calvo, P. Briones, A. Aracil, M. Galván, C. Espinós, et al., Cerebellar ataxia with coenzyme Q10 deficiency: diagnosis and follow-up after coenzyme Q10 supplementation, J. Neurol. Sci. 246 (1–2) (2006) 153–158.

[162] M. Furtado, M.A. Katzman, Neuroinflammatory pathways in anxiety, posttraumatic stress, and obsessive compulsive disorders, Psychiatry Res. 229 (1–2) (2015) 37–48.

[163] A.N. Kaczkurkin, T.M. Moore, M.E. Calkins, R. Ciric, J.A. Detre, M.A. Elliott, et al., Common and dissociable regional cerebral blood flow differences associate with dimensions of psychopathology across categorical diagnoses, Mol. Psychiatry 23 (10) (2018) 1981–1989.

[164] L.M. Jenkins, A. Barba, M. Campbell, M. Lamar, S.A. Shankman, A.D. Leow, et al., Shared white matter alterations across emotional disorders: a voxel-based meta-analysis of fractional anisotropy, NeuroImage Clin. 12 (2016) 1022–1034.

[165] M. Chiappedi, S. de Vincenzi, M. Bejor, Nutraceuticals in psychiatric practice, Rec. Pat. CNS Drug Discov. 7 (2) (2012) 163–172.

[166] K.P. van der Burg, L. Cribb, J. Firth, D. Karmacoska, J. Sarris, Nutrient and genetic biomarkers of nutraceutical treatment response in mood and psychotic disorders: a systematic review, Nutr. Neurosci. 1–17 (2019).

[167] M. Omidian, M. Mahmoudi, M. Abshirini, M.R. Eshraghian, M.H. Javanbakht, M. Zarei, et al., Effects of vitamin D supplementation on depressive symptoms in type 2 diabetes mellitus patients: randomized placebo-controlled double-blind clinical trial, Diabetes Metab. Syndr. 13 (4) (2019) 2375–2380.

[168] M.S. Trudeau, R.F. Madden, J.A. Parnell, G.W. Ben, J. Shearer, Dietary and supplement-based complementary and alternative medicine use in pediatric autism spectrum disorder, Nutrients 11 (8) (2019).

[169] D. Fraguas, C.M. Díaz-Caneja, L. Pina-Camacho, C. Moreno, M. Durán-Cutilla, M. Ayora, et al., Dietary interventions for autism spectrum disorder: a meta-analysis, Pediatrics 144 (5) (2019).

[170] R.G. Lande, Nutraceutical augmentation strategies for depression: a narrative review, J. Am. Osteopath. Assoc. 120 (2) (2020) 100–106.

[171] L. Jahangard, F. Yasrebifar, M. Haghighi, A. Ranjbar, M. Mehrpooya, Influence of adjuvant Coenzyme Q10 on inflammatory and oxidative stress biomarkers in patients with bipolar disorders during the depressive episode, Mol. Biol. Rep. 46 (5) (2019) 5333–5343.

[172] M. Mehrpooya, F. Yasrebifar, M. Haghighi, Y. Mohammadi, L. Jahangard, Evaluating the effect of coenzyme Q10 augmentation on treatment of bipolar depression: a double-blind controlled clinical trial, J. Clin. Psychopharmacol. 38 (5) (2018) 460–466.

[173] K.K. Goh, Y.-W. Liu, P.-H. Kuo, Y.-C.E. Chung, M.-L. Lu, C.-H. Chen, Effect of probiotics on depressive symptoms: a meta-analysis of human studies, Psychiatry Res. 282 (2019), 112568.

[174] K. Nishida, D. Sawada, Y. Kuwano, H. Tanaka, K. Rokutan, Health benefits of Lactobacillus gasseri CP2305 tablets in young adults exposed to chronic stress: a randomized, double-blind, placebo-controlled study, Nutrients 11 (8) (2019).
[175] E. Stefańska, A. Wendołowicz, M. Lech, B. Konarzewska, J. Zapolska, N. Waszkiewicz, et al., Does the usual dietary intake of schizophrenia patients require supplementation with vitamins and minerals? Psychiatr. Pol. 53 (3) (2019) 599–612.
[176] J. Firth, S.B. Teasdale, K. Allott, D. Siskind, W. Marx, J. Cotter, et al., The efficacy and safety of nutrient supplements in the treatment of mental disorders: a meta-review of meta-analyses of randomized controlled trials, World Psychiatry 18 (3) (2019) 308–324.
[177] M. Heinrich, P. Bremner, Ethnobotany and ethnopharmacy—their role for anticancer drug development, Curr. Drug Targets 7 (3) (2006) 239–245.
[178] M. Heinrich, S. Gibbons, Ethnopharmacology in drug discovery: an analysis of its role and potential contribution, J. Pharm. Pharmacol. 53 (4) (2001) 425–432.
[179] H.P.D. Fogang, F. Maggi, L.A. Tapondjou, H.M. Womeni, F. Papa, L. Quassinti, et al., In vitro biological activities of seed essential oils from the cameroonian spices afrostyrax lepidophyllus mildbr. and scorodophloeus zenkeri harms rich in sulfur-containing compounds, Chem. Biodivers. 11 (1) (2014) 161–169.
[180] B. Bayala, I.H.N. Bassole, C. Gnoula, R. Nebie, A. Yonli, L. Morel, et al., Chemical composition, antioxidant, anti-inflammatory and anti-proliferative activities of essential oils of plants from Burkina Faso, PLoS One 9 (3) (2014) 1–11.
[181] N. Robson, L. Quassinti, G. Lupidi, F. Maggi, Antioxidant and antiproliferative activity of Hypericum hircinum L. subsp majus (Aiton) N. Robson essential oil, Nat. Prod. Res. (2013) 37–41.
[182] C.B. Detoni, D.M. De Oliveira, I.E. Santo, A.S. Pedro, R. El-Bacha, V.E. Da Silva, et al., Evaluation of thermal-oxidative stability and antiglioma activity of Zanthoxylum tingoassuiba essential oil entrapped into multi- and unilamellar liposomes, J. Liposome Res. 22 (1) (2012) 1–7.
[183] A. Desai, T. Vyas, M. Amiji, Cytotoxicity and apoptosis enhancement in brain tumor cells upon coadministration of paclitaxel and ceramide in nanoemulsion formulations, J. Pharm. Sci. 97 (7) (2008) 2745–2756.
[184] D.P. Bezerra, J.D.B. Marinho Filho, A.P.N.N. Alves, C. Pessoa, M.O. De Moraes, O.D.L. Pessoa, et al., Antitumor activity of the essential oil from the leaves of Croton regelianus and its component ascaridole, Chem. Biodivers. 6 (8) (2009) 1224–1231.
[185] Y.C. Lin, C.M. Hung, J.C. Tsai, J.C. Lee, Y.L.S. Chen, C.W. Wei, et al., Hispidulin potently inhibits human glioblastoma multiforme cells through activation of AMP-activated protein kinase (AMPK), J. Agric. Food Chem. 58 (17) (2010) 9511–9517.
[186] J. Fernandes, C.O. Da Fonseca, A. Teixeira, C.R. Gattass, Perillyl alcohol induces apoptosis in human glioblastoma multiforme cells, Oncol. Rep. 13 (5) (2005) 943–947.
[187] C.O. Da Fonseca, M. Simão, I.R. Lins, R.O. Caetano, D. Futuro, T. Quirico-Santos, Efficacy of monoterpene perillyl alcohol upon survival rate of patients with recurrent glioblastoma, J. Cancer Res. Clin. Oncol. 137 (2) (2011) 287–293.
[188] I. Teruszkin Balassiano, S. Alves de Paulo, N. Henriques Silva, M. Curié Cabral, D. Gibaldi, M. Bozza, et al., Effects of perillyl alcohol in glial C6 cell line in vitro and anti-metastatic activity in chorioallantoic membrane model, Int. J. Mol. Med. 10 (6) (2002) 785–788.
[189] C.O.P. da Fonseca, Effects of in vitro and in vivo treatment of monoterpene perillyl alcohol on proliferation and gene expression control of high grade gliomas, Arq. Neuropsiquiatr. 62 (4) (2004) 1117–1118.
[190] H.Y. Cho, W. Wang, N. Jhaveri, S. Torres, J. Tseng, M.N. Leong, et al., Perillyl alcohol for the treatment of temozolomide-resistant gliomas, Mol. Cancer Ther. 11 (11) (2012) 2462–2472.

[191] W.L. Chen, A. Barszczyk, E. Turlova, M. Deurloo, B. Liu, B.B. Yang, et al., Inhibition of TRPM7 by carvacrol suppresses glioblastoma cell proliferation, migration and invasion, Oncotarget 6 (18) (2015) 16321–16340.
[192] G. Musumeci, G. Magro, V. Cardile, M. Coco, R. Marzagalli, P. Castrogiovanni, et al., Characterization of matrix metalloproteinase-2 and -9, ADAM-10 and N-cadherin expression in human glioblastoma multiforme, Cell Tissue Res. 362 (1) (2015) 45–60.
[193] S.S. Ambegaokar, L. Wu, K. Alamshahi, J. Lau, L. Jazayeri, S. Chan, et al., Curcumin inhibits dose-dependently and time-dependently neuroglial cell proliferation and growth, Neuroendocrinol. Lett. 24 (6) (2003) 469–473.
[194] P.M. Luthra, R. Kumar, A. Prakash, Demethoxycurcumin induces Bcl-2 mediated G2/M arrest and apoptosis in human glioma U87 cells, Biochem. Biophys. Res. Commun. 384 (4) (2009) 420–425.
[195] M.C. Perry, M. Demeule, A. Régina, R. Moumdjian, R. Béliveau, Curcumin inhibits tumor growth and angiogenesis in glioblastoma xenografts, Mol. Nutr. Food Res. 54 (8) (2010) 1192–1201.
[196] P. Langone, P.R. Debata, J.D.R. Inigo, S. Dolai, S. Mukherjee, P. Halat, et al., Coupling to a glioblastoma-directed antibody potentiates antitumor activity of curcumin, Int. J. Cancer 135 (3) (2014) 710–719.
[197] H. Pérez, D. de la Ossa, M. Lorente, M.E. Gil-Alegre, S. Torres, E. García-Taboada, M.R. del Aberturas, et al., Local delivery of cannabinoid-loaded microparticles inhibits tumor growth in a murine xenograft model of glioblastoma multiforme, PLoS One 8 (1) (2013) 2–9.
[198] S. Torres, M. Lorente, F. Rodríguez-Fornés, S. Hernández-Tiedra, M. Salazar, E. García-Taboada, et al., A combined preclinical therapy of cannabinoids and temozolomide against glioma, Mol. Cancer Ther. 10 (1) (2011) 90–103.
[199] M. Solinas, P. Massi, V. Cinquina, M. Valenti, D. Bolognini, M. Gariboldi, et al., Cannabidiol, a non-psychoactive cannabinoid compound, inhibits proliferation and invasion in U87-MG and T98G glioma cells through a multitarget effect, PLoS One 8 (10) (2013).
[200] G. Wang, F. Dai, K. Yu, Z. Jia, A. Zhang, Q. Huang, et al., Resveratrol inhibits glioma cell growth via targeting oncogenic microRNAs and multiple signaling pathways, Int. J. Oncol. 46 (4) (2015) 1739–1747.
[201] Y. Jiao, H. Li, Y. Liu, A. Guo, X. Xu, X. Qu, et al., Resveratrol inhibits the invasion of glioblastoma-initiating cells via down-regulation of the PI3K/Akt/NF-κB signaling pathway, Nutrients 7 (6) (2015) 4383–4402.
[202] A. Kermanizadeh, K. Jantzen, M.B. Ward, J.A. Durhuus, L. Juel Rasmussen, S. Loft, et al., Nanomaterial-induced cell death in pulmonary and hepatic cells following exposure to three different metallic materials: the role of autophagy and apoptosis, Nanotoxicology 11 (2) (2017) 184–200.
[203] M. Chakrabarti, S.K. Ray, Anti-tumor activities of luteolin and silibinin in glioblastoma cells: overexpression of miR-7-1-3p augmented luteolin and silibinin to inhibit autophagy and induce apoptosis in glioblastoma in vivo, Apoptosis 21 (3) (2016) 312–328.
[204] J.C. Chen, Y. Chen, J.H. Lin, J.M. Wu, S.H. Tseng, Resveratrol suppresses angiogenesis in gliomas: evaluation by color Doppler ultrasound, Anticancer Res. 26 (2A) (2006) 1237–1245.
[205] P. Massi, M. Valenti, A. Vaccani, V. Gasperi, G. Perletti, E. Marras, et al., 5-Lipoxygenase and anandamide hydrolase (FAAH) mediate the antitumor activity of cannabidiol, a non-psychoactive cannabinoid, J. Neurochem. 104 (4) (2008) 1091–1100.
[206] F. Limanaqi, F. Biagioni, C.L. Busceti, L. Ryskalin, M. Polzella, A. Frati, et al., Phytochemicals bridging autophagy induction and alpha-synuclein degradation in parkinsonism, Int. J. Mol. Sci. 20 (13) (2019) 3274.

[207] M. Hatami, M. Abdolahi, N. Soveyd, M. Djalali, M. Togha, N.M. Honarvar, Molecular mechanisms of curcumin in neuroinflammatory disorders: a mini review of current evidences, Endocr. Metab. Disord. 19 (3) (2019) 247–258.
[208] H.-F. Chiu, K. Venkatakrishnan, C.-K. Wang, The role of nutraceuticals as a complementary therapy against various neurodegenerative diseases: a mini-review, J. Tradit. Complement. Med. 10 (5) (2020) 434–439. Available from: https://www.sciencedirect.com/science/article/pii/S2225411020301425.
[209] M. Maes, A.P. Kallaur, J. Lopes, S.R. Oliveira, D. Ramon, E.M.V. Reiche, Immune-inflammatory and oxidative and nitrosative stress (IO & NS) pathways in depression and multiple sclerosis (MS): shared IO & NS pathways but less hyper-acute neuro-inflammation explain the increased incidence of depression in MS, Neurol. Psychiatry Brain Res. 1 (22) (2016) 16–17.
[210] F.M. Gutierrez-Mariscal, E.M. Yubero-Serrano, J.M. Villalba, J. Lopez-Miranda, Co-enzyme Q10: From bench to clinic in aging diseases, a translational review, Crit. Rev. Food Sci. Nutr. 59 (14) (2019) 2240–2257.
[211] X. Yang, Y. Zhang, H. Xu, X. Luo, J. Yu, J. Liu, et al., Neuroprotection of coenzyme Q10 in neurodegenerative diseases, Curr. Top. Med. Chem. 16 (8) (2016) 858–866.
[212] C. Moussa, M. Hebron, X. Huang, J. Ahn, R.A. Rissman, P.S. Aisen, et al., Resveratrol regulates neuro-inflammation and induces adaptive immunity in Alzheimer's disease, J. Neuroinflammation 14 (1) (2017) 1.
[213] Y. Wu, X. Li, J.X. Zhu, W. Xie, W. Le, Z. Fan, et al., Resveratrol-activated AMPK/SIRT1/autophagy in cellular models of Parkinson's disease, Neurosignals 19 (3) (2011) 163–174.
[214] B.A.Q. Gomes, J.P.B. Silva, C.F.R. Romeiro, S.M. Dos Santos, C.A. Rodrigues, P.R. Gonçalves, et al., Neuroprotective mechanisms of resveratrol in Alzheimer's disease: role of SIRT1, Oxidative Med. Cell. Longev. 2018 (2018).
[215] R. Avallone, G. Vitale, M. Bertolotti, Omega-3 fatty acids and neurodegenerative diseases: new evidence in clinical trials, Int. J. Mol. Sci. 20 (17) (2019) 4256.
[216] G.P. Eckert, U. Lipka, W.E. Muller, Omega-3 fatty acids in neurodegenerative diseases: focus on mitochondria, Prostaglandins Leukot. Essent. Fat. Acids 88 (1) (2013) 105–114.

CHAPTER 6

Phytonutrients in the management of glucose metabolism

Hammad Ullah[a] **and Maria Daglia**[a,b]
[a]Department of Pharmacy, School of Medicine and Surgery, University of Naples Federico II, Naples, Italy
[b]International Research Center for Food Nutrition and Safety, Jiangsu University, Zhenjiang, China

1. Introduction

Energy is required by cells to perform and maintain normal physiological functions, with the brain and blood cells only using glucose to produce this energy, unlike other cells which utilize glucose, proteins, and fats. Glucose is mainly stored as glycogen in the liver, which can be converted to glucose molecules in response to hypoglycemia. Glucose can also be produced from noncarbohydrate sources such as amino acids, pyruvate, lactic acid, and glycerol, through a process known as gluconeogenesis. Insulin, glucagon, amylin, glucagon-like peptide-1 (*GLP-1*), glucose-dependent insulinotropic peptide (GIP), growth hormone, cortisol, and epinephrine are glucoregulatory hormones maintaining a balance in the blood glucose concentration, keeping it within a narrow range. In a bi-hormonal model, insulin and glucagon are the two major hormones responsible for glucose disappearance and glucose appearance, respectively.

Insulin, also known as an anabolic hormone, is secreted by pancreatic β-cells and regulates the metabolism of carbohydrates, proteins, and fats by enhancing the uptake of glucose the from blood into the liver, adipose tissues, and skeletal muscles, where the glucose molecules may be converted either into glycogen via glycogenesis, or triglycerides via lipogenesis. Increased circulating levels of insulin in the blood decrease hepatic glucose production and secretion. As β-cells are sensitive to blood glucose concentration, they secrete insulin in response to high blood glucose concentration, which tends to increase the absorption of glucose by insulin-dependent tissues or may directly suppress endogenous glucose production. Glucose stimulates insulin secretion by triggering and amplifying signals in β-cells, which involves several sequential events including entry of glucose into β-cells,

https://doi.org/10.1016/B978-0-12-824356-5.00011-4

oxidative glycolysis, increase in ATP-to-ADP ratio, closure of K_{ATP} channels (ATP-sensitive K^+ channels), membrane depolarization, opening of voltage gated Ca^{2+} channels, Ca^{2+} influx, increase in cytoplasmic free Ca^{2+} concentration and stimulation of the exocytotic machinery [1].

In contrast, glucagon is the hormone secreted by α-cells in cases of low blood glucose, increasing blood glucose levels by stimulating hepatic glycogenolysis and gluconeogenesis. Glucagon can also decrease fatty acid synthesis and increase lipolysis in the liver and adipose tissues, which may lead to an enhanced release of fatty acids into circulation to generate energy in tissues like skeletal muscles. Other hormones of note include amylin, which suppresses postprandial glucose secretion and slows gastric emptying, GLP-1, which enhances glucose-dependent insulin secretion, suppresses postprandial glucose secretion, slows gastric emptying, and promotes β-cell health, and somatostatin, which inhibits the secretion of pancreatic hormones (insulin and glucagon) [2,3]. Neurotransmitters also possess glucoregulatory effects, such as adrenaline suppressing insulin secretion via α2-adrenergic receptors, while acetylcholine stimulates insulin secretion via activating M3 muscarinic receptors [3]. The metabolic imbalance triggered by chronic hyperglycemia and hyperlipidemia may result in the impairment of glucose-induced insulin secretion and eventually result in the development of diabetes mellitus (DM).

2. Diabetes mellitus

DM is a metabolic disease characterized by chronic hyperglycemia, resulting from a defect in insulin secretion, action, or both. Several mechanisms explain the pathogenesis of DM, including the destruction of pancreatic β-cells or factors associated with insulin resistance. Resistance in the activities of insulin may affect the metabolism of carbohydrates, proteins, and fats. Furthermore, in the majority of DM cases, impaired insulin secretion and insulin resistance may exist concomitantly, which may make it difficult to identify the primary cause of hyperglycemia. According to the World Health Organization, the incidence of DM is significantly increasing worldwide, with the number of diabetic people rising from 108 million in 1980 to 422 million in 2014 [4]. Persistent or chronic cases of DM can silently lead to serious complications such as autonomic neuropathy, peripheral neuropathy, nephropathy, atherosclerotic cardiovascular disease (CVD), retinopathy, peripheral arterial disease (PAD), cerebrovascular events, and increased susceptibility to infection. Fig. 1 has illustrated the risk factors for developing DM.

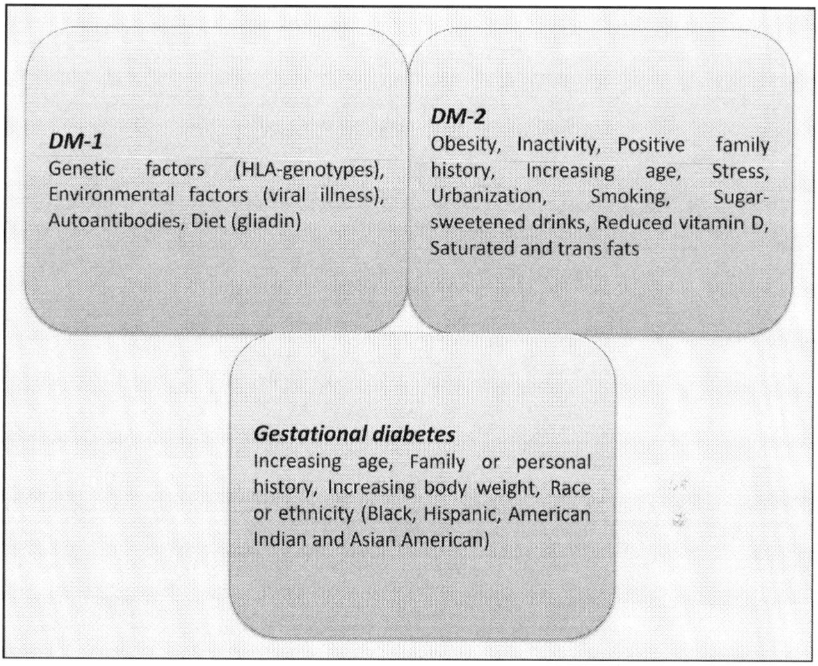

Fig. 1 Risk factors for developing Diabetes mellitus. Several factors are known to contribute to the pathogenesis of DM, like genetic factors, environmental factors, autoantibodies, dietary concerns, obesity, positive family history, old age, stress, sedentary lifestyle, and race or ethnicity.

2.1 Types of DM

The American Diabetes Association (ADA) has classified DM into four main types, comprising type 1 diabetes mellitus (DM1), type 2 diabetes mellitus (DM2), other specific types of diabetes, and gestational diabetes Table 1 [5].

2.1.1 Diabetes mellitus type 1

DM1 is characterized by insulin deficiency due to the loss of pancreatic β-cells and may be further classified into idiopathic and immune-mediated groups. The majority of cases of DM1 fall under immune-mediated diabetes, caused by T-cell-related autoimmunity, resulting in the progressive loss of insulin producing β-cells and ultimately in insulin deficiency. Its onset frequently appears in childhood, and thus may be referred to as juvenile diabetes. Moreover, insulin response and sensitivity usually remain normal, especially in the early stages of the disease [6]. The terms brittle diabetes or

Table 1 Classification of diabetes mellitus.

S. No.	DM class	Description
1	DM1	Idiopathic or autoimmune β-cell dysfunction and absolute insulin deficiency
2	DM2	Unknown etiology. Insulin resistance and/or relative insulin deficiency
3	Other specific types	Genetic defects in β-cell function MODY (Mutations in HNF-1, HNF-4, glucokinase and others). Genetic defects in insulin action. Pathologies of exocrine pancreas, Endocrinopathies (impaired insulin secretion or insulin resistance) Drug or chemical induced (glucocorticoids, thiazide diuretics, β-adrenergic agonists, protease inhibitors, atypical antipsychotics, and statins). Infections induced. Unknown forms of immune-mediated DM (antiinsulin receptor antibodies). Other genetic syndromes associated with DM such as Down syndrome
4	Gestational diabetes	Increased insulin resistance superimposed on β-cell dysfunction or loss

labile diabetes can also be used because of the occurrence of dramatic and recurrent swings in the blood glucose levels, though these terms have no biological basis [7,8]. A significant proportion of DM1 can also be diagnosed in adulthood, known as latent autoimmune diabetes of adults (LADA), with a slower onset compared to the same condition in children, and which might be misdiagnosed as DM2 based on the age rather than the cause [9]. Multiple genes, including HLA-genotypes, are known to influence the risk of diabetes, which is partly inherited in nature. Environmental factors like viral infections (cytomegalovirus, mumps, rubella, and rotavirus) or diet (gliadin, a protein present in gluten) can also trigger the pathogenesis of DM1 [10–13]. Patients with DM1 are more prone to the development of diabetic ketoacidosis, infections, impaired counter-regulatory responses to low blood sugar levels, gastroparesis, and endocrinopathies such as Addison's disease.

2.1.2 Diabetes mellitus type 2

DM2 is the most common type of diabetes, characterized by insulin resistance accompanied by reduced insulin secretion, especially at advanced stages of the disease. Most commonly, people show evidence of prediabetic symptoms, such as impaired fasting glucose or glucose tolerance before meeting the criteria for DM2. The progression of prediabetes to diabetes can be reversed or slowed down by the intervention of lifestyle modifications or medications that can improve insulin sensitivity or reduce hepatic glucose production. Lifestyle and genetics are primary factors involved in the pathogenesis of DM2. High risk factors include obesity, sedentary lifestyle, stress, urbanization, smoking, sugar-sweetened drinks, reduced vitamin D, and increased intake of saturated and trans fats [14]. In contrast, high intake of mono- or polyunsaturated fats may improve insulin sensitivity and thus can decrease the risk of development of the disease [15]. Abuse, neglect, or household difficulties in childhood may increase the likelihood of DM2 later in life by almost 32% [16]. Chronic hyperglycemia in patients with DM2 is associated with the development of both microvascular and macrovascular complications.

2.1.3 Other specific types

Maturity onset diabetes of young (MODY) is a rare autosomal dominant inherited form of DM, characterized by a defect in insulin production due to multiple single gene mutations such as of hepatocyte nuclear factor-1α (HNF-1 α) and glucokinase gene. It is often referred to as monogenic diabetes to distinguish it from DM1 and DM2. MODY has 13 subtypes and can occur at different ages and with different degrees of severity, depending on the specific gene defect. The onset of hyperglycemia usually occurs at an early age, such as before 25 years. Insulin therapy is a central element of MODY therapeutics [17,18]. Genetic defects in insulin action at the receptor level is rare form of diabetes, which can be further classified as type A insulin resistance, characterized by severe insulin resistance, acanthosis nigricans and hyperandrogenism in females, however glucose intolerance and diabetes might not be present, and type B insulin resistance characterized by insulin resistance and hyperinsulinemia due to the presence of antibodies to insulin receptors [19]. Diseases associated with extensive harm to the pancreas, such as chronic pancreatitis and cystic fibrosis, may lead to diabetes [20,21]. Some conditions such as tumors promote the increased production of insulin antagonists such as cortisol, growth hormone, glucagon, and catecholamines, antagonizing the action of insulin. Importantly, the amelioration of diabetes largely depends on the removal of underlying tumors [19]. The intake of certain drugs, the most common of which are glucocorticoids, thiazide diuretics, β-adrenergic agonists, protease inhibitors, atypical antipsychotics, and statins, can cause hyperglycemia and diabetes [22,23].

2.1.4 Gestational diabetes

Gestational diabetes resembles DM2 in several aspects and is characterized by a combination of inadequate insulin secretion and responsiveness. Approximately 1%–14% of all pregnancies experience gestational diabetes, which may improve after delivery [24]. It is generally recommended that all pregnant women should be tested for diabetes at around 24–28 weeks of gestation. It is usually diagnosed in the second or third trimester because of the increased levels of the insulin antagonist hormone [25]. Gestational diabetes can be treated with dietary changes, blood glucose monitoring or insulin therapy in some cases. Untreated cases may result in damage to the health of the fetus and the mother. Macrosomia, congenital heart disease, central nervous system abnormalities and skeletal muscle malformations are some of the potential risks to the baby. High levels of insulin in the fetus's blood may inhibit fetal surfactant production, causing infant respiratory distress syndrome [26–28]. Perinatal death may occur in severe cases due to vascular impairment and poor placental perfusion [29].

2.2 Pharmacologic treatment and limitations

The selection of pharmacological agents for the treatment of DM depends on its specific type. Multiple daily injections of prandial and basal insulin or continuous insulin infusion are the mainstay of the treatment of DM1, depending on the severity of the condition. In combination with lifestyle measures, metformin is the preferred initial choice in all patients with DM2 if tolerated and not contraindicated, which works by reducing the hepatic production of glucose. Other therapeutic entities include insulin secretagogues (sulfonylureas and meglitinides), amylin mimetics (Pramlintide), glucagon-like peptide-1 receptor (GLP-1) agonists (exenatide), α-glucosidase inhibitors (acarbose), dipeptidyl peptidase-4 (DPP-4) inhibitors (sitagliptin), peroxisome proliferator-activated receptor gamma (PPAR-γ) activators (thiazolidinediones), and sodium-glucose transport protein 2 (SGLT2) inhibitors (gliflozins). Table 2 summarizes the available pharmacologic options for the treatment of DM.

3. Phytonutrients and DM

Phytonutrients can play a vital role in the maintenance of health and wellness by protecting against chronic degenerative disorders such as CVD, cancer, neurodegenerative disorders, inflammatory conditions, metabolic

Table 2 Summary of the available pharmacologic options for the treatment of DM.

Pharmacological class	Drugs	Mechanism of action	Therapeutic response	Common ADRs	Cost
Insulin	Rapid acting (Lispro, Aspart, Glulisine), Short-acting (Human Regular insulin), Intermediate-acting (NPH insulin), Basal insulin analogs (Glargine, Detemir, Degludec), Premixed insulin products (NPH/Regular 70/30)	Activation of insulin receptors	↑ Peripheral glucose uptake, ↓ hepatic glucose production, suppresses lipolysis, and proteolysis	Hypoglycemia, weight gain, and lipodystrophy	High
Sulfonylureas (2nd generation)	Glipizide, Glyburide, Glimepiride	Closes KATP channels on β-cell plasma membranes, resulting in direct stimulation of insulin release from the β-cells	↑ Insulin secretion	Hypoglycemia and weight gain	Low
Biguanides	Metformin	Activation of AMPK	↑ Insulin sensitivity. ↓ hepatic glucose production, and ↑ peripheral glucose uptake	Lactic acidosis, GIT disturbances (nausea, diarrhea, abdominal cramps), Vitamin B12 deficiency	Low

Continued

Table 2 Summary of the available pharmacologic options for the treatment of DM—cont'd

Pharmacological class	Drugs	Mechanism of action	Therapeutic response	Common ADRs	Cost
Meglitinides	Repaglinide, Nateglinide	Closes KATP channels on β-cell plasma membranes, resulting in direct stimulation of insulin release from the β-cells. Glucose-dependent action	↓ Postprandial glucose excursions	Hypoglycemia and weight gain	Moderate
Amylinomimetics	Pramlintide	Activation of amylin receptors which suppresses glucagon, slows gastric emptying, and regulates appetite	↓ Postprandial glucose excursions, ↓ body weight	GIT disturbances (nausea. vomiting), hypoglycemia	High
GLP-1 agonists	Exenatide, Liraglutide, Lixisenatide, Dulaglutide	Activates GLP-1 receptors	↑ Insulin secretion, ↓ glucagon secretion, slows gastric emptying, ↑ satiety. Glucose-dependent action	GIT disturbances (nausea. vomiting, diarrhea), tachycardia, acute pancreatitis	High
α-glucosidase inhibitors	Acarbose, Miglitol	Inhibits intestinal α-glucosidase	Slows intestinal carbohydrates digestion and absorption. ↓ Postprandial glucose excursions	GIT disturbances (flatulence, diarrhea)	Low-moderate

DPP-4 inhibitors	Sitagliptin, Saxagliptin, Linagliptin	Inhibits DPP-4 activity, ↑ postprandial incretin concentrations	↑ Insulin secretion and ↓ glucagon secretion. Glucose-dependent action	Immune-mediated skin reactions, acute pancreatitis, ↑ heart failure	High
Thiazolidinediones	Pioglitazone, Rosiglitazone	Activates the nuclear transcription factor PPAR-γ	↑ Insulin sensitivity	Weight gain, edema, cardiac failure, bone fractures	Low
SGLT2 inhibitors	Canagliflozin, Empagliflozin	Inhibits SGLT2 in the proximal nephron	Increasing glucosuria by suppressing renal glucose reabsorption	UTIs, polyuria, volume depletion resulting in hypotension, and dizziness, ↑ LDL, DKA, AKI, angioedema	High

disorders including diabetes, infections, psychiatric illnesses, and GI pathologies. Having favorable safety profiles and low costs, they can be used effectively either in the form of extracts or as isolated compounds, serving as alternative therapeutic agents in glucose metabolic disorders. Thousands of herbs have been implicated in the treatment of DM, and a plethora of these products, mostly in combination, are marketed to lower blood glucose levels and for treatment of diabetes-associated comorbid conditions [30,31]. With increases in the available literature, it is possible that one or more of these agents may become a part of conventional antidiabetic therapies. Metformin, the most widely used antidiabetic medicine, is one example of such a transition, as it was discovered from the use of *Galega officinalis* L. for the treatment of DM [32]. Fig. 2 highlights the mechanistic targets of phytonutrients in the improvement of glucose metabolism.

3.1 Phenolic compounds

An important link has been established between oxidative stress, inflammatory processes, and insulin activity. Growing evidence suggests that hyperglycemia provokes the production of reactive oxygen species, resulting

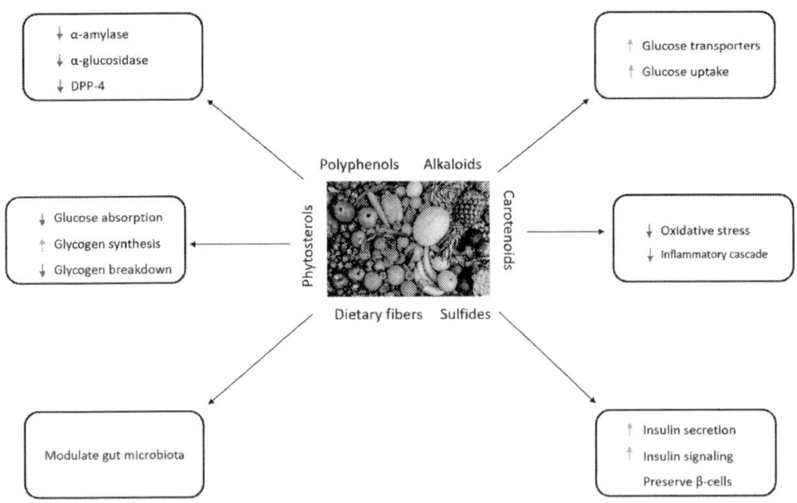

Fig. 2 Mechanistic targets of phytonutrients in the improvement of glucose metabolism. Different classes of phytonutrients possess hypoglycemic effects via inhibition of glucose metabolizing enzymes, reducing glucose absorption, increasing glycogen synthesis, and decreasing glycogen breakdown, enhancing expression of glucose transporters, decreasing oxidative and inflammatory stresses, increasing insulin secretion and signaling, preserving pancreatic β-cells, and modulating gut microbiota.

in increased oxidative stress in tissues including the vascular system. The ability of natural antioxidants, including phenolic compounds, may protect against the lethal effects of hyperglycemia through an improvement of glucose metabolism. Individual phenolic compounds may vary in their antioxidant response based on the number and position of hydroxyl groups present [33]. The literature data shows that foods and beverages containing polyphenols, such as berries, nuts, dark chocolate, grape seeds, red wine, and green tea, are associated with considerable effects on the varied aspects of metabolic dysfunction. Phenolic compounds may possess a positive impact on metabolic health through decreased glucose absorption, improved insulin signaling, decreased oxidative stress, and modulation of gut microbiota [34,35]. The potential roles of each individual class of polyphenols in DM have been described below.

3.1.1 Flavonoids

Flavonoids are known to interact with several biological targets at the molecular level, involving different physiological processes. They most commonly occur in dietary sources such as tea, cocoa, red wine, fruits, vegetables, and legumes. Their antioxidant potential makes them a valuable therapeutic choice in the management of distinct pathological conditions. Since 1980, flavonoids evaluated for their hypoglycemic effects showed relevant results [36]. In vitro and in vivo studies have demonstrated significant antidiabetic effects with flavones (eupatilin, wogonin and 5,7-Dihydroxy-6,8-dimethyl-4′-methoxyflavone), flavonols (fisetin, quercetin, myricetin), catechins ((−)-epigallocatechin-3-gallate and (−)-epicatechin), isoflavones (daidzein, genistein, and biochanin A), isoflavanes (glabridin), flavanones (naringenin), anthocyanins (pelargonidin), flavanone glycosides (naringin and hesperidin), flavonol glycosides (rutin and kaempferitrin), and chalcones (phloridzin, xanthoangelol, 4-hydroxyderricin, licochalcone E) [37].

A meta-analysis of prospective cohort studies showed a reduced risk of DM2 with regular consumption of dietary total flavonoids. Six prospective cohorts involving 284,806 participants were evaluated and the relative risk of DM2 for the lowest intake of flavonoids was compared with the highest intake. Total flavonoid intake of up to 500 mg/day was associated with a 5% reduction in risk for the development of DM2 [38]. A large prospective study across European countries exhibited an inverse relation between the risk of DM2 and the intake of individual flavonols and flavanols [39]. Flavan-3-ol monomers, proanthocyanidin dimers, and myricetin were found to be associated with a decreased incidence of DM2, highlighting the importance of flavonoid subclasses in the management of diabetes. Treatment of postmenopausal women with metabolic syndrome, in a randomized clinical trial of genistein (54 mg/day) for 1 year, revealed decreased fasting levels of glucose and insulin, homeostasis model assessment for insulin resistance (HOMA-IR), low-density lipoprotein (LDL), adiponectin, triglycerides, and homocysteine levels with an increase in high-density lipoprotein (HDL) [40].

The reported antidiabetic mechanisms of flavonoid-based polyphenols include inhibition of α-amylase (luteolin, kaempferol, and myricetin), inhibition of α-glucosidase (quercetin, luteolin, naringenin, apigenin-6-C-glucosyl-7-*O*-glucoside, kaempferol-3-*O*-rutinoside, isoquercetin, and rutin), protection of pancreatic β-cells (quercetin, kaempferol, apigenin, genistein, and (−)-epicatechin), preservation of β-cell mass (quercetin), stimulation of glycogen synthesis (quercetin and myricetin), reduction of glycogen breakdown (genistein, daidzein, hesperidin, naringin, and rutin), increase in glucose uptake (myricetin, baicalein, tangeritin, eriodictyol, kaempferitrin, rutin, and isorhamnetin-3-*O*-glucoside), upregulation of insulin secretion (eupatilin and genistein), insulin receptor signaling (genistein, kakkalide, and rutin), and downstream regulation of glucose-6-phosphatase (genistein, hesperidin, and naringin) [37]. Despite multiple therapeutic benefits, flavonoids are not used as a part of regular clinical practice due to their poor solubility, low bioavailability, and extensive first pass metabolism. Nanoparticulate systems of flavonoids have been proposed to improve their pharmacokinetic profile, which may enhance their antidiabetic efficacy [41].

3.1.2 Phenolic acids

Phenolic acids are a subgroup of polyphenols with strong antioxidant properties, owing to their radical scavenging, electron donation, and singlet oxygen quenching mechanisms [33]. They have been detected in many plant species, but dried fruits are their most common dietary source. Phenolic acids also strengthen endogenous antidiabetic defenses, such as glutathione peroxidase (GPx) and glutathione reductase (GR), by upregulating transcription factor nuclear factor erythroid 2-related factor 2 (Nrf2) via c-Jun N-terminal kinase (JNK)—mediated phosphorylation [42]. This could explain the possible role of phenolic acids in combating diabetic pathogenesis, as evident from a wide range of studies. More interestingly, these compounds are ubiquitous in edible fruits, vegetables, and nuts, and it is estimated that they may be consumed in the human diet with an average of 1–2 g/day [43].

Enough studies have reported the inhibition of key enzymes (α-amylase and α-glucosidase) related to DM by phenolic acids. They may also alter the expression of glucose and insulin receptors, augment the expression of glucose transporter GLUT2 in pancreatic β-cells producing insulin, and promote the translocation of GLUT2 via phosphoinositide 3-kinase/protein kinase B PI3K/Akt and 5′ AMP-activated protein kinase (AMPK) pathways. Ferulic and chlorogenic acids showed antidiabetic effects through the stimulation of glucose transporters via the same mechanism [33]. There is much evidence of the beneficial effects of coffee consumption by type 2 diabetics [44,45], mainly due to the presence of chlorogenic acid. Chlorogenic acid likely inhibits Na^+-dependent glucose transporters, SGLT1 and SGLT2, interacting with glucose absorption from the intestine.

Sinapic and ferulic acids demonstrate significant hypoglycemic effects in diabetic rats through increases in glucokinase activity and glycogen production in the liver, along with elevation of plasma insulin levels [46,47]. Phenolic acids also possess the capacity to regulate postprandial glycemia by upregulating the insulin response and attenuation of the secretion of GIP and GLP-1 [48]. Stimulation of ATP synthesis by phenolic acids through oxidative phosphorylation by inhibition of Na^+-Ca^{2+} exchangers has also been evident, which may consume forward glucose and stimulate insulin secretion [49].

3.1.3 Coumarins

Essential oils including cinnamon bark oil, cassia leaf oil and lavender oil are the richest sources of coumarins; however, some fruits, green tea, and chicory also contain lesser amounts. They are well known for their antithrombotic and anticoagulation effects; however, over the past two decades, there has been increasing interest in evaluating any protective effects of coumarins in diabetes and related complications. Osthole and esculin were found to significantly lower fasting blood glucose levels, HOMA-IR, total cholesterol (TC), total triglycerides (TG) and free fatty acids (FFAs), with increased insulin levels in high-fat diet, ICR mice [50]. In the same study, fraxetin was only found to decrease FFAs and increase insulin levels. Researchers observed antioxidant effects in the pancreas with osthole and esculin, by increasing the activities of GPx, catalase, and superoxide dismutase (SOD), while fraxetin only affects catalase activity.

Pari and colleagues examined the modulating effects of coumarins on the key hepatic enzymes involved in the glucose metabolism in chemical-induced DM2 rats, including enhanced hexokinase and glucose-6-phophate dehydrogenase (G6PD) levels, and decreased levels of glucose-6-phosphatase and fructose-1,6-bisphosphatase, which indicate that coumarins can alter the glucose metabolism through modulation of glucose metabolizing enzymes [51]. Other mechanistic targets include the upregulation of PPAR-γ, PPAR-α, GLUT-4 expression/translocation and AMPK, and inhibition of α-amylase, α-glucosidase, nuclear factor-kappa B (NF-kβ) expression, caspase-3, inflammatory gene expression (Ccl6, Il6, and Mcp1) and p-JNK [52].

3.1.4 Xanthones

Xanthones have been identified in 20 families of higher plants, mainly in the *Bonnetiaceae and Clusiaceae* families. As with other polyphenols, xanthones have not been explored much for their hypoglycemic effects. In vitro studies have shown weak to moderate antioxidant activities with virgataxanthone-A, griffipavixanthone, 1,5,8-trihydroxy-3-methoxyxanthone, 6-hydroxy-3,5-dimethoxy-1-[(6-O-β-D-xylopyranosyl-β-D-glucopyranosyl) oxy] xanthone and 1,8-Dihydroxy3,5-dimethoxyxanthone, while xanthone molecules like 1,3,5-trihydroxy-2-(2′,2′-dimethyl-4′-isopropenyl) cyclopentanylxanthone (126) and 5-*O*-demethylpaxanthonin have shown potent radical scavenging activity [53]. Their antidiabetic effects are mainly mediated by delaying carbohydrate absorption from the gastrointestinal tract (GIT) via inhibition of the α-glucosidase enzyme.

Macluraxanthone-B, cudratricusxanthone-A, cudratricusxanthone-F, cudraxanthone-L, cudraxanthone-M, 1,3,7-trihydroxy-4-(1,1-dimethyl-2-propenyl)-5,6-(2–2-dimethylchromeno)-xanthone, and 1,3,6,7-tetrahydroxy-2-(3-methylbut-2-enyl)-8-(2-methylbut-3-en-2-yl) xanthone have all been found to exert moderate α-glucosidase inhibition activity with IC50 values of 31.7, 16.2, 35.8, 37.7, 32.0, 24.9, and 38.2 μM respectively [54]. Mangiferin (xanthone glucoside) showed hypoglycemic and hypolipidemic effects in an experimental model of diabetic rats, with an in vitro inhibition of α-amylase and α-glucosidase enzymes. Treatment of diabetic rats with mangiferin resulted in decreasing fasting blood glucose, TC, TG, LDL, and VLDL and increasing HDL levels [55]. Short-term administration of xanthones isolated from *Garcinia mangostana* L. fruit pericarp to DM2 rats significantly reformed kidney and hepatic histological alterations [56].

3.1.5 Stilbenes

Stilbenes are compounds with proven efficacy against age-related disorders, mainly by targeting oxidative defense mechanisms. They are present at low concentrations in a limited number of human foods, with red wine being the most abundant dietary source, followed by grape berries and grape juice. Growing evidence from preclinical and clinical studies suggests that resveratrol improves biochemical and clinical parameters in diabetes type 1 and 2 by affecting both insulin action and pancreatic β-cells, and thus it could be useful in protecting against diabetes and its complications [57]. In in vivo experimental models of diabetes, resveratrol improved glucose homeostasis, decreased insulin resistance, enhanced insulin secretion, protected pancreatic β-cells, and ameliorated metabolic dysregulations. Its cellular targets include the enhanced expression of AMPK and sirtuin 1 (SIRT1) in several tissues of diabetic subjects [58].

Resveratrol also induces the secretion of gut incretin hormones and GLP-1 and activation of sirtuin 2 (SIRT2). The latter may mimic the benefits of calorie restriction [59]. Kerem et al. [60] evaluated the antioxidant and α-glucosidase inhibition activity of trans-resveratrol, piceid, and rumexoid isolated from the roots of Israeli *Rumex bucephalophorus* L [60]. *trans*-Resveratrol showed the highest Trolox equivalent antioxidant capacity (TEAC) and rumexoid showed the lowest. *Trans*-Resveratrol and rumexoid demonstrated the most potent α-glucosidase inhibitory activities with IC50 values of < 0.1 and < 0.5 mM, respectively. Piceatannol is another natural stilbene found in fruits and vegetables, and it is known for its beneficial effects on hyperglycemia, insulin resistance, hyperlipidemia, adipogenesis, and fatty acid-induced oxidative and inflammatory stresses; however, investigation regarding its positive impact on metabolic health is still in its infancy [61].

Studies also linked the antidiabetic effects of resveratrol with its antioxidant and antiinflammatory potential. Resveratrol has been associated with increased activity of GPx, resulting in decreasing the oxidative damage of the hepatic tissues [62]. It is also capable of reducing the expression of proinflammatory cytokines in the liver [63] and decreasing microphage infiltration in the hepatic tissues of animals on a high-fat diet [64]. A meta-analysis of clinical trials conducted by Zhu et al. [65] showed an improvement in glycemic control and insulin resistance under resveratrol in patients with DM2 [65]. However, this compound is still under investigation because of certain limitations, including poor pharmacokinetic parameters such as low aqueous solubility and extensive first pass metabolism. Nanoformulation techniques have recently been employed to improve the targetability and bioavailability of resveratrol [66].

3.1.6 Lignans

Lignans (a type of phytoestrogens) have been a part of diets and medicines for centuries, though they have gained attention from pharmacologists in recent decades due to their potential health benefits. Fruits and vegetables such as apricot, strawberry, peach, pear, brassica, and kale are dietary sources of lignans. They have been shown to possess a positive impact on the relative risk factors of CVD including diabetes [67]. Flaxseed is the richest dietary source of lignans, containing secoisolariciresinol in the highest amount, in addition to lariciresinol, matairesinol, and pinoresinol [68]. A modulation of C-reactive protein levels was noted in diabetic patients (men and postmenopausal women) with mild hypercholesterolemia, when supplemented with flaxseed-derived lignan capsules (360 mg/day) or for 12 weeks in a randomized, double-blind, placebo-controlled, and cross-over trial [69].

The total lignan from Fructus arctii (*Arctium lap*pa L.) was evaluated by Xu et al. [70] for its antidiabetic activity in alloxan-induced diabetes in mice and rats [70]. Hypoglycemia, hypocholesterolemia, and hypotriglyceridemia were observed in both species treated with total lignan from *A. lappa*, while the serum insulin level, glucose tolerance, and HDL levels were raised without the risk of hypoglycemia. Sesame oil contains sesamin, sesaminol, and sesamolin lignan fractions, which are known for their potent antioxidant activity, and thus can promote the health benefits of these foods regarding metabolic health, hypertension, hypercholesterolemia, cancer, neurodegenerative diseases, and aging [71]. An in vitro study demonstrated a decrease in lipid peroxidation in diabetic control blood treated with *sesamol* and sesame lignans (*sesamin and episesamin*), suggesting that they may be effective in protecting plasma, LDL, and the erythrocyte membrane from oxidation, thus reducing the risk of coronary heart disease in diabetic individuals [72].

3.1.7 Curcuminoids

Curcumin, the active principle of turmeric (*Curcuma longa* L.), has been the most widely studied phytochemical for its physiological and pharmacological properties such as antioxidant, antiinflammatory, neuroprotective, cardioprotective, anticancer, hepatoprotective, nephroprotective, antidiabetic, and antiinfective activities [73]. It has gained scientific attention for the treatment of diabetes and its complications because of its potential to reduce plasma glucose and cholesterol levels in rodent models of diabetes. The first report of the hypoglycemic effects of curcumin in diabetic individuals was published in 1972 [74]. Most of the therapeutic effects of curcumin can be attributed to its strong antioxidant and antiinflammatory activities, in view of oxidative stress and inflammatory cascades as possible and progressive pathogenic mechanisms of diabetes, and curcumin could thus be considered a suitable alternative in the prevention and amelioration of diabetes and associated complications.

A reduction in glucose tolerance has been reported with the administration of theracurmin (a more bioavailable curcumin formulation) in rats [75]. In vivo studies have shown a decrease in insulin resistance with curcumin treatment through upregulation of the IRS/PI3K/Akt pathway and enhanced expression of GLUT1 and GLUT3 [76,77], a mechanism that is normally activated by insulin on its receptors and is responsible for glucose metabolism and transport [76]. PI3K/Akt/GSK-3β is another mechanism dealing with glucose metabolism, and it is potentially an important therapeutic target in the treatment of metabolic diseases. A simulated docking experiment demonstrated that curcumin fits in the binding pocket of GSK-3β, the enzyme which inhibits glycogen synthase by phosphorylation [78]. This binding results in increased hepatic glycogen synthesis through the inhibition of GSK-3β in fasting mice in a dose-dependent manner. Curcumin administration to male Sprague-Dawley rats prevented diabetes-associated abnormalities in kidneys by inhibition of oxidative stress, mesangial expansion, p300 and NF-kβ expression [79]. Curcumin also improved diabetes-induced cerebral infarction by enhancing the expression of glucose transporters (GLUT1 and GLUT3) in male Sprague-Dawley rats [80].

A meta-analysis of randomized clinical trials' "metabolic benefits of curcumin supplementation in patients with metabolic syndrome" revealed a significant reduction in fasting blood glucose and TG levels, with a considerable increase in HDL levels, while the effects of curcumin on waist circumference and systolic blood pressure were not significant when compared to placebo [81]. It is worth mentioning that the efficacy and potency of curcumin has rarely been compared with the available antidiabetic agents, most probably due to the bioavailability issues of curcumin which may thus require higher doses to produce similar results. A study performed by El-Moselhy et al. [82] using high-fat diet rats showed oral doses of 80 mg/kg/day curcumin to be as effective as 1 mg/kg/day rosiglitazone in reducing fasting insulin levels, blood glucose concentration, and tumor necrosis factor-alpha (TNF-α) levels [82]. Abdel Aziz and colleagues developed a novel water-soluble derivative of curcumin with an increased in vivo bioavailability profile, which possessed antidiabetic effects in rats at relatively small doses, through decreasing oxidative stress by reducing malondialdehyde in the pancreas, liver, and aorta [83].

3.1.8 Chalcones

Chalcones, precursors of flavonoids and isoflavonoids, have been reported in a restricted number of foods (apples and cherry tomatoes). They are recognized for their multiple biological activities, including in DM, though the mechanisms of most of these activities are yet to be elucidated. With regard to diabetes, chalcones may modulate numerous therapeutic targets including PPAR-γ, DPP-4, α-glucosidase, protein-tyrosine phosphatase 1B (PTP1B), aldose reductase, and insulin secretion and sensitivity [84]. Chalcones from *Angelica keiskei* (Miq.) Koidz. (4-hydroxyderricin and xanthoangelol) showed potent insulin-like activity in diabetic KK-Ay/Ta mice, reflecting a decrease in blood glucose levels and increase in glucose uptake through a PPAR-γ-independent pathway [85]. In another study, 4-hydroxyderricin and xanthoangelol inhibited adipocyte differentiation via AMPK and mitogen-activated protein kinase (MAPK) pathways, which resulted in a reduced expression of adipocyte-specific transcription factors [86]. A group of chalcone substitutes were tested against glucose metabolism enzymes α-amylase and α-glucosidase by Rocha et al. [87], and the results indicated that the substitution pattern and type of substitution alter the inhibitory activity of compounds, with the presence of hydroxy groups being the most favorable substitution for the intended effect [87]. Butein was the most active compound among all substitutes, with moderate inhibition of both enzymes.

3.1.9 Secoiridoids

Olea europaea L. (olive) is the richest source of secoiridoids and has been a main component of healthy diets for many populations over the centuries. The reported pharmacological effects of secoiridoids include antidiabetic, antiinflammatory, immunosuppressive, neuroprotective, anticancer, antiobesity, and cardioprotective effects [88]. Oleuropein and hydroxytyrosol-rich extracts from olive leaf significantly decreased blood glucose and cholesterol levels and restored antioxidant perturbation when administered to diabetic rats for 4-weeks [89]. In another study, an oleuropein-rich diet (35% *w*/w) attenuated hyperglycemia and impaired glucose tolerance in diabetic mice [90]. Khalili et al. observed an improvement in glucose tolerance and serum lipid profiles in male Sprague-Dawley rats with simultaneous renovascular hypertension and DM2 when they were treated with oleuropein for 4-weeks [91]. A reduction in blood pressure, blood glucose levels, TC, LDL, TG, and malondialdehyde, and an increase in HDL levels and erythrocyte SOD, with improved glucose tolerance, were noted in rats treated with oleuropein.

Oral administration of swertiamarin, a secoiridoid glycoside, in doses of 15, 25, and 50 mg/kg body weight to diabetic rats for 4-weeks significantly decreased fasting blood glucose level, HbA1c, TC, TG, LDL, and increased levels of plasma insulin, hemoglobin, body weight, and HDL. Histopathological analysis revealed the regeneration of pancreatic islets in rats treated with swertiamarin, compared to streptozotocin-treated diabetic rats [92]. Amarogentin, another secoiridoid glycoside, activated AMPK, increased endothelial nitric oxide synthase (eNOS), and inhibited TNF-α-induced endothelial inflammation in an in vitro study model, exerting beneficial vasculo-metabolic effects reflected by hypoglycemia, hypolipidemia, and antiatherosclerotic effects in diabetic mice [93]. Moreover, amarogentin treatment reduced levels of hepatic enzymes (alanine aminotransferase and aspartate aminotransferase), increased basal AMPK Thr^{172} phosphorylation in the hepatic tissues of the diabetic mice and decreased liver fibrosis.

3.2 Alkaloids

Alkaloids are widespread in terrestrial and marine life including plants and animals. Many alkaloids have been found to improve insulin signaling and glucose metabolism, and these can be used as lead molecules to develop novel antidiabetic agents with improved efficacy and safety profiles. Alteration of multiple targets has been reported for a range of alkaloids from different botanical sources, including inhibition of carbohydrate-hydrolyzing enzymes, protein tyrosine phosphate 1B inhibition, AMPK activation, DPP-4 inhibition, GLUT4 translocation activation, increased insulin secretion, regeneration of pancreatic β-cells [94]. Indole alkaloids, aminoalkaloids, isoquinoline alkaloids, and terpenoidal alkaloids are four classes that have shown antidiabetic efficacy in in vitro and in vivo studies ([95]). Piperumbellactam A–C (*Piper umbellatum L.*) [96], schulzeine A–C (*Penares schulzei* Dendy) [97], 1,4-Dideoxy-1,4-imino-D-arabinitol (*Morus alba* L.) [98], Mahanimbine (*Murraya koenigii* (L.) Spreng.) [99], Radicamine A and B (*Lobelia chinensis* Lour.) [100], and Vindogentianine (*Catharanthus roseus* (L.) G.Don) [101] are alkaloids with weak to moderate α-*glucosidase inhibition activity.*

An in vitro study revealed the reversible inhibition of sucrase by vasicine and vasicinol isolated from *Justicia adhatoda* L., with IC50 values of 125 and 250 μM, respectively [102]. Chelerythrine and sanguinarine completely inhibited porcine pancreatic α-amylase at concentrations of 250 μM with IC50 values of 111.1 and 119.4 μM, respectively. However, poor activity of both alkaloids against human salivary α-amylase was found, up to a concentration of 2500 μM with percentage inhibition of 23% and 48%, respectively [103]. Mahanimbine [99] demonstrated remarkable activity against α-amylase, while vindogentianine [101] showed weak activity. Treatment of mice with mahanimbine resulted in the upregulation of expression of insulin-responsive genes, improvement in glucose clearance, and hyperlipidemia and prevention of fat accumulation in adipose tissues [110].

Preclinical studies revealed the alteration of insulin signaling and related cascades in pancreatic β-cells, hepatocytes, myocytes, and adipocytes by berberine, vindoneline, trigonelline, oxymatrine, piperine, neferine, and evodiamine, though influencing associated receptors, β-cell functioning, oxidative stress, and inflammatory pathways [107]. Berberine demonstrated antidiabetic effects by suppressing hepatic gluconeogenesis though regulation of the liver kinase (LK) B1-AMPK-CREB-regulated transcription coactivator (TORC2) signaling pathway in a rodent model of diabetes [111]. The LKB1-AMPK-TORC2 signaling pathway is a core regulator of hepatic gluconeogenesis, where LKB1 stimulates AMPK, which may lead to TORC2 phosphorylation resulting in the inhibition of TORC2 translocation. Hypoglycemic effects of berberine have also been linked with GLUT1, PPAR α/γ, SIRT1, and mitochondrial biogenesis [105].

Canthinone alkaloids (picrasidine L, eurycomine E, 5-methoxy-canthin-6-one, 5-acethoxy-canthin-6-one, 4-ethyl-3-methyl-canthin-5,6-dione, and 3,4-dimethyl-canthin-5,6-dione) have been found to inhibit PTP1B [122], a negative regulator of the insulin signaling pathway, where PTP dephosphorylates the insulin receptors, the deregulation of which can lead to impaired insulin signaling. Trigonelline (isolated from *Trigonella foenum-graecum* L.) at a dose of 75 mg/kg for 28-days [123] and L-ephedrine (isolated from *Ephedra sinica* Stapf) at a dose of 0.62 mg/kg for 14-days [127] enhanced the regeneration of pancreatic β-cells with significant hypoglycemia in rodent models of diabetes.

3.3 Sulfides

Sulfides are organosulfur compounds, most commonly found in Allium vegetables such as *Allium sativum* L. (garlic) and *Allium cepa* L. (onion). This class of phytonutrients has gained much attention because of their ability to alter molecular signaling pathways, and they are best known for their potential to fight infections, DM, cardiotoxicities, and cancers. Their antioxidant, antiinflammatory, hypoglycemic, and immunomodulatory effects may contribute to the manner in which these compounds modulate microvascular and macrovascular complications in DM2 [117]. A meta-analysis of the available studies was conducted by Kook et al. to evaluate the antidiabetic potential of onion and garlic involving experimental diabetic rats, where the animals were either supplemented with onion or garlic extract or with single components such as diallyl trisulfide, S-allylcysteine sulfoxide, and *S*-methylcysteine sulfoxide [112]. The onion extract and single components were found to be significant in lowering glucose concentration and body weight, but the garlic extract was not.

Several studies have demonstrated a reduction of insulin resistance and blood glucose by garlic in chemical-induced diabetes in mice and rats [117]. A combination of onion peel and garlic peel extracts significantly lowered blood glucose concentration in healthy rats with induced diabetes [116]. Allicin (diallylthiosulfinate) ameliorated diabetes-induced morphological alterations of the kidney with decreased fasting blood glucose concentration, blood urea nitrogen, serum creatinine and TG levels in diabetic rats. The downstream regulation of collagen 1, transforming growth factor beta 1 (TGF-β1) and phospho—extracellular signal-regulated kinase 1/2 (p-ERK1/2) was observed in rats treated with allicin. Allicin administration to diabetic rats also prevented DM-induced cardiac complications via inhibition of B-cell lymphoma 2 (*Bcl-2*), cluster of differentiation 95 (*CD95*), connective tissue growth factor (CTGF), and TGF-β1 protein expression, which resulted in the suppression of the progression of myocardial fibrosis [115]. Treatment of H9c2 cells and male Wistar rats with diallyl trisulfide indicated protection against hyperglycemia-induced oxidative stress-mediated apoptosis through the upregulation of the PI3K/Akt/Nrf2 pathway, leading to the activation of Nrf2- regulated antioxidant enzymes in cardiomyocytes [125].

3.4 Phytosterols

Stigmasterol, sitosterol, and campesterol are the most abundant phytosterols present in cereal grains, grain legumes, nuts, vegetable oils, and pecans. They have been reported to be useful in the management of several disorders. The first ever therapeutic activity of phytosterols was reported in 1951 in the management of hypercholesterolemia [126]. Studies have recently identified some phytosterols acting as key regulators of glucose metabolism, through AMPK and PPARs activation. Tanaka et al. [124] identified five phytosterols from *Aloe vera* (L.) Burm. f. gel as potential antidiabetic compounds, including lophenol, 24-ethyl-lophenol, 24-methyl-lophenol, cycloartanol, and 24-methylene-cycloartanol. Treatment of diabetic BKS.Cg-m^{+}/$^{+}$Lepr$^{db/J}$

(*db/db*) mice with 1 μg of either sterol resulted in a reduction of HbA1c and blood glucose levels, with no significant differences in the hypoglycemic efficacy between the individual sterols [124].

Oral ingestion of phytosterols lophenol and cycloartanol, isolated from *Aloe vera* (L.) Burm. f., altered hepatic gene expression (gluconeogenic enzymes, lipogenic enzymes, and sterol regulatory element-binding protein 1 or *SREBP-1*) in Zucker diabetic fatty rats and ameliorated obesity-associated metabolic changes, including decreased fasting and random blood glucose levels, visceral fat weights, and serum/hepatic TC, TG, and nonesterified fatty acid concentrations [118]. Moreover, the mRNA levels of glycolysis enzymes in the liver as well as PPAR-α expression increased in rats treated with *Aloe* sterols. Conversely, one study did not show any improvement in insulin resistance, susceptibility to obesity and diabetes in high-fat diet fed mice, after the intake of a phytosterol-rich Western-type diet (41% β-sitosterol, 20% campesterol, and 22% stigmasterol) for 32-weeks [106]. A meta-analysis of randomized clinical trials demonstrated an improvement of the lipid profile, reflected by reduced TC and LDL levels, and increased HDL levels in patients with DM2. No apparent effect was seen on TG concentration [104].

3.5 Dietary fibers

Dietary fibers are most abundantly found in fruits and vegetables, ranging from 1 g/100 g in grapes or lettuce to more than 10 g/100 g in guava. Studies have shown an inverse relation between the daily intake of fruits, legumes, and fibers and metabolic consequences, as a general observation of the obese and diabetic population of North America lacking an adequate amount of dietary fiber in their diet. Though there is no special recommendation regarding the daily intake of dietary fibers in individuals at a high risk for diabetes, ADA recommends a daily intake of 38 g of fiber for men and 25 g of fiber for women [109]. A daily consumption of fiber in sufficient amounts modulates the gut microbiota and may improve insulin sensitivity, glucose/lipids homeostasis, endothelial dysfunction, and inflammatory markers [109]. Li et al. [113] observed a significant reduction in body weight, fasting, blood glucose concentration, HbA1c levels, plasma lipopolysaccharide, and alterations in inflammatory mediators (increased IL-10 and decreased IL-6, TNF-α, and IL-17A) in genetically modified mice when treated with inulin for 6-weeks [113]. Gut microbiota analysis revealed a reduction of *Deferribacteres*, *Mucispirillum*, *Ruminiclostridium_6*, and *Tenericutes*, with an elevation of *Bacteroides* and *Cyanobacteria* in inulin-treated groups. Furthermore, the results showed a close correlation of *Bacteroides* and *Cyanobacteria* with IL-10, and similarly *Deferribacteres, Mucispirillum, Ruminiclostridium_6, and Tenericutes*, with TNF-α, IL-6, and IL-17A.

3.6 Carotenoids

Carotenoids are a group of antioxidant phytonutrients, found in a variety of fruits and vegetables, i.e., green vegetables (broccoli, spinach, and green beans) containing xanthophylls and carotenes, yellow and red fruits/vegetables (plums, carrots, melons, and tomatoes) containing primarily carotenes, and yellow or orange fruits (pumpkins, peaches, and oranges) containing xanthophyll esters. To date, a large number of studies have reported the protective effects of carotenoids against cancer, DM2, CVD, and neurodegenerative disorders. A daily intake of a diet higher in carotenoid contents (α- and β-carotenoids) may be associated with reduced DM2 incidence in healthy men and women [119]. A population-based study conducted in Queensland, Australia justified the above statement with the conclusion that serum carotenoids (α-carotene, β-carotene, β-cryptoxanthin, lutein/zeaxanthin, and lycopene) can be inversely related to impaired glucose metabolism and DM2 [108]. However, a randomized clinical trial showed no benefits of β-carotene supplementation for an average of 12 months on the relative risk of DM2 development in a healthy male population [114].

The antidiabetic effects of carotenoids may be attributed to their ability to enhance insulin sensitivity and decrease insulin resistance through upregulating PPAR-γ gene expression (bixin), inhibiting JNK and IKKβ signaling pathways (crocetin), stimulating antioxidant defense mechanisms (bixin, astaxanthin, α-tocopherol, β-carotene, and lycopene), and altering immune-modulation pathways (astaxanthin, bixin, lutein, fucoxanthin, and lycopene) [121]. Some studies also report a direct association between carotenoids and glucose metabolizing enzymes with astaxanthin and fucoxanthin, such as hexokinase, glucose-6-phosphatase, fructose-1,6-bisphosphatase, pyruvate kinase, and glycogen phosphorylase. Fucoxanthin has been found to increase the insulin receptor and GLUT4 expression, Akt phosphorylation, and PGC-1α in the muscles of mice [120].

4. Concluding remarks

Although many effective drugs exist for the treatment of metabolic disorders, none can control the rapidly increasing trends of diabetic morbidity and mortality. Phytonutrients possess significant hypoglycemic potential, evident from preclinical and clinical studies, owing to their multiple mechanistic targets. The relatively low cost of food supplements containing phytonutrients may be an advantage for people living with diabetes. Conversely, there are certain limitations in considering phytonutrients for their clinical use in DM, including poor pharmacokinetic profiles, safety concerns, and the risk of drug interactions. Mislabeling, misidentification, adulteration with other herbs, and contamination with mycotoxins and heavy metals (i.e., mercury, lead, and arsenic) could lead to serious events, although phytonutrients are perceived to be effective and safe. More in-depth studies are needed to evaluate the efficacy and safety of phytonutrients in subjects with diabetes. The advancement of pharmacological assessment techniques and analytical techniques will enhance the quality of these agents for use in diabetic patients. Moreover, the development of novel formulation techniques could improve their pharmacokinetic profile and targeted delivery.

References

[1] J.C. Henquin, Triggering and amplifying pathways of regulation of insulin secretion by glucose, Diabetes 49 (2000) 1751–1760.
[2] S.L. Aronoff, K. Berkowitz, B. Shreiner, L. Want, Glucose metabolism and regulation: beyond insulin and glucagon, Diabetes Spectr. 17 (2004) 183–190.
[3] P. Rorsman, M. Braun, Regulation of insulin secretion in human pancreatic islets, Annu. Rev. Physiol. 75 (2013) 155–179.
[4] World Health Organization, Global Report on Diabetes, World Health Organization, 2016. ISBN 9789241565257.
[5] American Diabetes Association, Classification and diagnosis of diabetes: standards of medical care in diabetesd-2019, Diabetes Care 42 (2019) S13–S28.
[6] J.L. Chiang, M.S. Kirkman, L.M.B. Laffel, A.L. Peters, Type 1 diabetes through the life span: a position statement of the American Diabetes Association, Diabetes Care 37 (2014) 2034–2054.
[7] C.J. Garrett, P. Choudhary, S.A. Amiel, P. Fonagy, K. Ismail, Recurrent diabetic ketoacidosis and a brief history of brittle diabetes research: contemporary and past evidence in diabetic ketoacidosis research including mortality, mental health and prevention, Diabet. Med. 36 (2019) 1329–1335.
[8] I.B. Hirsch, L.M. Gaudiani, A new look at brittle diabetes, J. Diabetes Complications 35 (2020), 107646.
[9] E. Laugesen, J.A. Østergaard, R.D.G. Leslie, Latent autoimmune diabetes of the adult: current knowledge and uncertainty, Diabet. Med. 32 (2015) 843–852.
[10] S. Butalia, G.G. Kaplan, B. Khokhar, D.M. Rabi, Environmental risk factors and type 1 diabetes: past, present, and future, Can. J. Diabetes 40 (2016) 586–593.
[11] A. Petzold, M. Solimena, K.P. Knoch, Mechanisms of beta cell dysfunction associated with viral infection, Curr. Diab. Rep. 15 (2015) 73.
[12] G. Serena, S. Camhi, C. Sturgeon, S. Yan, A. Fasano, The role of gluten in celiac disease and type 1 diabetes, Nutrients 7 (2015) 7143–7162.
[13] J. Visser, J. Rozing, A. Sapone, K. Lammers, A. Fasano, Tight junctions, intestinal permeability, and autoimmunity: celiac disease and type 1 diabetes paradigms, Ann. N.Y. Acad. Sci. 1165 (2009) 195.

[14] V. Bellou, L. Belbasis, I. Tzoulaki, E. Evangelou, Risk factors for type 2 diabetes mellitus: an exposure-wide umbrella review of meta-analyses, PLoS One 13 (2018), e0194127.

[15] U. Risérus, W.C. Willett, F.B. Hu, Dietary fats and prevention of type 2 diabetes, Prog. Lipid Res. 48 (2009) 44–51.

[16] H. Huang, P. Yan, Z. Shan, S. Chen, M. Li, C. Luo, H. Gao, L. Hao, L. Liu, Adverse childhood experiences and risk of type 2 diabetes: a systematic review and meta-analysis, Metab. Clin. Exp. 64 (2015) 1408–1418.

[17] B.M. Shields, S. Hicks, M.H. Shepherd, K. Colclough, A.T. Hattersley, S. Ellard, Maturity-onset diabetes of the young (MODY): how many cases are we missing? Diabetologia 53 (2010) 2504–2508.

[18] G. Thanabalasingham, K.R. Owen, Diagnosis and management of maturity onset diabetes of the young (MODY), BMJ 343 (2011), d6044.

[19] J.F. de Maraschin, Classification of diabetes, in: S.I. Ahmad (Ed.), Diabeteses, Springer, New York, 2013, pp. 12–19.

[20] D.K. Andersen, M. Korc, G.M. Petersen, G. Eibl, D. Li, M.R. Rickels, S.T. Chari, J.L. Abbruzzese, Diabetes, pancreatogenic diabetes, and pancreatic cancer, Diabetes 66 (2017) 1103–1110.

[21] S.M. Blackman, C.W. Commander, C. Watson, K.M. Arcara, L.J. Strug, J.R. Stonebraker, F.A. Wright, J.M. Rommens, L. Sun, R.G. Pace, S.A. Norris, P.R. Durie, M.L. Drumm, M.R. Knowles, G.R. Cutting, Genetic modifiers of cystic fibrosis-related diabetes, Diabetes 62 (2013) 3627–3635.

[22] B. Luna, M.N. Feinglos, Drug-induced hyperglycemia, JAMA 286 (2001) 1945–1948.

[23] N. Sattar, D. Preiss, H.M. Murray, P. Welsh, B.M. Buckley, A.J. de Craen, S.R.K. Seshasai, J.J. McMurray, D.J. Freeman, J.W. Jukema, P.W. Macfarlane, C.J. Packard, D.J. Stott, R.G. Westendorp, J. Shepherd, B.R. Davis, S.L. Pressel, R. Marchioli, R.M. Marfisi, A.P. Maggioni, L. Tavazzi, G. Tognoni, J. Kjekshus, T.R. Pedersen, T.J. Cook, A.M. Gotto, M.B. Clearfield, J.R. Downs, H. Nakamura, Y. Ohashi, K. Mizuno, K.K. Ray, I. Ford, Statins and risk of incident diabetes: a collaborative meta-analysis of randomised statin trials, Lancet 375 (2010) 735–742.

[24] American Diabetes Association, Diagnosis and classification of diabetes mellitus, Diabetes Care 37 (2014) S81–S90.

[25] J. Soldavini, Krause's food & the nutrition care process, J. Nutr. Educ. Behav. 51 (2019) 1225.

[26] C.P. Chen, Congenital malformations associated with maternal diabetes, Taiwan. J. Obstet. Gynecol. 44 (2005) 1–7.

[27] K. Kc, S. Shakya, H. Zhang, Gestational diabetes mellitus and macrosomia: a literature review, Ann. Nutr. Metab. 66 (2015) 14–20.

[28] E.S. Ogata, Problems of the infant of the diabetic mother, NeoReviews 11 (2010) e627–e631.

[29] C. Billionnet, D. Mitanchez, A. Weill, J. Nizard, F. Alla, A. Hartemann, S. Jacqueminet, Gestational diabetes and adverse perinatal outcomes from 716,152 births in France in 2012, Diabetologia 60 (2017) 636–644.

[30] K. Shapiro, W.C. Gong, Natural products used for diabetes, J. Am. Pharm. Assoc. 42 (2002) (1996) 217–262.

[31] V. Vuksan, J.L. Sievenpiper, Herbal remedies in the management of diabetes: lessons learned from the study of ginseng, Nutr. Metab. Cardiovasc. Dis. 15 (2005) 149–160.

[32] J.D. Smith, V.B. Clinard, Natural products for the management of type 2 diabetes mellitus and comorbid conditions, J. Am. Pharm. Assoc. 54 (2014) e304–e321.

[33] N. Kumar, N. Goel, Phenolic acids: natural versatile molecules with promising therapeutic applications, Biotechnol. Rep. 24 (2019), e00370.

[34] H. Cao, J. Ou, L. Chen, Y. Zhang, T. Szkudelski, D. Delmas, M. Daglia, J. Xiao, Dietary polyphenols and type 2 diabetes: human study and clinical trial, Crit. Rev. Food Sci. Nutr. 59 (2019) 3371–3379.

[35] F. Francini-Pesenti, P. Spinella, L.A. Calò, Potential role of phytochemicals in metabolic syndrome prevention and therapy, Diabetes Metab. Syndr. Obes. 12 (2019) 1987–2002.

[36] E. Nicolle, F. Souard, P. Faure, A. Boumendjel, Flavonoids as promising lead compounds in type 2 diabetes mellitus: molecules of interest and structure-activity relationship, Curr. Med. Chem. 18 (2011) 2661–2672.

[37] J. Chen, S. Mangelinckx, A. Adams, Z.T. Wang, W.L. Li, N. de Kimpe, Natural flavonoids as potential herbal medication for the treatment of diabetes mellitus and its complications, Nat. Prod. Commun. 10 (2015) 187–200.

[38] Y.J. Liu, J. Zhan, X.L. Liu, Y. Wang, J. Ji, Q.Q. He, Dietary flavonoids intake and risk of type 2 diabetes: a meta-analysis of prospective cohort studies, Clin. Nutr. 33 (2014) 59–63.

[39] R. Zamora-Ros, N.G. Forouhi, S.J. Sharp, C.A. González, B. Buijsse, M. Guevara, Y.T. van der Schouw, P. Amiano, H. Boeing, L. Bredsdorff, G. Fagherazzi, E.J. Feskens, P.W. Franks, S. Grioni, V. Katzke, T.J. Key, K.T. Khaw, T. Kühn, G. Masala, A. Mattiello, E. Molina-Montes, P.M. Nilsson, K. Overvad, F. Perquier, M.L. Redondo, F. Ricceri, O. Rolandsson, I. Romieu, N. Roswall, A. Scalbert, M. Schulze, N. Slimani, A.M.W. Spijkerman, A. Tjonneland, M.J. Tormo, M. Touillaud, R. Tumino, L.A. van der Daphne, G.J. van Woudenbergh, C. Langenberg, E. Riboli, N.J. Wareham, Dietary intakes of individual flavanols and flavonols are inversely associated with incident type 2 diabetes in European populations, J. Nutr. 144 (2014) 335–343.

[40] F. Squadrito, H. Marini, A. Bitto, D. Altavilla, F. Polito, E.B. Adamo, R. D'Anna, V. Arcoraci, B.P. Burnett, L. Minutoli, A. di Benedetto, G. di Vieste, D. Cucinotta, C. de Gregorio, S. Russo, F. Corrado, A. Saitta, C. Irace, S. Corrao, G. Licata, Genistein in the metabolic syndrome: results of a randomized clinical trial, J. Clin. Endocrinol. Metab. 98 (2013) 3366–3374.

[41] S. Mohan, L. Nandhakumar, Role of various flavonoids: hypotheses on novel approach to treat diabetes, J. Med. Hypotheses Ideas 8 (2014) 1–6.

[42] V. Saibabu, Z. Fatima, L.A. Khan, S. Hameed, Therapeutic potential of dietary phenolic acids, Adv. Pharmacol. Sci. 2015 (2015) 1–10.

[43] R. Vinayagam, M. Jayachandran, B. Xu, Antidiabetic effects of simple phenolic acids: a comprehensive review, Phytother. Res. 30 (2016) 184–199.

[44] J.A. Greenberg, C.N. Boozer, A. Geliebter, Coffee, diabetes, and weight control, Am. J. Clin. Nutr. 84 (2006) 682–693.

[45] M.F. McCarty, Nutraceutical resources for diabetes prevention—an update, Med. Hypotheses 64 (2005) 151–158.

[46] Y.G. Cherng, C.C. Tsai, H.H. Chung, Y.W. Lai, S.C. Kuo, J.T. Cheng, Antihyperglycemic action of sinapic acid in diabetic rats, J. Agric. Food Chem. 61 (2013) 12053–12059.

[47] H.J. Eun, R.K. Sung, K.H. In, Y.H. Tae, Hypoglycemic effects of a phenolic acid fraction of rice bran and ferulic acid in C57BL/KsJ-db/db mice, J. Agric. Food Chem. 55 (2007) 9800–9804.

[48] S. Meng, J. Cao, Q. Feng, J. Peng, Y. Hu, Roles of chlorogenic acid on regulating glucose and lipids metabolism: a review, Evid. Based Complement. Alternat. Med. 2013 (2013), 801457.

[49] L. Vetterli, T. Brun, L. Giovannoni, D. Bosco, P. Maechler, Resveratrol potentiates glucose-stimulated insulin secretion in INS-1E β-cells and human islets through a SIRT1-dependent mechanism, J. Biol. Chem. 286 (2011) 6049–6060.

[50] Y.Yao, X. Zhao, J. Xin, Y. Wu, H. Li, Coumarins improved type 2 diabetes induced by high-fat diet and streptozotocin in mice via antioxidation, Can. J. Physiol. Pharmacol. 96 (2018) 765–771.

[51] L. Pari, N. Rajarajeswari, Efficacy of coumarin on hepatic key enzymes of glucose metabolism in chemical induced type 2 diabetic rats, Chem. Biol. Interact. 181 (2009) 292–296.

[52] H. Li, Y. Yao, L. Li, Coumarins as potential antidiabetic agents, J. Pharm. Pharmacol. 69 (2017) 1253–1264.

[53] H. El-Seedi, M. El-Barbary, D. El-Ghorab, L. Bohlin, A.-K. Borg-Karlson, U. Goransson, R. Verpoorte, Recent insights into the biosynthesis and biological activities of natural xanthones, Curr. Med. Chem. 17 (2010) 854–901.

[54] E.J. Seo, M.J. Curtis-Long, B.W. Lee, H.Y. Kim, Y.B. Ryu, T.S. Jeong, W.S. Lee, K.H. Park, Xanthones from Cudrania tricuspidata displaying potent α-glucosidase inhibition, Bioorg. Med. Chem. Lett. 17 (2007) 6421–6424.

[55] B. Dineshkumar, A. Mitra, M. Manjunatha, Studies on the anti-diabetic and hypolipidemic potentials of mangiferin (xanthone glucoside) in streptozotocin-induced type 1 and type 2 diabetic model rats, Int. J. Adv. Pharm. Res. 1 (2010) 75–85.

[56] N. Karim, M.A. Rahman, S. Changlek, J. Tangpong, Short-time administration of xanthone from Garcinia mangostana fruit pericarp attenuates the hepatotoxicity and renotoxicity of type II diabetes mice, J. Am. Coll. Nutr. 39 (2020) 501–510.

[57] E. Öztürk, A.K.K. Arslan, M.B. Yerer, A. Bishayee, Resveratrol and diabetes: a critical review of clinical studies, Biomed. Pharmacother. 95 (2017) 230–234.

[58] T. Szkudelski, K. Szkudelska, Resveratrol and diabetes: from animal to human studies, Biochim. Biophys. Acta Mol. Basis Dis. 1852 (2015) 1145–1154.

[59] N.G. Vallianou, A. Evangelopoulos, C. Kazazis, Resveratrol and diabetes, Rev. Diabet. Stud. 10 (2013) 236–242.

[60] Z. Kerem, I. Bilkis, M.A. Flaishman, L. Sivan, Antioxidant activity and inhibition of α-glucosidase by trans-resveratrol, piceid, and a novel trans-stilbene from the roots of Israeli Rumex bucephalophorus L, J. Agric. Food Chem. 54 (2006) 1243–1247.

[61] J. Kershaw, K.H. Kim, The therapeutic potential of Piceatannol, a natural stilbene, in metabolic diseases: a review, J. Med. Food 20 (2017) 1–12.

[62] W. Zhu, S. Chen, Z. Li, X. Zhao, W. Li, Y. Sun, Z. Zhang, W. Ling, X. Feng, Effects and mechanisms of resveratrol on the amelioration of oxidative stress and hepatic steatosis in KKAy mice, Nutr. Metab. 11 (2014) 1–11.

[63] S.J. Yang, Y. Lim, Resveratrol ameliorates hepatic metaflammation and inhibits NLRP3 inflammasome activation, Metab. Clin. Exp. 63 (2014) 693–701.

[64] B.T. Jeon, E.A. Jeong, H.J. Shin, Y. Lee, D.H. Lee, H.J. Kim, S.S. Kang, G.J. Cho, W.S. Choi, G.S. Roh, Resveratrol attenuates obesity-associated peripheral and central inflammation and improves memory deficit in mice fed a high-fat diet, Diabetes 61 (2012) 1444–1454.

[65] X. Zhu, C. Wu, S. Qiu, X. Yuan, L. Li, Effects of resveratrol on glucose control and insulin sensitivity in subjects with type 2 diabetes: systematic review and meta-analysis, Nutr. Metab. 14 (2017) 60.

[66] N. Pannu, A. Bhatnagar, Resveratrol: from enhanced biosynthesis and bioavailability to multitargeting chronic diseases, Biomed. Pharmacother. 109 (2019) 2237–2251.

[67] N.D. Westcott, A.D. Muir, Flax seed lignan in disease prevention and health promotion, Phytochem. Rev. 2 (2003) 401–417.

[68] C. Andres-Lacueva, A. Medina-Remon, R. Llorach, M. Urpi-Sarda, N. Khan, G. Chiva-Blanch, R. Zamora-Ros, M. Rotches-Ribalta, R.M. Lamuela-Raventos, Phenolic compounds: chemistry and occurrence in fruits and vegetables, in: L.A. de la Rosa, E. Alvarez-Parrilla, G.A. Gonzalez-Aguilar (Eds.), Fruit and Vegetable

Phytochemicals: Chemistry, Nutritional Value and Stability, John Wiley & Sons, New Delhi, India, 2010, pp. 53–88.

[69] A. Pan, W. Demark-Wahnefried, X. Ye, Z. Yu, H. Li, Q. Qi, J. Sun, Y. Chen, X. Chen, Y. Liu, X. Lin, Effects of a flaxseed-derived lignan supplement on C-reactive protein, IL-6 and retinol-binding protein 4 in type 2 diabetic patients, Br. J. Nutr. 101 (2009) 1145–1149.

[70] Z. Xu, X. Wang, M. Zhou, L. Ma, Y. Deng, H. Zhang, A. Zhao, Y. Zhang, W. Jia, The antidiabetic activity of total lignan from Fructus Arctii against alloxan-induced diabetes in mice and rats, Phytother. Res. 22 (2008) 97–101.

[71] P. Kanu, J. Bahsoon, J. Kanu, J. Kandeh, Nutraceutical importance of sesame seed and oil: a review of the contribution of their lignans, Sierra Leone J. Biomed. Res. 2 (2010) 4–16.

[72] P. Dhar, K. Chattopadhyay, D. Bhattacharyya, S. Ghosh, Antioxidative effect of sesame lignans in diabetes mellitus blood: an in vitro study, J. Oleo Sci. 54 (2005) 39–43.

[73] H. Khan, H. Ullah, S.M. Nabavi, Mechanistic insights of hepatoprotective effects of curcumin: therapeutic updates and future prospects, Food Chem. Toxicol. 124 (2019) 182–191.

[74] D.W. Zhang, M. Fu, S.H. Gao, J.L. Liu, Curcumin and diabetes: a systematic review, Evid. Based Complement. Alternat. Med. 2013 (2013) 1–16.

[75] H. Sasaki, Y. Sunagawa, K. Takahashi, A. Imaizumi, H. Fukuda, T. Hashimoto, H. Wada, Y. Katanasaka, H. Kakeya, M. Fujita, K. Hasegawa, T. Morimoto, Innovative preparation of curcumin for improved oral bioavailability, Biol. Pharm. Bull. 34 (2011) 660–665.

[76] R.V. Farese, Insulin-sensitive phospholipid signaling systems and glucose transport. Update II, Exp. Biol. Med. 226 (2001) 283–295.

[77] P. Wang, C. Su, H. Feng, X. Chen, Y. Dong, Y. Rao, Y. Ren, J. Yang, J. Shi, J. Tian, S. Jiang, Curcumin regulates insulin pathways and glucose metabolism in the brains of APPswe/PS1dE9 mice, Int. J. Immunopathol. Pharmacol. 30 (2017) 25–43.

[78] Y. Bustanji, M.O. Taha, I.M. Almasri, M.A.S. Al-Ghussein, M.K. Mohammad, H.S. Alkhatib, Inhibition of glycogen synthase kinase by curcumin: investigation by simulated molecular docking and subsequent in vitro/in vivo evaluation, J. Enzyme Inhib. Med. Chem. 24 (2009) 771–778.

[79] J. Chiu, Z.A. Khan, H. Farhangkhoee, S. Chakrabarti, Curcumin prevents diabetes-associated abnormalities in the kidneys by inhibiting p300 and nuclear factor-κB, Nutrition 25 (2009) 964–972.

[80] M. Xia, Z. Ye, Y. Shi, L. Zhou, Y. Hua, Curcumin improves diabetes mellitus-associated cerebral infarction by increasing the expression of GLUT1 and GLUT3, Mol. Med. Rep. 17 (2018) 1963–1969.

[81] M. Azhdari, M. Karandish, A. Mansoori, Metabolic benefits of curcumin supplementation in patients with metabolic syndrome: a systematic review and meta-analysis of randomized controlled trials, Phytother. Res. 33 (2019) 1289–1301.

[82] M.A. El-Moselhy, A. Taye, S.S. Sharkawi, S.F.I. El-Sisi, A.F. Ahmed, The antihyperglycemic effect of curcumin in high fat diet fed rats. Role of TNF-α and free fatty acids, Food Chem. Toxicol. 49 (2011) 1129–1140.

[83] M.T. Abdel Aziz, M.F. El-Asmar, I.N. El-Ibrashy, A.M. Rezq, A.L. Al-Malki, M.A. Wassef, H.H. Fouad, H.H. Ahmed, F.M. Taha, A.A. Hassouna, H.M. Morsi, Effect of novel water soluble curcumin derivative on experimental type-1 diabetes mellitus (short term study), Diabetol. Metab. Syndr. 4 (2012) 30.

[84] D.K. Mahapatra, V. Asati, S.K. Bharti, Chalcones and their therapeutic targets for the management of diabetes: structural and pharmacological perspectives, Eur. J. Med. Chem. 92 (2015) 839–865.

[85] T. Enoki, H. Ohnogi, K. Nagamine, Y. Kudo, K. Sugiyama, M. Tanabe, E. Kobayashi, H. Sagawa, I. Kato, Antidiabetic activities of chalcones isolated from a Japanese herb, Angelica keiskei, J. Agric. Food Chem. 55 (2007) 6013–6017.

[86] T. Zhang, K. Sawada, N. Yamamoto, H. Ashida, 4-Hydroxyderricin and xanthoangelol from Ashitaba (Angelica keiskei) suppress differentiation of preadiopocytes to adipocytes via AMPK and MAPK pathways, Mol. Nutr. Food Res. 57 (2013) 1729–1740.
[87] S. Rocha, A. Sousa, D. Ribeiro, C.M. Correia, V.L.M. Silva, C.M.M. Santos, A.M.S. Silva, A.N. Araújo, E. Fernandes, M. Freitas, A study towards drug discovery for the management of type 2 diabetes mellitus through inhibition of the carbohydrate-hydrolyzing enzymes α-amylase and α-glucosidase by chalcone derivatives, Food Funct. 10 (2019) 5510–5520.
[88] Y.L. Huang, M.B. Oppong, Y. Guo, L.Z. Wang, S.M. Fang, Y.R. Deng, X.M. Gao, The Oleaceae family: a source of secoiridoids with multiple biological activities, Fitoterapia 136 (2019), 104155.
[89] H. Jemai, A.E.L. Feki, S. Sayadi, Antidiabetic and antioxidant effects of hydroxytyrosol and oleuropein from olive leaves in alloxan-diabetic rats, J. Agric. Food Chem. 57 (2009) 8798–8804.
[90] K. Murotomi, A. Umeno, M. Yasunaga, M. Shichiri, N. Ishida, T. Koike, T. Matsuo, H. Abe, Y. Yoshida, Y. Nakajima, Oleuropein-rich diet attenuates hyperglycemia and impaired glucose tolerance in type 2 diabetes model mouse, J. Agric. Food Chem. 63 (2015) 6715–6722.
[91] A. Khalili, A.A. Nekooeian, M.B. Khosravi, Oleuropein improves glucose tolerance and lipid profile in rats with simultaneous renovascular hypertension and type 2 diabetes, J. Asian Nat. Prod. Res. 19 (2017) 1011–1021.
[92] G. Dhanavathy, Immunohistochemistry, histopathology, and biomarker studies of swertiamarin, a secoiridoid glycoside, prevents and protects streptozotocin-induced β-cell damage in Wistar rat pancreas, J. Endocrinol. Invest. 38 (2015) 669–684.
[93] U.R. Potunuru, K.V. Priya, M.K.N.S. Varsha, N. Mehta, S. Chandel, N. Manoj, T. Raman, M. Ramar, M.M. Gromiha, M. Dixit, Amarogentin, a secoiridoid glycoside, activates AMP-activated protein kinase (AMPK)to exert beneficial vasculo-metabolic effects, Biochim. Biophys. Acta Gen. Subj. 1863 (2019) 1270–1282.
[94] A. Kumar, S. Aswal, R.B. Semwal, A. Chauhan, S.K. Joshi, D.K. Semwal, Role of plant-derived alkaloids against diabetes and diabetes-related complications: a mechanism-based approach, Phytochem. Rev. 18 (2019) 1277–1298.
[95] R. Singh, A mini review on antidiabetic plant derived alkaloids, Indian J. Sci. Res. 10 (2) (2020) 137–142.
[96] T.K. Tabopda, J. Ngoupayo, J. Liu, A.C. Mitaine-Offer, S.A.K. Tanoli, S.N. Khan, M.S. Ali, B.T. Ngadjui, E. Tsamo, M.A. Lacaille-Dubois, B. Luu, Bioactive aristolactams from Piper umbellatum, Phytochemistry 69 (2008) 1726–1731.
[97] K. Takada, T. Uehara, Y. Nakao, S. Matsunaga, R.W.M. van Soest, N. Fusetani, Schulzeines A-C, new α-glucosidase inhibitors from the marine sponge Penares schulzei, J. Am. Chem. Soc. 126 (2004) 187–193.
[98] N. Asano, T. Yamashita, K. Yasuda, K. Ikeda, H. Kizu, Y. Kameda, A. Kato, R.J. Nash, H.S. Lee, K.S. Ryu, Polyhydroxylated alkaloids isolated from mulberry trees (Morus alba L.) and silkworms (Bombyx mori L.), J. Agric. Food Chem. 49 (2001) 4208–4213.
[99] B. Dineshkumar, A. Mitra, M. Mahadevappa, Antidiabetic and hypolipidemic effects of mahanimbine (carbazole alkaloid) from Murraya koenigii (rutaceae) leaves, Int. J. Phytomedicine 2 (2010) 22–30.
[100] M. Shibano, D. Tsukamoto, A. Masuda, Y. Tanaka, G. Kusano, Two new pyrrolidine alkaloids, radicamines A and B, as inhibitors of α-glucosidase from Lobelia chinensis Lour, Chem. Pharm. Bull. 49 (2001) 1362–1365.
[101] S.H. Tiong, C.Y. Looi, A. Arya, W.F. Wong, H. Hazni, M.R. Mustafa, K. Awang, Vindogentianine, a hypoglycemic alkaloid from Catharanthus roseus (L.) G. Don (Apocynaceae), Fitoterapia 102 (2015) 182–188.

[102] H. Gao, Y.N. Huang, B. Gao, P. Li, C. Inagaki, J. Kawabata, Inhibitory effect on α-glucosidase by Adhatoda vasica Nees, Food Chem. 108 (2008) 965–972.
[103] L. Zajoncova, P. Kosina, J. Vicar, J. Ulrichová, P. Pec, Study of the inhibition of alpha-amylase by the benzo[c]phenanthridine alkaloids sanguinarine and chelerythrine, J. Enzyme Inhib. Med. Chem. 20 (2005) 261–267.
[104] W.L. Baker, E.L. Baker, C.I. Coleman, The effect of plant sterols or stanols on lipid parameters in patients with type 2 diabetes: a meta-analysis, Diabetes Res. Clin. Pract. 84 (2009) e33–e37.
[105] T. Belwal, A. Bisht, H.P. Devkota, H. Ullah, H. Khan, A. Pandey, I.D. Bhatt, J. Echeverría, Phytopharmacology and clinical updates of Berberis species against diabetes and other metabolic diseases, Front. Pharmacol. 11 (2020) 41.
[106] L. Calpe-Berdiel, J.C. Escolà-Gil, N. Rotllan, F. Blanco-Vaca, Phytosterols do not change susceptibility to obesity, insulin resistance, and diabetes induced by a high-fat diet in mice, Metab. Clin. Exp. 57 (2008) 1497–1501.
[107] M.-I. Christodoulou, J. Tchoumtchoua, A.-L. Skaltsounis, A. Scorilas, M. Halabalaki, Natural alkaloids intervening the insulin pathway: new hopes for anti-diabetic agents? Curr. Med. Chem. 26 (2018) 5982–6015.
[108] T. Coyne, T.I. Ibiebele, P.D. Baade, A. Dobson, C. McClintock, S. Dunn, D. Leonard, J. Shaw, Diabetes mellitus and serum carotenoids: findings of a population-based study in Queensland, Australia, Am. J. Clin. Nutr. 82 (2005) 685–693.
[109] A. de Filippis, H. Ullah, A. Baldi, M. Dacrema, C. Esposito, E.U. Garzarella, C. Santarcangelo, A. Tantipongpiradet, M. Daglia, Gastrointestinal disorders and metabolic syndrome: Dysbiosis as a key link and common bioactive dietary components useful for their treatment, Int. J. Mol. Sci. 21 (2020) 4929.
[110] S. Jagtap, P. Khare, P. Mangal, K.K. Kondepudi, M. Bishnoi, K.K. Bhutani, Effect of mahanimbine, an alkaloid from curry leaves, on high-fat diet-induced adiposity, insulin resistance, and inflammatory alterations, Biofactors 43 (2017) 220–231.
[111] S.J. Jiang, H. Dong, J.B. Li, L.J. Xu, X. Zou, K.F. Wang, F.E. Lu, P. Yi, Berberine inhibits hepatic gluconeogenesis via the LKB1-AMPK-TORC2 signaling pathway in streptozotocin-induced diabetic rats, World J. Gastroenterol. 21 (2015) 7777–7785.
[112] S. Kook, G.H. Kim, K. Choi, The antidiabetic effect of onion and garlic in experimental diabetic rats: meta-analysis, J. Med. Food 12 (2009) 552–560.
[113] K. Li, L. Zhang, J. Xue, X. Yang, X. Dong, L. Sha, H. Lei, X. Zhang, L. Zhu, Z. Wang, X. Li, H. Wang, P. Liu, Y. Dong, L. He, Dietary inulin alleviates diverse stages of type 2 diabetes mellitus: via anti-inflammation and modulating gut microbiota in db/db mice, Food Funct. 10 (2019) 1915–1927.
[114] S. Liu, U. Ajani, C. Chae, C. Hennekens, J.E. Buring, J.A.E. Manson, Long-term β-carotene supplementation and risk of type 2 diabetes mellitus: a randomized controlled trial, JAMA 282 (1999) 1073–1075.
[115] Y. Liu, H. Qi, Y. Wang, M. Wu, Y. Cao, W. Huang, L. Li, Z. Ji, H. Sun, Allicin protects against myocardial apoptosis and fibrosis in streptozotocin-induced diabetic rats, Phytomedicine 19 (2012) 693–698.
[116] N. Lolok, H.M. Mashar, I. Annah, A. Saleh, W.O. Yuliastri, M. Isrul, Antidiabetic effect of the combination of garlic peel extract (Allium sativum) and onion peel (Allium cepa) in rats with oral-glucose tolerance method, Res. J. Pharm. Technol. 12 (2019) 2153–2156.
[117] S. Melino, S. Leo, V.T. Papajani, Natural hydrogen sulfide donors from Allium sp. as a nutraceutical approach in type 2 diabetes prevention and therapy, Nutrients 11 (2019) 1581.
[118] E. Misawa, M. Tanaka, K. Nomaguchi, K. Nabeshima, M. Yamada, T. Toida, K. Iwatsuki, Oral ingestion of Aloe vera phytosterols alters hepatic gene expression profiles

and ameliorates obesity-associated metabolic disorders in Zucker diabetic fatty rats, J. Agric. Food Chem. 60 (2012) 2799–2806.

[119] J. Montonen, P. Knekt, R. Järvinen, A. Reunanen, Dietary antioxidant intake and risk of type 2 diabetes, Diabetes Care 27 (2004) 362–366.

[120] S. Nishikawa, M. Hosokawa, K. Miyashita, Fucoxanthin promotes translocation and induction of glucose transporter 4 in skeletal muscles of diabetic/obese KK-Ay mice, Phytomedicine 19 (2012) 389–394.

[121] A. Roohbakhsh, G. Karimi, M. Iranshahi, Carotenoids in the treatment of diabetes mellitus and its complications: a mechanistic review, Biomed. Pharmacother. 91 (2017) 31–42.

[122] T. Sasaki, W. Li, K. Higai, K. Koike, Canthinone alkaloids are novel protein tyrosine phosphatase 1B inhibitors, Bioorg. Med. Chem. Lett. 25 (2015) 1979–1981.

[123] S.N. Shah, S.L. Bodhankar, S.L. Badole, H.V. Kamble, V. Mohan, Effect of trigonelline: an active compound from Trigonella foenumgraecum Linn. in alloxan induced diabetes in mice, Cell Tissue Res. 6 (2006) 585.

[124] M. Tanaka, E. Misawa, Y. Ito, N. Habara, K. Nomaguchi, M. Yamada, T. Toida, H. Hayasawa, M. Takase, M. Inagaki, R. Higuchi, Identification of five phytosterols from Aloe vera gel as anti-diabetic compounds, Biol. Pharm. Bull. 29 (2006) 1418–1422.

[125] C.-Y. Tsai, C.-C. Wang, T.-Y. Lai, H.-N. Tsu, C.-H. Wang, H.-Y. Liang, W.-W. Kuo, Antioxidant effects of diallyl trisulfide on high glucose-induced apoptosis are mediated by the PI3K Akt-dependent activation of Nrf2 in cardiomyocytes, Int. J. Cardiol. 168 (2013) 1286–1297.

[126] H. Ullah, A. Khan, N.U. Rehman, S.A. Halim, H. Khan, I. Khan, R. Csuk, A. Al-Rawahi, S. Al-Hatmi, A. Al-Harrasi, Lophenol and lathosterol from resin of Commiphora kua possess hepatoprotective effects in vivo, J. Ethnopharmacol. 252 (2020), 112558.

[127] L.M. Xiu, A.B. Miura, K. Yamamoto, T. Kobayashi, Q.H. Song, H. Kitamura, J.C. Cyong, Pancreatic islet regeneration by ephedrine in mice with streptozotocin-induced diabetes, Am. J. Chin. Med. 29 (2001) 493–500.

CHAPTER 7

Phytonutrients in the management of lipids metabolism

Shabana Bibi[a,b], Mohammad Mehedi Hasan[c], Partha Biswas[d], Anastasiia Shkodina[e], Muhammad Ajmal Shah[f], Ghulam Mujtaba Shah[f,g], Ajmal Khan[h], and Ahmed Al-Harrasi[h]

[a]Yunnan Herbal Laboratory, School of Ecology and Environmental Sciences, Yunnan University, Kunming, China
[b]Research Center for Sustainable Utilization of Cordyceps Bioresources in China and Southeast Asia, Yunnan University, Kunming, China
[c]Department of Biochemistry and Molecular Biology, Mawlana Bhashani Science and Technology University, Tangail, Bangladesh
[d]Department of Genetic Engineering and Biotechnology, Faculty of Biological Science and Technology, Jashore University of Science and Technology (JUST), Jashore, Bangladesh
[e]Poltava State Medical University, Poltava, Ukraine
[f]Department of Pharmacy, Hazara University, Mansehra, Pakistan
[g]Department of Botany, Hazara University, Mansehra, Pakistan
[h]Natural and Medical Sciences Research Centre, University of Nizwa, Nizwa, Oman

1. Introduction

The metabolism of lipid is a complicated strategical process in which several steps are involved, including the consumption of lipids in the body through the diet (exogenous) and the transformation of these lipids inside the body (endogenous) into various compounds catalyzing by several catabolic or anabolic enzymes of lipid metabolism [1]. Mainly, lipids are a source of energy and can also be stored in body cells for proper cellular functions. They are a heterogeneous category of fats or fat-containing compounds known as fatty acids, waxes, neutral fats, and steroids. When they are degraded, they can also produce lipoproteins, phospholipids, and glycolipids. In the body, lipids can travel in the bloodstream as lipoproteins, also as apoproteins. The lipoprotein complexes also act as ligands to the distinct receptors for their signal transduction and regulate enzymatic activity [2].

When abnormal lipid metabolism occurs in our body, it causes various metabolic difficulties including diseases like obesity, hypertension, cardiovascular diseases, insulin resistance-related disorders, and atherogenic dyslipidemia, which are the most common and severe health abnormalities in modern society [3]. In this modern world filled with food

The Role of Phytonutrients in Metabolic Disorders
https://doi.org/10.1016/B978-0-12-824356-5.00010-2

adulteration, people from different age groups are being affected with abnormal lipid-metabolism-associated diseases. A case-control study among the 51,462 patients with metabolic disorder related to cardiovascular disease (age within 62.6 years) have demonstrated that after about 3 years, 919 patients have died, about 1650 patients were hospitalized with atherosclerosis complications, and 1510 hospitalizations with heart stroke incidence [4].

The disorders of lipid metabolism are primarily of two types; one is hyperlipoproteinemia, which has been considered as single-gene-disorder (that can be transmitted through the mechanisms of autosomal dominant or recessive), and another is a type of multifactorial disorders that are caused by both genetic and environmental factors. These two categories of disorders are very significant for therapeutic reasons [5]. The xanthoma disorder can represent lipid diseases, which are important because they can help in the diagnosis and treatment of several types of hyperlipidemias [6].

Additionally, phytonutrients, which are conserved in the plant as edible food source, can play an essential part in controlling the critical functioning of the human body. The common phytonutrients, which are contained in plant-based food provide nutrients, including carbohydrates, vitamins, proteins, minerals, and lipids [7]. These phytonutrients have such a profound effect on human health and demonstrate high potential therapeutic activity for both the deterrence and treatment of several physiological disorders in humans [7].

Moreover, the phytonutrients can also regulate and maintain the body's immune function to suppress specific diseases and being natural products, they show potential clinical activities that are generally compared with chemotherapy or radiotherapy [8]. Several dietary carbohydrates from the plant can control lipidemia and triglyceridemia in both human and animal bodies [9]. The mechanisms of their serum lipid-lowering effect have been demonstrated. Oligofructose, which is the main ingredient of edible phytonutrients, can decrease triacylglycerol in VLDL when given to rats [10].

There is no significant information about the consumption of organic phytonutrients in the human diet because it is critical to obtain the ingredients from the food in the mixed diet and the crops which are enriched with specific types of phytonutrients [11]. More clinical research activities are required to effectively elucidate the strategy of absorption, function, and the role of several phytonutrients in human health and reveal how they regulate the disorders of lipid metabolism for implementing the therapeutic potential of several phytonutrients in metabolic disorders.

2. Disorders of lipid metabolism

Two main clinical disorders are mostly related to lipoprotein disorders in which a high level of triglyceride is the major cause of pancreatitis. Particularly, the high concentration of LDL and the low concentration of HDL facilitate coronary artery disease. Plasma lipid levels depend mostly on lifestyle such as high-fat diets that promote plasma cholesterol. In particular, NCEP (The National Cholesterol Education Program) prepared a standardized estimate of cholesterol levels and individuals at risk for cardiovascular disease (CVD) were classified accordingly. In 2001, NCEP categorized the concentrations of 200 mg/dL cholesterol as desirable, 200–240 mg/dL as moderately elevated, and more than 240 mg/dL as excessive [12]. The cholesterol level is lower in children because lipid level increases with age [13]. More than 500 mg/dL of triglyceride concentration poses a heightened likelihood of pancreatitis. When triglyceride levels are higher than 2000 mg/dL, this extreme hypertriglyceridemia can cause pancreatitis. [14]. Lipoproteins vary in metabolic pathways, physiology functions, and pathologic significance. Fig. 1, Depicts the common metabolic disorders of lipid metabolism.

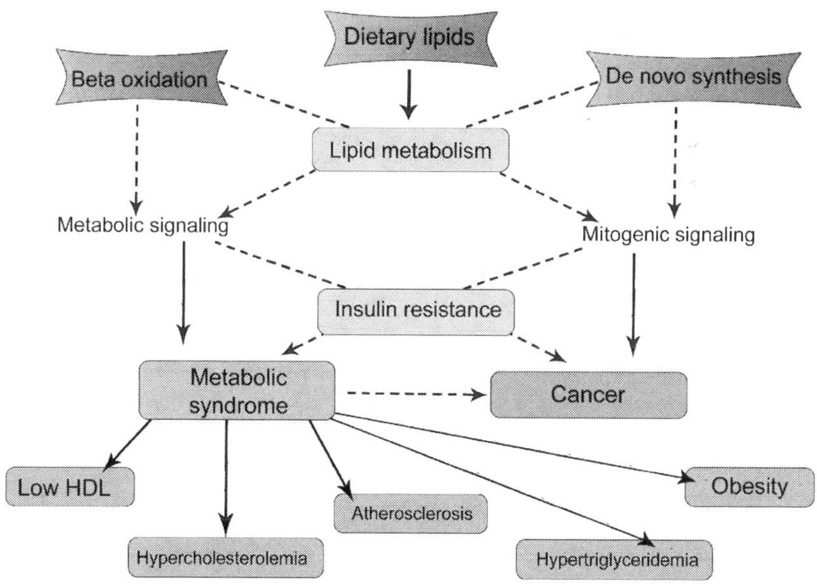

Fig. 1 Dysregulation of lipid metabolism can confer metabolic disorders and trigger cancer.

3. Hypertriglyceridemia

Fasting hyperchylomicronemia is a typical instance of acute hypertriglyceridemia. This may be caused by chylomicron metabolism defect and the lipoprotein lipase (LPL) saturation to catabolize triglycerides (TGs) into free fatty acids (FAs). When TG levels exceed 500 mg/dL, the LPL saturation occurs. Various dietary and environmental agents govern triglyceride production. Alcohol is the most common agent for triglyceride production. Fructose also plays a significant role in lipid production though it has less effect on triglyceride circulation [15].

Genetic defects in LPL have been reported in patients from diverse ethnicity and race, [16] and a particular alteration in gene level has been found as a common genetic defect in the Canadian French population. LPL defects are the primary reason in nearly 50% of the reported severe hypertriglyceridemia cases as it renders the LPL protein inactive, although abnormal protein production has also been identified in the patient body. This is because LPL has many regulator mechanisms that are not dependent on any catalytic activity and hence, an aggressive phenotype is seen in patients with severe defects. Moreover, the genetic complications exerted by LPL revealed that severe hyperchylomicronemia in adulthood is also regulated by LPL abnormalities or other causes [17]. In adults and aged peoples, the most common complication of these defects are obesity and type-2 diabetes, as abnormalities in lipoprotein also give rise to insulin resistance [18]. In addition, a major cause of diabetes is postprandial lipemia [19].

Diabetes mellitus is frequently observed in the cases of hypertriglyceridemia, in which a large proportion of people who are diabetic generally suffer from type-2 diabetes. Insulin lowers the concentration of FA in adipose tissue as well as apoB synthesis in liver, restricts de novo TG production, and ultimately advances the yield of LPL. The vigorous studies conducted on humans demonstrate that TG release increases and the removal of TG from the blood circulation is also lessened in patients with diabetes; most of the time both take place simultaneously [20]. There is also a strong correlation between diabetes and elevated postprandial lipidemia. Diabetic dyslipidemia, which is one of the most familiar form of hypertriglyceridemia, and it reduces the amount of HDL. The low amount of HDL arises from the enzyme hepatic lipase-mediated catalysis of TG-rich HDL via higher VLDL exchange for HDL, which confers rapid bloodstream cleansing of related HDLs [21]. HDL production from TG-rich lipoproteins led to the decrease in the amount of cholesterol that could result from defective lipolysis. The enzyme CETP also enhances the transport of LDL from TGs and facilitates these lipoproteins into probably more atherogenic forms by converting into smaller and denser elements. This type of lipoprotein feature is also found in nonhyperglycemic patients with metabolic disorders. [22]. While most diabetes patients do not have a higher amount of LDL, with better diabetes management, reduction in LDL can be achieved, if any. As discussed before, diabetes is strongly correlated to fatal chylomicronemia and due to heterozygous LPL deficiency, a significant amount of patients may have inherent dyslipidemia, while others cannot be characterized with lipid-metabolism abnormalities [23].

Renal failure is also linked with hypertriglyceridemia and low HDL levels. The connection is not understood yet, but probably it causes underlying insulin resistance and defects in the lipolysis of plasma triglycerides. Increased circulating levels of the LPL inhibitor angiopoietin-like protein 4 happen to have a link with hypertriglyceridemia in nephrotic syndrome [24].

4. Hypercholesterolemia

Since cholesterol is found in all lipoproteins, a dramatic rise of TGs will constantly contribute to higher blood cholesterol concentrations. However, the proportion of TG to cholesterol will be more than five. In this section, the link between primarily increased cholesterol and disorders are discussed. Hypercholesterolemia are discussed and the clinical appearance of hypercholesterolemia is confirmed. Even patients with serious disease conditions sometimes have cosmetic orthopedic or cosmetic complications linked to tendon xanthoma; hypercholesterolemia is normally hidden and revealed while regular blood evaluation during vascular disease screening [25].

The examination by the Brown and Goldstein laboratory investigates the reason of FH and reveals the harmony of the LDL receptor to explain cholesterol mechanism as the cause. This most common reason for fatal hypercholesterolemia leads to abnormalities in the production or function of the LDL receptor protein [26]. Patients who possess familial hypercholesterolemia (FH) with concentration of cholesterol up to 300 mg/dL demonstrate higher severity of the disease condition. The homozygous type of this disease increases cholesterol proportion and exhibits a more than twofold increase in the amount. The heterozygous type of the disease can be as regular as 1 among 200 people [27] and is a main culprit of premature coronary artery disorder. Moreover, stenosis and aortic valve calcification are also the outcome of homozygous and other types of LDL receptor deficiency. [28].

Generally, in this rare disorder dietary sitosterol and other plant sterols are usually absorbed in the intestine in large amounts. Consequently, premature atherosclerosis occurs, in their assortment in the plasma and peripheral tissues [29]. The mutant genes ABCG8 and ABCG5 are responsible for the secretion of absorbed plant sterols. In childhood, the presence of high plasma levels of LDL causes tendon xanthomas, and the diagnosis includes FH and cerebrotendinous xanthomatosis. Gas-liquid chromatography of plasma lipids can confirm the diagnosis that exhibits high levels of plant sterols. Restriction of plant sterols in the diet therapy consists of treatment with ezetimibe that impedes the exploitation of dietary sterols [30].

Most patients with high LDL cholesterol do not have FH; cholesterol levels over 300 mg/dL are not normally combined with xanthomas or defects in the LDL receptor [31]. Regarding the laboratory values, hypercholesterolemia shows a higher cholesterol value that overcomes the 95th percentile for the population whereas only 1–25 of these patients should have FH. Although diet and lifestyle influence LDL, the most exalted LDL cholesterol levels that are attached with the genetic and environmental factors are unknown and this type of hypercholesterolemia is alluded to as polygenic [32]. Generally, the increase of cholesterol levels has a higher risk of coronary artery disease. Increased LDL levels show LDL clearance with normal LDL receptors; sometimes it increases LDL production. This last type occurs in the setting of familial-associated hyperlipoproteinemia, which can be described as a primary exaltation of LDL. Greater LDL production is responsible for greater absorption of gut cholesterol and abnormalities in the adjustment of lipid-regulated nuclear transcription factors also [33].

When defect LDL binds with normal LDL receptors it leads to exalted plasma cholesterol. The LDL ligands that bind with the LDL receptor are apoB100 and apoE. LDL is increased by apoB100 and its phenotype is indistinguishable from that of FH and increased susceptibility to CHD also [34]. When glutamine substitutes for arginine at amino acid 3500 then it reduces LDL binding to the LDL receptor. Often, the LDL exaltation is less severe, then a partial receptor binding deficiency which is attributed to mutation or the continued ability of apoE to mediate lipoprotein elevation [35].

Hyperlipidemia is connected with nephrotic syndrome. Total cholesterol, VLDL, LDL-C, total triglycerides, and plasma apoB may all be exalted.

Liver production of apoB-containing lipoproteins is increased by the nephrotic syndrome. It also increases plasma LDL or VLDL, or both. It can be a response to hypoalbuminemia and a combined generalized increase in liver protein secretion [36].

Thyroid hormone deficiency causes hypercholesterolemia because hyperthyroidism and low levels of thyroid hormone predispose to statin-induced myositis [37]. Owing to reduced LDL clearance, hypothyroidism normally multiplies LDL-C and it can also be combined with high plasma triglyceride levels. In hyperthyroidism, HDL-C is normally unaltered or may be diminished. Hypercholesterolemia is caused by subclinical hypothyroidism that sometimes reacts to thyroid hormone replacement [38].

5. Low HDL-related abnormalities

In general, coronary artery disease is associated with low concentrations of the HDL. Genetic disorders can also mediate lower plasma levels of HDL in the body and impose the risk of coronary artery disease. In addition, these alterations can also lead to rare metabolic phenotypes and diseases, the pathophysiology and underlying mechanism of which are still unknown [39].

Defective conversion of cholesterol to cholesteryl ester is caused by low HDL led by LCAT deficiency. In a cohort of clinical patients, the free cholesterol to cholesteryl ester measurement ratio is diacritic; the percentage increases to more than 90% in LCAT deficiency while normally free cholesterol is approximately 30% of the total. LCAT activity can be determined with a sequencing approach [40]. LCAT deficiency leads to corneal arcus (sometimes directed to marked visual impairment), normochromic anemia, and, occasionally, renal failure in young adults. Despite low HDL concentration, the risk for coronary disease in patients with LCAT deficiency is not pronounced, this reflects the low levels of LDL found in many of these patients [41].

Mutations of the LCAT gene cause fish-eye disease, a variant of LCAT deficiency, and the complete LCAT deficiency is more severe than that seen in mutational phenotypes. Low plasma HDL-C levels and corneal opacities characterize fish-eye disease; renal disease and anemia do not occur. The phenotypic differences between LCAT deficiency and fish-eye disease have been attributed to whether mutations in the LCAT gene encode variants that fail to esterify cholesterol of both HDL and apoB-containing lipoproteins (LCAT deficiency) or of HDL only (fish-eye disease) [42].

Both liver and the small intestine, for complete synthesis of mature HDL, need ABCA1 transporter, a major element for producing HDL. Hypoalphalipoproteinemia is connected with several mutations in this receptor. Since the number of genetic mutations is high, assays also examine cholesterol "unloading" of fibroblasts to apoAI to demonstrate the defect. The most flagrant example of a defect in ABCA1 is Tangier disease [43]. Originally from Tangier Island in the Chesapeake Bay, these patients had hypocholesterolemia due to a marked reduction in plasma HDL as well as low LDL and a striking physical detection of orange tonsils. It is suspected that the orange tonsils originate from faulty reverse cholesterol transfer from reticuloendothelial system macrophages, with the color likely to be caused by carotenoids. With this syndrome, the probability of cardiovascular disease is unknown [44].

ApoAI gene mutations can minimize HDL formation and result in low levels of HDL-C in plasma. Point mutations in the apoAI gene or deletions or gene rearrangements at the gene locus of apoAI/CIII/AIV/AV may cause ApoAI deficiency. Plasma HDL-C levels smaller than 0.3 mmol/L (10 mg/dL) usually arise from ApoAI deficiency and the LCAT is badly triggered by such apoAI variants [42,43]. Protein examination indicating an altered apoAI scale and genetic sequencing are used to make the molecular diagnosis. Amyloidosis is associated with certain apoAI forms. Cysteine substitution of amino acid 173 causes the apoAI Milano version (apoAIMilano) for arginine This, without premature CHD, results in low plasma HDL-C levels. This HDL is also hypothesized to be antiatherogenic and has been used in a clinical trial in humans [44].

6. Atherosclerosis

Atherosclerosis presents complex chronic inflammatory complaints categorized via storage of lipid-loaded fibrous plagues inside the wall of arteries and damage the heart severely, proceeding by the increasing destruction of vessel walls, can conclude with atherosclerotic plague rupture and consequently formation of a thrombus [45]. Foremost, common clinical manifestations associated with it are myocardial infarction or stroke [46]. Initially, atherosclerosis progresses in the endothelium that is the inner layer of artery. The vascular endothelium is a discriminating semipermeable unremitting monolayer of endothelial cells, which is responsible for the management of vascular tone and vascular viscosity through combining a plethora of autocrine and paracrine substances, such as nitric oxide (NO), prostacyclin, histamine, angiotensin II, heparin, tissue plasminogen activator, and plasminogen activator inhibitor-1, and associated with the progression of vascular smooth muscle cell (VSMC), leukocyte migration, platelet accumulation, and adhesion [47,48].

Frequent universal and hemodynamic analysis relating to blood flow risk elements involved in the beginning of endothelial dysfunction, which is the start of plague development [49]. Endothelium incoherence aids the entry of cholesterol-containing low-density lipoprotein (LDL) particles in the inner layer of big arteries [48], a process facilitated by dealings between LDL apolipoprotein B100 and matrix proteoglycans. LDL management influences toward oxidative modification [50], and the resulting oxidized LDLs, by interacting with explicit receptor recognized as lectin-like oxidized LDLs receptor-1, might integrate expression levels of vascular cell adhesion molecule 1 and intercellular adhesion molecule 2 by endothelial cells [51,52]. These explicit adhesion molecules with chemotactic entities, for example monocyte chemo-attractant protine-1 secreted by endothelial cells and VSMC, enable the drifting of the movement of monocytes in the subendothelium, where they differentiate into macrophages. These later adopt an M1 proinflammatory phenotype and encode a wide range of scavenger receptors, beneficial for facilitating the endocytosis oxidized LDLs [53].

Furthermore, mast cells, T cells, and other inflammation mediators enter lesions and along with foam cells, endure a maladaptive proatherosclerotic inflammatory response. Foam cells secrete chemotactic growth factors and metallopeptidases that by the deprivation of the extracellular matrix, sustenance proliferation and migration of VSMC and leukocytes enter into the inner layer of artery [54]. In the inner layer of arteries, the VSMCs yield interstitial collagen and elastin and tolerate a fibrous cap development, which will perform as a shield to plaques. The cap superimposes the macrophage-derived foam cells; few of them pass away through an apoptotic procedure and discharge fats with extracellular storage succeeding the establishment of a lipid-rich pool called the "necrotic core," which progresses toward vulnerability of the plaque [45]. The permanence of the plaques is high in collagen. As a substitute, unsteady plaques have a thin covering on the large fatty core [55] and likely to split and move onwards toward the exposure of tissue factors to blood flow and the stimulation of coagulation cascade with consequential thrombus formation [45,56]. An intraluminal thrombus in the coronary arteries may reduce blood flow triggering ischemic cardiomyopathy and ultimately a complete vascular obstruction will lead to myocardial infarction [57].

7. Obesity

Lipids are fundamental in performing the cellular functions [58–60]. They are particularly involved in building structural features for providing the inflexibility and permeability to biological membranes. Lipids also help to distinguish the characteristics of various organelles by regulating molecular motions across membranes [61,62]. Additionally, they activate the precise biological events as instant messengers and support standby energy stored as lipid droplets [60].

Lipid metabolism (LM) is recognized to unswervingly encourage inflammatory procedures [60,63,64]. Thus, dysregulation in LM motivates the etiology of numerous ailments including diabetes mellitus (DM) and cardiovascular disease (CVD) that is activated by prolonged inflammation. This has provided insight to understand in what way LM is reconfigured in disease development and how it influences the immune responses [65,66]. Particularly, lipid efflux and TLR signaling are firmly related. Homeostatic reactions to cellular lipid loading are facilitated by the liver X receptors, and via transcriptional activity undertake transportation of lipid and its disposal. The natural chemicals for liver X receptors, oxysterols, are generated as a result of macrophage uptake of oxidized LDL [67,68]. Liver X receptors when activated generate the code for genes intricate in lipid efflux comprising ATP-binding cassette (ABC) transporters A1 (ABCA1), ABCD1, and phospholipid transfer protein [69]. While ABCG1 rich in lipids efflux to HDL, ABCA1 presents its function in terms of promoting LDL and phospholipid efflux toward apolipoproteins. Macrophages without the ABCA1 gene highlight the storage of lipids and that go together with the enhanced TLR-mediated proinflammatory signaling cascade. By convention the TLR3- and TLR4-mediated signaling by IRF3 transcription activates and decrease the liver X receptors-induced ABCA1 manifestation that could lead to inhibit the LDL efflux, and promote atherogenic activity [70,71]. Additionally, proinflammatory mediators are also linked with the downregulation of ABCA1. However, TNF-alpha and interleukin-6 are one of the primary cytokines released upon TLR stimulation and upregulation of macrophage ABCA1 by the regulation of NF-kB transcription [72–74]. NF-kB transcription factors might be associated with the progression and resolution of inflammatory mediators upon lipopolysaccharide exposure in vitro and inhibit inflammatory activity in mouse models of contact dermatitis along with inflammatory gene expression in the aortas of atherosclerotic mice [75]. The literature highlights the elaborate association between inflammatory events and lipid efflux that have life-threatening consequences in the context of a multiplicity of LDL-related malfunctioning including CVD [76].

8. Cancer

In mammalian cells, a major portion of the lipid comes from the blood circulation and such lipids are mostly acquired through food components. These lipids can also be synthesized in adipocytes or in liver as fatty-acids (FAs) and subsequently stored in lipid droplets. FAs are vital for various lipid biosynthesis including lipid in cellular membrane, signaling molecules such as Toll-like receptors (TLRs). Fatty acid synthase (FASN), stearoyl-CoA desaturases (SCD), adenosine triphosphate citrate lyase (ACLY), phospholipase D (PLD), phospholipase A2 (PLA2), diacylglycerol acyltransferase (DGAT), acetyl-CoA carboxylase (ACC), phosphatidic acid phosphatase (PAP), monoacylglycerol lipase (MAGL), and carnitine palmitoyl transferase 1 (CPT1) are the major enzymes responsible for FA biosynthesis and hence, critical for the pathogenesis of different forms of carcinoma [77]. Several investigations on cancer cells have explained mechanism of metastasis, which is significantly triggered by the upregulation of FASN [78–82]. Overexpression of FASN is found to be strongly correlated to the metastasis of hepatocellular carcinoma (HCC) and colorectal cancer (CRC) cells [82,83]. FASN was required for epithelial mesenchymal transition (EMT)-induced ovarian and brain carcinoma metastasis [78,81]. SCD is critical for lipid function. SCD1 and SCD5 are the characterized isoforms of SCD in human cells [84,85]. SCD1 expression promotes lymphatic metastasis and strong correlation has been observed between SCD1 upregulation and tumor-node-metastasis (TNM) stage in renal cell carcinoma (RCC). The knockdown of SCD1 gene overexpression limited tumor cell invasion and migration [86]. ACLY catalyzes the formation of cytosolic acetyl-CoA and oxaloacetate in the FA biosynthetic pathway and plays a vital role in tumor cell progression and metastasis by regulating the expression of a number of key target proteins [87,88]. Clinical data has shown that ACLY overexpression leads to the aggressive phenotype of cancer cells in gastric adenocarcinoma patients [89]. DGAT is responsible for converting diacylglycerol (DAG) and fatty acid-CoA to triglycerides (TGs). Lipid synthesis can occur in neoplastic tissues and high expression of DGAT can limit the proliferation of neoplastic cells by suppressing phospholipid synthesis and increasing TGs [90,91]. ACC converts acetyl-CoA to yield malonyl-CoA, which is responsible for lipogenesis and can be present as ACC1 and ACC2 isoforms in the cytosol [92]. Besides, ACC2 functions as a key regulator of FA β-oxidation via the allosteric inhibition of CPT1 [93]. Su et al. reported that in a cohort study of patients with head and neck cancer, ACC overexpression led to overall poor survival [94]. In addition, elevated expression of ACC1 has also demonstrated worse overall survival rate in patients with hepatocellular carcinoma (HCC) [95]. Lipin 1, lipin 2, and lipin 3 genes are critical for PAP activity. Lipins induce the dephosphorylation of phosphatidic acid (PA), which is positively correlated to the metastasis of tumor cells. Furthermore, lipins play a key role in lipid metabolism by regulating the expression of many transcription factors such as SREBP and PPAR [96]. MAGL is an important enzyme of the FA biosynthetic pathways, which catalyzes the synthesis of monoacylglycerols (MGs) from FAs. MAGL upregulation is associated with the cancer cell metastatic phenotype and it is required for the maintenance of the stemness characteristics of tumor cells [97]. In colorectal cancer, MAGL has shown to control cancer cell proliferation and migration via modulating the FA biosynthetic pathway [98]. PLA2 hydrolyzes glycerophospholipids to synthesize FAs and lysophospholipids [99]. Lysophosphatidic acid (LPA) produced by PLA2 is responsible for tumor proliferation. PLA2 stimulates the growth and invasion of ovarian cancer cells and triggers cancer metastasis in vivo [100]. PLD converts phosphatidylcholine (PC) to produce free choline and PA and exists as PLD1 and PLD2 isoforms in human cells and it has been observed to provide tumor cells with strong metastatic advantage [101–103]. Metastasis of lymphoma cells is exacerbated with increasing PLD activity and subsequently, suppression of tumor cell metastasis is evident with PLD2 inhibition [101]. CPT1 induces the conjugation of carnitine to FA and aids in mitochondrial transport. Besides, it also plays an important role in fatty acid oxidation (FAO) [104]. Three identified isoforms of CPT1 are CPT1A, CPT1B, CPT1C, which are localized in the liver, muscle, and brain, respectively [105]. It has been found that CPT1 provides metastatic advantage to hepatocellular carcinoma (HCC) cells in a FAO-dependent manner [95]. The role of lipid-metabolism enzymes involved in anabolic or catabolic lipid metabolism is represented in Fig. 2.

9. The role of phytonutrients in managing lipid-metabolism-associated disorders

Besides arterial hypertension the most frequent risk factor associated with human health is CVD and the main reason for these diseases is abnormal LM [106]. The major disorders due to imbalance of LM are LDL-hypercholesterolemia, hypertriglyceridemia, in a combination of hyperlipoproteinemia and other illnesses due to low HDL cholesterol [5]. The lipoprotein levels can be upgraded by the one or multiple-associated

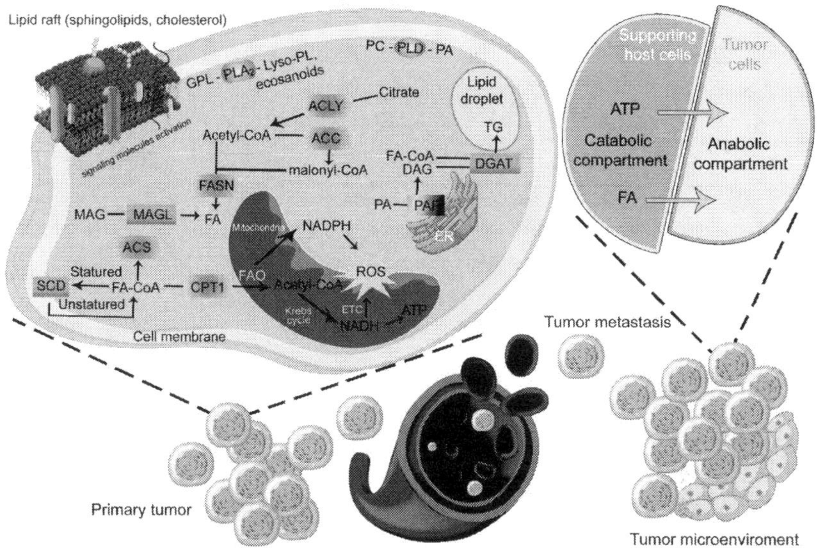

Fig. 2 Role of lipid enzymes in cancer metastasis. Anabolic or catabolic lipid-metabolism enzymes help in fulfilling the metabolic demand of cancer cells and exert metastatic advantage. To help tumors metastasize, cancer cells connect with supporting host cells with lipid biosynthetic pathways in the microenvironment.

disorders of LM because LDL-C is actually the main target to explain the overall risk of CVD; if the patients are on the high risk then atherosclerosis develops [5]. Lipid management is necessary to maintain the heart-related diseases, which is actually the foremost reason of death worldwide; the number of deaths due to CVD could reach 17.9 million deaths per year while it is estimated that it could be nearly 23.6 million deaths by the end of 2030 due to severe heart-related disorders [107,108]. Due to imbalance of cholesterol levels in the body, there is a high risk of chronic heart diseases, cerebrovascular diseases, peripheral artery disease, and aortic atherosclerosis which could lead to death if not properly managed [109,110]. Obesity is one of the most common causes of secondary hyperlipidemia; the evolution of dyslipidemia is associated with the increased levels of triglycerides (TG) and HDL level in the body, which is linked with visceral obesity and other metabolic disorders [111,112]. It is also suggested that diabetic patients also required lipid-lowering therapies to maintain both types of type 1 diabetes mellitus (T1DM) and type 2 diabetes mellitus (T2DM), because there is always the risk of other severe complications due to high LDL-C in diabetic patients [113].

Several phytonutrients isolated from natural sources have presented their broad spectrum of medicinal activities to modulate metabolic processes and also involved in LM and management of cholesterol levels in the body [109]. Bioactive compounds such as small molecular phytonutrients from plants suggested prospective treatments against several diseases such inflammation, oxidative stress, insulin resistance (IR), CVD, and dyslipidemia [114,115]. Green tea, nuts, red wine, vegetables, and fruits contain numerous medicinal monomeric flavanols and oligomeric proanthocyanidins [116].

Flavonoids are an important class of medicinal chemical compounds found in several vegetables, fruits, and plants. Subgroups of flavonoids are flavones, flavonols, flavanonols, catechins, anthocyanins, and chalcones [117]. Numerous flavonoids have proved themselves as remarkable medicinal components and have a high impact on lipid-metabolism-related diseases (Table 1).

Flavanones are essential components of several fruits mostly citrus fruits and present numerous pharmacological properties to treat inflammatory diseases, DM-, TG-, and LM-related diseases [117]. Abyssinone I, a substantial phytochemical derived from *Erythrina lysistemon*, demonstrated HDL-C synthesis and inhibit the development of cholesterol gallstone in a female rat without ovaries [118]. Eriodictyol is a dietary flavanone useful in lowering the cholesterol and lipid profile; the supplementation of eriodictyol has considerably alleviated dyslipidemia and adiposity, enhanced IR by inhibiting the gluconeogenesis in the liver, and inflammation in the diet-induced (DI) obese mice [119]. Nonalcoholic fatty liver disorder, obesity, DM, and cancer proliferation are markedly associated with the imbalanced LM, natural compounds such as eriodictyol are significant in preventing metabolic disorders associated with LM abnormalities [120]. Hesperidin is a major phytonutrient of grapefruit associated with biological activities for atherosclerosis management. Herperidin ameliorated high-fat DI weight gain, and improved IR and ameliorated hyperlipidemia in tested mice; it also suppressed high-fat DI liver abnormalities and atherosclerotic plaque [121]. Naringenin, along with apigenin, improve the regulation of glucose and LM with the amelioration of vascular dysfunction in T2DM [122]. Chemical structure and physicochemical information of abyssinone, eriodictyol, hesperidin, and naringenin flavanones are shown in Table 1.

Organosulfur compounds such as allicin, allyl mercaptan, diallyl disulfide, and diallyl sulfide usually found in garlic, onion, and leek have presented their impact in LM-related abnormalities such as nonalcoholic fatty liver disease (NFLD) in dose-dependent protected obese mice [123] and

Table 1 List of natural chemical compounds associated with the management of lipid-metabolism-related disorders.

Chemical names/ PubChem CID.	Chemical class	Chemical structures	Physiochemical properties	Source
Abyssinones I [CID: 442152]	Flavanone	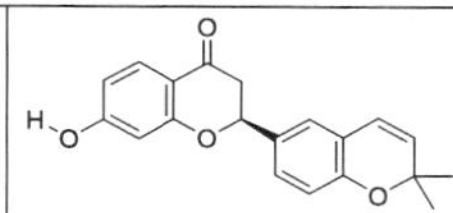	MW = 322.4 XlogP3 = 3.5 HBD = 1 HBA = 4 RB = 1 TPSA = 55.8	French bean seeds
Allicin [CID: 65036]	Organosulfur compound	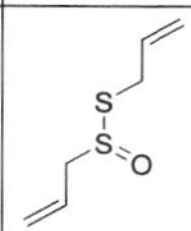	MW = 162.3 XlogP3 = 1.3 HBD = 0 HBA = 3 RB = 5 TPSA = 61.6	Garlic, onion, and leek
Allyl mercaptan [CID: 13367]	Organosulfur compound	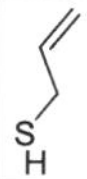	MW = 74.15 XlogP3 = 1.2 HBD = 1 HBA = 1 RB = 1 TPSA = 1	Garlic, onion, leek
Alpha-Carotene [CID:6419725]	Carotenoid	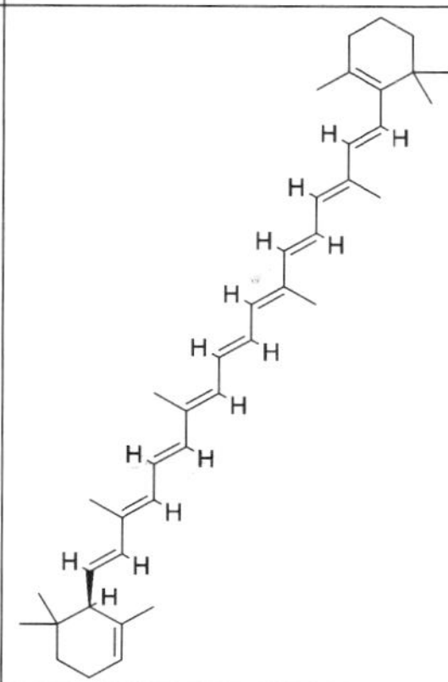	MW = 536.9 XlogP3 = 13.6 HBD = 0 HBA = 0 RB = 10 TPSA = 0	Fruits, vegetables, garlic, leek, maize, onion, pumpkin, tangerines, and cereals.

Continued

Table 1 List of natural chemical compounds associated with the management of lipid-metabolism-related disorders—cont'd

Chemical names/ PubChem CID.	Chemical class	Chemical structures	Physiochemical properties	Source
Apigenin [CID: 5280443]	Flavones	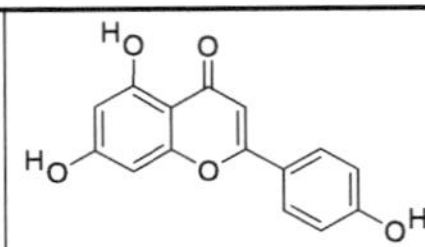	MW = 270.24 XlogP3 = 1.7 HBD = 3 HBA = 5 RB = 1 TPSA = 87	Fruits and vegetables, parsley, celery, celeriac, and chamomile tea
Benzyl (BITC) [CID: 123147]	Isothiocynates	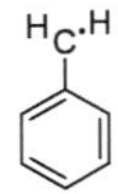	MW = 91.13 XlogP3 = 2.7 HBD = 0 HBA = 0 RB = 0 TPSA = 0	Cruciferous vegetables (e.g., watercress, broccoli)
Beta-Carotene [CID: 5280489]	Carotenoid	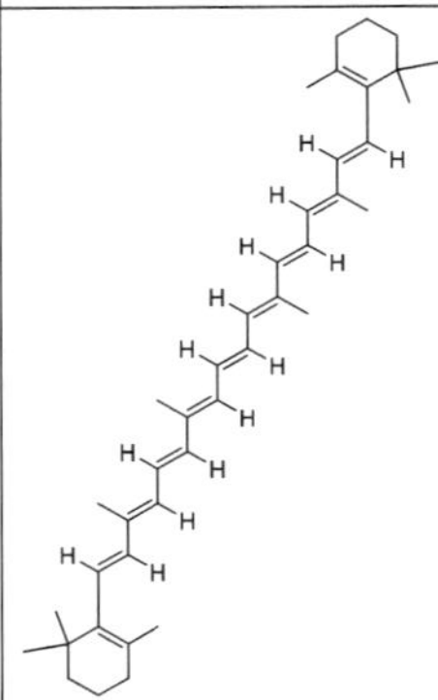	MW = 536.9 XlogP3 = 13.6 HBD = 0 HBA = 0 RB = 10 TPSA = 0	Fruits, vegetables, garlic, leek, maize, onion, pumpkin, tangerines, and cereals

Beta-Glucan [CID: 439262]	Soluble dietary fibers	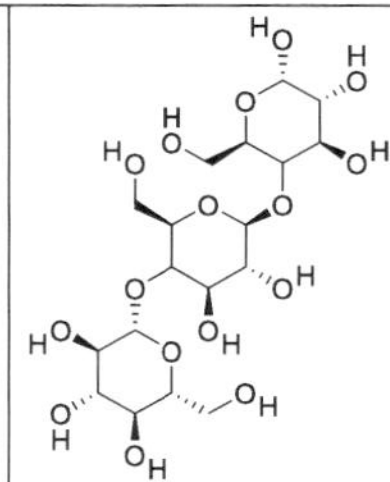	MW = 504.4 XlogP3 = − 6.9 HBD = 11 HBA = 16 RB = 7 TPSA = 269	Fruits, vegetables, legume, cereals, and grains.
Biochanin A [CID: 5280373]	Isoflavone	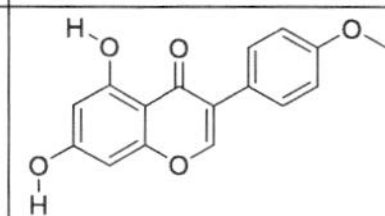	MW = 284.26 XlogP3 = 3 HBD = 2 HBA = 5 RB = 2 TPSA = 76	Red clover, soya, alfalfa sprouts, peanuts, chickpeas, and other legumes
Caffeic acid [CID: 689043]	Phenolic acids	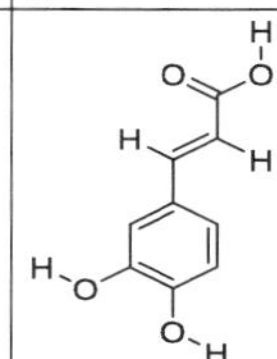	MW = 180.16 XlogP3 = 1.2 HBD = 3 HBA = 4 RB = 2 TPSA = 77.8	Extra virgin olive oil
Campesterol [CID: 173183]	Plant sterols	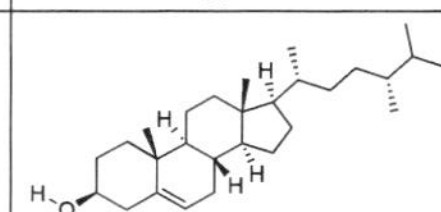	MW = 412.7 XlogP3 = 8.2 HBD = 1 HBA = 1 RB = 5 TPSA = 20.2	Tall oil, soybean oil, and rice bran oil
Catechin [CID: 731601]	Flavonol	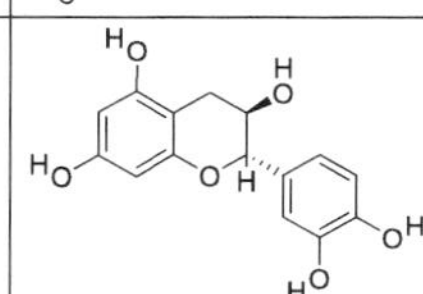	MW = 290.27 XlogP3 = 0.4 HBD = 5 HBA = 6 RB = 1 TPSA = 110	Apple, berries, broccoli, cocoa/chocolate, lettuce, olives, onion, and tea

Continued

Table 1 List of natural chemical compounds associated with the management of lipid-metabolism-related disorders—cont'd

Chemical names/ PubChem CID.	Chemical class	Chemical structures	Physiochemical properties	Source
Daidzein [CID: 5281708]	Isoflavone	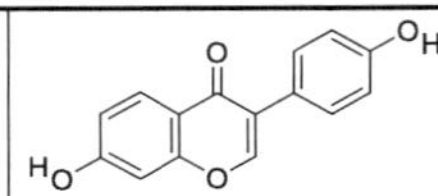	MW = 254.24 XlogP3 = 2.5 HBD = 2 HBA = 4 RB = 1 TPSA = 66.8	Soybeans, tofu, legumes
Delta-Carotene [CID: 5281230]	Carotenoid	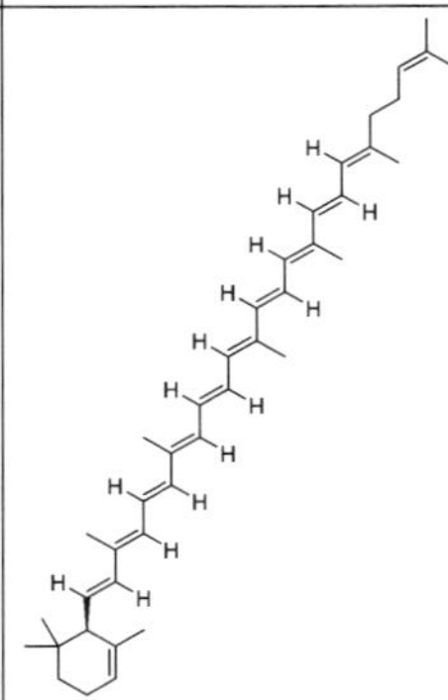	MW = 536.9 XlogP3 = 14.6 HBD = 0 HBA = 0 RB = 13 TPSA = 0	Fruits, vegetables, garlic, leek, maize, onion, pumpkin, tangerines, and cereals.
Diallyl disulfide [CID: 16590]	Organosulfur compound	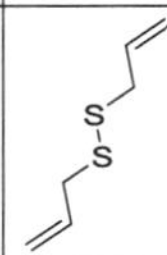	MW = 146.3 XlogP3 = 2.2 HBD = 0 HBA = 2 RB = 5 TPSA = 50.6	Garlic, onion, and leek
Diallyl sulfide [CID: 11617]	Organosulfur compound	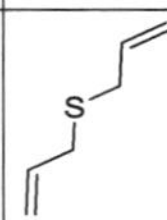	MW = 114.21 XlogP3 = 2.2 HBD = 0 HBA = 1 RB = 4 TPSA = 25.3	Garlic, onion, and leek

Diosmetin [CID: 5281612]	Flavone	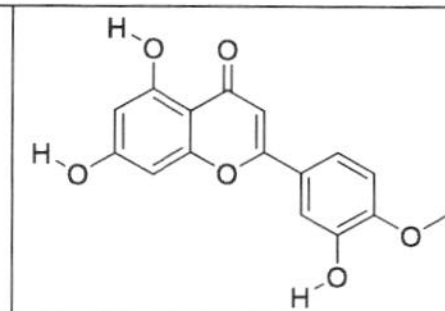	MW = 300.26 XlogP3 = 1.7 HBD = 3 HBA = 6 RB = 2 TPSA = 96.2	Vetch
Enterodiol [CID: 115089]	Lignan	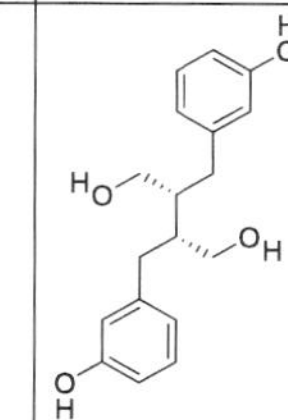	MW = 302.4 XlogP3 = 2.6 HBD = 4 HBA = 4 RB = 7 TPSA = 80.9	Flaxseed oil, Lucerne, and clover
Enterolactone [CID: 10685477]	Lignan	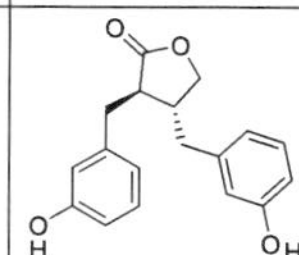	MW = 298.3 XlogP3 = 3.3 HBD = 2 HBA = 4 RB = 4 TPSA = 66.8	Flaxseed oil, Lucerne, and clover
Epicatechin-3-gallate [CID: 65056]	Flavonol/ catechins	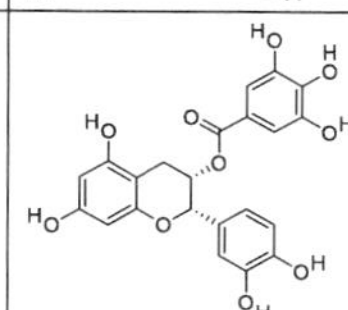	MW = 442.4 XlogP3 = 1.5 HBD = 7 HBA = 10 RB = 4 TPSA = 177	Green/black tea, cocoa/ chocolate
Epigallocatechin [CID: 72277]	Flavonol/ catechins	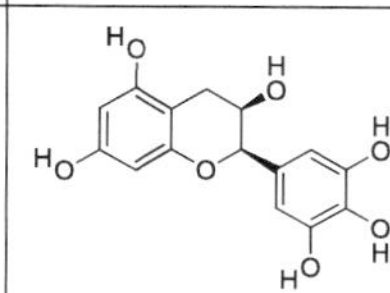	MW = 306 XlogP3 = 0 HBD = 6 HBA = 7 RB = 1 TPSA = 131	Green/black tea, cocoa/ chocolate

Continued

Table 1 List of natural chemical compounds associated with the management of lipid-metabolism-related disorders—cont'd

Chemical names/ PubChem CID.	Chemical class	Chemical structures	Physiochemical properties	Source
Epigallocatechin-3-gallate [CID: 65064]	Flavonol/ catechins	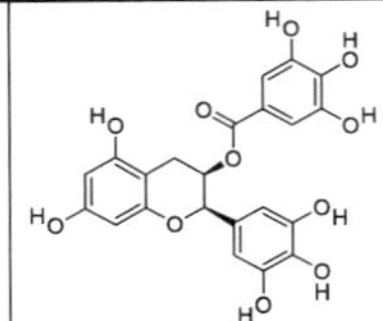	MW = 458.4 XlogP3 = 1.2 HBD = 8 HBA = 11 RB = 4 TPSA = 197	Green/black tea, cocoa/ chocolate
Eriodictyol [CID: 44073]	Flavanone	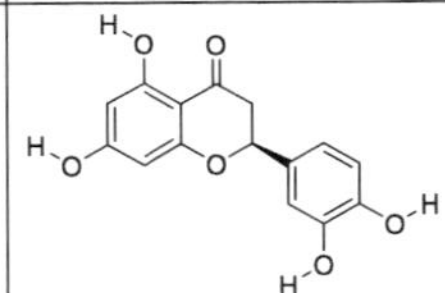	MW = 322.4 XlogP3 = 3.5 HBD = 1 HBA = 4 RB = 1 TPSA = 55.8	Lemons, rosehips
Fisetin [CID: 5281614]	Flavonol	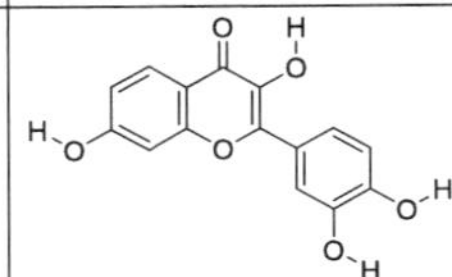	MW = 286.24 XlogP3 = 2 HBD = 4 HBA = 6 RB = 1 TPSA = 107	Strawberries, apples, persimmons, onions, and cucumbers
Gamma-Carotene [CID: 5280489]	Carotenoid	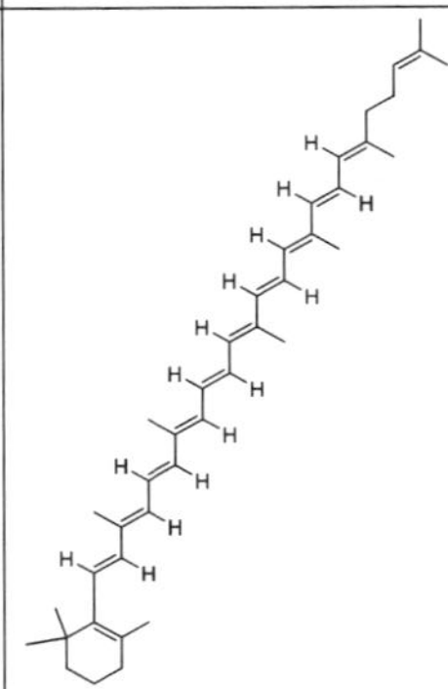	MW = 536.9 XlogP3 = 14.5 HBD = 0 HBA = 0 RB = 13 TPSA = 0	Carrots, pumpkins, maize, tangerine, orange and yellow fruits and vegetables, garlic, onion, and leek

Genistein [CID: 5280961]	Isoflavone	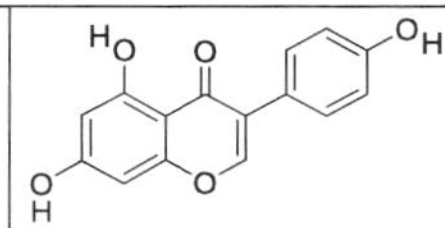	MW = 270.24 XlogP3 = 2.7 HBD = 3 HBA = 3 RB = 1 TPSA = 87	fava beans, psoralea, red clover, soybeans, and legumes
Hesperidin [CID: 10621]	Flavanone	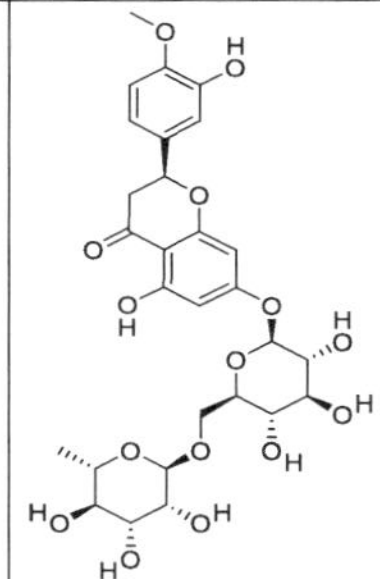	MW = 610.6 XlogP3 = − 1.1 HBD = 8 HBA = 15 RB = 7 TPSA = 234	Bitter orange, lemon, lime, and petit grain
Hydroxytyrosol [CID: 82755]	Phenolic acids	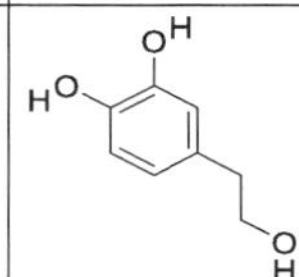	MW = 154.16 XlogP3 = − 0.7 HBD = 3 HBA = 3 RB = 2 TPSA = 60.7	Extra virgin olive oil
Kaempferol [CID: 5280863]	Flavonol	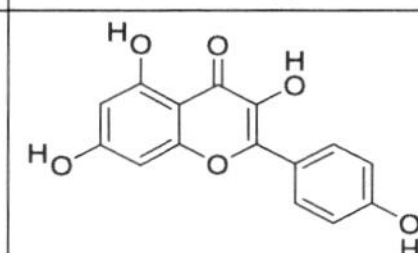	MW = 286.24 XlogP3 = 1.9 HBD = 4 HBA = 6 RB = 1 TPSA = 107	Apple, berries, broccoli, cocoa/chocolate, lettuce, olives, onion, and tea
Luteolin [CID: 5280445]	Flavones	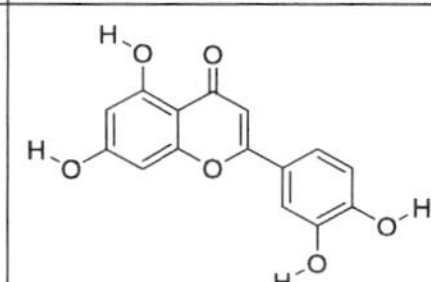	MW = 286.24 XlogP3 = 1.4 HBD = 4 HBA = 6 RB = 1 TPSA = 107	Broccoli, green pepper, celery, chamomile tea, carrots, dandelion, parsley, thyme, perilla, olive oil, peppermint, rosemary, and navel oranges

Continued

Table 1 List of natural chemical compounds associated with the management of lipid-metabolism-related disorders—cont'd

Chemical names/ PubChem CID.	Chemical class	Chemical structures	Physiochemical properties	Source
Lycopene [CID: 446925]	Carotenoid	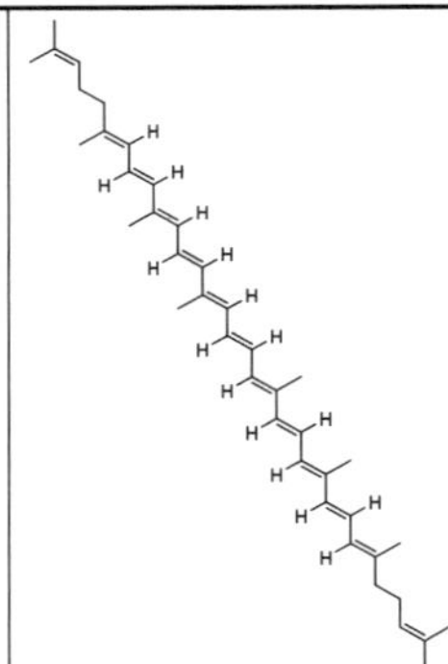	MW = 536.9 XlogP3 = 15.6 HBD = 0 HBA = 0 RB = 16 TPSA = 0	Tomatoes and tomato products
Myricetin [CID: 5281672]	Flavonols	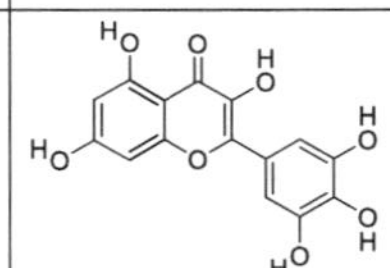	MW = 318.23 XlogP3 = 1.2 HBD = 6 HBA = 8 RB = 1 TPSA = 148	Vegetables, fruits, nuts, berries, tea, red wine, and citrus fruits.
Naringenin [CID: 932]	Flavanone	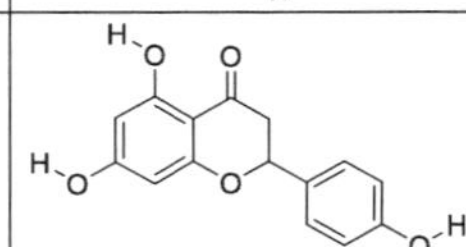	MW = 272.25 XlogP3 = 2.5 HBD = 3 HBA = 5 RB = 1 TPSA = 87	Grapes
Oleoeuropein [CID: 3789874]	Phenolic acids	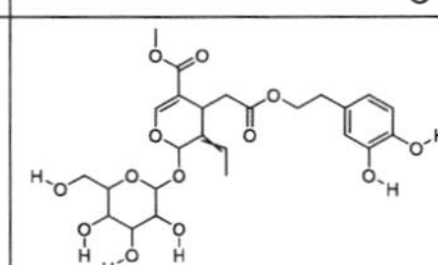	MW = 540.5 XlogP3 = −0.4 HBD = 6 HBA = 13 RB = 11 TPSA = 202	Extra virgin olive oil

P-coumaric acid [CID: 637542]	Phenolic acids	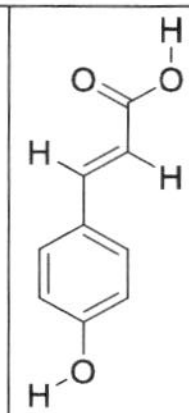	MW = 164.16 XlogP3 = 1.5 HBD = 2 HBA = 3 RB = 2 TPSA = 57.5	Extra virgin olive oil
Pectin [CID: 441476]	Soluble dietary fibers	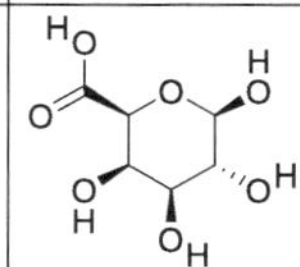	MW = 194.14 XlogP3 = −2.3 HBD = 5 HBA = 7 RB = 1 TPSA = 127	Barley, oats, fortified cereals, grains, fruits, vegetables, psyllium seeds, and yeast
Peonidin [CID: 441773]	Anthocyanidin	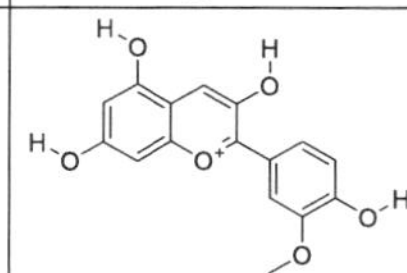	MW = 301.27 XlogP3 = not known HBD = 4 HBA = 5 RB = 2 TPSA = 91.2	Blueberries, cranberries, cherries, grapes, plums, and sweet potatoes
Phenethyl (PEITC) [CID: 146323]	Isothiocynates	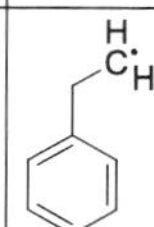	MW = 105.16 XlogP3 = 3.1 HBD = 0 HBA = 0 RB = 1 TPSA = 0	Cruciferous vegetables (e.g., watercress and broccoli)

Continued

Table 1 List of natural chemical compounds associated with the management of lipid-metabolism-related disorders—cont'd

Chemical names/ PubChem CID.	Chemical class	Chemical structures	Physiochemical properties	Source
Psyllium [CID: 181572]	Soluble dietary fibers	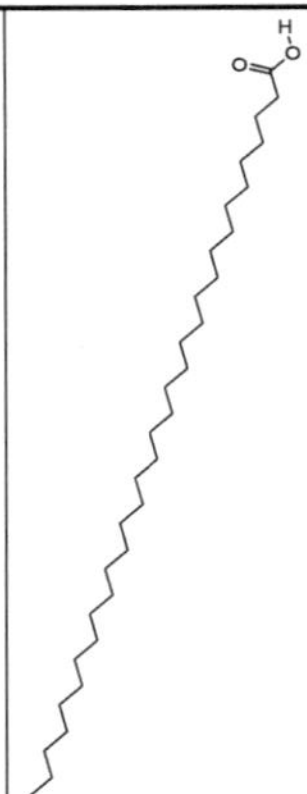	MW = 494.9 XlogP3 = 15.6 HBD = 1 HBA = 2 RB = 31 TPSA = 37.3	Fruits, vegetables, legume, cereals, and grains.
Quercetin [CID: 5280343]	Flavonol	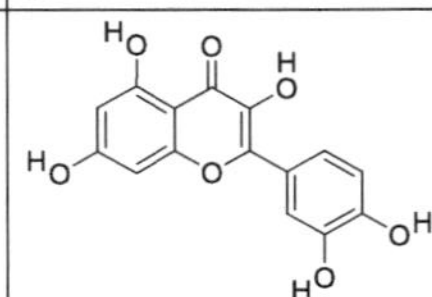	MW = 302.23 XlogP3 = 1.5 HBD = 5 HBA = 7 RB = 1 TPSA = 127	Apple, berries, broccoli, cocoa/chocolate, lettuce, olives, onion, and tea leaves

Resveratrol [CID: 445154]	Stilbenoids	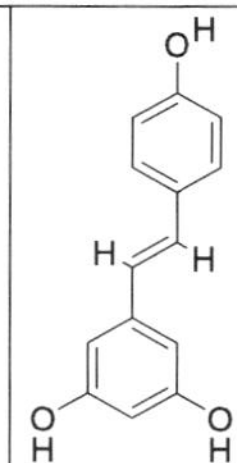	MW = 228.24 XlogP3 = 3.1 HBD = 3 HBA = 2 RB = 2 TPSA = 60.7	Grapes, peanuts, and red wine
Rutin [CID:5280805]	Flavonol	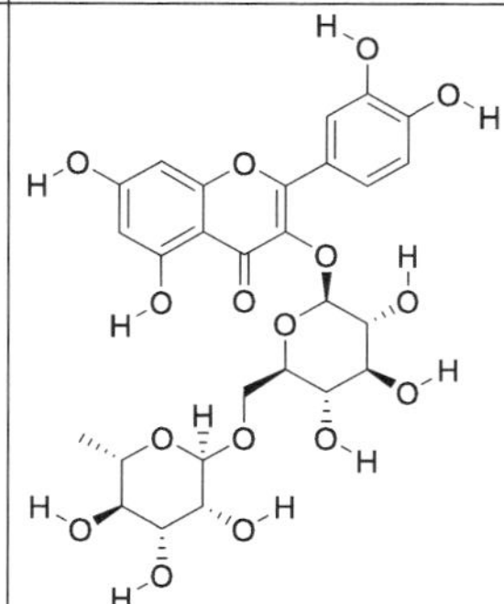	MW = 610.5 XlogP3 = – 1.3 HBD = 10 HBA = 16 RB = 6 TPSA = 266	Apple, berries, buckwheat, green tea, grape seeds, peaches, lemon, onion, and red pepper
Scopoletin [CID: 5280460]	Coumarin	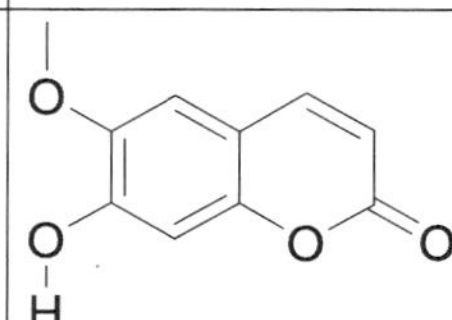	MW = 192.17 XlogP3 = 1.5 HBD = 1 HBA = 4 RB = 1 TPSA = 55.8	Dandelion coffee Vinegar

Continued

Table 1 List of natural chemical compounds associated with the management of lipid-metabolism-related disorders—cont'd

Chemical names/ PubChem CID.	Chemical class	Chemical structures	Physiochemical properties	Source
Sitostanol [CID: 241572]	Plant sterols	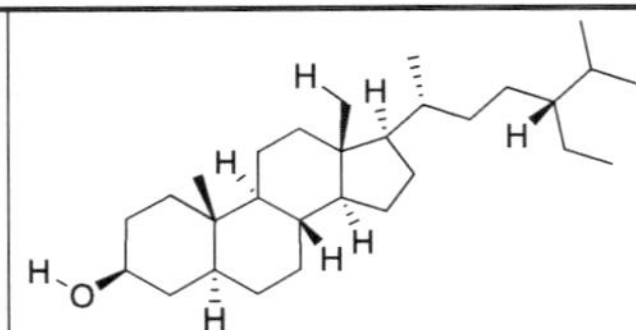	MW = 416.7 XlogP3 = 10.2 HBD = 1 HBA = 1 RB = 6 TPSA = 20.2	Tall oil, soybean oil, and rice bran oil
Stigmasterol [CID: 5280794]	Plant sterols	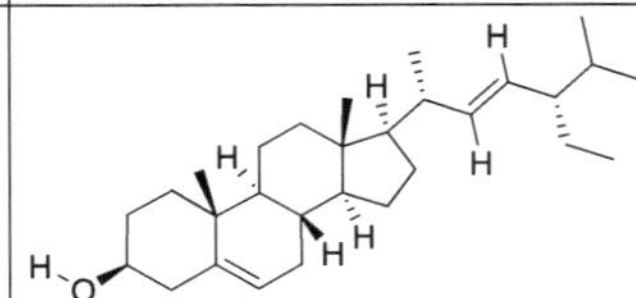	MW = 412.7 XlogP3 = 8.2 HBD = 1 HBA = 1 RB = 5 TPSA = 20.2	Tall oil, soybean oil, and rice bran oil
Sulforaphanes [CID: 5350]	Isothiocynates	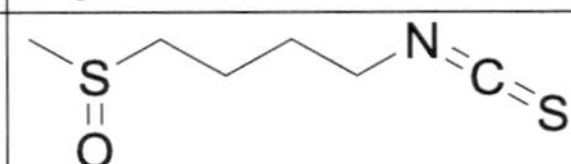	MW = 177.3 XlogP3 = 1.4 HBD = 0 HBA = 4 RB = 5 TPSA = 80.7	Cruciferous vegetables (e.g., watercress and broccoli)
Taxifolin [CID: 439533]	Flavanonol	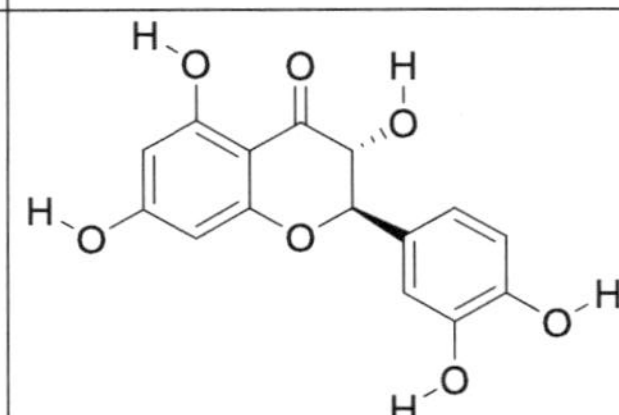	MW = 304.25 XlogP3 = 1.5 HBD = 5 HBA = 7 RB = 1 TPSA = 127	Several fruits and vegetables, citrus fruits grapes, olive oil, and onions

Theaflavin [CID: 135403798]	Catechins	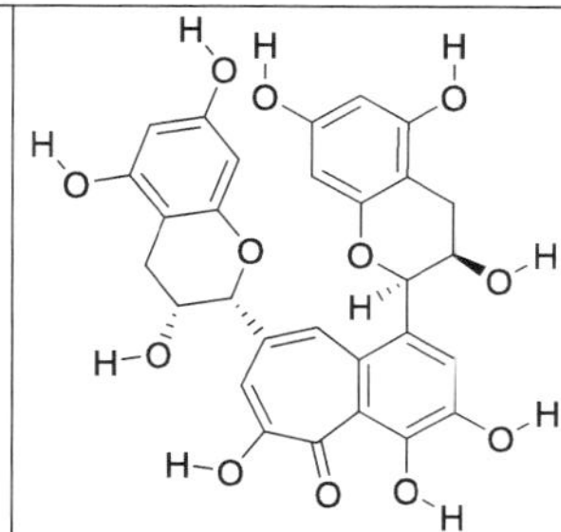	MW = 564.5 XlogP3 = 2.4 HBD9 HBA = 12 RB = 2 TPSA = 218	Tea leaves, black tea, and oolong tea
Tricin [CID: 5281702]	Flavone	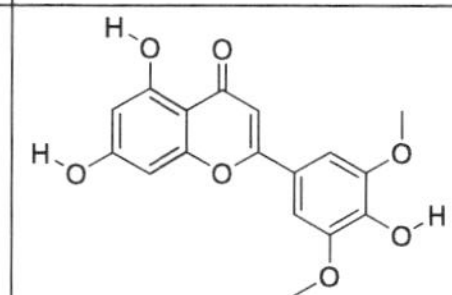	MW = 330.29 XlogP3 = 1.7 HBD = 3 HBA = 7 RB = 3 TPSA = 105	Rice bran
Tyrosol [CID: 10393]	Phenolic acids	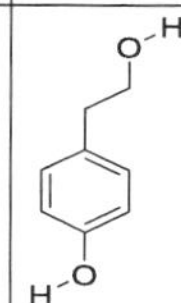	MW = 138.16 XlogP3 = 0.4 HBD = 2 HBA = 2 RB = 2 TPSA = 40.5	Extra virgin olive oil

prevent atherosclerosis [124]. The chemical structure and physicochemical information of allicin, allyl mercaptan, diallyl disulfide, and diallyl sulfide is shown in Table 1.

Carotenoids are lipophilic isoprenoid contents found in several vegetables, fruits, and medicinal plants. Both carotenoids and enzymatic cleavage of their chemicals are significantly known for the positive impact on human health; these are useful food constituents, essences, and other dietary supplements (DS). Alpha-carotene, beta-carotene, delta-carotene, gamma-carotene, and lycopene are important carotenoids involved in LM [124] (shown in Table 1), also involved in the regulation and suppression of signaling pathways; they also interact with transcription factors and activate specific genes [125,126]. Tomato products and lycopene decreased the risk of atherosclerosis and were involved in cholesterol metabolism, in experimental and human intervention trials; it is concluded that lycopene and tomato products could be important for reduction of plasma LDL-C depending on the dose and the time of administration [127].

Isothiocyanates found in cruciferous vegetables, e.g., watercress and broccoli, have presented antiobesity characteristics by the suppressing effects in the process of adipogensis and lipogenesis [128]. Benzyl (BITC), phenethyl (PEITC), and sulforaphane are dietary isothiocyanates; their chemical structures and physiochemical information are shown in Table 1.

Phytochemicals, known as soluble dietary fibers (SDF), are important as low-fats or no-fats supplementary food with medicinal properties. They interfere with the secondary absorption and reduce the solubility of chemicals while digestion and delay the absorption of food components; furthermore, they could be fermented in the intestine to create short chains of fatty acid (FA) which inhibit cholesterol synthesis and maintain the health of the gut [129]. The mechanism of LM regulation was studied by Huanhuan et al., in 2020, and indicated that micronized and nonmicronized extract from lotus root exposes adsorption and inhibitory activity of pancreatic lipase [130]. Another study revealed that SDF could affect the LM and improve the intestinal disaccharides in experimental rats [131]. Beta-glucan, pectin, and psyllium belong to the class of SDF and are involved in hypolipidemic activity, management of lipid profile, and induce a hypoglycemic effect, and also provide protection from LM-related diseases [124,130]. The chemical structure and physicochemical information of beta-glucan, pectin, and psyllium are shown in Table 1.

Isoflavones are class of flavonoids presenting profound lipid profile management properties by the modulation of signaling pathways. Biochanin A is well-known antidiabetic and cholesterol-lowering drug; its cholesterol-lowering effects in DM are achieved by the mechanism of activated peroxisome proliferation-activated receptor (PPAR)-alpha protein in the liver [132]. Daidzein, also known as soy isoflavone, affects impaired glucose (IG) and LM and vascular inflammation related with T2DM [133]. DS of daidzein along with the genistein also improved the plasma cholesterol (PC) levels, TG, HDL-C, and free FA, and have provided the evidence of a regulatory mechanism of glucose in the liver and LM in C57BL/KsJ-db/db mice [134]. The chemical structure and physicochemical information of biochanin A, daidzein, and genistein are shown in Table 1.

Phenolic acids are associated with excellent activities in terms of lowering liver and blood cholesterol levels in rats by the management of cholesterol metabolism; and caffeic acid and P-coumaric acid are antioxidant agents presenting scavenging free radicals [135,136]. Hydroxytyrosol improves metabolic pathways, and prevents CVD risk and liver damage in a model rat study with 20 mg/kg dose per day for 8 weeks, and concluded with reduced adiposity, establish IG, enhance insulin tolerance and endothelial functionalities by decline in the systolic blood pressure and reduced left ventricular fibrosis and results in diastolic toughness and decreasing the damage of liver in a DI model animal having LM abnormalities [137]. Oleoeuropein is found in olives and is significant for CVD and other metabolic syndromes such as cancer, inflammation, autoimmune disorders, and wound healing [138]. Hydroxytyrosol, tyrosol, and their derivatives are highly acceptable phytochemicals with cardioprotective, antiatherogenic, anticancer, and neuroprotective effects [139]. The chemical structure and physicochemical information of caffeic acid, hydroxytyrosol, oleoeuropein, P-coumaric acid, and tyrosol are shown in Table 1.

Phytosterols such as campesterol, sitostanol, and stigmasterol as shown in Table 1 are important natural products found in DS for the improvement of health, because they could inhibit cholesterol adsorption and fat-soluble plant esters help to lower the serum cholesterols level in functional foods; a short study has demonstrated a 20%–25% decrease in coronary heart disease (CHD) due to plant sterols [140]. Campesterol derivatives activate PPAR-alpha, and promote energy consumption and lower the fat deposit in the rat cells presenting the possibility that this molecule could be the active agent for the prevention of CHD by the improvement of obesity and imbalanced LM [141]. Sitostanol is beneficial for the improvement of lipid profile; dietary effects of sitostanol are proportionate to its concentration used in the formation of a phytosterol amalgam and in the DS, it could lower the TG and PC levels in hamsters [142].

Flavonol is an important class of flavonoids presenting 3-hydroxyfalvone in the structure of its compounds; fisetin is an essential content of DS and is found in various fruits and vegetables, and presents numerous biological activities, and also acts as an important cardioprotective agent and plays a role in atherosclerosis and lipid-metabolism-related diseases [143]. Fisetin has the ability to shelter against hepatosteatosis, which is closely associated with modulation of LM gene expression and miR-378 in mice [144]. Kaempferol is found abundantly in vegetables, fruits, herbs and in other plants [145,146]. Kaempferol presented antiobesity and antihyperlipidemic effects in the high-fat diet (HFD) treated rats by the mechanism of hepatic PPAR-alpha levels, reduced the triglyceride and cholesterols contents, and lowered the hepatic lipid droplet deposition and size of epididymal adipocytes in the HFD-fed rats [147]. Kaempferol shows the antiatherosclerotic effect by modulating the gene and protein expression of inflammatory molecules in high cholesterol-fed rabbits [148]. Kaempferol stimulated the Sp1 gene expression and activity of hepatic LDL in HepG2 cells [149].

Myricetin is a bioflavonoid that suppressed the weight gain and storage of fats by enhancing the oxidation of FA, which is monitored by the activation of PPAR-alpha and activation of hepatic sterol regulatory element-binding protein expression in the liver of HFD-fed rats [150]. Myricetin employs antiobesity properties by the activation of SIRT3 in adipose tissue; reduction of TG content is observed and amplified mitochondrial content with the consumption of oxygen in adipocytes during in vitro experiments in C57B6/J mice-induced HFD [151].

Quercetin is the main active phytonutrient in several plants; it is a low weight molecular compound presenting significant reduction of hyperlipidemia and atherosclerotic lesion generation, cholesterol entities transportation in a reverse manner and plays an important role in exporting LDL-C from peripheral cells, which is most beneficial in the prevention and management of atherosclerosis [152]. Quercetin decreases FA storage in mice treated with HFD and a high-sucrose diet [153,154]. Quercetin inhibited abdominal obesity in model animals that were treated with HFD added with 0.08% quercetin for a duration of 8 weeks [155]. It also reduced the chance of development of NFLD, partially due to exaggerated expression of adiponectin and decrease of inflammatory cytokine levels in ob/ob mice [156]. Quercetin manages very well with abdominal FA by the regulation of digestion and adsorption processes, breakdown of glycerophospholipids, regulation of AMP-activated protein kinases signaling pathway, and LM in broiler chickens [157].

Rutin is an excellent phytonutrient found in apple, berries, buckwheat, green tea, grape seeds, peaches, lemon, onion, and red peppers with antioxidative properties and its related consequences; rutin supplements-treated ischemic rats revealed reduction in lipid peroxidation in kidney [158]. Rutin is the mediator of LM and is associated with the cellular signaling pathways interacting in fibroblast alteration due to the induction of UVA (320–400 nm) and UVB (280–320 nm) radiation [159]. Rutin is helpful in the management of lipid profiles if 100 mg/kg is intaken solely or in amalgam with lovastatin it could significantly reduce LDL-C and efficiently inhibit the enzymes in the liver and also manage the animals' weight [160]. The chemical structure and physicochemical information of fisetin, kaempferol, myricetin, quercetin, and rutin are shown in Table 1.

Apigenin and luteolin are flavones commonly found in vegetables, parsley, celery, celeriac, fruits, and chamomile tea (shown in Table 1). Apigenin and naringenin together could be more significant in the regulation of glucose and LM by the admiration of 50 or 100 mg/kg once a day for 6 weeks. Results show that apigenin and naringenin significant reduced the blood glucose, serum lipid, malonaldehyde, IR, and enhanced superoxide dismutase activity and also improve the IG tolerance in the T2DM rats. In vitro studies shows that it could inhibit the NF-kB transcription factors initiation and ICAM-1 mRNA expression, also upgraded NO construction in the existence of insulin [122]. Another study has been conducted on apigenin to prove the modulation of the PPAR-gamma protein expression and also demonstrated that HFD-induced NFLD attenuation by regulation of hepatocyte LM with oxidative stress through Nrf2 signaling [161]. While luteolin when induced with hypoglycemic drug metformin hydrochloride, that results with the alleviation of LM-related diseases and regulate the intestinal flora composition in HFD mice [162].

Lignans such as enterodiol and enterolactone are dietary components found in flaxseed oil, lucerne, and clover (shown in Table 1). Lignans are very helpful in preventing DM and hypercholesterolemic atherosclerosis [163] and the study with respect to postmenopausal women demonstrated that lignan excretion is significant in lowering the urine level in women with breast cancer; enterodiol and enterolactone lignan designed by the intestinal microflora are present in fiber-rich food such as nuts, grains, and legumes [164]. Flaxseed lignan encouraged adiponectin mRNA expression and exhibited significant effects on LM in DI obesity in mice [163].

Anthocyanidins are abundantly found in blueberries, cranberries, cherries, grapes, plums, and sweet potatoes. Peonidin is a bioactive phytonutrient that belongs to the class of anthocyanidins, shown in Table 1, having anti-inflammatory and antioxidative activities and involved in the regulation of lipid-related metabolic processes [165]; most of all berries and their anthocyanidin extracts are important supplementary components having characteristics to improve the metabolic syndromes and lipid-metabolism-related diseases and also CVD, these might be due to the mechanism of inhibition of NF-kB transcription factor-dependent gene expressions associated with the innate immune response and improvement of PPAR-gamma protein expression [166].

Resveratrol is a remarkable dietary constituent that belongs to the class of stilbenoids that are hydroxylated derivatives of stilbene shown in Table 1. Resveratrol has the ability to alter the LM-related gene expression of mice on an atherogenic diet, increase the life span and improve metabolic disease [167]. Resveratrol supplementation also enhanced the IR, glucose, and LM very efficiently in the patients of NAFL disease [168]. Another study highlighted that resveratrol has altered the LM in cancer patients therefore affecting the storage of energy, cell signaling cascade, event of proliferation and progression with invasiveness of cancer cells; it concluded with the new therapeutic strategy of lipid pathways and signaling molecules that could monitor carcinogenesis by resveratrol supplementation [169].

Green tea is a rich source of catechins with multiple pharmacological characteristics [170]. Intake of green tea means taking abundant catechins with numerous other essential components such as polysaccharides isolated while processing the tea leaves could be prospective constituents for anti-DM and obesity management by inhibition of the lipid intestinal TG absorption and storage of fats in adipose tissues [171].

Theaflavin is an excellent bioactive phytonutrient isolated from tea leaves; it is involved in the regulatory mechanism of inflammatory signaling with the regulation of phosphorylated AMP-activated kinase, FA synthase, and carnitine palmitoyl transferase I that is highly recommended for the management of weight gain, and lower FAs, and triglyceride and total cholesterol levels increased in DM and obese patients [172]. It significantly decreased the interleukin-6 levels and also inhibited the iNOS and regulate LM-related proteins and also improve the health of the gastrointestinal tract [173,174]. Theaflavin, epicatechin-3-gallate, epigallocatechin, and epigallocatechin-3-gallate acknowledged as green tea catechins have presented numerous health benefits such as lower HDL-C levels, antiinflammation and antisteatotic impact on the liver, clear lipid profile along with stimulation of hepatic autophagy and also provide support to improve intestinal health [175,176]. Chemical structure and physicochemical information of theaflavin, epicatechin-3-gallate, epigallocatechin, and epigallocatechin-3-gallate are shown in Table 1.

10. Concluding remarks

Dietary supplements prescribed by the dieticians are necessary to control any LM-related disease, because a clear knowledge of food is necessary to keep the balance in the calories, food indicators are highly significant to regulate glucose and LM in patients with cholesterol, obesity, and DM. It is interesting to study the extensive range of bioactivities of phytonutrients such as flavonoids, catechins, isothiocyanates, plant sterols, phenolic acids, stilbenoids, and soluble dietary fibers, etc. isolated from vegetables, fruits, and plants, playing beneficial roles in the regulation of LM and its related disorders (shown in Table 1). It is highly recommended to add more vegetables, fruits, and legumes in the diet plans of cholesterol patients, because due to their low-fat contents, and soluble fractions of dietary fibers, it could be helpful in decreasing the concentration of LDL-C, TG levels, and maintain body weight. It could also mediate insulin resistance, which is important to manage LM. Consumption of dietary phytonutrients can be modified by additional contents such as cereal grains, cereal products, and olive oil with the recommended advantages as whole meal products. These products are good sources of essential nutrients and may also play a role in the prevention and management of other metabolic abnormalities closely associated with high cholesterol levels in the body such as cancer, obesity, neurodegenerative disorders, DM, hypoglycemia, NFLD, and many other lipid accumulation-related disorders.

References

[1] K.E. Suckling, B. Jackson, Animal models of human lipid metabolism, Prog. Lipid Res. 32 (1) (1993) 1–24.

[2] L. Chen, X.-W. Chen, X. Huang, B.-L. Song, Y. Wang, Y. Wang, Regulation of glucose and lipid metabolism in health and disease, Sci. China Life Sci. 62 (11) (2019) 1420–1458.

[3] J. Swierczynski, A. Hebanowska, T. Sledzinski, Role of abnormal lipid metabolism in development, progression, diagnosis and therapy of pancreatic cancer, World J Gastroenterol: WJG 20 (9) (2014) 2279.

[4] O. Cheung, A.J. Sanyal, Abnormalities of lipid metabolism in nonalcoholic fatty liver disease, in: Seminars in Liver Disease, Thieme Medical Publishers, 2008, pp. 351–359.

[5] K.G. Parhofer, The treatment of disorders of lipid metabolism, Dtsch. Arztebl. Int. 113 (15) (2016) 261.

[6] A. Zak, M. Zeman, A. Slaby, M. Vecka, Xanthomas: clinical and pathophysiological relations, in: Biomedical Papers of the Medical Faculty of Palacky University in Olomouc, 158, 2014. 2.
[7] A. Salter, H. Wiseman, G. Tucker, Phytonutrients, John Wiley & Sons, 2012.
[8] R. Orgeron II, J. Pope, V. Green, D. Erickson, Phytonutrient intake and body composition: considering colors, Funct. Foods Health Dis. 9 (2) (2019) 108–122.
[9] J. Zhao, Nutraceuticals, nutritional therapy, phytonutrients, and phytotherapy for improvement of human health: a perspective on plant biotechnology application, Recent Pat. Biotechnol. 1 (1) (2007) 75–97.
[10] A. Mastaloudis, S.M. Wood, Age-related changes in cellular protection, purification, and inflammation-related gene expression: role of dietary phytonutrients, Ann. N.Y. Acad. Sci. 1259 (1) (2012) 112–120.
[11] A.R. Williams, A.I. Andersen-Civil, L. Zhu, A. Blanchard, Dietary phytonutrients and animal health: regulation of immune function during gastrointestinal infections, J. Anim. Sci. 98 (4) (2020), skaa030.
[12] N.J. Stone, S. Bilek, S. Rosenbaum, Recent national cholesterol education program adult treatment panel III update: adjustments and options, Am. J. Cardiol. 96 (4) (2005) 53–59.
[13] R.-E.W. Kavey, S.R. Daniels, R.M. Lauer, D.L. Atkins, L.L. Hayman, K. Taubert, American Heart Association guidelines for primary prevention of atherosclerotic cardiovascular disease beginning in childhood, Circulation 107 (11) (2003) 1562–1566.
[14] L. Berglund, J.D. Brunzell, A.C. Goldberg, I.J. Goldberg, F. Sacks, M.H. Murad, et al., Evaluation and treatment of hypertriglyceridemia: an Endocrine Society clinical practice guideline, J. Clin. Endocrinol. Metabol. 97 (9) (2012) 2969–2989.
[15] A. Brahm, R.A. Hegele, Hypertriglyceridemia, Nutrients 5 (3) (2013) 981–1001.
[16] M. Merkel, R.H. Eckel, I.J. Goldberg, Lipoprotein lipase, J. Lipid Res. 43 (12) (2002) 1997–2006.
[17] D.M. Ng, A.J. Hooper, M.I. Bellgard, J.R. Burnett, The role of patient registries for rare genetic lipid disorders, Curr. Opin. Lipidol. 29 (2) (2018) 156–162.
[18] D.E. Wilson, A. Hata, L.K. Kwong, A. Lingam, J. Shuhua, D.N. Ridinger, et al., Mutations in exon 3 of the lipoprotein lipase gene segregating in a family with hypertriglyceridemia, pancreatitis, and non-insulin-dependent diabetes, J. Clin. Invest. 92 (1) (1993) 203–211.
[19] H.N. Ginsberg, Diabetic dyslipidemia: basic mechanisms underlying the common hypertriglyceridemia and low HDL cholesterol levels, Diabetes 45 (Supplement 3) (1996) S27–S30.
[20] M.-R. Taskinen, M. Adiels, J. Westerbacka, S. Söderlund, J. Kahri, N. Lundbom, et al., Dual metabolic defects are required to produce hypertriglyceridemia in obese subjects, Arterioscler. Thromb. Vasc. Biol. 31 (9) (2011) 2144–2150.
[21] C.D. Saudek, H.A. Eder, Lipid metabolism in diabetes mellitus, Am. J. Med. 66 (5) (1979) 843–852.
[22] E.L. Bierman, V.P. Dole, T.N. Roberts, An abnormality of nonesterified fatty acid metabolism in diabetes mellitus, Diabetes 6 (6) (1957) 475–479.
[23] L. Sun, N. Halaihel, W. Zhang, T. Rogers, M. Levi, Role of sterol regulatory element-binding protein 1 in regulation of renal lipid metabolism and glomerulosclerosis in diabetes mellitus, J. Biol. Chem. 277 (21) (2002) 18919–18927.
[24] L. Visconti, S. Benvenga, A. Lacquaniti, V. Cernaro, A. Bruzzese, G. Conti, et al., Lipid disorders in patients with renal failure: role in cardiovascular events and progression of chronic kidney disease, J. Clin. Transl. Endocrinol. 6 (2016) 8–14.
[25] S.M. Freier, R.M. Crooke, M.J. Graham, K.L. Lemonidis, S. Bhanot, D. Tribble, et al., Methods for Treating Hypercholesterolemia, Google Patents, 2012.

[26] A.K. Soutar, R.P. Naoumova, Mechanisms of disease: genetic causes of familial hypercholesterolemia, Nat. Clin. Pract. Cardiovasc. Med. 4 (4) (2007) 214–225.

[27] A.J. Vallejo-Vaz, S.R.K. Seshasai, D. Cole, G.K. Hovingh, J.J. Kastelein, P. Mata, et al., Familial hypercholesterolaemia: a global call to arms, Atherosclerosis 243 (1) (2015) 257–259.

[28] A. Kawaguchi, K. Miyatake, C. Yutani, S. Beppu, M. Tsushima, T. Yamamura, et al., Characteristic cardiovascular manifestation in homozygous and heterozygous familial hypercholesterolemia, Am. Heart J. 137 (3) (1999) 410–418.

[29] K.E. Berge, Sitosterolemia: a gateway to new knowledge about cholesterol metabolism, Ann. Med. 35 (7) (2003) 502–511.

[30] G. Salen, K. Von Bergmann, D.T. Lütjohann, P. Kwiterovich, J. Kane, S.B. Patel, et al., Ezetimibe effectively reduces plasma plant sterols in patients with sitosterolemia, Circulation 109 (8) (2004) 966–971.

[31] M. Sharifi, M. Futema, D. Nair, S.E. Humphries, Polygenic hypercholesterolemia and cardiovascular disease risk, Curr. Cardiol. Rep. 21 (6) (2019) 1–6.

[32] G. Ruiu, S. Pinach, F. Veglia, R. Gambino, S. Marena, B. Uberti, et al., Phytosterol-enriched yogurt increases LDL affinity and reduces CD36 expression in polygenic hypercholesterolemia, Lipids 44 (2) (2009) 153.

[33] M. Sharifi, E. Higginson, S. Bos, A. Gallivan, D. Harvey, K.W. Li, et al., Greater preclinical atherosclerosis in treated monogenic familial hypercholesterolemia vs. polygenic hypercholesterolemia, Atherosclerosis 263 (2017) 405–411.

[34] J. Borén, U. Ekström, B. Agren, P. Nilsson-Ehle, T.L. Innerarity, The molecular mechanism for the genetic disorder familial defective apolipoprotein B100, J. Biol. Chem. 276 (12) (2001) 9214–9218.

[35] L.F. Soria, E.H. Ludwig, H.R. Clarke, G.L. Vega, S.M. Grundy, B.J. McCarthy, Association between a specific apolipoprotein B mutation and familial defective apolipoprotein B-100, Proc. Natl. Acad. Sci. 86 (2) (1989) 587–591.

[36] M.A. Ibrahim, I. Jialal, Hypercholesterolemia, 2017.

[37] P.D. Thompson, P. Clarkson, R.H. Karas, Statin-associated myopathy, JAMA 289 (13) (2003) 1681–1690.

[38] T. Diekman, P.J. Lansberg, J.J. Kastelein, W.M. Wiersinga, Prevalence and correction of hypothyroidism in a large cohort of patients referred for dyslipidemia, Arch. Intern. Med. 155 (14) (1995) 1490–1495.

[39] J.L. Third, J. Montag, M. Flynn, J. Freidel, P. Laskarzewski, C.J. Glueck, Primary and familial hypoalphalipoproteinemia, Metabolism 33 (2) (1984) 136–146.

[40] B.F. Asztalos, E.J. Schaefer, K.V. Horvath, S. Yamashita, M. Miller, G. Franceschini, et al., Role of LCAT in HDL remodeling: investigation of LCAT deficiency states, J. Lipid Res. 48 (3) (2007) 592–599.

[41] J.A. Kuivenhoven, H. Pritchard, J. Hill, J. Frohlich, G. Assmann, J. Kastelein, The molecular pathology of lecithin: cholesterol acyltransferase (LCAT) deficiency syndromes, J. Lipid Res. 38 (2) (1997) 191–205.

[42] G. Utermann, W. Schoenborn, K.H. Langer, P. Dieker, Lipoproteins in LCAT-deficiency, Humangenetik 16 (4) (1972) 295–306.

[43] S.R. Bates, J.-Q. Tao, H.L. Collins, O.L. Francone, G.H. Rothblat, Pulmonary abnormalities due to ABCA1 deficiency in mice, Am. J. Physiol. Lung Cell. Mol. Physiol. 289 (6) (2005) L980–L989.

[44] V. Hirsch-Reinshagen, S. Zhou, B.L. Burgess, L. Bernier, S.A. McIsaac, J.Y. Chan, et al., Deficiency of ABCA1 impairs apolipoprotein E metabolism in brain, J. Biol. Chem. 279 (39) (2004) 41197–41207.

[45] L. Badimon, G. Vilahur, Thrombosis formation on atherosclerotic lesions and plaque rupture, J. Intern. Med. 276 (6) (2014) 618–632.

[46] P. Libby, P.M. Ridker, G.K. Hansson, Progress and challenges in translating the biology of atherosclerosis, Nature 473 (7347) (2011) 317–325.
[47] J.E. Deanfield, J.P. Halcox, T.J. Rabelink, Endothelial function and dysfunction: testing and clinical relevance, Circulation 115 (10) (2007) 1285–1295.
[48] D. Mehta, A.B. Malik, Signaling mechanisms regulating endothelial permeability, Physiol. Rev. 86 (2006) 279–367.
[49] R.J. Widmer, A. Lerman, Endothelial dysfunction and cardiovascular disease, Glob. Cardiol. Sci. Pract. 2014 (3) (2014) 43.
[50] K.J. Williams, I. Tabas, The response-to-retention hypothesis of early atherogenesis, Arterioscler. Thromb. Vasc. Biol. 15 (5) (1995) 551–561.
[51] S.D. Cushing, J.A. Berliner, A.J. Valente, M.C. Territo, M. Navab, F. Parhami, et al., Minimally modified low density lipoprotein induces monocyte chemotactic protein 1 in human endothelial cells and smooth muscle cells, Proc. Natl. Acad. Sci. 87 (13) (1990) 5134–5138.
[52] H.F. McMurray, S. Parthasarathy, D. Steinberg, et al., Oxidatively modified low density lipoprotein is a chemoattractant for human T lymphocytes, J. Clin. Invest. 92 (2) (1993) 1004–1008.
[53] K. Ley, Y.I. Miller, C.C. Hedrick, Monocyte and macrophage dynamics during atherogenesis, Arterioscler. Thromb. Vasc. Biol. 31 (7) (2011) 1506–1516.
[54] L.K. Jennings, Mechanisms of platelet activation: need for new strategies to protect against platelet-mediated atherothrombosis, Thromb. Haemost. 102 (08) (2009) 248–257.
[55] C.L. Lendon, M.J. Davies, G.V.R. Born, P.D. Richardson, Atherosclerotic plaque caps are locally weakened when macrophages density is increased, Atherosclerosis 87 (1) (1991) 87–90.
[56] M. Aikawa, P. Libby, The vulnerable atherosclerotic plaque: pathogenesis and therapeutic approach, Cardiovasc. Pathol. 13 (3) (2004) 125–138.
[57] G. Aquila, L. Marracino, V. Martino, D. Calabria, G. Campo, C. Caliceti, et al., The use of nutraceuticals to counteract atherosclerosis: the role of the notch pathway, Oxid. Med. Cell. Longev. 2019 (2019).
[58] M.B. Fessler, The intracellular cholesterol landscape: dynamic integrator of the immune response, Trends Immunol. 37 (12) (2016) 819–830.
[59] S. Munro, Lipid rafts: elusive or illusive? Cell 115 (4) (2003) 377–388.
[60] M.P. Wymann, R. Schneiter, Lipid signalling in disease, Nat. Rev. Mol. Cell Biol. 9 (2) (2008) 162–176.
[61] W.A. Prinz, Lipid trafficking sans vesicles: where, why, how? Cell 143 (6) (2010) 870–874.
[62] C.L. Jackson, L. Walch, J.-M. Verbavatz, Lipids and their trafficking: an integral part of cellular organization, Dev. Cell 39 (2) (2016) 139–153.
[63] S.-S. Im, L. Yousef, C. Blaschitz, J.Z. Liu, R.A. Edwards, S.G. Young, et al., Linking lipid metabolism to the innate immune response in macrophages through sterol regulatory element binding protein-1a, Cell Metab. 13 (5) (2011) 540–549.
[64] A.R. Tall, L. Yvan-Charvet, Cholesterol, inflammation and innate immunity, Nat. Rev. Immunol. 15 (2) (2015) 104–116.
[65] A.J. de Jong, M. Kloppenburg, R.E.M. Toes, A. Ioan-Facsinay, Fatty acids, lipid mediators, and T-cell function, Front. Immunol. 5 (2014) 483.
[66] M.J. Hubler, A.J. Kennedy, Role of lipids in the metabolism and activation of immune cells, J. Nutr. Biochem. 34 (2016) 1–7.
[67] J.M. Lehmann, S.A. Kliewer, L.B. Moore, T.A. Smith-Oliver, B.B. Oliver, J.-L. Su, et al., Activation of the nuclear receptor LXR by oxysterols defines a new hormone response pathway, J. Biol. Chem. 272 (6) (1997) 3137–3140.

[68] B.A. Janowski, P.J. Willy, T.R. Devi, J.R. Falck, D.J. Mangelsdorf, An oxysterol signalling pathway mediated by the nuclear receptor LXRα, Nature 383 (6602) (1996) 728–731.

[69] J.J. Repa, D.J. Mangelsdorf, The liver X receptor gene team: potential new players in atherosclerosis, Nat. Med. 8 (11) (2002) 1243–1248.

[70] A. Castrillo, S.B. Joseph, S.A. Vaidya, M. Haberland, A.M. Fogelman, G. Cheng, et al., Crosstalk between LXR and toll-like receptor signaling mediates bacterial and viral antagonism of cholesterol metabolism, Mol. Cell 12 (4) (2003) 805–816.

[71] W. Khovidhunkit, A.H. Moser, J.K. Shigenaga, C. Grunfeld, K.R. Feingold, Endotoxin down-regulates ABCG5 and ABCG8 in mouse liver and ABCA1 and ABCG1 in J774 murine macrophages: differential role of LXR, J. Lipid Res. 44 (9) (2003) 1728–1736.

[72] M.-C. Gerbod-Giannone, Y. Li, A. Holleboom, S. Han, L.-C. Hsu, I. Tabas, et al., TNFα induces ABCA1 through NF-κB in macrophages and in phagocytes ingesting apoptotic cells, Proc. Natl. Acad. Sci. 103 (9) (2006) 3112–3117.

[73] W. Khovidhunkit, M.-S. Kim, R.A. Memon, J.K. Shigenaga, A.H. Moser, K.R. Feingold, et al., Effects of infection and inflammation on lipid and lipoprotein metabolism: mechanisms and consequences to the host, J. Lipid Res. 45 (7) (2004) 1169–1196.

[74] E. Frisdal, P. Lesnik, M. Olivier, P. Robillard, M.J. Chapman, T. Huby, et al., Interleukin-6 protects human macrophages from cellular cholesterol accumulation and attenuates the proinflammatory response, J. Biol. Chem. 286 (35) (2011) 30926–30936.

[75] S.B. Joseph, A. Castrillo, B.A. Laffitte, D.J. Mangelsdorf, P. Tontonoz, Reciprocal regulation of inflammation and lipid metabolism by liver X receptors, Nat. Med. 9 (2) (2003) 213–219.

[76] R.K. Upadhyay, Emerging risk biomarkers in cardiovascular diseases and disorders, J. Lipids 2015 (2015).

[77] C.R. Santos, A. Schulze, Lipid metabolism in cancer, FEBS J. 279 (15) (2012) 2610–2623.

[78] L. Jiang, H. Wang, J. Li, X. Fang, H. Pan, X. Yuan, et al., Up-regulated FASN expression promotes transcoelomic metastasis of ovarian cancer cell through epithelial-mesenchymal transition, Int. J. Mol. Sci. 15 (7) (2014) 11539–11554.

[79] I. Ahmad, E. Mui, L. Galbraith, R. Patel, E.H. Tan, M. Salji, et al., Sleeping Beauty screen reveals Pparg activation in metastatic prostate cancer, Proc. Natl. Acad. Sci. U. S. A. 113 (29) (2016) 8290–8295.

[80] J. Li, L. Dong, D. Wei, X. Wang, S. Zhang, H. Li, Fatty acid synthase mediates the epithelial-mesenchymal transition of breast cancer cells, Int. J. Biol. Sci. 10 (2) (2014) 171–180.

[81] Y. Yasumoto, H. Miyazaki, L.K. Vaidyan, Y. Kagawa, M. Ebrahimi, Y. Yamamoto, et al., Inhibition of fatty acid synthase decreases expression of stemness markers in glioma stem cells, PLoS One 11 (1) (2016), e0147717.

[82] H. Wang, Q. Xi, G. Wu, Fatty acid synthase regulates invasion and metastasis of colorectal cancer via Wnt signaling pathway, Cancer Med. 5 (7) (2016) 1599–1606.

[83] Q. Hao, T. Li, X. Zhang, P. Gao, P. Qiao, S. Li, et al., Expression and roles of fatty acid synthase in hepatocellular carcinoma, Oncol. Rep. 32 (6) (2014) 2471–2476.

[84] J. Wang, L. Yu, R.E. Schmidt, C. Su, X. Huang, K. Gould, et al., Characterization of HSCD5, a novel human stearoyl-CoA desaturase unique to primates, Biochem. Biophys. Res. Commun. 332 (3) (2005) 735–742.

[85] R.A. Igal, Stearoyl-CoA desaturase-1: a novel key player in the mechanisms of cell proliferation, programmed cell death and transformation to cancer, Carcinogenesis 31 (9) (2010) 1509–1515.

[86] H. Wang, Y. Zhang, Y. Lu, J. Song, M. Huang, J. Zhang, et al., The role of stearoyl-coenzyme A desaturase 1 in clear cell renal cell carcinoma, Tumour Biol. 37 (1) (2016) 479–489.

[87] A. Varis, M. Wolf, O. Monni, M.-L. Vakkari, A. Kokkola, C. Moskaluk, et al., Targets of gene amplification and overexpression at 17q in gastric cancer, Cancer Res. 62 (9) (2002) 2625–2629.
[88] H.F. Yancy, J.A. Mason, S. Peters, C.E. Thompson, G.K. Littleton, M. Jett, et al., Metastatic progression and gene expression between breast cancer cell lines from African American and Caucasian women, J. Carcinog. 6 (2007) 8.
[89] X. Qian, J. Hu, J. Zhao, H. Chen, ATP citrate lyase expression is associated with advanced stage and prognosis in gastric adenocarcinoma, Int. J. Clin. Exp. Med. 8 (5) (2015) 7855–7860.
[90] G. Medes, A. Thomas, S. Weinhouse, Metabolism of neoplastic tissue. IV. A study of lipid synthesis in neoplastic tissue slices in vitro, Cancer Res. 13 (1) (1953) 27–29.
[91] C. Bagnato, R.A. Igal, Overexpression of diacylglycerol acyltransferase-1 reduces phospholipid synthesis, proliferation, and invasiveness in simian virus 40-transformed human lung fibroblasts, J. Biol. Chem. 278 (52) (2003) 52203–52211.
[92] S.J. Wakil, L.A. Abu-Elheiga, Fatty acid metabolism: target for metabolic syndrome, J. Lipid Res. 50 (Suppl) (2009) S138–S143.
[93] J.D.Y. Chow, R.T. Lawrence, M.E. Healy, J.E. Dominy, J.A. Liao, D.S. Breen, et al., Genetic inhibition of hepatic acetyl-CoA carboxylase activity increases liver fat and alters global protein acetylation, Mol. Metab. 3 (4) (2014) 419–431.
[94] Y.-W. Su, Y.-H. Lin, M.-H. Pai, A.-C. Lo, Y.-C. Lee, I.-C. Fang, et al., Association between phosphorylated AMP-activated protein kinase and acetyl-CoA carboxylase expression and outcome in patients with squamous cell carcinoma of the head and neck, PLoS One 9 (4) (2014), e96183.
[95] M.-D. Wang, H. Wu, G.-B. Fu, H.-L. Zhang, X. Zhou, L. Tang, et al., Acetyl-coenzyme A carboxylase alpha promotion of glucose-mediated fatty acid synthesis enhances survival of hepatocellular carcinoma in mice and patients, Hepatology 63 (4) (2016) 1272–1286.
[96] T.E. Harris, B.N. Finck, Dual function lipin proteins and glycerolipid metabolism, Trends Endocrinol. Metab. 22 (6) (2011) 226–233.
[97] D.K. Nomura, D.P. Lombardi, J.W. Chang, S. Niessen, A.M. Ward, J.Z. Long, et al., Monoacylglycerol lipase exerts dual control over endocannabinoid and fatty acid pathways to support prostate cancer, Chem. Biol. 18 (7) (2011) 846–856.
[98] M. Ma, J. Bai, Y. Ling, W. Chang, G. Xie, R. Li, et al., Monoacylglycerol lipase inhibitor JZL184 regulates apoptosis and migration of colorectal cancer cells, Mol. Med. Rep. 13 (3) (2016) 2850–2856.
[99] M. Murakami, Y. Taketomi, H. Sato, K. Yamamoto, Secreted phospholipase A2 revisited, J. Biochem. 150 (3) (2011) 233–255.
[100] Q. Cai, Z. Zhao, C. Antalis, L. Yan, G. Del Priore, A.H. Hamed, et al., Elevated and secreted phospholipase A_2 activities as new potential therapeutic targets in human epithelial ovarian cancer [Internet], FASEB J. 26 (2012). [cited 2021 Feb 1]. Available from: https://pubmed.ncbi.nlm.nih.gov/22767227/.
[101] S.M. Knoepp, M.S. Chahal, Y. Xie, Z. Zhang, D.J. Brauner, M.A. Hallman, et al., Effects of active and inactive phospholipase D2 on signal transduction, adhesion, migration, invasion, and metastasis in EL4 lymphoma cells [Internet], Mol. Pharmacol. 74 (2008). [cited 2021 Feb 1]. Available from: https://pubmed.ncbi.nlm.nih.gov/18523140/.
[102] J. Gomez-Cambronero, Phospholipase D in cell signaling: from a myriad of cell functions to cancer growth and metastasis, J. Biol. Chem. 289 (33) (2014) 22557–22566.
[103] K.M. Henkels, G.P. Boivin, E.S. Dudley, S.J. Berberich, J. Gomez-Cambronero, Phospholipase D (PLD) drives cell invasion, tumor growth and metastasis in a human breast cancer xenograph model, Oncogene 32 (49) (2013) 5551–5562.
[104] J. Kerner, C. Hoppel, Fatty acid import into mitochondria, Biochim. Biophys. Acta 1486 (1) (2000) 1–17.

[105] R.R. Ramsay, V.A. Zammit, Carnitine acyltransferases and their influence on CoA pools in health and disease, Mol. Aspects Med. 25 (5–6) (2004) 475–493.

[106] J. Reguła, The role of diet in treatment of lipid metabolism disorders, Acta Sci. Pol. Technol. Aliment. 8 (3) (2009) 97–113.

[107] I.I. Abubakar, T. Tillmann, A. Banerjee, Global, regional, and national age-sex specific all-cause and cause-specific mortality for 240 causes of death, 1990-2013: a systematic analysis for the global burden of disease study 2013, Lancet 385 (9963) (2015) 117–171.

[108] G.A. Roth, M.D. Huffman, A.E. Moran, V. Feigin, G.A. Mensah, M. Naghavi, et al., Global and regional patterns in cardiovascular mortality from 1990 to 2013, Circulation 132 (17) (2015) 1667–1678.

[109] G.R. Caponio, D.Q.-H. Wang, A. Di Ciaula, M. De Angelis, P. Portincasa, Regulation of cholesterol metabolism by bioactive components of soy proteins: novel translational evidence, Int. J. Mol. Sci. 22 (1) (2021) 227.

[110] E.D. Michos, J.W. McEvoy, R.S. Blumenthal, Lipid management for the prevention of atherosclerotic cardiovascular disease, N. Engl. J. Med. 381 (16) (2019) 1557–1567.

[111] P.G. O'Malley, M.J. Arnold, C. Kelley, L. Spacek, A. Buelt, S. Natarajan, et al., Management of dyslipidemia for cardiovascular disease risk reduction: synopsis of the 2020 updated US Department of Veterans Affairs and US Department of Defense clinical practice guideline, Ann. Intern. Med. 173 (10) (2020) 822–829.

[112] S. Tonstad, J.-P. Després, Treatment of lipid disorders in obesity, Expert Rev. Cardiovasc. Ther. 9 (8) (2011) 1069–1080.

[113] A. Sillars, N. Sattar, Management of lipid abnormalities in patients with diabetes, Curr. Cardiol. Rep. 21 (11) (2019) 1–8.

[114] F. Francini-Pesenti, P. Spinella, L.A. Calò, Potential role of phytochemicals in metabolic syndrome prevention and therapy, Diabetes Metab. Syndr. Obes. 12 (2019) 1987.

[115] B. Dinda, M. Dinda, A. Roy, S. Dinda, Dietary plant flavonoids in prevention of obesity and diabetes, Adv. Protein Chem. Struct. Biol. 120 (2020) 159–235.

[116] D. Del Rio, A. Rodriguez-Mateos, J.P.E. Spencer, M. Tognolini, G. Borges, A. Crozier, Dietary (poly) phenolics in human health: structures, bioavailability, and evidence of protective effects against chronic diseases, Antioxid. Redox Signal. 18 (14) (2013) 1818–1892.

[117] A.N. Panche, A.D. Diwan, S.R. Chandra, Flavonoids: an overview, J. Nutr. Sci. 5 (2016).

[118] M.A. Mvondo, D. Njamen, G. Kretzschmar, M. Imma Bader, S. Tanee Fomum, J. Wandji, et al., Alpinumisoflavone and abyssinone V 4′-methylether derived from E rythrina lysistemon (F abaceae) promote HDL-cholesterol synthesis and prevent cholesterol gallstone formation in ovariectomized rats, J. Pharm. Pharmacol. 67 (7) (2015) 990–996.

[119] E.-Y. Kwon, M.-S. Choi, Dietary eriodictyol alleviates adiposity, hepatic steatosis, insulin resistance, and inflammation in diet-induced obese mice, Int. J. Mol. Sci. 20 (5) (2019) 1227.

[120] C. Cheng, S. Zhuo, B. Zhang, X. Zhao, Y. Liu, C. Liao, et al., Treatment implications of natural compounds targeting lipid metabolism in nonalcoholic fatty liver disease, obesity and cancer, Int. J. Biol. Sci. 15 (8) (2019) 1654.

[121] Y.-Z. Sun, J.-F. Chen, L.-M. Shen, J. Zhou, C.-F. Wang, Anti-atherosclerotic effect of hesperidin in LDLr-/- mice and its possible mechanism, Eur. J. Pharmacol. 815 (2017) 109–117.

[122] B. Ren, W. Qin, F. Wu, S. Wang, C. Pan, L. Wang, et al., Apigenin and naringenin regulate glucose and lipid metabolism, and ameliorate vascular dysfunction in type 2 diabetic rats, Eur. J. Pharmacol. 773 (2016) 13–23.

[123] Y.-S. Lai, W.-C. Chen, C.-T. Ho, K.-H. Lu, S.-H. Lin, H.-C. Tseng, et al., Garlic essential oil protects against obesity-triggered nonalcoholic fatty liver disease through modulation of lipid metabolism and oxidative stress, J. Agric. Food Chem. 62 (25) (2014) 5897–5906.

[124] M. Massaro, E. Scoditti, M.A. Carluccio, R. De Caterina, Nutraceuticals and prevention of atherosclerosis: focus on ω-3 polyunsaturated fatty acids and mediterranean diet polyphenols, Cardiovasc. Ther. 28 (4) (2010) e13–e19.

[125] M.L. Bonet, J. Ribot, A. Palou, Lipid metabolism in mammalian tissues and its control by retinoic acid, Biochim. Biophys. Acta 1821 (1) (2012) 177–189.

[126] M. Rodriguez-Concepcion, J. Avalos, M.L. Bonet, A. Boronat, L. Gomez-Gomez, D. Hornero-Mendez, et al., A global perspective on carotenoids: metabolism, biotechnology, and benefits for nutrition and health, Prog. Lipid Res. 70 (2018) 62–93.

[127] P. Palozza, A. Catalano, R.E. Simone, M.C. Mele, A. Cittadini, Effect of lycopene and tomato products on cholesterol metabolism, Ann. Nutr. Metab. 61 (2) (2012) 126–134.

[128] Y.-J. Kim, D.-H. Lee, J. Ahn, W.-J. Chung, Y.J. Jang, K.-S. Seong, et al., Pharmacokinetics, tissue distribution, and anti-lipogenic/adipogenic effects of allyl-isothiocyanate metabolites, PLoS One 10 (8) (2015), e0132151.

[129] S.H. Duncan, A. Belenguer, G. Holtrop, A.M. Johnstone, H.J. Flint, G.E. Lobley, Reduced dietary intake of carbohydrates by obese subjects results in decreased concentrations of butyrate and butyrate-producing bacteria in feces, Appl. Environ. Microbiol. 73 (4) (2007) 1073–1078.

[130] H. Chen, J. Li, R. Yao, S. Yan, Q. Wang, Mechanism of lipid metabolism regulation by soluble dietary fibre from micronized and non-micronized powders of lotus root nodes as revealed by their adsorption and activity inhibition of pancreatic lipase, Food Chem. 305 (2020), 125435.

[131] Y.-S. Choi, S.-H. Cho, H.-J. Kim, H.-J. Lee, Effects of soluble dietary fibers on lipid metabolism and activities of intestinal disaccharidases in rats, J. Nutr. Sci. Vitaminol. 44 (5) (1998) 591–600.

[132] L. Qiu, B. Lin, Z. Lin, Y. Lin, M. Lin, X. Yang, Biochanin A ameliorates the cytokine secretion profile of lipopolysaccharide-stimulated macrophages by a PPARγ-dependent pathway, Mol. Med. Rep. 5 (1) (2012) 217–222.

[133] D. Das, S. Sarkar, J. Bordoloi, S.B. Wann, J. Kalita, P. Manna, Daidzein, its effects on impaired glucose and lipid metabolism and vascular inflammation associated with type 2 diabetes, Biofactors 44 (5) (2018) 407–417.

[134] S.A. Park, M.-S. Choi, S.-Y. Cho, J.-S. Seo, U.J. Jung, M.-J. Kim, et al., Genistein and daidzein modulate hepatic glucose and lipid regulating enzyme activities in C57BL/KsJ-db/db mice, Life Sci. 79 (12) (2006) 1207–1213.

[135] M.P. Andreas, Antioxidant Status, Diet, Nutrition and Health, CRC Press, Boca Raton, 1999.

[136] Y.-H. Yeh, Y.-T. Lee, H.-S. Hsieh, D.-F. Hwang, Dietary caffeic acid, ferulic acid and coumaric acid supplements on cholesterol metabolism and antioxidant activity in rats, J. Food Drug Anal. 17 (2) (2009).

[137] H. Poudyal, N. Lemonakis, P. Efentakis, E. Gikas, M. Halabalaki, I. Andreadou, et al., Hydroxytyrosol ameliorates metabolic, cardiovascular and liver changes in a rat model of diet-induced metabolic syndrome: pharmacological and metabolism-based investigation, Pharmacol. Res. 117 (2017) 32–45.

[138] C. La Lastra, M.D. Barranco, V. Motilva, J.M. Herrerias, Mediterrranean diet and health biological importance of olive oil, Curr. Pharm. Des. 7 (10) (2001) 933–950.

[139] A. Karković Marković, J. Torić, M. Barbarić, B.C. Jakobušić, Hydroxytyrosol, tyrosol and derivatives and their potential effects on human health, Molecules 24 (10) (2019) 2001.

[140] H. Gylling, T.A. Miettinen, The effect of plant stanol-and sterol-enriched foods on lipid metabolism, serum lipids and coronary heart disease, Ann. Clin. Biochem. 42 (4) (2005) 254–263.

[141] I. Ikeda, R. Konno, T. Shimizu, T. Ide, N. Takahashi, T. Kawada, et al., Campest-5-en-3-one, an oxidized derivative of campesterol, activates PPARα, promotes energy consumption and reduces visceral fat deposition in rats, Biochim. Biophys. Acta Gen. Subj. 1760 (5) (2006) 800–807.

[142] F.Y. Ntanios, P.J.H. Jones, Effects of variable dietary sitostanol concentrations on plasma lipid profile and phytosterol metabolism in hamsters, Biochim. Biophys. Acta 1390 (3) (1998) 237–244.
[143] H.C. Pal, R.L. Pearlman, F. Afaq, Fisetin and its role in chronic diseases, in: Anti-inflammatory Nutraceuticals and Chronic Diseases, 2016, pp. 213–244.
[144] T.-I. Jeon, J.W. Park, J. Ahn, C.H. Jung, T.Y. Ha, Fisetin protects against hepatosteatosis in mice by inhibiting mi R-378, Mol. Nutr. Food Res. 57 (11) (2013) 1931–1937.
[145] U. Justesen, P. Knuthsen, T. Leth, Quantitative analysis of flavonols, flavones, and flavanones in fruits, vegetables and beverages by high-performance liquid chromatography with photo-diode array and mass spectrometric detection, J. Chromatogr. A 799 (1–2) (1998) 101–110.
[146] S.H. Häkkinen, S.O. Kärenlampi, I.M. Heinonen, H.M. Mykkänen, A.R. Törrönen, Content of the flavonols quercetin, myricetin, and kaempferol in 25 edible berries, J. Agric. Food Chem. 47 (6) (1999) 2274–2279.
[147] C.J. Chang, T.-F. Tzeng, S.-S. Liou, Y.-S. Chang, I.-M. Liu, Kaempferol regulates the lipid-profile in high-fat diet-fed rats through an increase in hepatic PPARα levels, Planta Med. 77 (17) (2011) 1876–1882.
[148] L. Kong, C. Luo, X. Li, Y. Zhou, H. He, The anti-inflammatory effect of kaempferol on early atherosclerosis in high cholesterol fed rabbits, Lipids Health Dis. 12 (1) (2013) 1–12.
[149] A. Ochiai, S. Miyata, M. Iwase, M. Shimizu, J. Inoue, R. Sato, Kaempferol stimulates gene expression of low-density lipoprotein receptor through activation of Sp1 in cultured hepatocytes, Sci. Rep. 6 (1) (2016) 1–10.
[150] C.J. Chang, T.-F. Tzeng, S.-S. Liou, Y.-S. Chang, I.-M. Liu, Myricetin increases hepatic peroxisome proliferator-activated receptor α protein expression and decreases plasma lipids and adiposity in rats, Evid. Based Complement. Alternat. Med. 2012 (2012).
[151] S. Akindehin, Y.-S. Jung, S.-N. Kim, Y.-H. Son, I. Lee, J.K. Seong, et al., Myricetin exerts anti-obesity effects through upregulation of SIRT3 in adipose tissue, Nutrients 10 (12) (2018) 1962.
[152] Y. Cui, P. Hou, F. Li, Q. Liu, S. Qin, G. Zhou, et al., Quercetin improves macrophage reverse cholesterol transport in apolipoprotein E-deficient mice fed a high-fat diet, Lipids Health Dis. 16 (1) (2017) 1–7.
[153] Y. Li, W. Zhao, W.W. OuYang, M. Wang, F. Jin, Effect of quercetin on lipid metabolism in adipocytes, J. Northeast. Agric. Univ. 44 (3) (2013) 58–65.
[154] M. Kobori, S. Masumoto, Y. Akimoto, H. Oike, Chronic dietary intake of quercetin alleviates hepatic fat accumulation associated with consumption of a Western-style diet in C57/BL6J mice, Mol. Nutr. Food Res. 55 (4) (2011) 530–540.
[155] S.K. Panchal, H. Poudyal, L. Brown, Quercetin ameliorates cardiovascular, hepatic, and metabolic changes in diet-induced metabolic syndrome in rats, J. Nutr. 142 (6) (2012) 1026–1032.
[156] H.-N. Choi, S.-M. Jeong, G.H. Huh, J.-I. Kim, Quercetin ameliorates insulin sensitivity and liver steatosis partly by increasing adiponectin expression in ob/ob mice, Food Sci. Biotechnol. 24 (1) (2015) 273–279.
[157] M. Wang, Y. Mao, B. Wang, S. Wang, H. Lu, L. Ying, et al., Quercetin improving lipid metabolism by regulating lipid metabolism pathway of ileum mucosa in broilers, Oxid. Med. Cell. Longev. 2020 (2020).
[158] A. Korkmaz, D. Kolankaya, Protective effect of rutin on the ischemia/reperfusion induced damage in rat kidney, J. Surg. Res. 164 (2) (2010) 309–315.
[159] A. Gęgotek, P. Rybałtowska-Kawałko, E. Skrzydlewska, Rutin as a mediator of lipid metabolism and cellular signaling pathways interactions in fibroblasts altered by UVA and UVB radiation, Oxid. Med. Cell. Longev. 2017 (2017).
[160] A. Ziaee, F. Zamansoltani, M. Nassiri-Asl, E. Abbasi, Effects of rutin on lipid profile in hypercholesterolaemic rats, Basic Clin. Pharmacol. Toxicol. 104 (3) (2009) 253–258.

[161] X. Feng, W. Yu, X. Li, F. Zhou, W. Zhang, Q. Shen, et al., Apigenin, a modulator of PPARγ, attenuates HFD-induced NAFLD by regulating hepatocyte lipid metabolism and oxidative stress via Nrf2 activation, Biochem. Pharmacol. 136 (2017) 136–149.
[162] X. Ge, H. Chen, T. Liu, L. Chen, Y. Huang, F. Zeng, et al., Luteolin cooperated with metformin hydrochloride alleviates lipid metabolism disorders and optimizes intestinal flora compositions of high-fat diet mice, Food Funct. 11 (11) (2020) 10033–10046.
[163] S. Fukumitsu, K. Aida, N. Ueno, S. Ozawa, Y. Takahashi, M. Kobori, Flaxseed lignan attenuates high-fat diet-induced fat accumulation and induces adiponectin expression in mice, Br. J. Nutr. 100 (3) (2008) 669–676.
[164] H. Adlercreutz, R. Heikkinen, M. Woods, T. Fotsis, J.T. Dwyer, B.R. Goldin, et al., Excretion of the lignans enterolactone and enterodiol and of equol in omnivorous and vegetarian postmenopausal women and in women with breast cancer, Lancet 320 (8311) (1982) 1295–1299.
[165] T. Wu, L. Yang, X. Guo, M. Zhang, R. Liu, W. Sui, Raspberry anthocyanin consumption prevents diet-induced obesity by alleviating oxidative stress and modulating hepatic lipid metabolism, Food Funct. 9 (4) (2018) 2112–2120.
[166] A. Aboonabi, A. Aboonabi, Anthocyanins reduce inflammation and improve glucose and lipid metabolism associated with inhibiting nuclear factor-kappaB activation and increasing PPAR-γ gene expression in metabolic syndrome subjects, Free Radic. Biol. Med. 150 (2020) 30–39.
[167] J. Ahn, I. Cho, S. Kim, D. Kwon, T. Ha, Dietary resveratrol alters lipid metabolism-related gene expression of mice on an atherogenic diet, J. Hepatol. 49 (6) (2008) 1019–1028.
[168] S. Chen, X. Zhao, L. Ran, J. Wan, X. Wang, Y. Qin, et al., Resveratrol improves insulin resistance, glucose and lipid metabolism in patients with non-alcoholic fatty liver disease: a randomized controlled trial, Dig. Liver Dis. 47 (3) (2015) 226–232.
[169] T. Kisková, M. Kassayová, Resveratrol action on lipid metabolism in cancer, Int. J. Mol. Sci. 20 (11) (2019) 2704.
[170] V. Crespy, G. Williamson, A review of the health effects of green tea catechins in in vivo animal models, J. Nutr. 134 (12) (2004) 3431S–3440S.
[171] S.-H. Yoo, Y.-E. Lee, J.-O. Chung, C.-S. Rha, Y.-D. Hong, M.-Y. Park, et al., Enhancing the effect of catechins with green tea flavonol and polysaccharides on preventing lipid absorption and accumulation, LWT 134 (2020), 110032.
[172] D.J. Maron, G.P. Lu, N.S. Cai, Z.G. Wu, Y.H. Li, H. Chen, et al., Cholesterol-lowering effect of a theaflavin-enriched green tea extract: a randomized controlled trial, Arch. Intern. Med. 163 (12) (2003) 1448–1453.
[173] C. Liu, Y. Guo, L. Sun, X. Lai, Q. Li, W. Zhang, et al., Six types of tea reduce high-fat-diet-induced fat accumulation in mice by increasing lipid metabolism and suppressing inflammation, Food Funct. 10 (4) (2019) 2061–2074.
[174] G. Pereira-Caro, J.M. Moreno-Rojas, N. Brindani, D. Del Rio, M.E.J. Lean, Y. Hara, et al., Bioavailability of black tea theaflavins: absorption, metabolism, and colonic catabolism, J. Agric. Food Chem. 65 (26) (2017) 5365–5374.
[175] Q.Y. Zhu, A. Zhang, D. Tsang, Y. Huang, Z.-Y. Chen, Stability of green tea catechins, J. Agric. Food Chem. 45 (12) (1997) 4624–4628.
[176] J. Zhou, B.L. Farah, R.A. Sinha, Y. Wu, B.K. Singh, B.-H. Bay, et al., Epigallocatechin-3-gallate (EGCG), a green tea polyphenol, stimulates hepatic autophagy and lipid clearance, PLoS One 9 (1) (2014), e87161.

CHAPTER 8

Cancer metabolism regulation by phytonutrients

Ammara Riaz[a,*], Rabia Zara[a,*], Gul Bushra[b], Nazia Kanwal[a], Ayesha Sadiqa[a], Farzana Shareef[a], Iqra Sarfraz[a], Muhammad Ajmal Shah[c], Ilknur Ucak[d], Shazia Anwer Bukhari[e], and Azhar Rasul[a]

[a]Department of Life Sciences, Khwaja Fareed University of Engineering and Information Technology, Rahim Yar Khan, Pakistan
[b]Department of Bioinformatics and Biotechnology, Faculty of Life Sciences, Government College University, Faisalabad, Pakistan
[c]Department of Pharmacognosy, Faculty of Pharmaceutical Sciences, Government College University, Faisalabad, Pakistan
[d]Nigde Omer Halisdemir University, Nigde, Turkey
[e]Department of Biochemistry, Government College University, Faisalabad, Pakistan

1. Introduction

Cancer has been documented as the second leading cause of mortality all over the world and it has been expected that its prevalence will increase in the future [1]. It accounted for 9.6 million deaths and 18.1 million newly diagnosed cancer cases all over the world during the year 2018 [2]. In spite of the growing area of research in the arena of cancer biology, cancer has been emerging as a complicated and diverse set of disorders [3]. Cancer can be defined as a multifaceted abnormality characterized by the aberrant cell signaling cascades leading to abnormal cellular proliferation, angiogenesis, tumor progression, deregulated cell cycle, and apoptosis [4].

Cellular proliferation is an eminent hallmark of cancer which is triggered when a cell switches its metabolism to the deregulated state due to the remarkable mutations in cell signaling cascades [5]. The cellular proliferation ultimately paves its way toward tumorigenesis while enabling the cells to acquire greater malignant potential [6]. Metabolic alterations help the cancer cells to fulfill their energetics and anabolic demands for enhanced proliferation and abrupt growth. To achieve sustainable progression, cancer cells activate various metabolic pathways, a process termed as metabolic reprogramming [7]. At this stage, metabolic pathways need a lot of energy

*Authors who contributed equally in publication.

The Role of Phytonutrients in Metabolic Disorders
https://doi.org/10.1016/B978-0-12-824356-5.00002-3

to satisfy their infinitely growing energy demands which they fulfilled by utilizing the cellular nutrients to produce metabolic precursors for anabolic reactions and maintain an equilibrium during redox reactions in the cell [8]. Metastasis is the last stage of cancer development which is referred to as the overgrowth and invasiveness of tumor cells [9].

Lipids, proteins, and nucleotides constitute the dry mass of mammalian cells. Inside the cells, these macromolecules are manufactured by their respective metabolic precursors, e.g., the precursor of lipids is acetyl-CoA, whereas amino acids play their part in the synthesis of proteins and nucleotides are synthesized by purines and pyrimidines. All of these precursors are prepared by the nutrients available in the cell by several metabolic processes carried out inside the cell [10]. As has already been mentioned, cancer cells undergo cellular reprogramming and have a different metabolism compared to normal cells. Otto Warburg elaborated a peculiar type of cancer cell metabolism in the 1920s, and his findings about the reprogrammed cell metabolism were named the "Warburg effect." He explained that glucose, even in the presence of oxygen, incompletely metabolized and converted into carbon dioxide and water and led to lactic acid accumulation inside the cell [11].

This process was called aerobic glycolysis as opposed to anaerobic glycolysis, because it also takes place in the presence of adequate oxygen concentrations. A scientific discussion was pivoted around this concept for the next 50 years after this discovery. It was noticed that tumor cells undergo metabolic reprogramming on the basis of availability of oxygen and changes in the tumor microenvironment [12]. Tumor cells meet their energy requirements by making ATP and NADPH through the breakdown of glucose and glutamine, so the increased rate of glycolysis not only helps the tumor cell to fulfill its elevated energy demands but also helps in the production of proteins, lipids, and amino acids via glucose metabolism, lipid metabolism, and serine metabolism [13]. Mitochondria play significant roles in the production and synthesis of ATP, several metabolites in addition to controlling the production of reactive oxygen species (ROS). Apoptosis, the programmed cell death, also triggers in mitochondria. In case of tumor cells, there is an increased risk of mitochondrial dysfunction, thereby increasing the ROS levels inside the cell which favors the process of tumorigenesis and retards apoptosis [14].

In this chapter, we briefly describe the metabolic pathways with special reference to glucose as the starting materials due to its abundance inside the cell and its fundamental status in metabolism reprogramming in mammalian cells. After that glutamine is discussed (subject to its consumption) followed by the metabolism of serine as well as other amino acids. In addition, there is also an illustration of the role of fatty acid synthesis and functions of oxygen, both as the source of ROS generation and the electron acceptor.

1.1 Aerobic glycolysis

In healthy cells, most of the glucose is catabolized to pyruvate by undergoing the glycolysis process. As a result of glycolysis, pyruvate can be obtained as a by-product which is further transported into mitochondria. Here the tricarboxylic acid cycle (TCA cycle) and electron transport chain [15] are utilized to carry out aerobic respiration. The breakdown of glucose coupled with oxidative phosphorylation results in a higher output of energy obtained as ATP units [16]. In contrast to the process of glycolysis in normal cells, cancer cells convert the pyruvate into lactate utilizing lactate transporters. The catabolism of glucose into lactate generates a very low amount of energy, and the cancer cells have to consume more and more glucose to carry out their routine metabolism and continue the process of proliferation and metastasis [17]. Fig. 1 elaborates the difference in the process of glycolysis in normal and cancer cells.

A glucose transporter such as GLUT-1 helps in the high consumption of glucose by the cancer cells during the process of synthesis of acetyl-Co-A

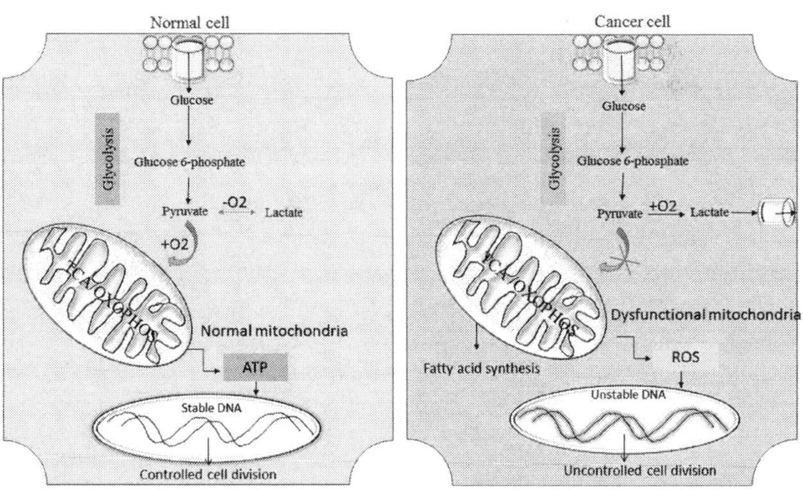

Fig. 1 Normal cells undergo the process of aerobic glycolysis leading to end product pyruvate while cancer cells alter their metabolic machinery and perform anaerobic glycolysis leading to the end product, lactic acid.

from pyruvate, a precursor of fatty acid, cholesterol, and lipids [18]. Glucose 6-phosphate (G6P) is produced during glycolysis. G6P is a point of convergence among the pentose phosphate pathway (PPP) and glycolysis. PPP plays a significant role in NADPH production, and it also produces the ribose group. This group is the prerequisite for nucleotides synthesis. Glycolysis provides a key process to the tumor cells in terms of generating high-energy compounds, e.g., NADPH, by the utilization of glucose as their starting material [19].

1.2 Glycolysis

Glycolysis is a metabolic process which involves the conversion of glucose into pyruvate and alongside the production of ATP and NADH [20]. In the presence of adequate amounts of oxygen, pyruvate (the end product of glucose metabolism) is actively transported to mitochondria for metabolism through tricarboxylic acid cycle [15] cycle which produces energy precursors for oxidative phosphorylation. On the other side, in the absence of oxygen, pyruvate is converted into lactate and glycolysis remains the main source of ATP production [21]. The whole process of glycolysis consists of 20 steps of chemical reactions and each step is catalyzed by a specific enzyme, which was discovered in the 1940s [22]. Under hypoxic conditions, pyruvate is converted into lactate both in normal and cancer cells, but tumor cells prefer the conversion of pyruvate into lactate instead of entering into the TCA cycle, even in the availability of sufficient oxygen [23]. This section of the chapter aims to explain the role of glycolytic enzymes in the cancer metabolism and progression and their role as therapeutic agents in cancer therapy by targeting through phytonutrients.

1.3 Targeting glycolysis by phytonutrients

1.3.1 Hexokinase

The first step of the process of glycolysis is catalyzed by the enzyme Hexokinase [22]. It is a tissue-specific enzyme which catalyzes the conversion of glucose-to-glucose 6 phosphate (G6P). HK is categorized as a rate-limiting enzyme of glucose oxidation reaction [24]. There are four isoforms of HK in a mammalian cell. HK1/A is considered as the housekeeping enzyme as it is found in all mammalian tissues. HKII/B is considered as the principal regulated isoform with overexpression in a number of cancer cells. HKIII/C is a substrate inhibited form at physiologic concentrations, and finally HKIV is referred to as glucokinase. In the glucose catabolism, HKII/B plays a principal role [25]. Many research reports have mentioned that HKII functions as cancer's double-edged sword because it acts as both the gatekeeper enzyme and facilitator of tumor malignancy when bound to mitochondria [24].

Moreover, the functional study of HK has reported that the glucose dependence of the antiapoptotic effects of growth factors and protein kinase B showed a significant correlation between AKT-regulated mitochondrial HK association and survival of cancer cells. So it can be summarized that the interactions between HK and mitochondria are not only essential to facilitate and maintain a high rate of glycolysis in malignant cells but are also crucial for tumor survival [26]. Overexpression of HK has been reported in various cancers such as ovarian cancer [27], breast cancer [28], liver cancer [29], gastric cancer [30], cervical cancer [31], and colon cancer [32]. Due to the significant role of HK in the cancer metabolism, it is regarded as a potential therapeutic target of cancer therapy. Some studies have reported the targeting of HK by phytonutrients which are mentioned as follows:

Resveratrol is a major polyphenol naturally found in raspberries, grapes, and peanuts. It has a wide range of antioxidant, anticancer, and antiinflammatory pharmacological properties. It modulates several pathways which are involved in cell progression and proliferation. Resveratrol can subdue the expression of ROS and miRNA in pancreatic cancer cells by the disruption of HK-II/B [33]. Another dietary inhibitor is capsaicin which is the main component of capsicum. Capsaicin has been involved in the treatments of a variety of cancers. It can suppress the activity of HK-II in esophageal squamous cell carcinoma. Capsaicin enhances the level of PTEN expression, which acts as a tumor suppressor gene and inhibits the activity of HK-II with an IC50 value of 30 μM [34].

1.3.2 GPI

Phosphoglucose isomerase (GPI) is another enzyme of glucose metabolism, which has a characteristic dual nature. It not only catalyzes the conversion of G6P into fructose-6-phospahte (F6P), but also acts as an extracellular cytokine under the name of autocrine motility factor (AMF) [35]. The cytokine role of AMF/GPI has a direct link with cell differentiation and survival. AMF/GPI cytokine function in tumor cell motility is dependent on interaction with its receptor, gp78/AMFR. gp78/AMFR, like its ligand, has multiple roles dictated by its cellular localization [36].

Phosphoglucose isomerase is another enzyme which plays a great role in glycolysis and glycogenesis pathways. Emerging evidence has reported that it encodes the glucose 6 phosphate isomerase in humans and catalyzes the conversion of G6P into fructose 6 phosphate (F6P). It was first reported in 1933 by Ohm who discovered it in skeletal muscles. He further described that its activity is relatively higher in body tissue than in plasma [37].

The aberrant action of this enzyme has been reported in different kinds of cancers like glioblastoma [38], lung cancer [39], breast cancer [40,41], gastrointestinal cancer [41,42], head and neck carcinoma [43], colorectal cancer [44], and gastric cancer [45]. In different types of cancers, the up-regulation of glycolysis has been identified. Overexpression of AMF/GPI contributes to tumor progression and metastasis. It also acts as a paracrine factor in normal cells. The higher level of AMF/GPI may act as a prognostic factor in cancer identification [46].

Various reports have provided us with the targeting of GPI with anticancer phytonutrients obtained from natural sources. Ursolic acid is the major bioactive component and a pentacyclic triterpenoid. Apple skin is a promising source of ursolic acid. This pentacyclic triterpenoid exhibits functional properties in suppression of cancer cells [47]. The emerging evidences indicate that ursolic acid had a potent effect against hepatocellular carcinoma by the suppression of AMF/GPI. In HCC, it restrains the aberrant activity of GPI and MMP-3 secretions protect against the TGF-β-induced apoptosis and phosphorylates Akt, p85, Bad, and Stat3. So ursolic acid is a novel dietary inhibitor for the suppression of GPI and inhibits the PI3 kinase activity in the Huh-7 cell line [48].

1.3.3 PFK

Phosphofructokinase (PFK) is designated as the gatekeeper enzyme of glucose metabolism and catalyzes the transformation of G6P into fructose 1,6-bisphosphate. In mammalian tissues, it is found in three isoforms such as the PFKL (liver), PFKP (platelet), and PFKM (muscle) [49]. PFK is activated by AMP, ADP, and inorganic phosphate and is inhibited by ATP, fatty acids, and citrate. Phosphofructokinase has great importance in cell proliferation and cancer progression [50]. Expression of PFK has been reported in bladder cancer [51], nasopharyngeal carcinoma [52], breast carcinoma [53,54], pancreatic cancer [55], and renal carcinoma [56]. Tap 73 is a homologue of the tumor suppressor gene p53 and is upregulated in different cancers. PFKL is the most important site of regulation and Tap73 has a critical role in PFKL because its aberrant effect enhances the glucose consumption level and increases the lactate production. So Tap73 and the PFKL axis represent a significant way through which the growth signals coupled with the glucose metabolism. These growth signals help in cancer cell proliferation [57].

Targeting of PFK by epigallocatechin-3-gallate (EGCG), which is mainly found in green tea, apple peels, and plums, proved to be effective in cancer therapy. EGCG lowers the abnormal expression of Phosphofructokinase in hepatocellular carcinoma cell lines HepG2 and Huh-7 with an IC50 value of 50 μM via the downregulation of the mitochondrial membrane potential ($\Delta\psi m$) [58].

1.3.4 Aldolase

Aldolase is a glycolytic enzyme which is responsible for the conversion of fructose 1,6-bisphosphate into glyceraldehyde-3-phosphate and dihydroxyacetone phosphate (DHAP). Aldolase is a family of enzymes which have three isoforms, ALDOA, ALDOB, and ALDOC [59]. All these isoforms have variable functions in different bodily tissues such as ALDOB, which is found in the kidney, liver, and erythrocytes, and ALDOC, which has high expression in brain tissues. ALDOB is involved in both glycolysis and gluconeogenesis, whereas ALDOA and ALDOC are mainly involved in glycolysis [60]. Among all isoforms, ALDOA is a highly conserved enzyme and its upregulation has been reported in various types of cancers such as colon cancer [46], lung cancer [61], gastric cancer [62], pancreatic cancer [63], and colorectal cancer [64]. It presents in all types of cells, especially in the liver and brain [59]. In colon cancer, Aldolase shows aggressive behavior and causes metastasis at both the mRNA and protein level [46].

Due to the overexpression of ALDOA in various reported cancers, it can be a potential therapeutic anticancer target. The application of shikonin, a bioactive compound from plants, proved to be useful in the treatment of various cancer cell lines. It has the ability to treat breast cancer. Shikonin give its anticancer results by reducing the aberrant expression of ALDOA against the MCF-7 cells. So it is designated as a novel compound to treat breast cancer via lowering the activity of ALDOA [65].

1.3.5 TPI (triose-phosphate isomerase)

This particular enzyme functions to derive the catalysis of DHAP to glyceraldehyde-3-phosphate [66]. Its structure consists of a homodimer with two units weighing 27 kDa. TPI expression has been reported to enhance in hypoxic tumors, which are regulated by the HIF-1 signaling cascade [67]. It is also known to be involved in the migration as well as invasion of tumor cells in different types of cancers, e.g., gastric cancer [68], lung cancer [69], prostate cancer [70], and kidney cancer [71]. Depending upon the expression and role of TPI in cancer development, it is thought to be an attractive therapeutic target as well as a cancer-related biomarker for the diagnosis of malignancy. Caffeic acid phenethyl ester, a compound from propolis, is a natural phenolic antioxidant which is known to exert anticancer effects against colorectal (CRC) cells by downregulating TPI in cancer cells [72].

1.3.6 GAPDH

The addition of one phosphate group in glyceraldeyde-3-phosphate converts into 1,3-bisphosphoglycerate with simultaneous reduction of NAD+ to NADH. This process is usually catalyzed by glyceraldehyde-3-phosphate dehydrogenase (GAPDH). It is regarded as a housekeeping gene that is expressed in a majority of cells where it participates in multiple cellular functions such as DNA replication and repair, endocytosis, exocytosis cell death, and many more; however, the expression of GAPDH is upregulated in only tumor cells. Cancer aggressiveness and drug resistance are associated with the overexpression of GAPDH. GAPDH has been reported to upregulate in several types of cancer including breast cancer [73], lung cancer, esophageal squamous cell carcinoma [74], liver cancer [75], ovarian cancer [76], and colorectal cancer [77].

Koningic acid, also known as avocettin, is derived from a fungus *Trichoderma koningii*, which covalently binds to the Cys 149 residue in the active pocket of GAPDH, thus inhibiting the enzyme activity [78]. Upregulated-glycolytic tumor cells are significantly killed when exposed to koningic acid at the $\mu g\,mL^{-1}$ concentration via glucose-dependent active ATP depletion, and a $1\,mg\,kg^{-1}$ dose of this compound was reported to be effective in vivo, inhibiting the tumor growth of Erlich ascites in mice [79]. Shikonin, vitamin K3, and vitamin K5 are major naphthaquinones which have been reported as efficient inhibitors of glycolysis [80]. Shikonin and vitamin K5 have been revealed to significantly inhibit the GAPDH activity in MCF-7 breast cancer cell lines [65].

1.3.7 PGK

Phosphoglycerate kinase (PGK) is known as a central enzyme of glycolysis, which is present in all somatic cells, where it is responsible to supply energy via a reversible phosphor-transfer reaction from substrate 1,3-bisphosphoglycerate (1,3-BPG) to ADP in order to form 3-phosphoglycerate (3-PG) and ATP in the presence of free magnesium. Human PGK is a monomer of 48 kDa present in two isoforms: PGK1, which is expressed in all somatic and tumor cells and exposed to HIF-1 upregulation, and PGK2, which is only found in spermatozoids for normal motility and fertility of mammalian spermatozoa [81].

PGK1 exhibits many oncogenic features promoting cancer cell proliferation, invasion, and migration and is reported to overexpress in a variety of cancers including breast cancer [82], lung cancer [83], prostate cancer [84], pancreatic ductal adenocarcinoma [85], gastric cancer [86,87], hepatocellular carcinoma [88–90], glioma [91], and colorectal cancer [92]. In addition to acting as a glycolytic enzyme, PGK1 is also involved in extracellular secretion and regulation of angiogenesis in cancer cells by serving as a disulfide reductase. Furthermore, overexpression of this enzyme seems to be associated with the development of a multidrug-resistance phenotype in various cancers, by means of an MDR-1 independent mechanism. So PGK1 is a highly important molecular target for cancer therapy, which has also become a research hotspot in recent years [93].

Curcumin, a dietary phytochemical naturally derived from the rhizome of *Curcuma longa*, modulates a variety of signaling pathways associated with cell proliferation, progression, inflammation, apoptosis, and androgen signaling [94]. Emerging evidences indicate that curcumin also alters specific miRNA expression in a variety of cancers. MicroRNAs (miRNAs) are a class of noncoding small RNAs that posttranscriptionally regulate a large array of biological processes [84]. PGK1 is also a common target of miRNAs. Curcumin treatment in DU145 prostate cancer cells significantly decreases cell proliferation by inhibiting the activity of PGK1 via increasing the expression of FOXD3. In summary, curcumin restores the expression of miR-143 in prostate cancer by downregulating the expression of PGK1 [95].

1.3.8 PGAM

Phosphoglycerate mutase was initially discovered in yeast [96] and later on in many other organisms (with crystal structure determination and amino acid sequencing) including humans, rats [97], and bacteria. Phosphoglycerate mutases are a group of enzymes which play a crucial role in glucose and the 2, 3-bisphosphoglycerate (2, 3-BPG) metabolism. These enzymes are responsible for the conversion of phosphate groups into phosphoglycerates. The PGAM family can be subdivided into two distinct classes, monophosphoglycerate mutase (mPGAM) and bisphosphoglycerate mutase (BPGAM); mPGAM primarily catalyzes the reversible transformation of 3-PG into 2-PG, whereas the conversion of 1,3-bisphosphoglycerate (BPG) into 2,3-BPG in the presence of 3-PG is usually catalyzed by BPGAM [98].

Phosphoglycerate mutase 1 (PGAM1) is an important nonrate-limiting enzyme responsible for catalyzing the reversible transformation of

3-phosphoglycerate to 2-phosphoglycerate in the latter stage of glycolysis [99]. PGAM1 is not only associated with the progression of tumor cells via its metabolic performance but also drives metastasis through its nonmetabolic networks. PGAM1 directly binds with ACTA2 (α-smooth muscle actin 2) that converts globular actin into filamentous actin which is involved in cytoskeleton remodeling. Actin subtleties and their arrangement show a basic role in the migration of colorectal cancer cells and many other aggressive types of cancer [100]. In the previous few years, growing attention is given to PGAM1 because it is overexpressed in numerous kinds of human aggressive cancer, mainly breast cancer [101], prostate cancer [102,103], lung cancer [104,105], colorectal cancer [106], hepatocellular carcinoma [107], oral squamous cell carcinoma (OSCC) [108], and pancreatic ductal adenocarcinoma (PDAC) [109,110] with higher enzymatic activity than in adjacent healthy tissues. Previous studies indicated that PGAM1-mediated glycolysis is interrelated with tumor development, propagation, survival, and migration of cancer cells [104].

Although PGAM1 has become an emerging and promising target for cancer therapy, only a few small molecules are currently reported as representative of PGAM1 inhibitors [109]. Epigallocatechin-3-gallate (EGCG), a major natural catechin that is extracted from green tea, is discovered to be a PGAM1 inhibitor immensely more potent than other known PGAM1 inhibitors. EGCG inhibits PGAM1 with IC50 values of $0.49 \pm 0.17\,\mu M$, which shows that it is 30 times more potent than PGMI-004A (a previously known PGAM1 inhibitor). EGCG modulated the intracellular level of 2-phosphoglycerate, decreased the rate of glycolysis and the PPP pathway, and inhibited the proliferation of human nonsmall cell lung carcinoma NCI-H1299 and breast cancer MDA-MB-231 cell lines [111].

1.3.9 ENO

The ninth step of glycolysis is catalyzed by Enolase (ENO) in which reversible dehydration of 2-phosphoglycerate (2-PGA) takes place into phosphoenolpyruvate (PEP). Enolase contributes in both glycolysis and gluconeogenesis two metabolic pathways that are very important for cellular function [112]. Enolase has three dimeric isoenzymes in humans: ENO1 which is found in the liver, spleen, kidney, and adipose tissue; ENO2 (neuron-specific) and ENO3 (muscle-specific). Enolase1 is overexpressed in more than 20 different types of cancer [113] such as gastric cancer [114], breast cancer [115], liver cancer [116], endometrial carcinoma [117], pancreatic cancer [118], lung cancer [119], and colorectal cancer [120].

1.3.10 Pyruvate kinase

In the glycolytic pathway, pyruvate kinase is a complex enzyme. It is an irreversible step which converts the phosphoenolpyruvate to pyruvate and produces one molecule of ATP [121]. In the presence of oxygen, pyruvate enters the mitochondria and is converted into acetyl-Co-A by the help of the pyruvate dehydrogenase complex, or if there is a low level of oxygen, then pyruvate converts into lactic acid [122] as pyruvate kinase has both dimeric and tetrameric forms. In mammals, there are four isoforms of PK which are encoded by two genes. PKL encoded by the *PKRL* gene is expressed in some cells of the pancreas, kidney, and liver [123]. But the PKM2 is highly expressed in different types of cancers, as reported by the data since the last 40 years [124]. It is overexpressed in multiple cancers like thyroid cancer [125], ovarian cancer [126], renal carcinoma [127], breast cancer [128], and lung cancer [129].

Apigenin is a flavonoid that is derived from fruits and vegetables like parsley, celery, and grapefruits. It is a phytonutrient which proved to exert different antioxidant, antiinflammatory, and anticancer activities. It is reported that apigenin exerts its effect in signaling pathways against cancer cells [130]. Apigenin is capable of smoothening the role of PKM2 in tumor cells like in colon cancer it inhibits B-catenin and c-Myc [131]. Furthermore, Quercetin, which is another flavonoid, is found in red onion or cabbage leaves. It has a significant role in the regulation of PKM2 against the breast cancer cell line MCF-7. Quercetin inhibits the Akt-mTOR pathway, which is responsible for the regulation of the cell cycle, and it is related to cellular quiescence with an IC50 value of 30 μM [132]. In addition, to further regulate the normal PKM2 activity, shikonin and oleanolic acid exhibit the ability to treat breast cancer, bladder cancer, and prostate cancer via maintaining the expression of PKM2 in cancer cell lines [133,134] Table 1.

2. Pentose phosphate pathway (PPP)

Monohexose shunt or PPP is a glucose-consuming metabolic pathway which is divided into two biochemical phases: oxidative phase and nonoxidative phase [138]. In the oxidative branch, G6P is converted into 6-phosphogluconate, while in the nonoxidative branch reversible carbon-exchanging reactions occur leading to the production of F6P and G3P (22580150). Oxidative branch reactions are catalyzed by G6PD and 6-PGD while nonoxidative branch reactions catalyzation is the responsibility of TKT and TALDO [139].

Table 1 Phytonutrients as metabolic regulators of glycolytic enzymes.

Metabolic Enzyme	Phytonutrients modulators			Cancer type	Cell line	EC50/IC50	Molecular mechanism	References
	Name of compound	Class	Source					
Hexokinase 2	Resveratrol	Phenol	Grapes, peanuts, mulberries, and raspberries	Pancreatic cancer	Panc-1	–	miR-21↓, PTEN↑, and ROS↓	[135]
	EGCG	Catechins	Green tea, apple skin, and plums	Tongue cancer	Tca8113 and TSCCa	40 μM	Akt⊥	[136]
	Capsaicin	–	Capsicum	Esophageal squamous cell carcinoma	KYSE150	30 μM	PTEN↑, RACα↓	[137]
Phosphogluco Isomerase	Ursolic acid	Triterpenoid	Peals of apple and bilberries	Hepatocellular carcinoma	Huh-7 and Hep3B	9.5 μM	PI3-kinase↓	[48]
Phosphofructo-kinase	EGCG	Catechins	Green tea, apple skin, and plums	Hepatocellular carcinoma	HepG2 and Huh-7	50 μM	Bcl2, Bad⊥, and Δψm↓	[58]
Aldolase	Shikonin	Naphtho-quinones	*Lithospermum erythrorhizon*	Breast cancer		–	–	[65]

PKM2	Apigenin	Flavonoid		Colon cancer	HCT116 and HT29	27.9 ± 2.45 and 48.2 ± 3.01 μM	B-catenin/c-Myc/PTBP1⊥	[131]
	Quercetin	Flavonoid	Red onion and cabbage leaf	Breast cancer	MDA-MB-231	30 μM	MMP-2, MMP-9↓, and Akt-mTOR⊥	[132]
	Oleanolic acid	Triterpenoid saponins	Olive oil	Prostate cancer and breast cancer	PC-3 and MCF-7	–	mTOR⊥, cMYC↓	[133]
	Shikonin	Naphtho-quinones	*L. erythrorhizon*	Bladder cancer	T24 and SW870	15.41 and 18.04 μM	Bcl-2 and Bax↓	[134]

Previously, PPP has been viewed as a defensive and biosynthetic pathway with respect to counteracting oxidative stress and nucleotide synthesis. But recent studies have focused on its importance in cancer cells from various aspects such as growth, invasion, metastasis, apoptosis, and drug resistance. PPP enzymes are regulated allosterically via their catalytic products and metabolites. This allosteric regulation of enzymes in coordination with the reversible nonoxidative branch allows PPP to modify itself according to the cellular demands [140]. Cancer cells have the potential to modulate PPP flux either directly or indirectly in order to meet their energy and biosynthetic demands via targeting enzymatic machineries [141]. These studies revealed that PPP is critical for the cancer metabolism and a potential target for the development of chemotherapeutics.

2.1 Targeting enzymes of PPP by phytonutrients

2.1.1 G6PD

G6PD is an X-linked gene having a cytogenetic location as Xq2.8 [142]. This gene is comprised of 12 introns and 13 exons with a total length of 18.5 kb [143]. It has been observed that G6PD exists in dimer and tetramer forms. Current studies revealed that the dimeric form is essential for its activity and the tetramer form is not required [144], while the monomeric form remains inactive [145]. The *G6PD* gene represents the most polymorphic locus having approximately 400 variants in humans as a result of different mutations [146]. G6PD is required for the normal metabolism, but its deficiency is present in common enzymopathy leading to hemolytic anemia [147].

Glucose 6 phosphate dehydrogenase (G6PD) is quoted as the first and rate-limiting enzyme of PPP [148] that catalyzes the dehydrogenation of G6P to 6-phosphogluconate (6-PG) along with NADP reduction to NADPH [149]. This enzyme acts as a gatekeeper in PPP. Therefore, it is involved in determining the PPP flux [150]. G6PD has been found to be hyperactivated in several cancers (lung, liver, and breast) [151–153] and is associated with poor prognosis in cancer patients [154]. G6PD is activated by glycosylation. O-linked β-*N*-acetylglucosamine is a sugar that is involved in the enzymatic activation of G6PD as well as in enhancing glucose flux through PPP. In in vitro and in vivo experimentation G6PD inhibition strongly affected cancer cell growth, thus presenting G6PD as a strong anticancer target [155].

An in vitro polyphenol-based investigation suggested the inhibitory effects of several compounds like caffeic acid, ferulic acid, naringenin, hesperidin, polydatin, and ellagic acid on G6PD. The IC_{50} values for these compounds were described as 0.481, 0.693, 0.403, 0.572, 0.383, and 0.072, respectively [156]. Resveratrol is a well-known polyphenol that works by targeting several signaling cascades [157]. Polydatin is a resveratrol glucoside that is a member of class polyphenols. It holds several biological properties including apoptotic cancer cell death [158]. An in vitro experimentation by polydatin in head and neck carcinoma cells resulted in suppression of cancer cells growth, an increase in cell cycle arrest, and cells invasion. Moreover, this small molecule inhibited the G6PD activity by increasing the oxidative stress [159]. Epigallocatechin gallate (EGCG) is the main catechin of green tea that carries a tumor suppressive potential against different cancers via different signaling cascades regulation [160]. An in silico and in vitro G6PD enzymatic assay-based screening of 250 selected compounds identified EGCG as a potential $NADP^+$ competitive G6PD inhibitor [161]. Resveratrol is a potent chemopreventive stilbenoid. This phytoalexin treatment reduced the cell cycle progression in colon cancer cells by attenuating the G6PD level [162]. Rosmarinic acid is a caffic acid ester that is rewarded with several biological activities. In vitro screening of G6PD (purified from sheep brain) inhibition by Rosmarinic acid showed that this compound has the potential to inhibit G6PD activity in a concentration-dependent manner [163].

2.1.2 PGD

6PGD is the third enzyme of monohexose shunt that is involved in the catalyzation of 6PG to ribulose-5-phosphate (Ru5P) amid NADPH generation [164]. This enzyme is critical for cancer cells growth as it coordinates lipogenesis, oxidative PPP, and tumor growth [165]. 6PGD is overexpressed in different cancers such as breast cancer, ovarian cancer, leukemia (myeloid), and lung cancer [166]. Lysine acetylation of 6PGD is responsible for its activation in cancer cells. This acetylation endorses the binding of $NADP^+$ to 6PGD in order to form active 6PGD dimers [167]. Studies revealed that 6PGD inhibition not only repressed the cancer cells growth and mediated cell death but also enhanced the chemosensitivity of cancer cells [168]. These findings demonstrate 6PGD as a promising chemotherapeutic target.

Phenols derived from dietary sources present a diverse class of natural compounds that display valuable medicinal, biological, and pharmacological properties [169]. In vitro evaluation of polyphenols to understand their impact on 6PGD (human erythrocytes) activity revealed that caffeic acid, ferulic acid, naringenin, sinapic acid, ellagic acid, and chrysin hold an inhibitory potential against 6-PGD. The inhibition constant of these polyphenols was estimated within the range of 3.68–120.65 μM [156]. EGCG is a well-studied anticancer catechin. An in silico and conventional enzymatic screening of 250 compounds for G6PD inhibition suggested that EGCG holds an inhibitory potential against $NADP^+$-dependent enzymes such as 6PGD [161]. Physcion, an anthraquinone, is a well-known 6PGD inhibitor. In vitro studies in cancer cells such as H1299 and K562 suggested that Physcion and its derivative S3 effectively suppressed the cancer cells proliferation with low nonspecific toxicity [165]. Moreover, Physcion treatment in leukemia cells exhibited synergistic effects with dihydroartemisinin to inhibit cancer cells growth via AMPK activation. This combined therapy also attenuated in vivo K562 tumor growth in mice proposing this therapy as a novel antileukemic treatment with minimum toxicity to normal cells [170].

2.1.3 Transaldolase

Transaldolase (TALDO) is a ubiquitous enzyme that works as a dimmer [171]. The *TALDO1* gene encodes this enzyme in humans. The core structure of the enzyme is made up of 8 α/β sheets while the single transaldolase domain is 337 residues long in humans [172]. The cytogenetic location of human TALDO1 is mapped as 11p15.4–p15.5 [173].

TALDO is one of the main enzymes of the nonoxidative PPP branch [174]. TALDO helps in the carbon swap between glyceraldehydes-3-phosphate (G3P) and seduhepulose-7-phosphate to generate erythrose-4-phosphate and fructose-6-phosphate [175]. TALDO is an enzyme without any cofactor; instead, it has essential lysine residues present in its active region that are conserved in some bacteria and humans [171]. Lack of TALDO1 is associated with overexpression of seduhepulose-7-phosphate while downregulation of glutathione and NADPH [176]. TALDO1 deficiency results in different enzymopathies in patients characterized as hemolytic anemia, hepatosplenomegaly, cardiomyopathy, hydrops fetalis, and kidney failure [177]. Additionally, overexpression of TALDO1 has been observed in several cancers including breast cancer [178], head and neck carcinoma [179], and bladder cancer [180]. TALDO1 contributes to enhance cancer cells proliferation by supplying ribose-5-phosphate for nucleotide synthesis and NADPH to maintain their viability and fatty acid synthesis [181]. Although all these observations provide us with the insight into the critical role of TALDO1 in cancer, literature surveys have revealed that no natural inhibitor of TALDO/phytonutrient against TALDO has been reported to date. Further, its enzymatic inhibition has been achieved by antibodies as well as site-directed mutagenesis. Antibody 12,484 that was raised against the full length of h-TALDO suppressed the h-TALDO activity in a dose-dependent manner with the maximum inhibition at 300 μg/mL. Site-directed mutagenesis was performed by replacing lysine 142, which resulted in complete inhibition of enzymatic activity [182] (Table 2).

2.1.4 Transketolase

Transketolase is a homodimer, thiamine diphosphate-dependent enzyme which accelerates the nonoxidative arm of the hexose monophosphate shunt by catalyzing the reversible transfer of two carbon units to form 3 and 7 carbon compounds [188]. There are three isolated isoforms of TKT, TKT, TKTL1, and TKTL2 with different coenzyme affinity, subcellular location, and chromosomal region. TKT is found in various organs, whereas TKTL1 and TKTL2 are primarily expressed in testis [189]. The muted form of TKTL1, which endorses tumor cell proliferation and invasion, was first identified by Coy et al. in 2005. TKTL1 with 38-amino acid substitution at the N-terminal lacks conserved histidine residue and chromosomal locality Xq28 that activate during carcinogenesis, which made it different from hTKT and TKTL2 [190]. Transketolase enzyme-mediated reactions empowered the oxygen-independent glucose degradation, rerouting the carbon directly from glycolysis, crucial for synthesis of the RNA ribose moiety in tumor cells [191]. Overexpression of TKTL1 and Akt activation switched tumor cell metastasis which in turn favored enriched lactate production along with the mitochondrial independent-ATP generation [192–194]. The foregoing investigation has revealed that TKTL1 is overexpressed in the transketolase family in multiple human cancers including breast cancer [195], ovarian cancer [196], noncell small lung cancer [197], prostate cancer [198], renal cancer [199], and bladder cancer [200,201]. The biologically aggressive phenotype of TKT is overexpressed upon the accumulation of the hypoxia-inducible Factor 1 alpha and competitively snatched binding site of transcription repressor BTB and CNC homology 1 (BACH1) by NRF2, which is not ubiquitinated due to the inactivation of Kelch-like ECH-associated protein under normoxic condition [191,202].

Resveratrol (RSV), a stilbenoid found in grapes and peanuts, has been reported to inhibit the upper quartile range of TKT in colon cancer. The molecular mechanism insight revealed that the synergetic effects of IGF-1 and RSV remolded the insulin-like growth factor receptor IGE-IR activity

Table 2 Phytonutrients as metabolic regulators of PPP enzymes.

Metabolic Enzyme	Phytonutrients modulators: Name of compound	Class	Source	Cancer type	Cell line	EC50/IC50	Molecular mechanism	References
G6PD	Resveratrol	Stilbenoid	Peanuts, Red grapes	Colon	HT-29	150 μM	p-FAK↓	[183]
	Polydatin	Polyphenol	*Polygonum cuspidatum*	Head and neck carcinoma	HNSCC	22 μM		[159]
	Rosmarinic acid	Polyphenol	*Echium vulgare L.*			1.50 ± 0.0005 mM		[163]
	EGCG	Catechin	*Green tea*			0.25 ± 0.02 μlmol/L		[161]
	Caffeic acid	Polyphenol				0.481 mM		[156]
	Ferulic acid					0.693 mM		
	Naringenin					0.403 mM		
	Hesperidin					0.572 mM		
	Polydatin					0.383 mM		
	Ellagic acid					0.072 mM		
6PGD	Physcion	Anthraquinone	*Rheum Palmatum*	Lung carcinoma	H1299	38.5 μM		[165]
				Leukemia	K562			
	EGCG	Catechin	*Green tea*			0.72 ± 0.07 μlmol/L		[161]
	Caffeic acid	Phenol				0.486 mM		[156]
	Ferulic acid					0.888 mM		
	Naringenin					0.047 mM		
	Sinapic acid					0.614 mM		
	Ellagic acid					0.188 mM		
	Chrysin					0.198 mM		

TKT	Resveratrol	Stilbenoids	Grapes and peanut	Colon cancer	HT-29		Inhibit cell proliferation and closing of G_0/G_1 gate of cell cycle via activation of p53 and p27—Remodeling of IGF-1 receptor and downstreams PI3K/Akt, Wnt/β-catenin signaling targets	[164,183–187]

and its downstream target P13K/Akt/Wnt/β-catenin pathways that inhibit cell proliferation. Downregulation of the IGF-IR protein inhibits Akt phosphorylation that constrains the inactivated glycogen synthase kinase 3β (GSK-3β) mediated β-catenin/TCF complex that converts Wnt effectors into activators. RSV substitute (the phosphate molecule) from fork head transcriptional factor enables it to bind with cyclin D and hinders cancer cells to proliferate. RSV also downregulates the mammalian target of rapamycin mTOR involved in cell physiology alteration, leading to PPP suppression [183,185–187]. The synergistic effects of pharmaceutical drugs such as sorafenib with oxythiamine (OT), tert-Butyl hydroperoxide (tBHP) with OT, and OT with dehydroepiandrosterone effectively downregulate the TKT expressions due to NAPDH reduction and ROS accumulation that delay the cell cycle in tumor cells, which resulted in reduced proliferation ability [203,204]. A study on nasophyrangeal carcinoma showed that another chemotherapeutic drug, Cisplatin, damages tumor cells DNA by decreasing NADPH and ribose-5-phosphate levels. Therefore, less fuel for cell proliferation is unable to meet the energy demands of tumor cells [195]. A genetic inhibitor such as miR-497 directly binds with the 3-ultraslated region of TKT to antagonize the TKT function. Modulation in the gene expression of TKT through microRNA improves the cisplatin, chemotherapeutic drug resistance in cervical cancer cell lines [205,206]. Moreover, RNA interference (RNAi) that inhibits TKTL1 is associated with the reduction of cancer proliferation and cell cycle arrest at G0/G1 in hepatoma cells [198]. Oxythiamine is a thiamine antagonist, antimetabolite that alters Redox homeostasis, inhibits tumor cells invasiveness and metastasis. The interaction of the TKTL1 residue such as the nitrogen atom of His 160, hydrogen binding of Ser49 with aminopyrimidine and Lys 218 with the N-terminus hydroxyl group of oxythiamine stimulates the TKTL1 inhibitory mechanism. Moreover, the combined administration of oxythiamine and dehydroepiandrosterone arrests G1 arrest, salvages nucleic acid production in tumor cells [207,208].

3. Serine pathway

Serine metabolism is one of the metabolic aberrations reported in tumor cells. Serine, a nonessential amino acid, is synthesized from a glycolytic intermediate 3-phosphoglycerate (3PG). In a normal cell, serine is responsible for the production of cysteine and glycine [209]. The initial step of serine synthesis is catalyzed by 3PG dehydrogenase (PHGDH). High levels of PHGDH have been recorded in several types of cancer; hence, PHGDH has become an attractive target of cancer therapy. Serine is the third most utilized metabolite in tumor cells (after glucose and glutamine) [210]. High amounts of serine are converted into glycine by the activity of mitochondrial and cytosolic serine hydromethyltranferases enzymes (SHMT1 and SHMT2). Glycine synthesized by serine is directly incorporated into glutathione and purine nucleotide bases [211]. The need of serine biosynthesis in tumor cells was first reported during the observation of activity of 3-phosphoglycerate dehydrogenase in xenograft models having the fastest rate of cell growth [212]. Later on, the experimental studies revealed that activation of the p53 gene during serine starvation halts the process of nucleotide synthesis in case of colorectal cells, and as a result of this the need of serine resources is cut down for dependent pathways and serine is utilized in less amounts. Moreover, it has also been recorded that the functional metabolites, which are the critical imperatives in cell biology, are subsequently associated with serine/glycine and THF-dependent one-carbon metabolism, e.g., adenosine, S-adenosyl methionine, guanosine, nicotinamide, and glutathione [213].

3.1 Targeting enzymes of the serine pathway by phytonutrients

3.1.1 Phosphoserine aminotransferase 1

Phosphoserine aminotransferase 1 (PSAT1) catalyzes the second step of the serine-glycine biosynthetic pathway, i.e., transamination reaction utilizing glutamate-derived nitrogen, and produces α-ketoglutarate (α-KG). Moreover, this enzyme also converts 3PHP into 3-phosphoserine (3PS) in a glutamate (Glu)-dependent transamination reaction [13]. PSAT1 was reported as an upregulated enzyme characterizing the poor prognosis, cellular growth, proliferation, metastasis as well as chemoresistance in case of several cancers, e.g., nonsmall cell lung cancer (NSCLC), metastatic lung cancer, ovarian cancer, colon cancer, triple negative breast cancer (TNBC), nasopharyngeal carcinoma (NPC), lower grade gliomas, and esophageal squamous cell carcinoma (ESCC) [15,214–218]. In case of ER-negative breast cancer, this enzyme was found to be regulated under the action of Activating transcription factor 4 (ATF4), thereby potentiating the GSK-3β/β-catenin signaling cascade. The action mechanism was found to enhance the expression of cyclin D1 and promote cellular proliferation [214]. In case of TNBC, PSAT1 functions to promote the migration, invasion, and metastasis of cancerous cells [15]. Experimental evidences show that the knockdown of PSAT1 increased the sensitivity of NSCLC cells to glutamate-limiting conditions as well as ionizing radiations [219]. Thus, we can conclude that PSAT1 inhibitors may act as effective strategies against various types of cancers [218,220]. Contrary to that, recent data supports the mechanistic insights of regorafenib-induced autophagy arrest by overexpression of PSAT1 in glioblastoma multiforme, thereby suggesting a novel paradigm for the treatment of brain cancer [221].

3.1.2 Hydroxymethyltransferase

Hydroxymethyltransferase (SHMT) is a tetrahydrofolate-dependent enzyme of the serine metabolism that is involved in the conversion of serine to glycine, which is derived from the diet or from endogenous synthesis from glutamate and glucose. SHMT produces 5,10-methylenetetrahydrofolate (CH2-THF) after donating a one-carbon unit to tetrahydrofolate [222]. In the mammalian cell, it is found both in the cytoplasm and mitochondria [223]. Depending upon the occurrence, SHMT has variable metabolic functions, like mitochondrial SHMT (mSHMT or SHMT2) is abundant in most cells and is responsible for the bulk of glycine synthesis, whereas cytosolic SHMT (c SHMT or SHMT1) is mainly found in the liver and kidney cells and is less active in the conversion of serine to glycine than SHMT2 [224].

Advances in research studies have revealed the link between the serine one-carbon metabolism and nucleotide synthesis. CH2-THF, a direct product of serine to glycine conversion, acts as a substrate of cytosolic or mitochondrial methylenetetrahydrofolate dehydrogenase (MTHFD) to ultimately produce formate [224]. In most of the cells, SHMT1 operates glycine to serine direction, but in some cells it can produce CH2-THF and NADPH. Reaction catalyzed by SHMT involved the transfer of the C1 unit from C-3 of serine to tetrahydrofolate, yielding glycine and N5-N10 methylene tetrahydrofolate. The latter is a source of the methyl group for some methylation reactions [225].

One-carbon metabolism is critical for maintaining the genomic stability and epigenetic control of DNA and histone protein, the altered expression of which is a characteristic attribute of tumor cells. SHMT-mediated serine metabolism is a therapeutic target in cancer therapy as its expression has been reported in various human cancers, such as breast cancer [226], lung cancer [227], colon cancer [228], colorectal cancer [229], and gastric cancer [230]. Overexpression of SHMT1 and SHMT2 in numerous cancers makes these enzymes attractive targets for cancer therapy. There is no reported natural inhibitor of SHMT to date. Beyond this, the structural and kinetic analysis of hSHMT2 with antifolates revealed that the antifolates lometrexol and pemetrexed are inhibitors of SHMT2. Lometrexol was found to be the best hSHMT1/2 inhibitor from a panel of antifolates. Comparison of apo hSHMT1 with antifolate-bound hSHMT2 indicates a highly conserved active site architecture. This structural information offers insights as to how these compounds could be improved to produce more potent and specific inhibitors of this emerging anticancer drug target [231].

3.1.3 Citric acid cycle (TCA)

Citric acid cycle was proposed by Hans Adolf Krebs in 1937. It is the primary metabolic pathway for all aerobic processes in animal tissues [232]. The tricarboxylic acid cycle is one of the major biochemical routes of oxidative phosphorylation in a cell. It acts as a key regulator of bioenergetics, biosynthetic and redox balance requirements [233]. In the presence of a terminal electron acceptor, TCA oxidizes the substrate to CO_2 and generates NADH for the process of respiration. When there is no terminal electron acceptor, TCA does not work in a cycle, but it functions as a two-branch system; one is the oxidative branch from citrate to 2-oxo-glutarate and the other is the reductive branch from oxaloacetate to succinyl-co-enzyme A [234]. The citric acid cycle is the final common pathway for the oxidation of carbohydrate, protein, and lipids. TCA plays an important role in gluconeogenesis, transamination, deamination, and lipogenesis. TCA plays its role through the oxidative catabolism of carbohydrates, fatty acids, and amino acids and this cyclic process provides us precursors for various other biosynthetic pathways [235]. Different enzymes of the TCA cycle provide a unique approach regarding the proliferation and energy metabolism of cancer cells. The following section provides insights about the roles of different enzymes of the TCA cycle and targeting those enzymes by the use of phytonutrients.

4. Targeting enzymes of TCA by phytonutrients

4.1 PDH

Pyruvate dehydrogenase (PDH) is an enzyme that catalyzes an irreversible step in the metabolic pathway between glucose and fatty acid oxidation. PDH increases the acetyl-CoA influx from glycolysis into the TCA cycle through conversion of pyruvate into acetyl-CoA [236]. Control of PDH activity is regulated by the covalent modification via dephosphorylation of its substrates [237].

Pyruvate dehydrogenase complex (PDC) and pyruvate dehydrogenase kinases (PDKs) are significant mitochondrial enzymes which play a key role in the metabolic pathway of glucose and their interaction actively regulates the rate of reaction among aerobic respiration and the Warburg effect [238].

PDC is present in the mitochondrial intermembrane, which offers a link between glycolysis and oxidative phosphorylation via catalyzing the rate-limiting step in oxidative decarboxylation of pyruvate to acetyl-Co-A [239]. PDC has a crucial role in glucose metabolism and ATP production. Low levels of PDC tend to reduce the aerobic oxidation of pyruvate and endorse its transformation into lactate inside the cytoplasm [240]. The decreased influx of pyruvate results in a low amount of acetyl-CoA entering into the TCA cycle [241]. PDKs control the activity of PDC, i.e., stimulation in PDKs could suppress the expression of PDC, consequently detaining the pyruvate from entering into the mitochondrion, increasing pyruvate phosphorylation, and intensifying the Warburg effect in cancer cells [242]. Therefore, PDC and PDKs are the chief gatekeeping enzymes which govern the critical switch between glycolysis and the TCA cycle. Subsequently, inhibition of PDKs could be a promising approach to reverse the Warburg effect in cancer cells [21].

PDKs have been reported to be deregulated in multiple human cancers including colon cancer [243], breast cancer [244], gastric cancer [245], lung cancer, and hepatocellular carcinoma [246]. PDKs could be used as cancer biomarkers as the hyperactivity of PDKs, low PDC level, and their dependence on the glycolytic pathway correlates with increased tumorigenicity. PDK upregulation results in the inactivation of PDC in tumor cells and thrusts more pyruvate to be reduced into lactate rather than its oxidation in mitochondrial respiration. This metabolic change of low oxidative phosphorylation and higher lactate formation is strongly associated with the poor prognosis of multiple cancers [247].

Due to all previously described roles of PDKs, they are promising targets in cancer therapy. Various chemical agents targeting PDKs have been reported to date, but their efficacy needs to be validated clinically [248]. So far, resveratrol and ellagic acid are well-documented phytonutrients. Resveratrol can be obtained from natural sources and their in vitro treatment has been observed to modify the lipid profile by increasing the oxidative capacity and decreasing glycolysis as it directly targets the PDH complex leading to enhanced PDH activity [157]. Ellagic acid, another naturally obtained phytonutrient, has been noticed to induce cytotoxicity and antiproliferative activity by targeting PDK3, a member of the PDK family. The conformational dynamics of the EA-PDK3 complex during molecular dynamics simulation revealed that a stable complex was maintained by a significant number of hydrogen bonds throughout the 100 ns trajectories [249].

4.2 CS

Citrate synthase (CS) is a one of the chief enzyme of the TCA cycle, which derives the rate-limiting step of the TCA cycle [818082]. This enzyme has been found in mitochondria and functions to catalyze the synthesis of citrate from acetyl-CoA and oxaloacetate. Citrate, which is present in the mitochondria and cytosol, is cleaved into oxaloacetate and acetyl-CoA by the action of ATP-citrate lyase [250]. It has been reported that this enzyme constitutes an upregulated expression in cancers, e.g., hepatocellular carcinoma, pancreatic cancer, and ovarian cancer [251].

4.3 Aco

Acetyl-coenzyme A (acetyl-CoA) is a molecule responsible for the entry of glycolytic pyruvate into the TCA cycle. It acts as a significant precursor of lipid synthesis as well as being the only donor of acetyl groups for acetylation [252]. Acetyl-CoA is a membrane transient molecule constituted by an acetyl moiety (CH3CO) linked to coenzyme A (CoA), a derivative of vitamin B5 and cysteine, through a thioester bond. The distribution and abundance of this enzyme varies considerably depending upon the pathological and physiological states of subcellular or pericellular compartments of the cell [211].

There are different ways for the production of acetyl-CoA in mammalian cells. It is generated in the mitochondrial matrix through multiple metabolic circuits like ß-oxidation, glycolysis, and breakdown of branched amino acids [20]. A cell under normal conditions produces cytosolic acetyl-CoA by two pervasive metabolic circuits. The first includes reductive carboxylation of glutamine under hypoxic conditions, when glycolysis is blocked or due to mitochondrial defects [253]. The second source of production includes the role of the cytosolic acyl-CoA synthetase short chain family member 2 (ACSS2), which employs acetate to generate acetyl-CoA in an ATP-dependent manner [211].

Acetyl CoA is a starting material for fatty acid synthesis in the cytoplasm. In cancer cells, it is regenerated from citrate, which is a product of acetyl CoA in mitochondria [254]. As discussed earlier, cancer cells have activated glycolysis over mitochondrial respiration, so the entry of acetyl CoA in the truncated TCA cycle results in its conversion to citrate, which in turn shuttled out of the mitochondria into the cytoplasm [211]. Under non-hypoxic conditions, tumor cells predominantly generate lipogenic acetyl-CoA from glucose-derived pyruvate via the activity of pyruvate dehydrogenase [255]. Additionally, the activation of various oncogene products, such as MYC and KRAS, contributes to the acetyl-CoA metabolic phenotype with enhanced fatty acid synthesis.

4.4 IDH

Isocitrate dehydrogenase (IDH) is an indispensable enzyme of the TCA cycle, which is involved in cellular respiration [256]. There are three isozymes of IDH found in mammalian cells, namely IDH1, IDH2, and IDH3. IDH1 and IDH2 are homodimeric NADP-dependent enzymes located in the cytosol and mitochondrial matrix, respectively. IDH3 is a heterotetrameric NADP-dependent enzyme (consisting of two alpha subunits, one beta subunit, and one gamma subunit) located in the mitochondrial matrix [257]. IDH1 and IDH2 mutations are generally reported in glioblastoma [135], acute myeloid leukemia, and prostate cancer [258]. IDH1 and IDH2 mutations in cancers are mostly heterozygous with a wild-type allele and found to be a neomorphic enzyme activity that converts α-ketoglutarate into 2-hydroxyglutarate. 2-hydroxyglutarate inhibits the activity of the cytochrome *c* complex and ATP synthase of the TCA cycle in cancer cells. These findings suggest that the accumulation of 2-hydroxyglutarate contributes to the alterations in energy metabolism in cancer cells[259].

IDH mutation in cancer presents a unique phenomenon in which a metabolic enzyme contributes to tumor development by playing the role of an oncogene. In comparison to mutated IDH, wild-type IDH1 and IDH2 catalyze the reversible oxidative decarboxylation of isocitrate to alpha-ketoglutarate and CO_2, while mutant IDH1 and IDH2 in case of cancer cells catalyze the reduction of alpha-ketoglutarate by converting it into D-2-hydroxyglutarate [260]. As a result, D-2HG accumulation in cancer cells expressing mutant IDH results in the hypermethylation of histones and CpG islands in DNA [21130701]. These epigenetic changes caused by D-2HG contribute to cancer phenotypes and have been proposed to promote oncogenesis by preventing normal cellular differentiation [261]. Due to its aberrant role in cancer cells, IDH may act as a useful therapeutic target in cancer therapy but limited data is available on its natural inhibitors. A well-documented report on IDH inhibition through phytonutrient present the data of its targeting by a naturally occurring phenolic compound in extra-virgin olive oil (EVOO) selectively inhibits the production of 2HG by neomorphic IDH1 mutations. In in silico docking, molecular dynamics, including steered simulations, predicted the ability of the oleoside decarboxymethyl oleuropein aglycone (DOA) to preferentially occupy the allosteric pocket of mutant IDH1. DOA selectively blocked the colony formation of IDH1 mutant cells while sparing the wild-type IDH1 isogenic counterparts. In sum, the EVOO-derived oleoside DOA is a new, naturally occurring chemotype of mutant IDH1 inhibitors [262].

4.5 KGDH

α-ketoglutarate dehydrogenase (KGDH) is a tightly regulated key enzyme of Kreb's cycle which converts α-ketoglutarate to succinyl-CoA producing NADH, thereby providing electrons for the respiratory chain [263]. This enzyme is regarded as an integral component of the mitochondrial antioxidant system which may function to reprogram cellular metabolic systems to hinder oxidative damages by means of overtaking energy production via changing the mitochondrial as well as cellular ROS stress. This key enzyme of Kreb's cycle has been reported to be downregulated in pathological abnormalities, e.g., cardiovascular and neurological abnormalities, and ROS-related malignancies [264]. KGDH comprises three components: α-KG dehydrogenase (OGDH), dihydrolipoamide S-succinyltransferase (DLST), and dihydrolipoamide dehydrogenase (DLD). OGDH is reported to be downregulated due to hypermethylation in case of esophageal, lung, colorectal, breast, pancreatic, and cervical cancers. This component of KGDH is regulated by calcium, NADH, and adenine nucleotides. The oncogenic isoforms lack sensitivity against calcium ions. Moreover, DLST has been reported to be upregulated in case of T-cell acute lymphoblastic leukemia (T-ALL) [265].

Galangin (3,5,7-trihydroxyflavone), a natural flavonoid from *Alpinia officinarum Hance* root and honey, has been reported to possess certain anticancer, antioxidant, antiinflammatory, antiischemic, antiviral, and anticlastogenic therapeutic properties. The experimental results conducted on streptozotocin-induced diabetic rats show that this particular enzyme downregulates mitochondrial enzymes, namely isocitrate dehydrogenase (ICDH), alpha-ketoglutarate dehydrogenase (α-KGDH), succinate dehydrogenase (SDH), and malate dehydrogenase (MDH), in addition to decreasing the enzymatic (TBARS) as well as nonenzymatic (SOD, GPx) antioxidant levels [266]. In addition to that, CPI-613, a lipoic acid analog, has been reported to halt PDH and KGDH and induces a burst of mitochondrial ROS by acting on DLD and suppression of DLST. This compound is currently in clinical trials

(NCT02168140, NCT01902381, NCT02232152, and NCT01766219) for the treatment of cancer either alone or in combination with standard chemotherapeutic drugs [265].

4.6 SDH

Succinate dehydrogenase (SDH) is a unique enzyme of mitochondria in that it participates both in the citric acid cycle and electron transport chain. The structure of this protein comprises four subunits encoded by a nuclear genome. The hydrophilic (head) portion, consisting of SDHA (flavoprotein) and SDHB (iron sulfur containing) proteins, acts as the catalytic core. The membrane domain, consisting of SDHC and SDHD subunits, acts as a binding site for ubiquinone [267].

The deficiency of this enzyme is linked to pathological deformities like paragangliomas (autonomic nervous system neoplasms), gastrointestinal stromal disorders, infantile leukoencephalopathy, cardiomyopathy, thyroid tumors, testicular seminoma, neuroblastomas, renal cell cancers, Cowden syndrome, and related neurodegenerative disorders. [267,268]. It has been reported that a deficiency of this enzyme leads to the increased expression of various oncogenic factors leading to tumorigenesis as well as angiogenesis.

Castasterone, from *Brassica juncea*, has been reported to be involved in modulating the expression of several key enzymes taking part in carbon fixation (RUBISCO), Krebs cycle (CS, SUCLG1, SDH, FH), ROS generation (RBO), antioxidative enzymes (SOD, CAT, POD, DHAR, GR, GST) [269]. Another compound, malonate, is a well-known modulator of the succinate dehydrogenase enzyme [270]. It can be found naturally in legumes [271]. Moreover, vitamin *E*-derived compounds (α-tocopheryl succinate targets vitamin E succinate in mitochondria) provide a novel rationale to exert anticancer effects in various neoplasms. Several lines of evidences suggest that SDH serves as a potent target against lung, breast, and colon cancers as well as melanomas and mesotheliomas.

4.7 FH

Fumarate hydratase (FH) or fumarase is a highly conserved homotetrameric enzyme with two isoforms: mitochondrial and cystolic. The generation of both of these isoforms depends on the differential mRNA processing [272]. This is the energy-producing step and involves the production of significant molecular precursors. On the other hand, it produces fumarate in the cytosolic pathway, involving the nucleotide cycle as well as the urea cycle [273]. FH also functions as a tumor suppressor gene. The loss of FH can lead to carcinogenesis. The cells with decreased levels of FH have an elevated glycolytic function and instead of glucose oxidation, the cells shunt into lactic acid production as well as other glycolytic branches, e.g., pentose phosphate pathway [274].

Mutations in the activation of FH are associated with the accumulation of fumarate, characterizing the main feature of hereditary leiomyomatosis and renal cell carcinoma (HLRCC). This enzyme is also found to be deregulated in case of breast, bladder, testicular, Leydig cell tumors, cutaneous, and uterine cancers [268,275]. The major genetic abnormalities in FH include missense mutations (57%), frameshift as well as nonsense mutations (27%). Moreover, large-scale deletions, duplications, and insertions may also occur [276].

A sesquiterpene, Englerin A, isolated from *Phyllanthus engleri* (stems and root bark) functions to selectively inhibit the growth of renal cell carcinoma. This particular compound activates protein kinase C-θ (PKCθ) by binding with it and triggers the insulin-resistant phenotype, thereby cutting down the glucose access to the tumor cells. Moreover, it is also reported to be involved in killing the cancer cells by starving FH-deficient cells [277].

4.8 MDH

Malate dehydrogenases (MDH) exist as multimeric enzymes comprising similar subunits organized into dimeric or tetrameric subunits, with molecular weight ranging from 30 to 35 kDa molecules in most of the organisms [278]. MDH plays a key role in the malate/aspartate shuttle across the mitochondrial membrane as well as in Kreb's cycle inside the mitochondrial matrix. It functions to catalyze the NAD/NADH-dependent interconversion of malate and oxaloacetate [279,280]. There are two main forms of MDH which have been reported in most of the organisms, namely MDH1 and MDH2. Both of these forms are encoded by different genes and are functionally specific for NAD+/NADH, and exist as identical subunits in physiological conditions [88]. MDH2 is found in humans and plays a significant role in the TCA cycle [281].

Deregulations in both isoforms MDH1 and MDH2 are linked with several cancer types, e.g., prostate, uterine, nonsmall lung, breast, paragangliomas, and pheochromocytoma [282–285]. Moreover, their overexpression has been reported to be a significant cause of drug resistance in uterine cancer patients and their downregulation enhances the drug sensitivity to the patients by knocking down the production of ATP. Hence, it can be concluded that MDH can be an effective therapeutic target to control the cancer growth and enhance drug sensitivity [283]. Experimental evidences are lacking regarding the role of phytonutrients in the modulation of MDH. Hence, researches are encouraged by the scientists and research community on the role of phytonutrients in controlling cancer.

4.9 Malic enzyme (ME)

Malic enzymes (MEs) constitute tetrameric proteins which possess a dual dimeric structure. Each monomeric unit structure comprises four structural domains. MEs function as oxidative carboxylases and can be found in many species and have an analogous structure. MEs catalyze the oxidation of malate to pyruvate and CO2 with concomitant reduction of NAD(P) + to NAD(*P*)H. MEs are considered as the crucial enzymes in the processes like glycolysis, gluconeogenesis, and fatty acid metabolism due to their regulatory behavior regarding the bioenergetics, cellular synthesis, and oxidation/reduction balance. Mammalian cells constitute three isoforms of MEs, namely, malic enzyme 1 (cytosolic isoform), malic enzyme (NADP (+)-dependent mitochondrial isoform), and malic enzyme 3 (NADP(+)-dependent malic enzyme). Of all these forms, ME1 and ME2 are studied extensively [286].

ME1 is reported to be involved in the growth as well as migration of gastric cancer (SGC7901) cells marked by a poor survival rate of patients [230]. Furthermore, it was also documented that upregulated ME1 expression was associated with hepatocellular carcinoma (HCC) metastasis and epithelial and mesenchymal transition leading to poor prognosis and a reduced survival rate 25753478. Moreover, this enzyme has been reported to be upregulated in combined hepatocellular cholangiocarcinoma, nonsmall lung cancer, oral squamous cell carcinomas, and colorectal cancer [287–290]. ME1 can be used as an effective therapeutic target for cancer, as the expression of this enzyme plays a fundamental role in glycolysis inhibition [251].

ME2 has been reported to be overexpressed in various cancer types, e.g., lung cancer, glioblastoma multiforme, hepatomas, cutaneous melanoma, osteosarcoma, and erythroleukemia. ME2 knockdown impairs the proliferation and the growth of different cancer cell lines [286]. A little data is available on the role of phytonutrients in ME modulation. To date, no phytonutrient has been reported to regulate malic enzymes.

5. Lactic acid fermentation

5.1 LDH

Lactate dehydrogenase A (LDHA) is the last glycolytic enzyme which is responsible for catalyzing the reduction of pyruvate into lactate and transforming NADH to NAD+. LDHA is located in the cytosol, mitochondria, and nucleus. LDHA exhibits an overexpression profile in the number of cancers such as pancreatic cancer [291–293], prostate cancer [294], breast cancer [295], ovarian cancer [296], hepatocellular carcinoma [297], oral squamous cell carcinoma [298], gastric cancer [300], and renal carcinoma [343, 344].

There are many explanations for the molecular mechanisms underlying the proliferation and survival of cancer cells with overexpression of LDHA. First, LDHA supplies sufficient ATP for cancer cells [299]. Second, LDHA is involved in promoting the cancer stem cells (CSCs) phenotype by activating the octamer-binding transcription factor 4 (Oct-4), which critically involves in the self-renewal of embryonic stem cells [300]. Thirdly, LDHA indirectly favors tumor survival by protecting cancer cells from reactive oxygen species (ROS) damage [301]. Moreover, LDHA may also be directly involved in the inhibition of apoptosis via activation of antiapoptotic proteins [302]. Therefore, LDHA is regarded as a promising target for cancer prevention and cure. A natural phenolic compound known as Gossypol, isolated from cotton seeds oil, inhibits LDHA by competing with NADH. Gossypol showed dose-dependent cytotoxic activity in a variety of cancer cells, including small-cell lung cancer (H69), melanoma (SK-mel-19, SK-mel28), breast cancer (Walker), cervical cancer (Sihas), myelogenous leukemia (K562), and glioma (HS683, U373, U87, and U138). [303–305] (Table 3).

6. Other mechanisms involved in cancer metabolism and their modulation by phytonutrients

6.1 Glutaminolysis

Glutamine along with alanine serves to reallocate nitrogen and carbons between the source and sink organs of the respective elements. In tumor cells, glutamine performs many functions like ROS scavenging, metabolite production, and the synthesis of nonessential amino acids as well as fatty acids for cell signaling activation and replication [311]. Numerous in vitro studies prove that glutamine is the second most preferred substrate of glycolysis, the first one being glucose, in cancer cells and the need of this substrate increases in cancer cells with the synthesis of proteins in cancer cells [312]. This glutamine is consumed by the cell, deaminated, and released in the form of glutamate. Thus, glutamine reprogramming occurs due to the binding of c-Myc (proto-oncogene) to the promoter regions of glutamine importers, such as isoforms of system N, and binding of sodium-dependent neutral amino acid transporter type-2. As a result of this, glutamine is consumed by

Table 3 Metabolic enzymes as phytonutrient modulators.

Metabolic Enzyme	Phytonutrients modulators: Name of compound	Class	Source	Cancer type	Cell line	EC50/IC50	Molecular mechanism (Act/inh)	References
GLUT1	phloretin	Polyphenol	apple	Colon and breast cancer	SW620 K562	24.88 nM 20.4 nM	–	[306]
	Naringenin	Flavonoid	grapefruits	Breast cancer	MCF-7	–	PI3K↓, MAPK↓	[307]
	Resveratrol	Polyphenol	grape skins and peanuts	Myeloma	U937 and HL-60	73 μM 75 μM	–	[308]
GAPDH	Koningic acid		*Trichoderma koningii*					[79]
	Shikonin	naphtho-quinones	*Lithospermum erythrorhizon*	Breast cancer	MCF-7	1052.0 μM	–	[65]
PGK1	Curcumin	Polyphenol	*Curcuma longa*	prostate cancer	DU145	10-μM	FOXD3↑ miR-143↑	[95]
PGAM1	EGCG	Catchin	Green tea and apple peel	Human nonsmall cell lung carcinoma and breast cancer	NCI-H1299 and MDA-MB-231	0.49 ± 0.17 μM	–	[111]
LDHA	Gossypol	Polyphenol	Cotton seeds	Glioma	C6 and HS 683	18 μM 25 μM	–	[303]
	Ellagic acid	Polyphenol	Berries grapes and nuts	Dalton's lymphoma	–	–	–	[309]
	Eugenol		Bay, cinnamon, and clove leaves	Cervical cancer	HeLa cells	–	–	[310]

the tumor cells in high quantities [313]. Downregulation of the phosphatidyl 3-kinase/Akt pathway is reported to affect the glutamine metabolism in various cancers. Glutamine reprogramming directly influences the cellular apoptosis and induces drug resistance [314]

6.2 Fatty acid metabolism

Fatty acids are essentially required by the rapidly proliferating tumor cells to accomplish various biological activities, e.g., membrane formation, protein modification, and several other bioenergetic requirements [211]. Acetyl-CoA (ACC) acts as a precursor of fatty acids and cholesterol. The formation of ACC is accompanied by glucose, glutamate, and acetate in several cancers, e.g., liver, prostate, breast, and brain cancers. It has been observed that some cancerous tissues convert acetate into fatty acids for the production of biomass, while some other researchers have proposed that acetate is used during the TCA cycle [315].

Moreover, tumor cells show lipogenic phenotypes by using different types of proteins involved in the synthesis of fatty acids. Overexpression of fatty acid synthase (FASN) has also been recorded in various tumors, which cause poor prognosis of certain cancers [316]. This correlates with the expression of certain other enzymes such as ACC and ATP citrate lyase in cancer cells. As we know, fatty acid synthesis involves the signaling cascades (PI3K/Akt and MAPK) in cancer cells, the elevated levels of ACL, ACC, and FASN and their subsequent activities lead to the survival and proliferation of cancer cells [317].

7. Clinical trials

Many phytonutrients have been channelized in the different phases of clinical trials due to their anticancer, antioxidant, and antiinflammatory activities [318]. Various experimental evidences are available to describe the efficacy of phytonutrients as health promoters and immunomodulators [319].

In a clinical trial to determine the DNA protection and antioxidant capacity of phytonutrients, it was proved that different phytonutrients from plants like grape, blueberry, black currant, grapefruit, spinach, acerola, alfalfa, kelp, mandarin orange, onion, parsley, tomato, watercress, peppermint, turmeric, marigold, and orange possess significant DNA protection activity and are acting as ROS scavengers [319]. Curcumin, the bioactive polyphenol from *C. longa*, has been reported to alleviate the tumor initiation, progression, and metastasis. It has been documented as a bio-safe phytonutrient during human clinical trials with no dose-limiting toxicity even at the maximum dose of 10 g/day [320].

8. Bioavailability of phytonutrients

Although phytonutrients are regarded as marvel compounds regarding their efficacy and multidimensional therapeutic properties, yet their bioavailability puts a question mark on their dosage and efficacy against a certain disease [321]. It has been discovered by extensive researches in the area of phytotherapy that most of the phytonutrients are poorly bioavailable to the body, and hence they should be modified so that they can be channelized as effective medicinal drug candidates.

Numerous in vitro, in vivo, and preclinical trials provide evidences against the poor bioavailability of curcumin due to its less solubility, poor stability, low serum levels, and rapid metabolism after oral administration. In order to improve its efficacy and bioavailability in living systems, several approaches have been designed, e.g., modifications in the chemical structure, nano-formulations, development of curcumin prodrugs and administration in combination with metabolic inhibitors [321]. Likewise, another phytonutrient, quercetin, has been proved to be a poorly bioavailable phytochemical. The glucoside forms of quercetin are more bioavailable than the aglycone form [322,323]. Due to this reason, the use of this compound is recommended at high dosage levels. To improve it bioavailability, nano-quercetin formulations are in experimental trials [324]. Likewise, Allicin is another compound found to possess poor bioavailability. Its sensitivity toward alkaline media and thermal instability hinder its bioactivity and efficacy in living systems [325]. To improve its stability and enhance its bioavailability, liposome-mediated allicin administration is favored [322]. Resveratrol is a multitargeted phytonutrient but it is also poorly bioavailable to its experimental animals. The oral bioavailability of resveratrol has been improved by loading it into liposomes [326], solid lipid nanoparticles [327], mesoporous silica nanoparticles [328], and metallic nanoparticles [329]. The results from these studies are satisfactory in terms of improving the stabilization of the trans-isomer, protection against UV, and increased aqueous solubility. Hence, we can assume that the anticancer as well as antioxidant potential of resveratrol can be enhanced to improve its therapeutic targets [330]. The clinical use of EGCG is still limited due to its poor oral bioavailability. Recent experiments to prepare EGCG-loaded albumin nanoparticles concluded that such modifications to EGCG increased the solubility of this bioactive compound, thus increasing the bioavailability and improving the therapeutic potential of EGCG [331].

Biochanin A and B are potentially effective isoflavones with their therapeutic action against cancer and other metabolic disorders. Due to the good permeability and lipophilic nature, both biochanin A and biochanin B are quickly absorbed into the gut [332]. However, biochanin A is poorly bioavailable than biochanin B. Biochanin B shows slower intestinal glucuronidation and higher membrane permeability as compared to biochanin A [333]. Another study showed that the lower bioavailability (4.6%) of biochanin A is due to the rapid phase I and phase II hepatic and intestinal metabolism [333]. Biochanin A combined administration with EGCG and quercetin increases the bioavailability of biochanin A. Coadministration also enhanced the urinary excretion of biochanin A by approximately 2.97-folds, which is another effective method to increase its bioavailability [334].

9. Synergistic effects of phytonutrients

Risk of cancer recurrence as well as several other chronic disorders can be reduced significantly by regular consumption of vegetables and fruits [335,336]. Synergy is a process which describes that the combination of two or more bioactive substances produces a more pronounced biological effect than the effect caused by a single substance [337]. For example, the synergy of phytonutrients from different sources and their combination with anticancer drugs enhance the benefits conferred by the individual phytonutrient or the drug [338,339].

The combined treatment of curcumin and citral effectively kills breast cancer cells in vitro and causes cell death without disturbing normal breast epithelial tissues. The synergistic effects caused by this combination result in apoptosis induction by the hypergeneration of ROS along with the activation of p53 and cell cycle arrest at the G0/G1 stage. The results of this study provided the evidences in favor of the synergistic behavior of curcumin and citral against breast cancer [340]. Likewise, the combination of 6-gingerol (6-G) and γ-tocotrienol exhibits promising anticancer effects in colorectal cells by modulating gene expression pathways and downregulating the Wnt signaling pathway. This combination also induces apoptosis through caspase-independent programmed cell death in a synergistic manner [341]. The mixture of curcumin with silymarin provides effective synergistic effects in terms of chemoprevention. The in vitro application of curcumin and silymarin simultaneously induces apoptosis in colorectal cancer cells by suppressing NF-κB activity [342].

10. Conclusions

Cancer metabolism or metabolic rewiring is the fundamental step in the initiation of cancer. This critical step fulfills the energy demands for cancer progression and ultimately leads toward the deadly pathogenesis. Despite all the advancements in the treatment of this disease, it has been prevailing all around the globe at a constant pace. The side effects, high cost, and recurrence of cancer in the case of synthetic anticancer drugs demand alternative treatment strategies. In this regard, phytochemicals offer promising results in terms of the cost-effectiveness, biosafety profiling, and multitargeted approach. Phytonutrients are efficient modulators of cell signaling pathways (NF-κB, STAT3, PI33K/Akt/mTOR, and HIFα) as elaborated by the experimental evidences in this book chapter. Although several phytonutrients are in the phase of clinical trials, yet the exact action mechanism and the pharmacokinetics of these phytonutrients are still a topic of debate. Moreover, most of the phytonutrients in our diet hold efficient biosafety levels while having poor bioavailability. One of the most studied polyphenol curcumin is also in the stage of clinical trials but its poor bioavailability hinders its to become an anticancer compound. Likewise, catechins from green tea also possess poor bioavailability in the human body. All these issues need to be addressed to potentiate the bioactive phytonutrients as effective anticancer drug candidates.

References

[1] L.A. Torre, et al., Global cancer statistics, 2012, CA Cancer J. Clin. 65 (2) (2015) 87–108.

[2] J. Ferlay, et al., Estimating the global cancer incidence and mortality in 2018: GLOBOCAN sources and methods, Int. J. Cancer 144 (8) (2019) 1941–1953.

[3] A.R. Guerra, M.F. Duarte, I.F. Duarte, Targeting tumor metabolism with plant-derived natural products: emerging trends in cancer therapy, J. Agric. Food Chem. 66 (41) (2018) 10663–10685.

[4] M. Zafar, et al., Tubeimoside-1, triterpenoid saponin, as a potential natural cancer killer, Nat. Prod. Commun. 13 (5) (2018), 1934578X1801300.

[5] A. Vazquez, et al., Cancer metabolism at a glance, J. Cell Sci. 129 (18) (2016) 3367–3373.

[6] C.V. Dang, Cancer metabolism: the known, unknowns, Biochim. Biophys. Acta Rev. Cancer 1870 (1) (2018) 1.

[7] E. Enzo, et al., Aerobic glycolysis tunes YAP/TAZ transcriptional activity, EMBO J. 34 (10) (2015) 1349–1370.

[8] M.A. Zmijewski, Vitamin D and human health, Int. J. Mol. Sci. 20 (1) (2019).

[9] S.R. Nielsen, M.C. Schmid, Macrophages as key drivers of cancer progression and metastasis, Mediators Inflamm. 2017 (2017) 9624760.

[10] D.J.R. Lane, et al., Coupling of the polyamine and iron metabolism pathways in the regulation of proliferation: mechanistic links to alterations in key polyamine biosynthetic and catabolic enzymes, Biochim. Biophys. Acta, Mol. Basis Dis. **1864** (9 Pt B) (2018) 2793–2813.

[11] O. Warburg, On the origin of cancer cells, Science 123 (3191) (1956) 309–314.
[12] L. Li, et al., Transcriptional regulation of the Warburg effect in cancer by SIX1, Cancer Cell 33 (3) (2018) 368–385 e7.
[13] M. Yang, K.H. Vousden, Serine and one-carbon metabolism in cancer, Nat. Rev. Cancer 16 (10) (2016) 650–662.
[14] W.H. Koppenol, P.L. Bounds, C.V. Dang, Otto Warburg's contributions to current concepts of cancer metabolism, Nat. Rev. Cancer 11 (5) (2011) 325–337.
[15] S. Metcalf, et al., Selective loss of phosphoserine aminotransferase 1 (PSAT1) suppresses migration, invasion, and experimental metastasis in triple negative breast cancer, Clin. Exp. Metastasis 37 (1) (2020) 187–197.
[16] J.R. Doherty, J.L. Cleveland, Targeting lactate metabolism for cancer therapeutics, J. Clin. Invest. 123 (9) (2013) 3685–3692.
[17] M. Yu, et al., The prognostic value of GLUT1 in cancers: a systematic review and meta-analysis, Oncotarget 8 (26) (2017) 43356–43367.
[18] R. Stienstra, M.G. Netea, Firing up glycolysis: BCG vaccination effects on type 1 diabetes mellitus, Trends Endocrinol. Metab. 29 (12) (2018) 813–814.
[19] E.S. Cho, et al., The pentose phosphate pathway as a potential target for cancer therapy, Biomol. Ther. (Seoul) 26 (1) (2018) 29–38.
[20] S. Herzig, et al., Identification and functional expression of the mitochondrial pyruvate carrier, Science 337 (6090) (2012) 93–96.
[21] I. Papandreou, et al., HIF-1 mediates adaptation to hypoxia by actively downregulating mitochondrial oxygen consumption, Cell Metab. 3 (3) (2006) 187–197.
[22] W. Zwerschke, et al., Metabolic analysis of senescent human fibroblasts reveals a role for AMP in cellular senescence, Biochem. J. 376 (Pt 2) (2003) 403–411.
[23] M.G. Vander Heiden, L.C. Cantley, C.B. Thompson, Understanding the Warburg effect: the metabolic requirements of cell proliferation, Science 324 (5930) (2009) 1029–1033.
[24] S.P. Mathupala, Y.H. Ko, P.L. Pedersen, Hexokinase II: cancer's double-edged sword acting as both facilitator and gatekeeper of malignancy when bound to mitochondria, Oncogene 25 (34) (2006) 4777–4786.
[25] N.S. Akins, T.C. Nielson, H.V. Le, Inhibition of glycolysis and glutaminolysis: an emerging drug discovery approach to combat cancer, Curr. Top. Med. Chem. 18 (6) (2018) 494–504.
[26] R.B. Robey, N. Hay, Mitochondrial hexokinases, novel mediators of the antiapoptotic effects of growth factors and Akt, Oncogene 25 (34) (2006) 4683–4696.
[27] J. Zou, et al., Euxanthone inhibits glycolysis and triggers mitochondria-mediated apoptosis by targeting hexokinase 2 in epithelial ovarian cancer, Cell Biochem. Funct. 36 (6) (2018) 303–311.
[28] L. Tao, et al., Gen-27, a newly synthesized flavonoid, inhibits glycolysis and induces cell apoptosis via suppression of hexokinase II in human breast cancer cells, Biochem. Pharmacol. 125 (2017) 12–25.
[29] W. Guo, et al., MiR-199a-5p is negatively associated with malignancies and regulates glycolysis and lactate production by targeting hexokinase 2 in liver cancer, Hepatology 62 (4) (2015) 1132–1144.
[30] J. Wu, et al., Licochalcone A suppresses hexokinase 2-mediated tumor glycolysis in gastric cancer via downregulation of the Akt signaling pathway, Oncol. Rep. 39 (3) (2018) 1181–1190.
[31] L. Fan, et al., Long noncoding RNA urothelial cancer associated 1 regulates radioresistance via the hexokinase 2/glycolytic pathway in cervical cancer, Int. J. Mol. Med. 42 (4) (2018) 2247–2259.
[32] Y. Qin, et al., miR-4458 suppresses glycolysis and lactate production by directly targeting hexokinase2 in colon cancer cells, Biochem. Biophys. Res. Commun. 469 (1) (2016) 37–43.

[33] B.Yan, et al., Resveratrol inhibits ROS-promoted activation and glycolysis of pancreatic stellate cells via suppression of miR-21, Oxid. Med. Cell. Longev. 2018 (2018) 1346958.
[34] H. Li, et al., Capsaicin and piperine can overcome multidrug resistance in cancer cells to doxorubicin, Molecules 23 (3) (2018).
[35] C.G. Chiu, et al., Autocrine motility factor receptor: a clinical review, Expert Rev. Anticancer Ther. 8 (2) (2008) 207–217.
[36] J.W. Kim, C.V. Dang, Multifaceted roles of glycolytic enzymes, Trends Biochem. Sci. 30 (3) (2005) 142–150.
[37] P.C.Verma, et al., Study of serum phosphohexose isomerase (PHI) levels in the management of head and neck malignancies, Indian J. Otolaryngol. Head Neck Surg. 53 (1) (2001) 40–46.
[38] Y. Li, et al., Silencing of phosphoglucose isomerase/autocrine motility factor decreases U87 human glioblastoma cell migration, Int. J. Mol. Med. 37 (4) (2016) 998–1004.
[39] P.S. Patel, et al., Comparison between serum levels of carcinoembryonic antigen, sialic acid and phosphohexose isomerase in lung cancer, Neoplasma 42 (5) (1995) 271–274.
[40] T. Funasaka, V. Hogan, A. Raz, Phosphoglucose isomerase/autocrine motility factor mediates epithelial and mesenchymal phenotype conversions in breast cancer, Cancer Res. 69 (13) (2009) 5349–5356.
[41] M. Baumann, et al., The diagnostic validity of the serum tumor marker phosphohexose isomerase (PHI) in patients with gastrointestinal, kidney, and breast cancer, Cancer Invest. 8 (3-4) (1990) 351–356.
[42] M. Baumann, et al., Significance of serum phosphohexose isomerase in gastrointestinal cancer at different stages, Oncology 45 (3) (1988) 153–158.
[43] H. Goel, G.S. Kohli, H. Lal, Serum phosphohexose isomerase levels in patients with head and neck cancer, J. Laryngol. Otol. 100 (5) (1986) 581–585.
[44] S. Tsutsumi, et al., Phosphoglucose isomerase enhances colorectal cancer metastasis, Int. J. Oncol. 35 (5) (2009) 1117–1121.
[45] H.C. Huang, et al., Phosphoglucose isomerase gene expression as a prognostic biomarker of gastric cancer, Chin. J. Cancer Res. 31 (5) (2019) 771–784.
[46] F.Ye, et al., Aldolase A overexpression is associated with poor prognosis and promotes tumor progression by the epithelial-mesenchymal transition in colon cancer, Biochem. Biophys. Res. Commun. 497 (2) (2018) 639–645.
[47] S.T. Cargnin, S.B. Gnoatto, Ursolic acid from apple pomace and traditional plants: a valuable triterpenoid with functional properties, Food Chem. 220 (2017) 477–489.
[48] W.L. Shih, et al., Suppression of AMF/PGI-mediated tumorigenic activities by ursolic acid in cultured hepatoma cells and in a mouse model, Mol. Carcinog. 52 (10) (2013) 800–812.
[49] H. Pelicano, et al., Glycolysis inhibition for anticancer treatment, Oncogene 25 (34) (2006) 4633–4646.
[50] B.A. Webb, et al., Structures of human phosphofructokinase-1 and atomic basis of cancer-associated mutations, Nature 523 (7558) (2015) 111–114.
[51] C.M. Sun, et al., Genetic alteration in phosphofructokinase family promotes growth of muscle-invasive bladder cancer, Int. J. Biol. Markers 31 (3) (2016) e286–e293.
[52] S. Li, et al., Expression of phosphofructokinase 1 protein and it's enzyme activity on nasopharyngeal carcinoma, Lin Chung Er Bi Yan Hou Tou Jing Wai Ke Za Zhi 29 (16) (2015) 1455–1457.
[53] R.G. Coelho, et al., Hexokinase and phosphofructokinase activity and intracellular distribution correlate with aggressiveness and invasiveness of human breast carcinoma, Oncotarget 6 (30) (2015) 29375–29387.
[54] P. Zancan, et al., Differential expression of phosphofructokinase-1 isoforms correlates with the glycolytic efficiency of breast cancer cells, Mol. Genet. Metab. 100 (4) (2010) 372–378.

[55] G. Wang, et al., Differential phosphofructokinase-1 isoenzyme patterns associated with glycolytic efficiency in human breast cancer and paracancer tissues, Oncol. Lett. 6 (6) (2013) 1701–1706.

[56] J. Wang, et al., The platelet isoform of phosphofructokinase contributes to metabolic reprogramming and maintains cell proliferation in clear cell renal cell carcinoma, Oncotarget 7 (19) (2016) 27142–27157.

[57] L. Li, et al., TAp73-induced phosphofructokinase-1 transcription promotes the Warburg effect and enhances cell proliferation, Nat. Commun. 9 (1) (2018) 4683.

[58] S. Li, et al., In vitro and in vivo study of epigallocatechin-3-gallate-induced apoptosis in aerobic glycolytic hepatocellular carcinoma cells involving inhibition of phosphofructokinase activity, Sci. Rep. 6 (2016) 28479.

[59] K. Taguchi, Y. Takagi, Aldolase, Rinsho Byori Suppl 116 (2001) 117–124.

[60] Y.C. Chang, et al., Feedback regulation of ALDOA activates the HIF-1alpha/MMP9 axis to promote lung cancer progression, Cancer Lett. 403 (2017) 28–36.

[61] Y.C. Chang, et al., Therapeutic targeting of aldolase A interactions inhibits lung cancer metastasis and prolongs survival, Cancer Res. 79 (18) (2019) 4754–4766.

[62] Z. Jiang, et al., Aldolase A as a prognostic factor and mediator of progression via inducing epithelial-mesenchymal transition in gastric cancer, J. Cell. Mol. Med. 22 (9) (2018) 4377–4386.

[63] S. Ji, et al., ALDOA functions as an oncogene in the highly metastatic pancreatic cancer, Cancer Lett. 374 (1) (2016) 127–135.

[64] Q. Li, et al., Aldolase B overexpression is associated with poor prognosis and promotes tumor progression by epithelial-mesenchymal transition in colorectal adenocarcinoma, Cell. Physiol. Biochem. 42 (1) (2017) 397–406.

[65] J. Chen, X. Hu, J. Cui, Shikonin, vitamin K3 and vitamin K5 inhibit multiple glycolytic enzymes in MCF-7 cells, Oncol. Lett. 15 (5) (2018) 7423–7432.

[66] A. Ationu, A. Humphries, The feasibility of replacement therapy for inherited disorder of glycolysis: triosephosphate isomerase deficiency (review), Int. J. Mol. Med. 2 (6) (1998) 701–704.

[67] C. Granchi, F. Minutolo, Anticancer agents that counteract tumor glycolysis, ChemMedChem 7 (8) (2012) 1318–1350.

[68] T. Chen, et al., Role of triosephosphate isomerase and downstream functional genes on gastric cancer, Oncol. Rep. 38 (3) (2017) 1822–1832.

[69] X.Z. Zhang, et al., Triosephosphate isomerase and peroxiredoxin 6, two novel serum markers for human lung squamous cell carcinoma, Cancer Sci. 100 (12) (2009) 2396–2401.

[70] G.J. van den Bemd, et al., Mass spectrometric identification of human prostate cancer-derived proteins in serum of xenograft-bearing mice, Mol. Cell. Proteomics 5 (10) (2006) 1830–1839.

[71] R. Lichtenfels, et al., Identification of metabolic enzymes in renal cell carcinoma utilizing PROTEOMEX analyses, Biochim. Biophys. Acta 1646 (1–2) (2003) 21–31.

[72] G. Pekel, F. Ari, Therapeutic targeting of cancer metabolism with triosephosphate isomerase, Chem. Biodivers. 17 (5) (2020), e2000012.

[73] Y. Higashimura, et al., Up-regulation of glyceraldehyde-3-phosphate dehydrogenase gene expression by HIF-1 activity depending on Sp1 in hypoxic breast cancer cells, Arch. Biochem. Biophys. 509 (1) (2011) 1–8.

[74] L. Hao, et al., Elevated GAPDH expression is associated with the proliferation and invasion of lung and esophageal squamous cell carcinomas, Proteomics 15 (17) (2015) 3087–3100.

[75] S. Liu, et al., Glyceraldehyde-3-phosphate dehydrogenase promotes liver tumorigenesis by modulating phosphoglycerate dehydrogenase, Hepatology 66 (2) (2017) 631–645.

[76] Q. Huang, et al., Akt2 kinase suppresses glyceraldehyde-3-phosphate dehydrogenase (GAPDH)-mediated apoptosis in ovarian cancer cells via phosphorylating GAPDH at threonine 237 and decreasing its nuclear translocation, J. Biol. Chem. 286 (49) (2011) 42211–42220.
[77] Z. Tang, et al., Over-expression of GAPDH in human colorectal carcinoma as a preferred target of 3-bromopyruvate propyl ester, J. Bioenerg. Biomembr. 44 (1) (2012) 117–125.
[78] M.V. Liberti, et al., A predictive model for selective targeting of the warburg effect through GAPDH inhibition with a natural product, Cell Metab. 26 (4) (2017) 648–659 e8.
[79] S. Kumagai, R. Narasaki, K. Hasumi, Glucose-dependent active ATP depletion by koningic acid kills high-glycolytic cells, Biochem. Biophys. Res. Commun. 365 (2) (2008) 362–368.
[80] J. Chen, et al., Shikonin and its analogs inhibit cancer cell glycolysis by targeting tumor pyruvate kinase-M2, Oncogene 30 (42) (2011) 4297–4306.
[81] A. Fiorillo, et al., The phosphoglycerate kinase 1 variants found in carcinoma cells display different catalytic activity and conformational stability compared to the native enzyme, PLoS One 13 (7) (2018), e0199191.
[82] B. Shashni, et al., Glycolytic enzymes PGK1 and PKM2 as novel transcriptional targets of PPARgamma in breast cancer pathophysiology, J. Drug Target. 21 (2) (2013) 161–174.
[83] S.J. Tang, et al., Phosphoglycerate kinase 1-overexpressing lung cancer cells reduce cyclooxygenase 2 expression and promote anti-tumor immunity in vivo, Int. J. Cancer 123 (12) (2008) 2840–2848.
[84] J. Wang, et al., Characterization of phosphoglycerate kinase-1 expression of stromal cells derived from tumor microenvironment in prostate cancer progression, Cancer Res. 70 (2) (2010) 471–480.
[85] T.L. Hwang, et al., Overexpression and elevated serum levels of phosphoglycerate kinase 1 in pancreatic ductal adenocarcinoma, Proteomics 6 (7) (2006) 2259–2272.
[86] D. Zieker, et al., Phosphoglycerate kinase 1 promoting tumor progression and metastasis in gastric cancer—detected in a tumor mouse model using positron emission tomography/magnetic resonance imaging, Cell. Physiol. Biochem. 26 (2) (2010) 147–154.
[87] D. Zieker, et al., Phosphoglycerate kinase 1 a promoting enzyme for peritoneal dissemination in gastric cancer, Int. J. Cancer 126 (6) (2010) 1513–1520.
[88] L. Zhang, et al., Influence of phosphoglycerate kinase 1 on metastasis and invasion of hepatoma cells and prognosis of liver cancer, Zhonghua Gan Zang Bing Za Zhi 25 (6) (2017) 446–451.
[89] H. Hu, et al., Acetylation of PGK1 promotes liver cancer cell proliferation and tumorigenesis, Hepatology 65 (2) (2017) 515–528.
[90] H. Xie, et al., PGK1 drives hepatocellular carcinoma metastasis by enhancing metabolic process, Int. J. Mol. Sci. 18 (8) (2017).
[91] H. Ding, et al., Phosphoglycerate kinase 1 promotes radioresistance in U251 human glioma cells, Oncol. Rep. 31 (2) (2014) 894–900.
[92] J. Ge, et al., miR-548c-5p inhibits colorectal cancer cell proliferation by targeting PGK1, J. Cell. Physiol. 234 (10) (2019) 18872–18878.
[93] Q. Fu, Z. Yu, Phosphoglycerate kinase 1 (PGK1) in cancer: a promising target for diagnosis and therapy, Life Sci. 256 (2020), 117863.
[94] H. Hatcher, et al., Curcumin: from ancient medicine to current clinical trials, Cell. Mol. Life Sci. 65 (11) (2008) 1631–1652.
[95] H. Cao, et al., Curcumin inhibits prostate cancer by targeting PGK1 in the FOXD3/miR-143 axis, Cancer Chemother. Pharmacol. 79 (5) (2017) 985–994.

[96] R. Rodicio, J. Heinisch, Isolation of the yeast phosphoglyceromutase gene and construction of deletion mutants, Mol. Gen. Genet. 206 (1) (1987) 133–140.
[97] A. Martinuzzi, et al., Developmental expression of the muscle-specific isozyme of phosphoglycerate mutase in human muscle cultured in monolayer and innervated by fetal rat spinal cord, Exp. Neurol. 96 (2) (1987) 365–375.
[98] L.A. Fothergill-Gilmore, H.C. Watson, The phosphoglycerate mutases, Adv. Enzymol. Relat. Areas Mol. Biol. 62 (1989) 227–313.
[99] T. Hitosugi, et al., Phosphoglycerate mutase 1 coordinates glycolysis and biosynthesis to promote tumor growth, Cancer Cell 22 (5) (2012) 585–600.
[100] D. Zhang, et al., Phosphoglycerate mutase 1 promotes cancer cell migration independent of its metabolic activity, Oncogene 36 (20) (2017) 2900–2909.
[101] N. Durany, et al., Phosphoglycerate mutase, 2,3-bisphosphoglycerate phosphatase, creatine kinase and enolase activity and isoenzymes in breast carcinoma, Br. J. Cancer 82 (1) (2000) 20–27.
[102] Y.A. Wen, et al., Phosphoglycerate mutase 1 knockdown inhibits prostate cancer cell growth, migration, and invasion, Asian J. Androl. 20 (2) (2018) 178–183.
[103] N.K. Narayanan, B.A. Narayanan, D.W. Nixon, Resveratrol-induced cell growth inhibition and apoptosis is associated with modulation of phosphoglycerate mutase B in human prostate cancer cells: two-dimensional sodium dodecyl sulfate-polyacrylamide gel electrophoresis and mass spectrometry evaluation, Cancer Detect. Prev. 28 (6) (2004) 443–452.
[104] K. Huang, et al., Synthesis and biological evaluation of anthraquinone derivatives as allosteric phosphoglycerate mutase 1 inhibitors for cancer treatment, Eur. J. Med. Chem. 168 (2019) 45–57.
[105] Q. Sun, et al., Phosphoglyceric acid mutase-1 contributes to oncogenic mTOR-mediated tumor growth and confers non-small cell lung cancer patients with poor prognosis, Cell Death Differ. 25 (6) (2018) 1160–1173.
[106] L. Liu, et al., Identification of potential genes/proteins regulated by Tiam1 in colorectal cancer by microarray analysis and proteome analysis, Cell Biol. Int. 32 (10) (2008) 1215–1222.
[107] F. Ren, et al., Quantitative proteomics identification of phosphoglycerate mutase 1 as a novel therapeutic target in hepatocellular carcinoma, Mol. Cancer 9 (2010) 81.
[108] D. Zhang, et al., Erratum: phosphoglycerate mutase 1 predicts the poor prognosis of oral squamous cell carcinoma and is associated with cell migration—erratum, J. Cancer 11 (7) (2020) 1913–1914.
[109] C.L. Wen, et al., An allosteric PGAM1 inhibitor effectively suppresses pancreatic ductal adenocarcinoma, Proc. Natl. Acad. Sci. U. S. A. 116 (46) (2019) 23264–23273.
[110] X. Liu, et al., Identification of PGAM1 as a putative therapeutic target for pancreatic ductal adenocarcinoma metastasis using quantitative proteomics, Onco. Targets. Ther. 11 (2018) 3345–3357.
[111] X. Li, et al., Identification of epigallocatechin-3- gallate as an inhibitor of phosphoglycerate mutase 1, Front. Pharmacol. 8 (2017) 325.
[112] L. Avilan, et al., Enolase: a key player in the metabolism and a probable virulence factor of trypanosomatid parasites-perspectives for its use as a therapeutic target, Enzyme Res. 2011 (2011), 932549.
[113] B. Altenberg, K.O. Greulich, Genes of glycolysis are ubiquitously overexpressed in 24 cancer classes, Genomics 84 (6) (2004) 1014–1020.
[114] H. Qiao, et al., Enolase1 overexpression regulates the growth of gastric cancer cells and predicts poor survival, J. Cell. Biochem. 120 (11) (2019) 18714–18723.
[115] J. Gao, et al., Role of enolase-1 in response to hypoxia in breast cancer: exploring the mechanisms of action, Oncol. Rep. 29 (4) (2013) 1322–1332.

[116] W. Zhu, et al., Enolase-1 serves as a biomarker of diagnosis and prognosis in hepatocellular carcinoma patients, Cancer Manag. Res. 10 (2018) 5735–5745.
[117] M. Zhao, et al., Enolase-1 is a therapeutic target in endometrial carcinoma, Oncotarget 6 (17) (2015) 15610–15627.
[118] L. Sun, et al., Over-expression of alpha-enolase as a prognostic biomarker in patients with pancreatic cancer, Int. J. Med. Sci. 14 (7) (2017) 655–661.
[119] L. Zhang, H. Wang, X. Dong, Diagnostic value of alpha-enolase expression and serum alpha-enolase autoantibody levels in lung cancer, J. Bras. Pneumol. 44 (1) (2018) 18–23.
[120] P. Zhan, et al., alpha-enolase promotes tumorigenesis and metastasis via regulating AMPK/mTOR pathway in colorectal cancer, Mol. Carcinog. 56 (5) (2017) 1427–1437.
[121] K.S. Gill, et al., Glycolysis inhibition as a cancer treatment and its role in an anti-tumour immune response, Biochim. Biophys. Acta 1866 (1) (2016) 87–105.
[122] S. Yeluri, et al., Cancer's craving for sugar: an opportunity for clinical exploitation, J. Cancer Res. Clin. Oncol. 135 (7) (2009) 867–877.
[123] T.L. Dayton, T. Jacks, M.G. Vander Heiden, PKM2, cancer metabolism, and the road ahead, EMBO Rep. 17 (12) (2016) 1721–1730.
[124] W.J. Israelsen, M.G. Vander Heiden, Pyruvate kinase: function, regulation and role in cancer, Semin. Cell Dev. Biol. 43 (2015) 43–51.
[125] C. Feng, et al., Aberrant overexpression of pyruvate kinase M2 is associated with aggressive tumor features and the BRAF mutation in papillary thyroid cancer, J. Clin. Endocrinol. Metab. 98 (9) (2013) E1524–E1533.
[126] B. Zheng, et al., Overexpression of pyruvate kinase type M2 (PKM2) promotes ovarian cancer cell growth and survival via regulation of cell cycle progression related with upregulated CCND1 and downregulated CDKN1A expression, Med. Sci. Monit. 24 (2018) 3103–3112.
[127] P. Dey, et al., Knockdown of pyruvate kinase M2 inhibits cell proliferation, metabolism, and migration in renal cell carcinoma, Int. J. Mol. Sci. 20 (22) (2019).
[128] Y. Qian, et al., Effect of pyruvate kinase M2-regulating aerobic glycolysis on chemotherapy resistance of estrogen receptor-positive breast cancer, Anticancer Drugs 29 (7) (2018) 616–627.
[129] Z. Zhang, et al., PKM2, function and expression and regulation, Cell Biosci. 9 (2019) 52.
[130] M. Venigalla, E. Gyengesi, G. Munch, Curcumin and Apigenin—novel and promising therapeutics against chronic neuroinflammation in Alzheimer's disease, Neural Regen. Res. 10 (8) (2015) 1181–1185.
[131] S. Shan, et al., Apigenin restrains colon cancer cell proliferation via targeted blocking of pyruvate kinase M2-dependent glycolysis, J. Agric. Food Chem. 65 (37) (2017) 8136–8144.
[132] L. Jia, et al., Quercetin suppresses the mobility of breast cancer by suppressing glycolysis through Akt-mTOR pathway mediated autophagy induction, Life Sci. 208 (2018) 123–130.
[133] J. Liu, et al., Oleanolic acid suppresses aerobic glycolysis in cancer cells by switching pyruvate kinase type M isoforms, PLoS One 9 (3) (2014), e91606.
[134] Y. Wang, et al., PKM2 inhibitor shikonin overcomes the cisplatin resistance in bladder cancer by inducing necroptosis, Int. J. Biol. Sci. 14 (13) (2018) 1883–1891.
[135] H. Yan, D.W. Parsons, G. Jin, R. McLendon, B.A. Rasheed, W. Yuan, I. Kos, I. Batinic-Haberle, S. Jones, G.J. Riggins, H. Friedman, A. Friedman, D. Reardon, J. Herndon, K.W. Kinzler, V.E. Velculescu, B. Vogelstein, D.D. Bigner, IDH1 and IDH2 mutations in gliomas, N. Engl. J. Med. 360 (8) (2009) 765–773.
[136] F. Gao, et al., Epigallocatechin gallate inhibits human tongue carcinoma cells via HK2 mediated glycolysis, Oncol. Rep. 33 (3) (2015) 1533–1539.

[137] X. Mao, et al., Capsaicin inhibits glycolysis in esophageal squamous cell carcinoma by regulating hexokinase2 expression, Mol. Med. Rep. 17 (4) (2018) 6116–6121.
[138] N.J. Kruger, A. von Schaewen, The oxidative pentose phosphate pathway: structure and organisation, Curr. Opin. Plant Biol. 6 (3) (2003) 236–246.
[139] W.M. Frederiks, et al., Elevated activity of the oxidative and non-oxidative pentose phosphate pathway in (pre)neoplastic lesions in rat liver, Int. J. Exp. Pathol. 89 (4) (2008) 232–240.
[140] L.V. Eggleston, H.A. Krebs, Regulation of the pentose phosphate cycle, Biochem. J. 138 (3) (1974) 425–435.
[141] K.C. Patra, N. Hay, The pentose phosphate pathway and cancer, Trends Biochem. Sci. 39 (8) (2014) 347–354.
[142] P. Szabo, et al., Cytological mapping of the human glucose-6-phosphate dehydrogenase gene distal to the fragile-X site suggests a high rate of meiotic recombination across this site, Proc. Natl. Acad. Sci. U. S. A. 81 (24) (1984) 7855–7859.
[143] M.G. Persico, et al., Isolation of human glucose-6-phosphate dehydrogenase (G6PD) cDNA clones: primary structure of the protein and unusual 5' non-coding region, Nucleic Acids Res. 14 (6) (1986) 2511–2522.
[144] X.T. Wang, et al., What is the role of the second "structural" NADP+-binding site in human glucose 6-phosphate dehydrogenase? Protein Sci. 17 (8) (2008) 1403–1411.
[145] H.N. Kirkman, E.M. Hendrickson, Glucose 6-phosphate dehydrogenase from human erythrocytes. II. Subactive states of the enzyme from normal persons, J. Biol. Chem. 237 (1962) 2371–2376.
[146] E. Capoluongo, B. Giardina, A. Minucci, Glucose-6-phosphate dehydrogenase (G6PD) deficiency, in: Brenner's Encyclopedia of Genetics, vol. 2, 2013, pp. 340–342.
[147] H.M. Yaish, Glucose-6-phosphate dehydrogenase deficiency, in: Textbook of Clinical Pediatrics, Springer, Berlin, Heidelberg, 2012. T.o.C. Pediatrics, Ed.
[148] Y. Xu, B.W. Osborne, R.C. Stanton, Diabetes causes inhibition of glucose-6-phosphate dehydrogenase via activation of PKA, which contributes to oxidative stress in rat kidney cortex, Am. J. Physiol. Renal Physiol. 289 (5) (2005) F1040–F1047.
[149] J.T. Prchal, X.T. Gregg, Red cell enzymes, Hematology Am. Soc. Hematol. Educ. Program (2005) 19–23.
[150] K. Fukuoka, et al., Fanconi's anemia with squamous cell carcinoma—a case report and a review of literature, Rinsho Ketsueki 30 (11) (1989) 1992–1996.
[151] R. Nagashio, et al., Prognostic significance of G6PD expression and localization in lung adenocarcinoma, Biochim. Biophys. Acta Proteins Proteomics 1867 (1) (2019) 38–46.
[152] M. Lu, et al., Elevated G6PD expression contributes to migration and invasion of hepatocellular carcinoma cells by inducing epithelial-mesenchymal transition, Acta Biochim. Biophys. Sin. Shanghai 50 (4) (2018) 370–380.
[153] T. Dong, et al., Altered glycometabolism affects both clinical features and prognosis of triple-negative and neoadjuvant chemotherapy-treated breast cancer, Tumour Biol. 37 (6) (2016) 8159–8168.
[154] X. Wang, et al., Glucose-6-phosphate dehydrogenase expression is correlated with poor clinical prognosis in esophageal squamous cell carcinoma, Eur. J. Surg. Oncol. 41 (10) (2015) 1293–1299.
[155] X. Rao, et al., O-GlcNAcylation of G6PD promotes the pentose phosphate pathway and tumor growth, Nat. Commun. 6 (2015) 8468.
[156] S. Adem, et al., Investigation of the effects of some phenolic compounds on the activities of glucose-6-phosphate dehydrogenase and 6-phosphogluconate dehydrogenase from human erythrocytes, J. Biochem. Mol. Toxicol. 28 (11) (2014) 510–514.
[157] E. Saunier, et al., Resveratrol reverses the Warburg effect by targeting the pyruvate dehydrogenase complex in colon cancer cells, Sci. Rep. 7 (1) (2017) 6945.

[158] H. Liu, et al., Reactive oxygen species-mediated endoplasmic reticulum stress and mitochondrial dysfunction contribute to polydatin-induced apoptosis in human nasopharyngeal carcinoma CNE cells, J. Cell. Biochem. 112 (12) (2011) 3695–3703.
[159] L. Mele, et al., A new inhibitor of glucose-6-phosphate dehydrogenase blocks pentose phosphate pathway and suppresses malignant proliferation and metastasis in vivo, Cell Death Dis. 9 (5) (2018) 572.
[160] S. Bimonte, et al., Current shreds of evidence on the anticancer role of EGCG in triple negative breast cancer: an update of the current state of knowledge, Infect. Agent Cancer 15 (2020) 2.
[161] E.S. Shin, et al., Catechin gallates are NADP+-competitive inhibitors of glucose-6-phosphate dehydrogenase and other enzymes that employ NADP+ as a coenzyme, Bioorg. Med. Chem. 16 (7) (2008) 3580–3586.
[162] J. Vanamala, et al., Resveratrol suppresses human colon cancer cell proliferation and induces apoptosis via targeting the pentose phosphate and the talin-FAK signaling pathways-A proteomic approach, Proteome Sci. 9 (1) (2011) 49.
[163] B. Tandogan, et al., In vitro effects of rosmarinic acid on glutathione reductase and glucose 6-phosphate dehydrogenase, Pharm. Biol. 49 (6) (2011) 587–594.
[164] T. Ge, et al., The role of the pentose phosphate pathway in diabetes and cancer, Front. Endocrinol. (Lausanne) 11 (2020) 365.
[165] R. Lin, et al., 6-Phosphogluconate dehydrogenase links oxidative PPP, lipogenesis and tumour growth by inhibiting LKB1-AMPK signalling, Nat. Cell Biol. 17 (11) (2015) 1484–1496.
[166] L. Jin, Y. Zhou, Crucial role of the pentose phosphate pathway in malignant tumors, Oncol. Lett. 17 (5) (2019) 4213–4221.
[167] C. Shan, et al., Lysine acetylation activates 6-phosphogluconate dehydrogenase to promote tumor growth, Mol. Cell 55 (4) (2014) 552–565.
[168] H. Chen, et al., 6PGD inhibition sensitizes hepatocellular carcinoma to chemotherapy via AMPK activation and metabolic reprogramming, Biomed. Pharmacother. 111 (2019) 1353–1358.
[169] C.A. Rice-Evans, N.J. Miller, G. Paganga, Structure-antioxidant activity relationships of flavonoids and phenolic acids, Free Radic. Biol. Med. 20 (7) (1996) 933–956.
[170] S. Elf, et al., Targeting 6-phosphogluconate dehydrogenase in the oxidative PPP sensitizes leukemia cells to antimalarial agent dihydroartemisinin, Oncogene 36 (2) (2017) 254–262.
[171] A.K. Samland, G.A. Sprenger, Transaldolase: from biochemistry to human disease, Int. J. Biochem. Cell Biol. 41 (7) (2009) 1482–1494.
[172] S. Thorell, et al., The three-dimensional structure of human transaldolase, FEBS Lett. 475 (3) (2000) 205–208.
[173] K. Banki, et al., The human transaldolase gene (TALDO1) is located on chromosome 11 at p15.4-p15.5, Genomics 45 (1) (1997) 233–238.
[174] I. Giacomini, et al., The pentose phosphate pathway and its involvement in cisplatin resistance, Int. J. Mol. Sci. 21 (3) (2020).
[175] J.W. Pelley, Minor carbohydrate pathways, in: Integrated Review Biochemistry, Saunders, 2012, pp. 75–79. Elsevier's, Ed.
[176] K. Banki, et al., Glutathione levels and sensitivity to apoptosis are regulated by changes in transaldolase expression, J. Biol. Chem. 271 (51) (1996) 32994–33001.
[177] M. Hatting, C. Trautwein, F.J. Cubero, TAL deficiency, all roads lead to oxidative stress? Hepatology 50 (3) (2009) 979–981.
[178] Y. Ding, et al., Synthetic lethality between HER2 and transaldolase in intrinsically resistant HER2-positive breast cancers, Nat. Commun. 9 (1) (2018) 4274.
[179] P.V. Basta, et al., Genetic variation in Transaldolase 1 and risk of squamous cell carcinoma of the head and neck, Cancer Detect. Prev. 32 (3) (2008) 200–208.

[180] M.A. Kowalik, A. Columbano, A. Perra, Emerging role of the pentose phosphate pathway in hepatocellular carcinoma, Front. Oncol. 7 (2017) 87.
[181] T. Moriyama, et al., Two isoforms of TALDO1 generated by alternative translational initiation show differential nucleocytoplasmic distribution to regulate the global metabolic network, Sci. Rep. 6 (2016) 34648.
[182] K. Banki, A. Perl, Inhibition of the catalytic activity of human transaldolase by antibodies and site-directed mutagenesis, FEBS Lett. 378 (2) (1996) 161–165.
[183] J. Vanamala, C.C. Tarver, P.S. Murano, Obesity-enhanced colon cancer: functional food compounds and their mechanisms of action, Curr. Cancer Drug Targets 8 (7) (2008) 611–633.
[184] C. Desbois-Mouthon, et al., Insulin and IGF-1 stimulate the beta-catenin pathway through two signalling cascades involving GSK-3beta inhibition and Ras activation, Oncogene 20 (2) (2001) 252–259.
[185] D. LeRoith, C.T. Roberts Jr., The insulin-like growth factor system and cancer, Cancer Lett. 195 (2) (2003) 127–137.
[186] J. Liang, J.M. Slingerland, Multiple roles of the PI3K/PKB (Akt) pathway in cell cycle progression, Cell Cycle 2 (4) (2003) 339–345.
[187] K. Duvel, et al., Activation of a metabolic gene regulatory network downstream of mTOR complex 1, Mol. Cell 39 (2) (2010) 171–183.
[188] O.N. Solovjeva, M.V. Kovina, G.A. Kochetov, Substrate inhibition of transketolase, Biochim. Biophys. Acta 1864 (3) (2016) 280–282.
[189] M. Prejano, F.E. Medina, P.A. Fernandes, N. Russo, M.J. Ramos, T. Marino, The Catalytic Mechanism of Human Transketolase, ChemPhysChem 20 (21) (2019) 2881–2886.
[190] A.O. Maslova, L.E. Meshalkina, G.A. Kochetov, Computer modeling of transketolase-like protein, TKTL1, a marker of certain tumor tissues, Biochemistry (Mosc.) 77 (3) (2012) 296–299.
[191] S. Langbein, M. Zerilli, A. Zur Hausen, W. Staiger, K. Rensch-Boschert, N. Lukan, J. Popa, M.P. Ternullo, A. Steidler, C. Weiss, R. Grobholz, F. Willeke, P. Alken, G. Stassi, P. Schubert, J.F. Coy, Expression of transketolase TKTL1 predicts colon and urothelial cancer patient survival: Warburg effect reinterpreted, Br. J. Cancer 94 (4) (2006) 578–585.
[192] L.G. Boros, J. Puigjaner, M. Cascante, W.N. Lee, J.L. Brandes, S. Bassilian, F.I. Yusuf, R.D. Williams, P. Muscarella, W.S. Melvin, W.J. Schirmer, Oxythiamine and dehydroepiandrosterone inhibit the nonoxidative synthesis of ribose and tumor cell proliferation, Cancer Res. 57 (19) (1997) 4242–4248.
[193] J.F. Coy, D. Dressler, J. Wilde, P. Schubert, Mutations in the transketolase-like gene TKTL1: clinical implications for neurodegenerative diseases, diabetes and cancer, Clin. Lab. 51 (5–6) (2005) 257–273.
[194] G.P. Deshpande, H.G. Patterton, M. Faadiel Essop, The human transketolase-like proteins TKTL1 and TKTL2 are bona fide transketolases, BMC Struct. Biol. 19 (1) (2019) 2.
[195] Y. Dong, M. Wang, Knockdown of TKTL1 additively complements cisplatin-induced cytotoxicity in nasopharyngeal carcinoma cells by regulating the levels of NADPH and ribose-5-phosphate, Biomed. Pharmacother. 85 (2017) 672–678.
[196] M. Zhao, M. Ye, J. Zhou, X. Zhu, Prognostic values of transketolase family genes in ovarian cancer, Oncol. Lett. 18 (5) (2019) 4845–4857.
[197] D. Djureinovic, B.M. Hallstrom, M. Horie, J.S.M. Mattsson, L. La Fleur, L. Fagerberg, H. Brunnstrom, C. Lindskog, K. Madjar, J. Rahnenfuhrer, S. Ekman, E. Stahle, H. Koyi, E. Branden, K. Edlund, J.G. Hengstler, M. Lambe, A. Saito, J. Botling, F. Ponten, M. Uhlen, P. Micke, Profiling cancer testis antigens in non-small-cell lung cancer, JCI Insight 1 (10) (2016), e86837.

[198] L. Boldrini, R. Bartoletti, M. Giordano, F. Manassero, C. Selli, M. Panichi, L. Galli, F. Farci, P. Faviana, C-MYC, HIF-1alpha, ERG, TKT, and GSTP1: an axis in prostate cancer? Pathol. Oncol. Res. 25 (4) (2019) 1423–1429.
[199] H. Chen, J.X. Yue, S.H. Yang, H. Ding, R.W. Zhao, S. Zhang, Overexpression of transketolase-like gene 1 is associated with cell proliferation in uterine cervix cancer, J. Exp. Clin. Cancer Res. 28 (2009) 43.
[200] S. Zhang, J.X. Yue, J.H. Yang, P.C. Cai, W.J. Kong, Overexpression of transketolase protein TKTL1 is associated with occurrence and progression in nasopharyngeal carcinoma: a potential therapeutic target in nasopharyngeal carcinoma, Cancer Biol. Ther. 7 (4) (2008) 517–522.
[201] W. Yuan, S. Wu, J. Guo, Z. Chen, J. Ge, P. Yang, B. Hu, Z. Chen, Silencing of TKTL1 by siRNA inhibits proliferation of human gastric cancer cells in vitro and in vivo, Cancer Biol. Ther. 9 (9) (2010) 710–716.
[202] H.J. Warnatz, D. Schmidt, T. Manke, I. Piccini, M. Sultan, T. Borodina, D. Balzereit, W. Wruck, A. Soldatov, M. Vingron, H. Lehrach, M.L. Yaspo, The BTB and CNC homology 1 (BACH1) target genes are involved in the oxidative stress response and in control of the cell cycle, J. Biol. Chem. 286 (26) (2011) 23521–23532.
[203] A. Ramos-Montoya, W.N. Lee, S. Bassilian, S. Lim, R.V. Trebukhina, M.V. Kazhyna, C.J. Ciudad, V. Noe, J.J. Centelles, M. Cascante, Pentose phosphate cycle oxidative and nonoxidative balance: A new vulnerable target for overcoming drug resistance in cancer, Int. J. Cancer 119 (12) (2006) 2733–2741.
[204] I.M. Xu, R.K. Lai, S.H. Lin, A.P. Tse, D.K. Chiu, H.Y. Koh, C.T. Law, C.M. Wong, Z. Cai, C.C. Wong, I.O. Ng, Transketolase counteracts oxidative stress to drive cancer development, Proc. Natl. Acad. Sci. USA 113 (6) (2016) E725–734.
[205] Z. Fan, H. Cui, X. Xu, Z. Lin, X. Zhang, L. Kang, B. Han, J. Meng, Z. Yan, X. Yan, S. Jiao, MiR-125a suppresses tumor growth, invasion and metastasis in cervical cancer by targeting STAT3, Oncotarget 6 (28) (2015) 25266–25280.
[206] H. Yang, X.L. Wu, K.H. Wu, R. Zhang, L.L. Ju, Y. Ji, Y.W. Zhang, S.L. Xue, Y.X. Zhang, Y.F. Yang, M.M. Yu, MicroRNA-497 regulates cisplatin chemosensitivity of cervical cancer by targeting transketolase, Am. J. Cancer Res. 6 (11) (2016) 2690–2699.
[207] R. Mariadasse, et al., Mechanical insights of oxythiamine compound as potent inhibitor for human transketolase-like protein 1 (TKTL1 protein), J. Recept. Signal Transduct. Res. 36 (3) (2016) 233–242.
[208] J.F. Coy, EDIM-TKTL1/Apo10 blood test: an innate immune system based liquid biopsy for the early detection, characterization and targeted treatment of cancer, Int. J. Mol. Sci. 18 (4) (2017).
[209] J.A. Combs, G.M. DeNicola, The non-essential amino acid cysteine becomes essential for tumor proliferation and survival, Cancers (Basel) 11 (5) (2019).
[210] S.C. Dolfi, et al., The metabolic demands of cancer cells are coupled to their size and protein synthesis rates, Cancer Metab. 1 (1) (2013) 20.
[211] From the American Association of Neurological Surgeons (AANS), et al., Multisociety consensus quality improvement revised consensus statement for endovascular therapy of acute ischemic stroke, Int. J. Stroke 13 (6) (2018) 612–632.
[212] S.R. Davis, et al., Tracer-derived total and folate-dependent homocysteine remethylation and synthesis rates in humans indicate that serine is the main one-carbon donor, Am. J. Physiol. Endocrinol. Metab. 286 (2) (2004) E272–E279.
[213] O.D. Maddocks, et al., Serine metabolism supports the methionine cycle and DNA/RNA methylation through de novo ATP synthesis in cancer cells, Mol. Cell 61 (2) (2016) 210–221.
[214] S. Gao, et al., PSAT1 is regulated by ATF4 and enhances cell proliferation via the GSK3beta/beta-catenin/cyclin D1 signaling pathway in ER-negative breast cancer, J. Exp. Clin. Cancer Res. 36 (1) (2017) 179.

[215] M.J. Zheng, et al., Identification of molecular marker associated with ovarian cancer prognosis using bioinformatics analysis and experiments, J. Cell. Physiol. 234 (7) (2019) 11023–11036.

[216] S.P. Huang, et al., Overexpression of PSAT1 gene is a favorable prognostic marker in lower-grade gliomas and predicts a favorable outcome in patients with IDH1 mutations and chromosome 1p19q codeletion, Cancers (Basel) 12 (1) (2019).

[217] K.M. Liao, et al., Overexpression of the PSAT1 gene in nasopharyngeal carcinoma is an indicator of poor prognosis, J. Cancer 7 (9) (2016) 1088–1094.

[218] Y.C. Chan, et al., Overexpression of PSAT1 promotes metastasis of lung adenocarcinoma by suppressing the IRF1-IFNgamma axis, Oncogene 39 (12) (2020) 2509–2522.

[219] H.O. Jin, et al., Knock-down of PSAT1 enhances sensitivity of NSCLC cells to glutamine-limiting conditions, Anticancer Res 39 (12) (2019) 6723–6730.

[220] Y. Zhang, et al., PSAT1 regulated oxidation-reduction balance affects the growth and prognosis of epithelial ovarian cancer, Onco. Targets. Ther. 13 (2020) 5443–5453.

[221] J. Jiang, et al., Regorafenib induces lethal autophagy arrest by stabilizing PSAT1 in glioblastoma, Autophagy 16 (1) (2020) 106–122.

[222] E. White, Exploiting the bad eating habits of Ras-driven cancers, Genes Dev. 27 (19) (2013) 2065–2071.

[223] S. Girgis, I.M. Nasrallah, J.R. Suh, E. Oppenheim, K.A. Zanetti, M.G. Mastri, P.J. Stover, Molecular cloning, characterization and alternative splicing of the human cytoplasmic serine hydroxymethyltransferase gene, Gene 210 (2) (1998) 315–324.

[224] P.J. Stover, L.H. Chen, J.R. Suh, D.M. Stover, K. Keyomarsi, B. Shane, Molecular cloning, characterization, and regulation of the human mitochondrial serine hydroxymethyltransferase gene, J. Biol. Chem. 272 (3) (1997) 1842–1848.

[225] S.H. Mudd, R. Cerone, M.C. Schiaffino, A.R. Fantasia, G. Minniti, U. Caruso, R. Lorini, D. Watkins, N. Matiaszuk, D.S. Rosenblatt, B. Schwahn, R. Rozen, L. LeGros, M. Kotb, A. Capdevila, Z. Luka, J.D. Finkelstein, A. Tangerman, S.P. Stabler, R.H. Allen, C. Wagner, Glycine N-methyltransferase deficiency: a novel inborn error causing persistent isolated hypermethioninaemia, J. Inherit. Metab. Dis. 24 (4) (2001) 448–464.

[226] S. Bernhardt, M. Bayerlova, M. Vetter, A. Wachter, D. Mitra, V. Hanf, T. Lantzsch, C. Uleer, S. Peschel, J. John, J. Buchmann, E. Weigert, K.F. Burrig, C. Thomssen, U. Korf, T. Beissbarth, S. Wiemann, E.J. Kantelhardt, Proteomic profiling of breast cancer metabolism identifies SHMT2 and ASCT2 as prognostic factors, Breast Cancer Res. 19 (1) (2017) 112.

[227] G. Giardina, A. Paone, A. Tramonti, R. Lucchi, M. Marani, M.C. Magnifico, A. Bouzidi, V. Pontecorvi, G. Guiducci, C. Zamparelli, S. Rinaldo, A. Paiardini, R. Contestabile, F. Cutruzzola, The catalytic activity of serine hydroxymethyltransferase is essential for de novo nuclear dTMP synthesis in lung cancer cells, FEBS J. 285 (17) (2018) 3238–3253.

[228] C. Lin, Y. Zhang, Y. Chen, Y. Bai, Y. Zhang, Long noncoding RNA LINC01234 promotes serine hydroxymethyltransferase 2 expression and proliferation by competitively binding miR-642a-5p in colon cancer, Cell Death Dis. 10 (2) (2019) 137.

[229] Z. Wei, J. Song, G. Wang, X. Cui, J. Zheng, Y. Tang, X. Chen, J. Li, L. Cui, C.Y. Liu, W. Yu, Deacetylation of serine hydroxymethyl-transferase 2 by SIRT3 promotes colorectal carcinogenesis, Nat. Commun. 9 (1) (2018) 4468.

[230] Y. Shi, S. Zhou, P. Wang, Y. Guo, B. Xie, S. Ding, Malic enzyme 1 (ME1) is a potential oncogene in gastric cancer cells and is associated with poor survival of gastric cancer patients, OncoTargets Ther. 12 (2019) 5589–5599.

[231] E. Scaletti, A.S. Jemth, T. Helleday, P. Stenmark, Structural basis of inhibition of the human serine hydroxymethyltransferase SHMT2 by antifolate drugs, FEBS Lett. 593 (14) (2019) 1863–1873.

[232] E. Melendez-Hevia, T.G. Waddell, M. Cascante, The puzzle of the Krebs citric acid cycle: assembling the pieces of chemically feasible reactions, and opportunism in the design of metabolic pathways during evolution, J. Mol. Evol. 43 (3) (1996) 293–303.
[233] P. Rustin, T. Bourgeron, B. Parfait, D. Chretien, A. Munnich, A. Rotig, Inborn errors of the Krebs cycle: a group of unusual mitochondrial diseases in human, Biochim. Biophys. Acta 1361 (2) (1997) 185–197.
[234] G.E. Gibson, A. Starkov, J.P. Blass, R.R. Ratan, M.F. Beal, Cause and consequence: mitochondrial dysfunction initiates and propagates neuronal dysfunction, neuronal death and behavioral abnormalities in age-associated neurodegenerative diseases, Biochim. Biophys. Acta 1802 (1) (2010) 122–134.
[235] L.D. Roberts, P. Bostrom, J.F. O'Sullivan, R.T. Schinzel, G.D. Lewis, A. Dejam, Y.K. Lee, M.J. Palma, S. Calhoun, A. Georgiadi, M.H. Chen, V.S. Ramachandran, M.G. Larson, C. Bouchard, T. Rankinen, A.L. Souza, C.B. Clish, T.J. Wang, J.L. Estall, A.A. Soukas, C.A. Cowan, B.M. Spiegelman, R.E. Gerszten, beta-Aminoisobutyric acid induces browning of white fat and hepatic beta-oxidation and is inversely correlated with cardiometabolic risk factors, Cell Metab. 19 (1) (2014) 96–108.
[236] C.A. Steginsky, K.J. Gruys, P.A. Frey, alpha-Ketoglutarate dehydrogenase complex of Escherichia coli. A hybrid complex containing pyruvate dehydrogenase subunits from pyruvate dehydrogenase complex, J. Biol. Chem. 260 (25) (1985) 13690–13693.
[237] I. Elia, M. Rossi, S. Stegen, D. Broekaert, G. Doglioni, M. van Gorsel, R. Boon, C. Escalona-Noguero, S. Torrekens, C. Verfaillie, E. Verbeken, G. Carmeliet, S.M. Fendt, Breast cancer cells rely on environmental pyruvate to shape the metastatic niche, Nature 568 (7750) (2019) 117–121.
[238] J. Kaplon, L. Zheng, K. Meissl, B. Chaneton, V.A. Selivanov, G. Mackay, S.H. van der Burg, E.M. Verdegaal, M. Cascante, T. Shlomi, E. Gottlieb, D.S. Peeper, A key role for mitochondrial gatekeeper pyruvate dehydrogenase in oncogene-induced senescence, Nature 498 (7452) (2013) 109–112.
[239] A.J. Levine, A.M. Puzio-Kuter, The control of the metabolic switch in cancers by oncogenes and tumor suppressor genes, Science 330 (6009) (2010) 1340–1344.
[240] E. Kolobova, A. Tuganova, I. Boulatnikov, K.M. Popov, Regulation of pyruvate dehydrogenase activity through phosphorylation at multiple sites, Biochem. J. 358 (Pt 1) (2001) 69–77.
[241] J. Fan, C. Shan, H.B. Kang, S. Elf, J. Xie, M. Tucker, T.L. Gu, M. Aguiar, S. Lonning, H. Chen, M. Mohammadi, L.M. Britton, B.A. Garcia, M. Aleckovic, Y. Kang, S. Kaluz, N. Devi, E.G. Van Meir, T. Hitosugi, J.H. Seo, S. Lonial, M. Gaddh, M. Arellano, H.J. Khoury, F.R. Khuri, T.J. Boggon, S. Kang, J. Chen, Tyr phosphorylation of PDP1 toggles recruitment between ACAT1 and SIRT3 to regulate the pyruvate dehydrogenase complex, Mol. Cell 53 (4) (2014) 534–548.
[242] M.J. Holness, M.C. Sugden, Regulation of pyruvate dehydrogenase complex activity by reversible phosphorylation, Biochem. Soc. Trans. 31 (Pt 6) (2003) 1143–1151.
[243] C.W. Lu, S.C. Lin, C.W. Chien, S.C. Lin, C.T. Lee, B.W. Lin, J.C. Lee, S.J. Tsai, Overexpression of pyruvate dehydrogenase kinase 3 increases drug resistance and early recurrence in colon cancer, Am. J. Pathol. 179 (3) (2011) 1405–1414.
[244] G. Sutendra, P. Dromparis, A. Kinnaird, T.H. Stenson, A. Haromy, J.M. Parker, M.S. McMurtry, E.D. Michelakis, Mitochondrial activation by inhibition of PDKII suppresses HIF1a signaling and angiogenesis in cancer, Oncogene 32 (13) (2013) 1638–1650.
[245] H. Hur, Y. Xuan, Y.B. Kim, G. Lee, W. Shim, J. Yun, I.H. Ham, S.U. Han, Expression of pyruvate dehydrogenase kinase-1 in gastric cancer as a potential therapeutic target, Int. J. Oncol. 42 (1) (2013) 44–54.
[246] M.I. Koukourakis, A. Giatromanolaki, E. Sivridis, K.C. Gatter, A.L. Harris, Tumor, G. Angiogenesis Research, Pyruvate dehydrogenase and pyruvate dehydrogenase kinase expression in non small cell lung cancer and tumor-associated stroma, Neoplasia 7 (1) (2005) 1–6.

[247] S.M. Wigfield, S.C. Winter, A. Giatromanolaki, J. Taylor, M.L. Koukourakis, A.L. Harris, PDK-1 regulates lactate production in hypoxia and is associated with poor prognosis in head and neck squamous cancer, Br. J. Cancer 98 (12) (2008) 1975–1984.

[248] E.M. Dunbar, B.S. Coats, A.L. Shroads, T. Langaee, A. Lew, J.R. Forder, J.J. Shuster, D.A. Wagner, P.W. Stacpoole, Phase 1 trial of dichloroacetate (DCA) in adults with recurrent malignant brain tumors, Invest New Drugs 32 (3) (2014) 452–464.

[249] R. Dahiya, T. Mohammad, P. Gupta, A. Haque, M.F. Alajmi, A. Hussain, M.I. Hassan, Molecular interaction studies on ellagic acid for its anticancer potential targeting pyruvate dehydrogenase kinase 3, RSC Adv. 9 (40) (2019) 23302–23315.

[250] A. Mukherjee, P.A. Srere, E.P. Frenkel, Studies of the mechanism by which hepatic citrate synthase activity increases in vitamin B12 deprivation, J. Biol. Chem. 251 (7) (1976) 2155–2160.

[251] S. Todisco, P. Convertini, V. Iacobazzi, V. Infantino, TCA cycle rewiring as emerging metabolic signature of hepatocellular carcinoma, Cancers (Basel) 12 (1) (2019).

[252] C. Choudhary, B.T. Weinert, Y. Nishida, E. Verdin, M. Mann, The growing landscape of lysine acetylation links metabolism and cell signalling, Nat. Rev. Mol. Cell Biol. 15 (8) (2014) 536–550.

[253] C.M. Metallo, P.A. Gameiro, E.L. Bell, K.R. Mattaini, J. Yang, K. Hiller, C.M. Jewell, Z.R. Johnson, D.J. Irvine, L. Guarente, J.K. Kelleher, M.G. Vander Heiden, O. Iliopoulos, G. Stephanopoulos, Reductive glutamine metabolism by IDH1 mediates lipogenesis under hypoxia, Nature 481 (7381) (2011) 380–384.

[254] D.E. Bauer, G. Hatzivassiliou, F. Zhao, C. Andreadis, C.B. Thompson, ATP citrate lyase is an important component of cell growth and transformation, Oncogene 24 (41) (2005) 6314–6322.

[255] G. Hatzivassiliou, F. Zhao, D.E. Bauer, C. Andreadis, A.N. Shaw, D. Dhanak, S.R. Hingorani, D.A. Tuveson, C.B. Thompson, ATP citrate lyase inhibition can suppress tumor cell growth, Cancer Cell 8 (4) (2005) 311–321.

[256] M.F. Amary, K. Bacsi, F. Maggiani, S. Damato, D. Halai, F. Berisha, R. Pollock, P. O'Donnell, A. Grigoriadis, T. Diss, M. Eskandarpour, N. Presneau, P.C. Hogendoorn, A. Futreal, R. Tirabosco, A.M. Flanagan, IDH1 and IDH2 mutations are frequent events in central chondrosarcoma and central and periosteal chondromas but not in other mesenchymal tumours, J. Pathol. 224 (3) (2011) 334–343.

[257] Z.J. Reitman, C.G. Duncan, E. Poteet, A. Winters, L.J. Yan, D.M. Gooden, I. Spasojevic, L.G. Boros, S.H. Yang, H. Yan, Cancer-associated isocitrate dehydrogenase 1 (IDH1) R132H mutation and d-2-hydroxyglutarate stimulate glutamine metabolism under hypoxia, J. Biol. Chem. 289 (34) (2014) 23318–23328.

[258] A. Latini, C.G. da Silva, G.C. Ferreira, P.F. Schuck, K. Scussiato, J.J. Sarkis, C.S. Dutra Filho, A.T. Wyse, C.M. Wannmacher, M. Wajner, Mitochondrial energy metabolism is markedly impaired by D-2-hydroxyglutaric acid in rat tissues, Mol. Genet. Metab. 86 (1–2) (2005) 188–199.

[259] S. Kolker, V. Pawlak, B. Ahlemeyer, J.G. Okun, F. Horster, E. Mayatepek, J. Krieglstein, G.F. Hoffmann, G. Kohr, NMDA receptor activation and respiratory chain complex V inhibition contribute to neurodegeneration in d-2-hydroxyglutaric aciduria, Eur. J. Neurosci. 16 (1) (2002) 21–28.

[260] L. Dang, D.W. White, S. Gross, B.D. Bennett, M.A. Bittinger, E.M. Driggers, V.R. Fantin, H.G. Jang, S. Jin, M.C. Keenan, K.M. Marks, R.M. Prins, P.S. Ward, K.E. Yen, L.M. Liau, J.D. Rabinowitz, L.C. Cantley, C.B. Thompson, M.G. Vander Heiden, S.M. Su, Cancer-associated IDH1 mutations produce 2-hydroxyglutarate, Nature 462 (7274) (2009) 739–744.

[261] F. Wang, J. Travins, B. DeLaBarre, V. Penard-Lacronique, S. Schalm, E. Hansen, K. Straley, A. Kernytsky, W. Liu, C. Gliser, H. Yang, S. Gross, E. Artin, V. Saada, E. Mylonas, C. Quivoron, J. Popovici-Muller, J.O. Saunders, F.G. Salituro, S. Yan, S. Murray, W. Wei, Y. Gao, L. Dang, M. Dorsch, S. Agresta, D.P. Schenkein, S.A. Biller, S.M. Su, S. de Botton, K.E. Yen, Targeted inhibition of mutant IDH2 in leukemia cells induces cellular differentiation, Science 340 (6132) (2013) 622–626.

[262] S. Verdura, E. Cuyas, J. Lozano-Sanchez, C. Bastidas-Velez, L. Llorach-Pares, S. Fernandez-Arroyo, A. Hernandez-Aguilera, J. Joven, A. Nonell-Canals, J. Bosch-Barrera, B. Martin-Castillo, L. Vellon, M. Sanchez-Martinez, A. Segura-Carretero, J.A. Menendez, An olive oil phenolic is a new chemotype of mutant isocitrate dehydrogenase 1 (IDH1) inhibitors, Carcinogenesis 40 (1) (2019) 27–40.
[263] L. Tretter, V. Adam-Vizi, Alpha-ketoglutarate dehydrogenase: a target and generator of oxidative stress, Philos. Trans. R Soc. Lond. B Biol. Sci. 360 (1464) (2005) 2335–2345.
[264] A.L. McLain, P.A. Szweda, L.I. Szweda, alpha-Ketoglutarate dehydrogenase: a mitochondrial redox sensor, Free Radic. Res. 45 (1) (2011) 29–36.
[265] N.M. Anderson, P. Mucka, J.G. Kern, H. Feng, The emerging role and targetability of the TCA cycle in cancer metabolism, Protein Cell 9 (2) (2018) 216–237.
[266] A.A. Aloud, C. Veeramani, C. Govindasamy, M.A. Alsaif, K.S. Al-Numair, Galangin, a natural flavonoid reduces mitochondrial oxidative damage in streptozotocin-induced diabetic rats, Redox Rep. 23 (1) (2018) 29–34.
[267] A.P. Aldera, D. Govender, Gene of the month: SDH, J. Clin. Pathol. 71 (2) (2018) 95–97.
[268] S. Cardaci, M.R. Ciriolo, TCA cycle defects and cancer: when metabolism tunes redox state, Int. J. Cell Biol. 2012 (2012) 161837.
[269] A. Sharma, H. Yuan, V. Kumar, M. Ramakrishnan, S.K. Kohli, R. Kaur, A.K. Thukral, R. Bhardwaj, B. Zheng, Castasterone attenuates insecticide induced phytotoxicity in mustard, Ecotoxicol. Environ. Saf. 179 (2019) 50–61.
[270] M. Akram, Citric acid cycle and role of its intermediates in metabolism, Cell Biochem. Biophys. 68 (3) (2014) 475–478.
[271] Y.S. Kim, Malonate metabolism: biochemistry, molecular biology, physiology, and industrial application, J. Biochem. Mol. Biol. 35 (5) (2002) 443–451.
[272] E. Sass, E. Blachinsky, S. Karniely, O. Pines, Mitochondrial and cytosolic isoforms of yeast fumarase are derivatives of a single translation product and have identical amino termini, J. Biol. Chem. 276 (49) (2001) 46111–46117.
[273] A.S. Qureshi, S. Ali, Warburg effect and renal cancer caused by errs in fumarate hydratase encoding gene, Pak. J. Pharm. Sci. 32 (2) (2019) 743–749.
[274] C. Schmidt, M. Sciacovelli, C. Frezza, Fumarate hydratase in cancer: a multifaceted tumour suppressor, Semin. Cell Dev. Biol. 98 (2020) 15–25.
[275] G. Laurenti, D.A. Tennant, Isocitrate dehydrogenase (IDH), succinate dehydrogenase (SDH), fumarate hydratase (FH): three players for one phenotype in cancer? Biochem. Soc. Trans. 44 (4) (2016) 1111–1116.
[276] N. Raimundo, B.E. Baysal, G.S. Shadel, Revisiting the TCA cycle: signaling to tumor formation, Trends Mol. Med. 17 (11) (2011) 641–649.
[277] C. Sourbier, B.T. Scroggins, R. Ratnayake, T.L. Prince, S. Lee, M.J. Lee, P.L. Nagy, Y.H. Lee, J.B. Trepel, J.A. Beutler, W.M. Linehan, L. Neckers, Englerin A stimulates PKCtheta to inhibit insulin signaling and to simultaneously activate HSF1: pharmacologically induced synthetic lethality, Cancer Cell 23 (2) (2013) 228–237.
[278] C.R. Goward, D.J. Nicholls, Malate dehydrogenase: a model for structure, evolution, and catalysis, Protein Sci. 3 (10) (1994) 1883–1888.
[279] R.A. Musrati, M. Kollarova, N. Mernik, D. Mikulasova, Malate dehydrogenase: distribution, function and properties, Gen. Physiol. Biophys. 17 (3) (1998) 193–210.
[280] P. Minarik, N. Tomaskova, M. Kollarova, M. Antalik, Malate dehydrogenases—structure and function, Gen. Physiol. Biophys. 21 (3) (2002) 257–265.
[281] G.G. Habets, R.A. van der Kammen, V. Willemsen, M. Balemans, J. Wiegant, J.G. Collard, Sublocalization of an invasion-inducing locus and other genes on human chromosome 7, Cytogenet. Cell Genet. 60 (3–4) (1992) 200–205.
[282] A. Cascon, I. Comino-Mendez, M. Curras-Freixes, A.A. de Cubas, L. Contreras, S. Richter, M. Peitzsch, V. Mancikova, L. Inglada-Perez, A. Perez-Barrios, M. Calatayud, S. Azriel, R. Villar-Vicente, J. Aller, F. Setien, S. Moran, J.F. Garcia, A. Rio-

Machin, R. Leton, A. Gomez-Grana, M. Apellaniz-Ruiz, G. Roncador, M. Esteller, C. Rodriguez-Antona, J. Satrustegui, G. Eisenhofer, M. Urioste, M. Robledo, Whole-exome sequencing identifies MDH2 as a new familial paraganglioma gene, J. Natl. Cancer Inst. 107 (5) (2015).
[283] Y.W. Lo, S.T. Lin, S.J. Chang, C.H. Chan, K.W. Lyu, J.F. Chang, E.W. May, D.Y. Lin, H.C. Chou, H.L. Chan, Mitochondrial proteomics with siRNA knockdown to reveal ACAT1 and MDH2 in the development of doxorubicin-resistant uterine cancer, J. Cell Mol. Med. 19 (4) (2015) 744–759.
[284] S. Mansouri, A. Shahriari, H. Kalantar, T. Moini Zanjani, M. Haghi Karamallah, Role of malate dehydrogenase in facilitating lactate dehydrogenase to support the glycolysis pathway in tumors, Biomed. Rep. 6 (4) (2017) 463–467.
[285] B. Zhang, J. Tornmalm, J. Widengren, H. Vakifahmetoglu-Norberg, E. Norberg, Characterization of the role of the malate dehydrogenases to lung tumor cell survival, J. Cancer 8 (11) (2017) 2088–2096.
[286] I. Sarfraz, A. Rasul, G. Hussain, S.M. Hussain, M. Ahmad, B. Nageen, F. Jabeen, Z. Selamoglu, M. Ali, Malic enzyme 2 as a potential therapeutic drug target for cancer, IUBMB Life 70 (11) (2018) 1076–1083.
[287] G. Chakrabarti, Mutant KRAS associated malic enzyme 1 expression is a predictive marker for radiation therapy response in non-small cell lung cancer, Radiat. Oncol. 10 (2015) 145.
[288] H. Shen, C. Xing, K. Cui, Y. Li, J. Zhang, R. Du, X. Zhang, Y. Li, MicroRNA-30a attenuates mutant KRAS-driven colorectal tumorigenesis via direct suppression of ME1, Cell Death Differ. 24 (7) (2017) 1253–1262.
[289] C. Nakashima, K. Yamamoto, R. Fujiwara-Tani, Y. Luo, S. Matsushima, K. Fujii, H. Ohmori, T. Sasahira, T. Sasaki, Y. Kitadai, T. Kirita, H. Kuniyasu, Expression of cytosolic malic enzyme (ME1) is associated with disease progression in human oral squamous cell carcinoma, Cancer Sci. 109 (6) (2018) 2036–2045.
[290] Y. Mihara, J. Akiba, S. Ogasawara, R. Kondo, H. Fukushima, H. Itadani, H. Obara, T. Kakuma, H. Kusano, Y. Naito, K. Okuda, O. Nakashima, H. Yano, Malic enzyme 1 is a potential marker of combined hepatocellular cholangiocarcinoma, subtype with stem-cell features, intermediate-cell type, Hepatol. Res. 49 (9) (2019) 1066–1075.
[291] Y. Rong, W. Wu, X. Ni, T. Kuang, D. Jin, D. Wang, W. Lou, Lactate dehydrogenase A is overexpressed in pancreatic cancer and promotes the growth of pancreatic cancer cells, Tumour Biol. 34 (3) (2013) 1523–1530.
[292] T.L. He, Y.J. Zhang, H. Jiang, X.H. Li, H. Zhu, K.L. Zheng, The c-Myc-LDHA axis positively regulates aerobic glycolysis and promotes tumor progression in pancreatic cancer, Med. Oncol. 32 (7) (2015) 187.
[293] X.G. Cui, Z.T. Han, S.H. He, X.D. Wu, T.R. Chen, C.H. Shao, D.L. Chen, N. Su, Y.M. Chen, T. Wang, J. Wang, D.W. Song, W.J. Yan, X.H. Yang, T. Liu, H.F. Wei, J. Xiao, HIF1/2alpha mediates hypoxia-induced LDHA expression in human pancreatic cancer cells, Oncotarget 8 (15) (2017) 24840–24852.
[294] Z.Y. Xian, J.M. Liu, Q.K. Chen, H.Z. Chen, C.J. Ye, J. Xue, H.Q. Yang, J.L. Li, X.F. Liu, S.J. Kuang, Inhibition of LDHA suppresses tumor progression in prostate cancer, Tumour Biol. 36 (10) (2015) 8093–8100.
[295] C.K. Das, A. Parekh, P.K. Parida, S.K. Bhutia, M. Mandal, Lactate dehydrogenase A regulates autophagy and tamoxifen resistance in breast cancer, Biochim. Biophys. Acta Mol. Cell Res. 1866 (6) (2019) 1004–1018.
[296] R.L. Han, F.P. Wang, P.A. Zhang, X.Y. Zhou, Y. Li, miR-383 inhibits ovarian cancer cell proliferation, invasion and aerobic glycolysis by targeting LDHA, Neoplasma 64 (2) (2017) 244–252.
[297] S. Hua, C. Liu, L. Liu, D. Wu, miR-142-3p inhibits aerobic glycolysis and cell proliferation in hepatocellular carcinoma via targeting LDHA, Biochem. Biophys. Res. Commun. 496 (3) (2018) 947–954.

[298] H. Cai, J. Li, Y. Zhang, Y. Liao, Y. Zhu, C. Wang, J. Hou, LDHA promotes oral squamous cell carcinoma progression through facilitating glycolysis and epithelial-mesenchymal transition, Front. Oncol. 9 (2019) 1446.

[299] V.R. Fantin, J. St-Pierre, P. Leder, Attenuation of LDH-A expression uncovers a link between glycolysis, mitochondrial physiology, and tumor maintenance, Cancer Cell 9 (6) (2006) 425–434.

[300] Y. Zhang, X. Zhang, X. Wang, L. Gan, G. Yu, Y. Chen, K. Liu, P. Li, J. Pan, J. Wang, S. Qin, Inhibition of LDH-A by lentivirus-mediated small interfering RNA suppresses intestinal-type gastric cancer tumorigenicity through the downregulation of Oct4, Cancer Lett. 321 (1) (2012) 45–54.

[301] D.W. Jeong, I.T. Cho, T.S. Kim, G.W. Bae, I.H. Kim, I.Y. Kim, Effects of lactate dehydrogenase suppression and glycerol-3-phosphate dehydrogenase overexpression on cellular metabolism, Mol. Cell. Biochem. 284 (1–2) (2006) 1–8.

[302] L. Zhuang, R.A. Scolyer, R. Murali, S.W. McCarthy, X.D. Zhang, J.F. Thompson, P. Hersey, Lactate dehydrogenase 5 expression in melanoma increases with disease progression and is associated with expression of Bcl-XL and Mcl-1, but not Bcl-2 proteins, Mod. Pathol. 23 (1) (2010) 45–53.

[303] T. Coyle, S. Levante, M. Shetler, J. Winfield, In vitro and in vivo cytotoxicity of gossypol against central nervous system tumor cell lines, J. Neurooncol. 19 (1) (1994) 25–35.

[304] P. Bushunow, M.M. Reidenberg, J. Wasenko, J. Winfield, B. Lorenzo, S. Lemke, B. Himpler, R. Corona, T. Coyle, Gossypol treatment of recurrent adult malignant gliomas, J. Neurooncol. 43 (1) (1999) 79–86.

[305] M.D. Shelley, L. Hartley, R.G. Fish, P. Groundwater, J.J. Morgan, D. Mort, M. Mason, A. Evans, Stereo-specific cytotoxic effects of gossypol enantiomers and gossypolone in tumour cell lines, Cancer Lett. 135 (2) (1999) 171–180.

[306] X. Cao, L. Fang, S. Gibbs, Y. Huang, Z. Dai, P. Wen, X. Zheng, W. Sadee, D. Sun, Glucose uptake inhibitor sensitizes cancer cells to daunorubicin and overcomes drug resistance in hypoxia, Cancer Chemother. Pharmacol. 59 (4) (2007) 495–505.

[307] A.W. Harmon, Y.M. Patel, Naringenin inhibits glucose uptake in MCF-7 breast cancer cells: a mechanism for impaired cellular proliferation, Breast Cancer Res. Treat. 85 (2) (2004) 103–110.

[308] J.B. Park, Inhibition of glucose and dehydroascorbic acid uptakes by resveratrol in human transformed myelocytic cells, J. Nat. Prod. 64 (3) (2001) 381–384.

[309] S. Mishra, M. Vinayak, Ellagic acid induces novel and atypical PKC isoforms and promotes caspase-3 dependent apoptosis by blocking energy metabolism, Nut. Cancer 66 (4) (2014) 675–681.

[310] M. Fathy, M.A. Fawzy, H. Hintzsche, T. Nikaido, T. Dandekar, E.M. Othman, Eugenol exerts apoptotic effect and modulates the sensitivity of HeLa cells to cisplatin and radiation, Molecules 24 (21) (2019).

[311] L. Yang, S. Venneti, D. Nagrath, Glutaminolysis: a hallmark of cancer metabolism, Annu. Rev. Biomed. Eng. 19 (2017) 163–194.

[312] M. Jain, et al., Metabolite profiling identifies a key role for glycine in rapid cancer cell proliferation, Science 336 (6084) (2012) 1040–1044.

[313] Y.D. Bhutia, V. Ganapathy, Glutamine transporters in mammalian cells and their functions in physiology and cancer, Biochim. Biophys. Acta 1863 (10) (2016) 2531–2539.

[314] J.C. Paquette, P.J. Guerin, E.R. Gauthier, Rapid induction of the intrinsic apoptotic pathway by L-glutamine starvation, J. Cell. Physiol. 202 (3) (2005) 912–921.

[315] E. Ahn, et al., Temporal fluxomics reveals oscillations in TCA cycle flux throughout the mammalian cell cycle, Mol. Syst. Biol. 13 (11) (2017) 953.

[316] P.L. Sulkowski, et al., Krebs-cycle-deficient hereditary cancer syndromes are defined by defects in homologous-recombination DNA repair, Nat. Genet. 50 (8) (2018) 1086–1092.

[317] T. Mashima, H. Seimiya, T. Tsuruo, De novo fatty-acid synthesis and related pathways as molecular targets for cancer therapy, Br. J. Cancer 100 (9) (2009) 1369–1372.
[318] B. Salehi, et al., Phytotherapeutics in cancer invasion and metastasis, Phytother. Res. 32 (8) (2018) 1425–1449.
[319] S. Kang, et al., Multivitamin and mineral supplementation containing phytonutrients scavenges reactive oxygen species in healthy subjects: a randomized, double-blinded, placebo-controlled trial, Nutrients 11 (1) (2019).
[320] B.B. Aggarwal, A. Kumar, A.C. Bharti, Anticancer potential of curcumin: preclinical and clinical studies, Anticancer Res 23 (1A) (2003) 363–398.
[321] P.R.N. Bhuket, et al., Enhancement of curcumin bioavailability via the prodrug approach: challenges and prospects, Eur. J. Drug Metab. Pharmacokinet. 42 (3) (2017) 341–353.
[322] A. Haghi, H. Azimi, R. Rahimi, A comprehensive review on pharmacotherapeutics of three phytochemicals, curcumin, quercetin, and allicin, in the treatment of gastric cancer, J. Gastrointest. Cancer 48 (4) (2017) 314–320.
[323] W. Wiczkowski, et al., Quercetin from shallots (Allium cepa L. var. aggregatum) is more bioavailable than its glucosides, J. Nutr. 138 (5) (2008) 885–888.
[324] S. Chakraborty, et al., The use of nano-quercetin to arrest mitochondrial damage and MMP-9 upregulation during prevention of gastric inflammation induced by ethanol in rat, Biomaterials 33 (10) (2012) 2991–3001.
[325] M. Iciek, I. Kwiecien, L. Wlodek, Biological properties of garlic and garlic-derived organosulfur compounds, Environ. Mol. Mutagen. 50 (3) (2009) 247–265.
[326] X.X. Wang, et al., The use of mitochondrial targeting resveratrol liposomes modified with a dequalinium polyethylene glycol-distearoylphosphatidyl ethanolamine conjugate to induce apoptosis in resistant lung cancer cells, Biomaterials 32 (24) (2011) 5673–5687.
[327] K. Teskac, J. Kristl, The evidence for solid lipid nanoparticles mediated cell uptake of resveratrol, Int. J. Pharm. 390 (1) (2010) 61–69.
[328] N. Summerlin, et al., Colloidal mesoporous silica nanoparticles enhance the biological activity of resveratrol, Colloids Surf. B Biointerfaces 144 (2016) 1–7.
[329] C.G. Kumar, Y. Poornachandra, S.K. Mamidyala, Green synthesis of bacterial gold nanoparticles conjugated to resveratrol as delivery vehicles, Colloids Surf. B Biointerfaces 123 (2014) 311–317.
[330] D. Vervandier-Fasseur, N. Latruffe, The potential use of resveratrol for cancer prevention, Molecules 24 (24) (2019).
[331] N. Ramesh, A.K.A. Mandal, Encapsulation of epigallocatechin-3-gallate into albumin nanoparticles improves pharmacokinetic and bioavailability in rat model, 3 Biotech 9 (6) (2019) 238.
[332] R. Zhou, et al., Extract from Astragalus membranaceus inhibit breast cancer cells proliferation via PI3K/AKT/mTOR signaling pathway, BMC Complement. Altern. Med. 18 (1) (2018) 83.
[333] L.Y. Luo, et al., Pharmacokinetics and bioavailability of the isoflavones formononetin and ononin and their in vitro absorption in using chamber and Caco-2 cell models, J. Agric. Food Chem. 66 (11) (2018) 2917–2924.
[334] Y.J. Moon, M.E. Morris, Pharmacokinetics and bioavailability of the bioflavonoid biochanin A: effects of quercetin and EGCG on biochanin A disposition in rats, Mol. Pharm. 4 (6) (2007) 865–872.
[335] J. Fang, Bioavailability of anthocyanins, Drug Metab. Rev. 46 (4) (2014) 508–520.
[336] M. Metzler, et al., Curcumin uptake and metabolism, Biofactors 39 (1) (2013) 14–20.
[337] A. Riaz, et al., Eriocalyxin B biological activity: a review on its mechanism of action, Nat. Prod. Commun. 14 (8) (2019), 1934578X19868598.
[338] H.W. Jiang, et al., The evaluation of antioxidant interactions among 4 common vegetables using isobolographic analysis, J. Food Sci. 80 (6) (2015) C1162–C1169.

[339] T. Efferth, E. Koch, Complex interactions between phytochemicals. The multi-target therapeutic concept of phytotherapy, Curr. Drug Targets 12 (1) (2011) 122–132.
[340] P.B. Patel, V.R. Thakkar, J.S. Patel, Cellular effect of curcumin and citral combination on breast cancer cells: induction of apoptosis and cell cycle arrest, J. Breast Cancer 18 (3) (2015) 225–234.
[341] K.M. Yusof, et al., Suppression of colorectal cancer cell growth by combined treatment of 6-gingerol and gamma-tocotrienol via alteration of multiple signalling pathways, J. Nat. Med. 73 (4) (2019) 745–760.
[342] A. Montgomery, et al., Curcumin sensitizes silymarin to exert synergistic anticancer activity in colon cancer cells, J. Cancer 7 (10) (2016) 1250–1257.
[343] X. Wang, L. Xu, Q. Wu, M. Liu, F. Tang, Y. Cai, W. Fan, H. Huang, X. Gu, Inhibition of LDHA deliver potential anticancer performance in renal cell carcinoma, Urol. Int. 99 (2) (2017) 237–244.
[344] J. Zhao, X. Huang, Z. Xu, J. Dai, H. He, Y. Zhu, H. Wang, LDHA promotes tumor metastasis by facilitating epithelialmesenchymal transition in renal cell carcinoma, Mol. Med. Rep. 16 (6) (2017) 8335–8344.

CHAPTER 9

Acid-base and electrolyte balance regulations with phytonutrients

Waqas Alam[a], Haroon Khan[a], and Imad Ahmad[a,b]
[a]Department of Pharmacy, Abdul Wali Khan University Mardan, Mardan, Pakistan
[b]Department of Pharmacy, Abasyn University Peshawar, Peshawar, Pakistan

1. Introduction

Homeostasis of electrolytes and acid-base is critical for the appropriate execution of various functions of the body and basal metabolic reactions. Different vital organs such as the liver and kidneys play a major role in the regulation and equilibrium of electrolytes and acid-base balance [1]. An adult produces daily about 0.8–1 mEq/kg body weight of nonvolatile acid (NVA) and 15,000 mEq of volatile acid (CO_2). A small percentage of CO_2 is absorbed as a weak acid (carbonic acid H_2CO_3) in the body fluids, probably depending on the partial pressure of carbon dioxide (pCO_2), whereas a significant proportion of CO_2 is removed by respiration. To avoid acute systemic pH disturbances, NVAs are balanced in the body. The main buffer mechanism that neutralizes NVA at the expense of bicarbonate (HCO_3^-) is the HCO_3^-/H_2CO_3 depot. In addition, plasma electrolytes, serum calcium, and proteins play a vital role in homeostasis [2]. In the routine discussion of physiology or biochemistry, sodium is regarded as the "king electrolyte" (being the most prominent electrolyte), while chloride as the 'queen of electrolytes.' Although the first electrolyte to be easily measured was chloride, its importance is sometime overshadowed by other major serum electrolytes [3].

There is a mutual relationship between nutrition, fluid, and electrolyte balance with the intake of natural or artificial food. In clinical practice, nutrients, water, minerals, and electrolyte balance are all involved in the treatment of diseases [4]. Since ancient times, natural herbs are being used as nutritional additives to enhance the taste of food as well as in conventional therapies. Currently, due to their wide range of therapeutic applications to convalesce the health-related problems, they are the subject of research, predominantly within the pharmaceutical industries as functional food ingredients [5]. It is a reality that fruits, vegetables, and a healthy balanced

The Role of Phytonutrients in Metabolic Disorders
https://doi.org/10.1016/B978-0-12-824356-5.00003-5

diet produce remarkable effects when medications and injections are unable to prevent illness. Over the decades, the remarkable efficacy of vegetables, fruits, and natural herbs in treating, not only common illnesses, but even life-threatening diseases such as kidney disorders and cancers have been reported by several famous naturopathic doctors and physicians [6].

Food is the fundamental requirement of human existence. Humans receive a certain amount of nutrients from the food they consume diurnally. Food provides all the necessary elements required for homeostasis. One of the important elements of these food substances are minerals. These minerals determine the fate of energetic biomacromolecules and so maintain healthy growth, development, and physical condition of humans [7]. Depending on the intake level, elements may be macrominerals and microminerals (trace elements) [8]. As per chemical properties, they can be classified further into metals (sodium, potassium, calcium, iron, etc.) and nonmetals (selenium, chloride, iodine, etc.). However, foods are not only the sources of essential elements, but toxic elements are also found. These toxicants have no positive role in humans' health and generate negative biochemistry. Toxicants from the metal class are called "heavy metals" (mercury, cadmium, lead, etc.) and metalloids (arsenic) [9,10].

Researchers have reported that natural herbs are a potent source of phytonutrients and are responsible for the wide range of pharmacological actions such as inflammation, cancers, infections, etc. Daily consumption of an optimal level of these phytonutrients is hence necessary to preserve ideal health [11]. This chapter is aimed to provide updated knowledge regarding the acid-base and electrolyte balance regulation with phytonutrients. To date, literature review and research findings have been utilized to summarize the idea. The main objective of this chapter is to showcase phytonutrients having the potential to maintain electrolyte balance. Some of the essential electrolytes, macrominerals (Na, K, Ca, Mg, etc.) are discussed having a known source from plant origin.

2. Acid-base balance regulations

The extent of alkalinity and acidity is an essential feature of blood. Whenever in the body, the quantity/concentration of acidic compounds increases due to more synthesis or less excretion from the body or if the levels of alkaline compounds decrease due to less synthesis or excessive excretion, this will cause increased acidity of the body and vice versa. The regulation of equilibrium in alkalinity and acidity is called acid-base balance. Acids are usually sour while bases are bitter in taste. The acid-base balance of the blood is carefully regulated in the body, since certain organs may be seriously damaged by just a slight variation in the normal pH range. Mostly three mechanisms are used by the body for regulating acid-base balance such as acid chemical buffers and excretion via the kidneys and the respiratory system.

Blood pH is regulated between 7.38 and 7.42; the pH of muscles is upheld to 7.0. The first and most important mechanism that controls blood pH is via buffer system. This mechanism is abruptly done and citrate or bicarbonate ions gain a proton and a neutral salt is formed. The second mechanism takes place in the respiratory system by the release of H^+ due to excessive respiratory gaseous exchange. In the respiratory gaseous exchanges, H^+ and HCO_3^- react and form CO_2 and H_2O and are excreted via exhalation. The acid-base regulation via the kidney is a long-term mechanism. Kidneys are unable to remove the acidic urine (pH 4.4) from the body and such acidic urine needs buffer systems to be excreted from the body. For the excretion of such type of acidic urine, NH_3 (ammonia) is used as a buffer which receives H^+ and eliminates in the form of the NH_4^+ ion (ammonium) [12].

2.1 Acid-base regulation through the kidneys

In normal physiology, the synthesis of acid in the body is balanced by the same amount of acid removed from the body via renal excretion. This acid-base regulation is achieved by the production and elimination of NH_3 as well as NH_4 ions, recovery of about 4500 mEq filtered bicarbonate ions, and tubular controlled titratable acids (urinary buffers). The proximal tubules reclaim roughly 80% of the filtered HCO_3^- back into the bloodstream. The remaining 16% are reabsorbed from the ascending loop of Henle and distal convoluted tubules whereas the leftover 4% is reabsorbed in the collecting duct. Intercalated cells in the collecting ducts play a key role in the transport of HCO_3^- and H^+ ions. The apical membrane possesses α-intercalated cells which bears proton ATPase and release acid. On the basolateral surface, bicarbonate and chloride antiporters excrete bicarbonate ions. Varying phenotypes of intercalated cells such as non-A and non-B cells do exist [13–15].

The primary titratable urinary acid is hydrogen phosphate (HPO_4^{2-}). HPO_4^{2-} is removed via urine in the form of $H_2PO_4^-$ along with salts. HCO_3^- is reabsorbed in compensation to each H^+ eliminated. Parathormone inhibits the reclamation of phosphate ions at proximal tubules resulting in the excessive secretion of H^+ ions [16]. In the proximal tubules, the metabolism of glutamine results in the synthesis of ammonia. Upon the metabolism of each glutamine molecule, two molecules of HCO_3^- and NH_4^+ are formed. Na^+/H^+ transporters in the proximal tubules exchange the NH_4^+ in compensation to H^+. In the loop of Henle, $Na^+/K^+/Cl^{2-}$ transporters substitute NH_4^+ reabsorption with K^+ release. Glycoproteins in the distal convoluted tubules are responsible for ammonia and ammonium ions' transportation. An equal mole of HCO_3^- is reabsorbed to compensate NH_4^+ release [17–19].

2.2 Effect of proteins on acid-base balance

Proteins are a vital component of bones and muscles, and extreme insufficiency of proteins triggers muscle loss. Researchers have found a strong correlation between protein ingestion and lean body weight. The loss of bones and muscles takes place with the passage of times. About 2 kg of bones and muscles are lost above 50 years of age in a decade [20,21]. Highly proteinaceous diets result in excessive acid load and elevated nitrogen levels in the body. This high acid load and elevated nitrogen levels signify muscle loss. Researchers have reported that diets rich in proteins are acidic in nature and cause metabolic acidosis, which leads to wastage of muscles. The metabolic acidosis induced by rich proteinaceous diets leads to high acid load in the kidneys.

The capacity of the kidneys to eliminate NH_4^+ is increased by rich proteinaceous diets to maintain acid-base equilibrium which in turn increases the excretion of renal nitrogen, released from muscle wastage. With growing age, the glomerular filtration rate decreases about 50%. Metabolic acidosis rises as the age increases. The serum level of H^+ elevates while the levels of PCO_2 and HCO_3^- decline due to respiratory acidosis. The ability of kidneys to eliminate acids from the body varies with age. The hydrogen ion level of serum is 6%–7% more while carbonate ion levels are 12%–16% less in older age (80 years) patients as compared to a young individual [22,23]. A balanced diet and nutraceuticals can treat the acid-base equilibrium. Age-associated metabolic acidosis can be managed through the intake of alkaline dietary material and preventing acidic diets [24]. Metabolic acidosis may cause kidney stones and muscle wastage. Elevated levels of $NaHCO_3$ (sodium bicarbonate) and $Na_3C_6H_5O_7$ (sodium citrate) in the blood have been reported to enhance athletes' performance. It has been reported that a 0.5 g/kg dose of $Na_3C_6H_5O_7$ and a 0.3 kg/g dose of sodium bicarbonate stimulates the release of H^+ ion from muscles and increases the working potential [25].

2.3 Effect of food on acid-base regulations

Diet may shift the value of pH and generate an increased acid load. With this acid load, the elimination of renal acid is increased, thus reducing plasma $NaHCO_3$ and rising acidic pH [26].

The acidic properties of dietary food depend upon various parameters. The absorption of salts via the gastrointestinal tract determines the pH values. During dietary absorption, 25% of the magnesium is absorbed from magnesium chloride while chloride is absorbed by approximately 90%. Thus, it is reported that diets rich in magnesium chloride will increase the chloride levels in the body. Pancreatic secretions composed of $NaHCO_3$ provide excessive Na^+ ions to the already available dietary chloride ions in the serum. Thus, sodium bicarbonate loss resulted in the acidic environment and plays vital role in acid-base regulation. Amino acids having sulfur in their structure are oxidized by $NaHCO_3$, thus generating H^+ and basic ions. Glutamine is formed in the blood by the reaction of $NaHCO_3$ and amino acids. This glutamine is further utilized by the kidneys for the synthesis of NH_3 that gain protons and eliminates in the form NH_4 [21,27]. Fig. 1 shows a brief overview of the electrolytes and acid-base controlling mechanisms.

3. Phytonutrients

A balanced diet plays an important part in keeping the human body functioning normally. With current developments in nutritional and medical sciences, both health-care practitioners and customers have given considerable consideration to natural products as nutritional foods. Biologically active nutraceutical and food supplements have been established as promising supplements in the cure and prophylaxis of various ailments. Nutraceuticals can be used by malnutrition patients as a complement, during pregnancy, and losing weight, to promote better health, during ailments, to postpone the emergence of age-related disorders, to recover athletic performance, for depression and to cure symptoms such as in arthritis, cold, cough, fever and flu, etc. [28,29].

Phytonutrients is a supplementary modern concept referring to a therapeutic science that uses a variety of natural products to be used as nutritional supplements and treated as foods containing several herbs along with their derivatives [30]. Phytonutrients are naturally derived and are effective in clinical therapy because of their lesser adverse effects relative to radiotherapy and chemotherapy and are effective in minimizing the cost of health

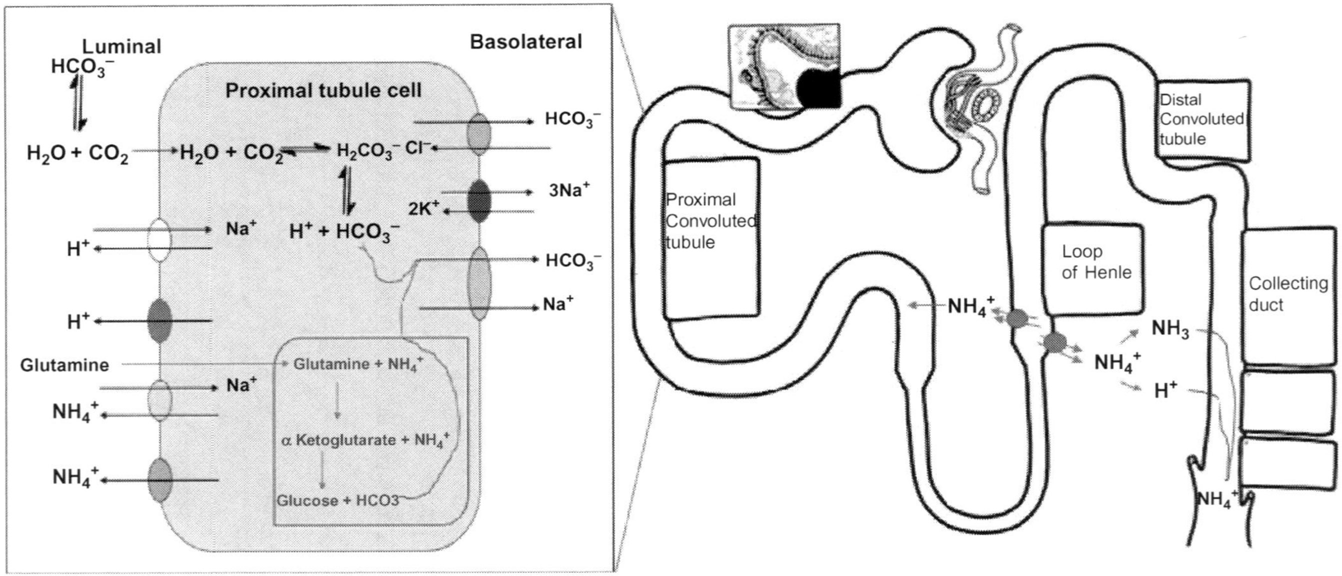

Fig. 1 A glimpse of acid-base and electrolytes movement in the urinary tubules. Sodium, potassium, bicarbonate, ammonium, and chloride ion transporters are visible. The proximal tubule generates ammonia, and relatively little ammonia is derived from glomerular filtration under basal conditions. This occurs via the metabolism of glutamine primarily, along with the generation of $NH4^+$ and HCO_3^- from each metabolized glutamine.

care [31]. The nutritional therapeutic applications of phytonutrients have been scientifically evidenced by different researchers from their mechanism of actions, clinical uses and efficacy, quality control, and biological properties [32]. Phytonutrients are found to be effective antibacterial, antiallergic, antifungal, antispasmodic, antioxidants, antiinflammatory, antihypertensive agents, neuroprotective agents, CNS stimulants, hepatoprotective, diuretic, hypolipidemic, carminative, analgesic, immuno-modulator, chemopreventive, and clinically safe in the treatment of osteoporosis, diabetes, and cardiac disorders [33–35].

Polyphenols, carotenoids, terpenoids, ascorbates, lipoic acids, and tocopherols are among the significant phytonutrients and are effective natural antioxidants having radical scavenging activity. They have reduced risk of neurodegenerative disorders. The nonsteroidal phytonutrients include phytoestrogens which have same functions as gonadal hormones. Phytoestrogens propose a surrogate treatment option for hormone replacement therapy, which has an advantageous impact on the cardiac system and can also mitigate the symptoms of menopause. The major group of phytonutrients found in foods and seeds are terpenoids, which provide a remedy against certain disorders, particularly those associated with severe disruption and deregulation of growth. Limonoids possess significant anticancer effect. Phytosterols are effective in the excretion of cholesterol. Glucosinolates activate liver microsomal enzymes which provides protection against cancer and mutagenesis [28,36].

Expertise in food science, clinical trials and nutrition offers a greater understanding of the biological features and applications of nutraceutics and their possible side effects. This knowledge and understanding contributes to the standardization of product development, clinical services, and significantly contributes to the nutraceuticals industry [37,38]. Phytonutrients and their pharmacological and nutraceutical actions are summarized in Table 1 [39–42].

4. Regulation of acid-base and electrolyte balance with phytonutrients

The nutritional and dietary demands of humans are obtained from naturals sources since ancient times. Research findings revealed that health deficiencies can considerably be reduced by dietary changes. Dietary foods regulate the acid-base and electrolyte balance due to the presence of different types of phytochemical constituents. Different elements are present in the food

Table 1 Summary of the therapeutic applications and origins of phytonutrients.

Phytonutrients	Therapeutic applications	Plant origin
Flavonoids	Antiviral, antiproliferative, antioxidant, antiinflammatory, antibacterial, analgesic, oxidative enzymes inhibitor	Grapes, vegetables, legumes, berries, peanuts, onion, olive oil, tea, cocoa, apple, walnuts
Polyphenols	Antiinflammatory, antidiabetic, antiallergic, Antioxidant, antineurodegenerative, antiplatelet, anticarcinogenic, cytoprotective, antiviral	Wheat, cereals, rice, flaxseed, sorghum, vegetables, beans, corn, olive seeds, barley, canola, pulses, oats, fruit juices, coffee, wine, cocoa
Carotene	Corneal protective effect, anticarcinogenic, stimulating DNA enzymes and increase the release of IL-1 and TNF-α	Pumpkin, oranges, carrots, leafy green vegetables
Limonoids	Insecticidal, antifungal, anticancer, antimalarial, antiviral and antibacterial	Citrus fruits
Terpenoids	Antiallergic, antifungal, antiinflammatory, antiviral, antimicrobial, antihyperglycemic, antispasmodic and antiparasitic	Vegetables, fruits, and cereals
ω-3-fatty acids	Hypolipidemics, fights wrinkles, antihypertensive, Osteoarthritis, decrease risk of heart attacks and skin disorders	Rainbow trout, herring, salmon fish, canola, soybean and flax oils
Anthocyanins	Antiinflammatory, antioxidants, and antiallergic	Cherry, raspberry, red grapes, orange, and blackberry
Resveratrol	Anticancer, antidiabetic, antioxidant	Peanuts, Grapes, red wine and Blueberry
Phytoestrogens	Osteoporosis, menopausal disorders, anticancer, and heart disorders	Barley, oats, soybeans, alfalfa, corn, and wheat
Isoflavonoids	Anticancer, antioxidant, and prevent osteoporosis	Family leguminosae and fabaceae members
Phytosterol (Stigmasterol)	Antihyperlipidemics, prevent osteoporosis and anticancer	Soybean
Quercetin	Vasodilator, antioxidant, anticoagulant, decreases LDL	Wheat, Grapes, apple pulp, green tea and onion
Glucosinolates	Prevent prostate and breast cancers, antioxidant and reduces damage to DNA	Cabbage, radish, cauliflower, broccoli, vegetables, and turnip

originating from plants. There is a large amount of scientific literature available on the use of these nutrients in relation with type of food substance, serum concentration, average dietary intake, their importance for medical perspective, food services, etc. [43–46]. The information on the role of phytonutrients in electrolyte imbalance is scattered in the literature. Here we are trying to funnel the phytonutrients to recommend some of the important sources. The medicinal and herbal sources of phytonutrients contributing to acid-base and electrolyte regulation have been summarized in Fig. 2.

4.1 Polyphenols (*Punica granatum*)

The regulation of plasma electrolytes by the natural polyphenols of pomegranate were reported by Achraf and his coresearchers. They established that pomegranate juice has significantly regulated the serum electrolyte levels of Na^+, K^+, Ca^{2+}, and Cl^- in intense resistant training sessions. They observed that after vigorous exercise the plasma electrolytes level was higher as compared to preexercise plasma electrolyte levels but does not induce hypernatremia [47]. To maintain normal functions of muscle contractions, it is mandatory to regulate the electrolyte balance [48]. It has been observed that during vigorous exercise the Na^+/K^+ transporters

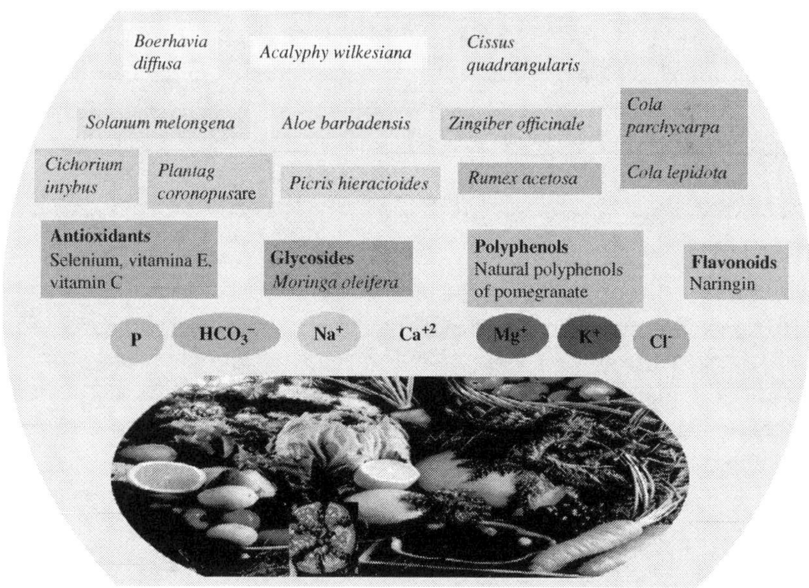

Fig. 2 Summary of the sources of phytonutrients contributing to electrolyte and acid-base balance.

across cell membranes activate the regulation of plasma electrolyte balance. The lactic acidosis formed during exercise stimulates the release of chloride ions, which is helpful in maintaining the excitability of muscles. Long term and aggressive exercise induce powerful muscle contractions due to electrolyte imbalance and thus cause muscle wastage and exhaustion [48–51].

Moreover, it has also been reported earlier that polyphenols isolated from pomegranate have inhibitory action on the Na^+/K^+ transport system of different organs (kidneys, brain, and cardiac muscles) [52,53]. Soluble polyphenols have been isolated from pomegranate and they have been proved to have lipid lowering and cardio-protective action [54,55]. Many other phytonutrients such as ellagitannin and anthocyanin have been reported to have antioxidant and free radical scavenging activity [56]. It has been confirmed that pomegranate juice has markedly regulated the electrolyte level in the body after vigorous exercise; however, the exact mechanism to regulate acid-base balance still needs to be evaluated.

4.2 Flavonoids (Naringin)

Alfred and his coresearchers reported that flavonoids like naringin improved the serum electrolytes and acid-base balance in diabetic ketoacidosis rats. They performed the study on type 1 diabetic rats induced by streptozotocin (STZ). They found that STZ completely damaged the β-cells of pancreas and ketoacidosis was induced in the rats leading to hyperglycemia. The hyperglycemia resulted in dehydration due to elevated osmolality. The elevated osmolality activated the osmoreceptors of the hypothalamus as a compensatory mechanism and enhanced the release of ADH hormone which, in turn, regulated the water electrolyte balance. Due to the failing of this compensatory mechanism the thirst center is activated which leads to excessive water intake (polydipsia and polyuria) [57]. Alfred and his coresearchers found that naringin significantly treated the polydipsia and thus recovered the electrolyte balance. In the diabetic rats, excessive synthesis and accumulation of ketone bodies were noticed with elevated ketogenesis, which are organic anions and upon dissociation produce H^+ ions. This H^+ ion has buffering capability and reacts with serum HCO_3^- and results in metabolic ketoacidosis. Alfred et al., found that naringin markedly regulated the blood pH and serum HCO_3^- level and thus scientifically provided a background to the acid-base regulation by naringin [58].

4.3 Antioxidants (selenium, vitamin E, and vitamin C)

The impact of selenium, vitamin E, and vitamin C were investigated for acid-base regulation in goats under heat stress conditions. The goats 1.5 years of age were grouped into three groups (control, antioxidant, and heat stress). Except for the control group, the remaining groups had been subjected for 21 days in a psychrometric compartment at a temperature of $40 \pm 2°C$ (humidity of 30%) for 5 h per day. Blood specimens had been taken to check the antioxidant effect of serum vitamin E and C. On every third day, blood specimens were collected for the estimation of acid-base balance. Respiratory rate and temperature were checked on a regular basis. They observed that the respiratory rate, temperature, partial pressure of oxygen and pH of the heat stress animals were elevated. The researchers reported that the acid-base balance of the antioxidant group was quite improved [59].

4.4 Glycosides (*Moringa oleifera*)

The electrolyte regulating effect of *M. oleifera* (*M. oleifera*) was reported earlier by Omolaso and his coresearchers. They established that the extract of *M. oleifera* had markedly reduced the serum electrolyte levels (Na^+, K^+, and Cl^-). It is established that *M. oleifera* has a remarkable variety of medicinal applications and has high nutrient content. In folkloric medicine, almost each section of this plant such as flowers, leaves, bark, roots, seeds, and fruits is being used for the management of various diseases [60,61]. The leaves of *M. oleifera* have been reported to have an antihypertensive effect and anticancer activity, and analgesic, antiinflammatory, antianemic, and antiulcer activities. The roots and flowers of *M. oleifera* possess diuretic activity and are used in the management of night blindness. The whole plant extract of *M. oleifera* lowers the elevated blood sugar level and is thus reported to have antidiabetic activity. The extract of *M. oleifera* has been reported to have glycosides, flavonoids, kaempferol, β-sitosterol, and quercetin [60,62–64].

Omolaso and his collaborators evaluated the electrolyte regulating effect of *M. oleifera* in humans. They administered 5 g of *M. oleifera* extract into each individual and calculated the serum electrolyte levels before and after dosing and reported that the extract of *M. oleifera* has markedly reduced the elevated serum electrolyte level. They assumed that the electrolyte regulating effect of *M. oleifera* was due to the presence of glycosides in *M. oleifera* as previously many researchers have reported that the glycosides of *M. oleifera* markedly lowered the elevated blood pressure by altering the serum electrolyte level [65,66]. However, still further detailed studies must be carried out to confirm the exact mechanism of acid-base and electrolyte regulation.

4.5 Saponins (*Solanum xanthocarpum*)

Solanum xanthocarpum (S. xanthocarpum), previously known as *Solanum surattense*, possesses the regulating potential of serum electrolytes and acid-base balance. Researchers established that *S. xanthocarpum* (methanolic extract) significantly regulated the serum electrolyte level by reducing the excessive plasma Ca^{2+}, Mg^{+}, K^{+}, Na^{+}, and blood urea nitrogen as well as excreting through urine the surplus Ca^{2+} and urinary electrolytes. Furthermore, they also evaluated that *S. xanthocarpum* regulates urinary pH by maintaining the bodily excretion of HCO_3^- ions [67]. *S. xanthocarpum* is conventionally used for the management of variety of disorders such as asthma, inflammation, and diuresis. Patel and his coresearchers also investigated that the methanolic extract of the fruits of *S. xanthocarpum* has a protective role in kidney stones and regulates the level of uric acid, oxalic acid, calcium, and magnesium [68–70].

Folkloric use of *S. xanthocarpum* is reported in the management of gonorrhea [71,72]. Researchers have also reported that *S. xanthocarpum* has a strong antioxidant potential in curing urinary tract infection and has antibacterial effect verses *Pseudomonas aeruginosa* [73–75]. Studies have shown that the seed extract of *S. xanthocarpum* possesses potent antitussive and antiasthmatic activities and has pronounced use as an expectorant while the leaf extract is used as an analgesic [69,70]. Scientific studies have reported the presence of alkaloidal glycosides and established the cardio-protective, wound healing and antidiabetic effect of the fruit extracts of *S. xanthocarpum* [71,76,77]. The phytochemical investigations showed that the fruits of *S. xanthocarpum* comprise of coumarins such as aesculin and aesculetin, β-sitosterol, solasurine, solamargine, solasonine, khasianine, aculeatiside A, torvoside K, solamargine, torvoside L, and caffeic acid [78–80].

The investigations of Ahmed and his co researcher established that the methanolic extract of *S. xanthocarpum* has prominent serum electrolytes and an acid-base regulating effect in a dose-dependent manner. They found that the *S. xanthocarpum* extract decreased the serum Na^{+}, Ca^{2+}, and K^{+} levels by enhancing their renal excretion from the body and elevated the plasma $NaHCO_3$ level. The phytochemicals accountable for the acid-base regulation and serum electrolytes balance are not yet scientifically recognized. The phytochemical screening of the *S. xanthocarpum* extract has shown the presence of different phytochemical groups such as saponins, terpenes, alkaloids, sterols, and phenols. Moreover, earlier studies have proved that tannins and saponins have a prominent role in electrolyte and acid-base regulation and have diuretic activity [81–83]. Therefore, it was suggested by Ahmed et al., that the acid-base and electrolyte regulation by *S. xanthocarpum* might be due to the presence of saponins. However, still further explication needs to be carried out to locate the phytonutrients involved in acid-base and electrolyte regulation and their precise mechanistic pathways.

4.6 Aqueous extract of *Ipomoea batatas*

I. batatas regulates the acid-base and electrolyte balance in diabetic patients. Research studies have shown that *I. batatas* (400 mg/kg aqueous extract) has regulated the serum levels of electrolytes such as Na^+, HCO_3^-, Ca^{2+}, K^+, PO_4^{3-}, and Cl^- in diabetic patients [84]. It has been reported that diabetic patients are often prone to electrolyte (Na^+, HCO_3^-, Mg^{2+}, Ca^{2+}, K^+, PO_4^{3-}, and Cl^-) disturbances as a result of ketoacidosis and hyper- or hypo-osmolar syndromes. In clinical practice, serum electrolytes and acid-base disturbances are common in diabetic patients [85,86]. The phytochemical analysis of *I. batatas* (both acetone and aqueous extract) has shown the existence of various phytonutrients such as terpenes, carbohydrates, flavonoids, balsam, resins, phenols, saponins, steroids, vitamin C, iron, calcium, phosphorus, tannins, vitamin A, dicaffeoylquinic, and caffeoylquinic acid derivatives [84,87–89]. *I. batatas* is traditionally used for the management of different disorders. *I. batatas* has antiinflammatory, antioxidant, antiulcer, antiproliferative, hepatoprotective, wound healing, antimicrobial, hypoglycemic, and cardio-protective activities [88].

Rafiu and his coresearchers observed that electrolytes and acid-base balance was disturbed in streptozotocin-induced diabetic patients. They administered the aqueous extract of *I. batatas* at a dose of 400 mg/kg and after investigating the plasma electrolyte level (Na^+, HCO_3^-, Mg^{2+}, Ca^{2+}, K^+, PO_4^{3-}, and Cl^-). They reported that the *I. batatas* extract has markedly increased the plasma electrolyte level. However, the phytochemical involved in the acid-base and electrolyte regulation was not identified yet. But it was assumed that the acid-base regulating effect must be due to the presence of phytochemicals available in *I. batatas*. Therefore, a detailed assay must be performed to unravel the acid-base and electrolyte activity of the phytonutrients present in *I. batatas* [84,90].

4.7 Medicinal plants as acid-base and electrolyte regulators

Aloe barbadensis (Asphodelaceae) contains sodium and potassium in the range of 5280 and 10,670 ppm, respectively. This shows the tendency of *A. barbadensis* to regulate or control the osmotic balance of the body fluids as well as the body pH. *A. barbadensis* is also rich in phosphorus 6657 ppm, which is the mainstay of bone formation. Magnesium is present as 325.8 ppm, which tends to lower the blood pressure. Other minerals such as calcium, zinc, manganese, copper, chromium, and iron are also the constituents of *A. barbadensis*. This makes *A. barbadensis* one of useful electrolyte replenishers [91]. The levels of calcium and potassium are higher in the round variety of *Solanum melongena* (Solanaceae) than in the oval variety. However, higher levels of phosphorus, magnesium, and sodium were found in the oval variety than in the round one [92]. The aqueous leaf extract of *Acalyphy wilkesiana* (Euphorbiacaece) contains sodium (2530 mg/L), potassium (390 mg/L), chloride (3550 mg/L), calcium (30.8855 mg/L), and magnesium (5.4068 mg/L) in moderate quantities [93].

The fresh *Zingiber officinale* (Zingiberanceae) rhizome was subjected to elemental analysis. The quantitative mineral analysis revealed the presence of different electrolytes: Na (38.96 μg/g), K (36.34 μg/g), Ca (34.55 μg/g), and P (26.70 μg/g) [94]. The pulverized dried roots of *Cissus quadrangularis* (Vitaceae), which is an edible Nigerian vegetable, constitute a rich source of mineral elements. The mg/100 g dry matter of the vegetable revealed approximately potassium 67.5, calcium 39.5, sodium 22.5, and magnesium 1.15. This promotes the use of *C. quadrangularis* in terms of its nutritive value and the public health implication of having it as part of their diet [95].

Macromineral content is also found in the two varieties of monkey kola, i.e., *Cola parchycarpa* (Sterculiaceae) and *Cola lepidota* (Sterculiaceae). The dried pulp extract is loaded with abundant minerals. Calcium content is significantly higher in *C. parchycarpa* (195–199 mg/100 g) than in *C. lepidota* (39–62 mg/100 g). The phosphorus content of *C. lepidota* is 34–58 mg/100 g while *C. parchycarpa* has 32–36 mg/100 g. *C. lepidota* had higher sodium content 61–62 mg/100 g) and potassium (204–209 mg/100 g) than *C. parchycarpa* (36–37 mg for sodium and 60–74 mg/100 g for potassium) [96].

The quantitative estimation of mineral composition of *Boerhavia diffusa* (Nyctaginaceae) revealed the presence sodium, potassium, magnesium, and calcium.The mineral contents in mg/100 g are, sodium 82.5 ± 2.5, potassium 61.35 ± 0.85, calcium 76.25 ± 0.65, and magnesium 145.9 ± 0.5 [97]. The various electrolytes present in medicinal plants which are responsible for acid-base and electrolyte regulations are summarized in Table 2.

Table 2 The quantities of different electrolytes in medicinal plants.

Medicinal plants	Electrolytes	Quantity
Aloe barbadensis	Sodium	5280 ppm
	Potassium	10,670 ppm
	Phosphorus	6657 ppm
	Magnesium	325.8 ppm
Acalyphy wilkesiana	Sodium	2530 mg/L
	Potassium	390 mg/L
	Chloride	3550 mg/L
	Calcium	30.8855 mg/L
	Magnesium	5.4068 mg/L
Zingiber officinale	Sodium	38.96 μg/g
	Potassium	36.34 μg/g
	Calcium	34.55 μg/g
	Phosphorus	26.70 μg/g
Cissus quadrangularis	Potassium	67.5 mg/100 g
	Calcium	39.5 mg/100 g
	Sodium	22.5 mg/100 g
	Magnesium	1.15 mg/100 g
Cola parchycarpa	Calcium	195–199 mg/100 g
	phosphorus	32–36 mg/100 g.
	Sodium	36–37 mg/100 g
	Potassium	60–74 mg/100 g
Cola lepidota	*Calcium*	39–62 mg/100 g
	Phosphorous	34–58 mg/100 g
	Sodium	61–62 mg/100 g
	Potassium	204–209 mg/100 g
Boerhavia diffusa	Sodium	82.5 ± 2.5 mg/100 g
	Potassium	61.35 ± 0.85 mg/100 g
	Calcium	76.25 ± 0.65 mg/100 g
	Magnesium	145.9 ± 0.5 mg/100 g

4.8 Wild herbs as acid-base and electrolyte regulators

Wild herbs are used as edibles commonly since ancient times. They improve the intake and annihilation of daily human minerals supply. Wild edible species such as *Rumex acetosa, Picris hieracioides, Cichorium intybus, and Plantago coronopus* are rich sources of minerals and consumed in various parts of the world. *R. acetosa* (Polygonaceae) contains Na 0.60 ± 0.04, K 3.35 ± 0.10, Ca 0.64 ± 0.02, and Mg 0.21 ± 0.01 mg/g (mean ± SD). *P. hieracioides* (Asteraceae) possesses Na 0.95 ± 0.04, K 6.02 ± 0.06, Ca 4.73 ± 0.65, and Mg 0.08 ± 0.05. Similarly, *C. intybus* (Asteraceae) contains Na 1.59 ± 0.25, K 4.05 ± 0.24, Ca 1.32 ± 0.10, and Mg 0.10 ± 0.01. *P. coronopus* (Plantaginaceae) has Na

Table 3 Different electrolytes and their quantities in wild herbs.

Wild herbs	Electrolytes	Quantities (mean ± SD)
Rumex acetosa	Na	0.60 ± 0.04 mg/g
	K	3.35 ± 0.10 mg/g
	Ca	0.64 ± 0.02 mg/g
	Mg	0.21 ± 0.01 mg/g
Picris hieracioides	Na	0.95 ± 0.04 mg/g
	K	6.02 ± 0.06 mg/g
	Ca	4.73 ± 0.65 mg/g
	Mg	0.08 ± 0.05 mg/g
Cichorium intybus	Na	1.59 ± 0.25 mg/g
	K	4.05 ± 0.24 mg/g
	Ca	1.32 ± 0.10 mg/g
	Mg	0.10 ± 0.01 mg/g
Plantago coronopus	Na	1.27 ± 0.26 mg/g
	K	2.46 ± 0.27 mg/g
	Ca	1.23 ± 0.11 mg/g
	Mg	0.08 ± 0.05 mg/g
Cynara scolymus	K	506.3 ± 1.5 mg/100 g
	P	414.0 ± 1.2 mg/100 g
	Ca	386.9 ± 13.0 mg/100 g
	Mg	220.7 ± 0.2 mg/100 g
	Na	194.4 ± 4.4 mg/100 g

content 1.27 ± 0.26, K 2.46 ± 0.27, Ca 1.23 ± 0.11, and Mg 0.08 ± 0.05. *Cynara scolymus* L. (Asteraceae) is the green globe cultivar of artichoke which is a herbaceous plant. The leaf extract possesses selected macroelements (K, Ca, P, Mg, and Na). *C. scolymus* contains K content of 506.3 ± 1.5 mg + SD, P 414.0 ± 1.2, Ca 386.9 ± 13.0, Mg 220.7 ± 0.2, and Na 194.4 ± 4.4 per 100 g of dry matter [98]. Table 3 presents the electrolyte composition and their quantities, which have acid-base and electrolyte regulating effects.

5. Conclusions

Electrolytes and acid-base are the key agents in the homeostasis of body systems and normal functioning of organs. To date, literature review was done to gather comprehensive knowledge about the acid-base and electrolyte regulation with phytonutrients. It was concluded from the detailed review that phytonutrients are necessary for the regulations of electrolytes and acid-base balance. It has been established that different phytonutrients such as polyphenols, glycosides, flavonoids, saponins, and some plant resources have contributed to the regulation of acid-base and electrolyte balance. Up till now, there is no literature available as such to confirm the precise mechanism of action of acid-base and electrolyte regulation by phytonutrients. Therefore, further elucidative research is strongly recommended to confirm the underlying mechanism and provide scientific background for the use of phytonutrients as acid-base and electrolyte regulators.

References

[1] T. Dhondup, Q. Qian, Acid-base and electrolyte disorders in patients with and without chronic kidney disease: an update, Kidney Dis. (Basel) 3 (4) (2017) 136–148.
[2] I. Kurtz, et al., Effect of diet on plasma acid-base composition in normal humans, Kidney Int. 24 (5) (1983) 670–680.
[3] K. Berend, L.H. van Hulsteijn, R.O. Gans, Chloride: the queen of electrolytes? Eur. J. Intern. Med. 23 (3) (2012) 203–211.
[4] D.N. Lobo, Fluid, electrolytes and nutrition: physiological and clinical aspects, Proc. Nutr. Soc. 63 (3) (2004) 453–466.
[5] M. Vranješ, et al., Effects of bearberry, parsley and corn silk extracts on diuresis, electrolytes composition, antioxidant capacity and histopathological features in mice kidneys, J. Funct. Foods 21 (2016) 272–282.
[6] M. Gautam, V. Gupta, The nutritive and health benefits of fresh raw fruits VS fruit juices, Int. J. Home Sci. 3 (2) (2017) 616–619.
[7] J. Barbaresko, et al., Dietary pattern analysis and biomarkers of low-grade inflammation: a systematic literature review, Nutr. Rev. 71 (8) (2013) 511–527.
[8] A.G. Godswill, et al., Health benefits of micronutrients (vitamins and minerals) and their Associated Deficiency Diseases: a systematic review, Int. J. Food Sci. 3 (1) (2020) 1–32.
[9] M. Edelstein, M. Ben-Hur, Heavy metals and metalloids: sources, risks and strategies to reduce their accumulation in horticultural crops, Sci. Hortic. 234 (2018) 431–444.
[10] K.H. Vardhan, P.S. Kumar, R.C. Panda, A review on heavy metal pollution, toxicity and remedial measures: current trends and future perspectives, J. Mol. Liq. 290 (2019) 111197.
[11] R.L. Prior, G. Cao, Antioxidant phytochemicals in fruits and vegetables: diet and health implications, HortScience 35 (4) (2000) 588–592.
[12] L.R. McNaughton, J. Siegler, A. Midgley, Ergogenic effects of sodium bicarbonate, Curr. Sports Med. Rep. 7 (4) (2008) 230–236.
[13] X. Gao, et al., Deletion of hensin/DMBT1 blocks conversion of β-to α-intercalated cells and induces distal renal tubular acidosis, Proc. Natl. Acad. Sci. 107 (50) (2010) 21872–21877.
[14] Y.-H. Kim, et al., Immunocytochemical localization of pendrin in intercalated cell subtypes in rat and mouse kidney, Am. J. Physiol. Renal Physiol. 283 (4) (2002) F744–F754.
[15] S.M. Wall, Y. Lazo-Fernandez, The role of pendrin in renal physiology, Annu. Rev. Physiol. 77 (2015) 363–378.
[16] J. Lemann Jr., D.A. Bushinsky, L.L. Hamm, Bone buffering of acid and base in humans, Am. J. Physiol. Renal Physiol. 285 (5) (2003) F811–F832.
[17] K.-H. Han, et al., Expression of the ammonia transporter family member, Rh B glycoprotein, in the human kidney, Am. J. Physiol. Renal Physiol. 304 (7) (2013) F972–F981.
[18] I.D. Weiner, J.W. Verlander, Ammonia transporters and their role in acid-base balance, Physiol. Rev. 97 (2) (2017) 465–494.

[19] A.-M. Marini, et al., The human Rhesus-associated RhAG protein and a kidney homologue promote ammonium transport in yeast, Nat. Genet. 26 (3) (2000) 341–344.
[20] L. Ceglia, et al., Potassium bicarbonate attenuates the urinary nitrogen excretion that accompanies an increase in dietary protein and may promote calcium absorption, J. Clin. Endocrinol. Metab. 94 (2) (2009) 645–653.
[21] B. Dawson-Hughes, S.S. Harris, L. Ceglia, Alkaline diets favor lean tissue mass in older adults, Am. J. Clin. Nutr. 87 (3) (2008) 662–665.
[22] L. Frassetto, A. Sebastian, Age and systemic acid-base equilibrium: analysis of published data, J. Gerontol. Ser. A Biol. Med. Sci. 51 (1) (1996) B91–B99.
[23] F. Manz, et al., Effects of a high protein intake on renal acid excretion in bodybuilders, Z. Ernahrungswiss. 34 (1) (1995) 10–15.
[24] T. Remer, ACID-BASE IN RENAL FAILURE: influence of diet on acid-base balance, in: Seminars in Dialysis, Wiley Online Library, 2000.
[25] B. Requena, et al., Sodium bicarbonate and sodium citrate: ergogenic aids? J. Strength Cond. Res. 19 (1) (2005) 213–224.
[26] L. Frassetto, R.C. Morris Jr., A. Sebastian, Potassium bicarbonate reduces urinary nitrogen excretion in postmenopausal women, J. Clin. Endocrinol. Metabol. 82 (1) (1997) 254–259.
[27] T. Remer, Influence of nutrition on acid-base balance-metabolic aspects, Eur. J. Nutr. 40 (5) (2001) 214–220.
[28] C. Gupta, D. Prakash, Phytonutrients as therapeutic agents, J. Complement. Integr. Med. 11 (3) (2014) 151–169.
[29] C. Gupta, D. Prakash, S. Gupta, Relationships between bioactive food components and their health benefits, in: Introduction to Functional Food Science Textbook, first ed., Create Space Independent Publishing Platform, USA, 2013, pp. 66–85.
[30] D. Bagchi, Nutraceutical and Functional Food Regulations in the United States and Around the world, Elsevier, 2014.
[31] C. Ramaa, et al., Nutraceuticals-an emerging era in the treatment and prevention of cardiovascular diseases, Curr. Pharm. Biotechnol. 7 (1) (2006) 15–23.
[32] V. Brower, Nutraceuticals: poised for a healthy slice of the healthcare market? Nat. Biotechnol. 16 (8) (1998) 728–731.
[33] D. Prakash, C. Gupta, Role of phytoestrogens asnutraceuticals in human health-a review, Biotechnology 5 (2011) 1–8.
[34] D. Prakash, K. Gupta, The antioxidant phytochemicals of nutraceutical importance, Open Nutraceuticals J. **2** (1) (2009).
[35] D. Prakash, C. Gupta, G. Sharma, Importance of phytochemicals in nutraceuticals, J. Chin. Med. Res. 1 (3) (2012) 70–78.
[36] M.M. Whitman, Understanding the perceived need for complementary and alternative nutraceuticals: lifestyle issues, Clin. J. Oncol. Nurs. **5** (5) (2001).
[37] E. Cieślik, A. Gręda, W. Adamus, Contents of polyphenols in fruit and vegetables, Food Chem. 94 (1) (2006) 135–142.
[38] M. Gidley, Naturally functional foods—challenges and opportunities, Asia Pac. J. Clin. Nutr. 13 (2004).
[39] N.J. Miller, M.B. Ruiz-Larrea, Flavonoids and other plant phenols in the diet: their significance as antioxidants, J. Nutr. Environ. Med. 12 (1) (2002) 39–51.
[40] A. Scalbert, et al., Dietary polyphenols and the prevention of diseases, Crit. Rev. Food Sci. Nutr. 45 (4) (2005) 287–306.
[41] V. Katalinic, et al., Screening of 70 medicinal plant extracts for antioxidant capacity and total phenols, Food Chem. 94 (4) (2006) 550–557.
[42] C.J. Dillard, J.B. German, Phytochemicals: nutraceuticals and human health, J. Sci. Food Agric. 80 (12) (2000) 1744–1756.

[43] W. Koch, et al., Dietary intake of metals by the young adult population of Eastern Poland: results from a market basket study, J. Trace Elem. Med. Biol. 35 (2016) 36–42.
[44] H.-S. Lee, et al., Dietary exposure of the Korean population to arsenic, cadmium, lead and mercury, J. Food Compos. Anal. 19 (2006) S31–S37.
[45] E. Babaali, et al., Dietary intakes of zinc, copper, magnesium, calcium, phosphorus, and sodium by the general adult population aged 20–50 years in shiraz, Iran: a total diet study approach, Nutrients 12 (11) (2020) 3370.
[46] T. Filippini, et al., Dietary estimated intake of trace elements: risk assessment in an Italian Population, Expos. Health (2019) 1–15.
[47] A. Ammar, et al., Effects of natural polyphenol-rich pomegranate juice supplementation on plasma ion and lipid profiles following resistance exercise: a placebo-controlled trial, Nutr. Metab. 17 (2020) 1–12.
[48] T. Clausen, Role of Na+, K+-pumps and transmembrane Na+, K+-distribution in muscle function: the FEPS Lecture-Bratislava 2007, Acta Physiol. 192 (3) (2008) 339–349.
[49] D.G. Allen, G.D. Lamb, H. Westerblad, Impaired calcium release during fatigue, J. Appl. Physiol. 104 (1) (2008) 296–305.
[50] R. McKelvie, et al., Renal responses to exercise-induced lactic acidosis, Am. J. Physiol. Regul. Integr. Comp. Physiol. 257 (1) (1989) R102–R108.
[51] M.J. McKenna, J. Bangsbo, J.-M. Renaud, Muscle K+, Na+, and Cl− disturbances and Na+-K+ pump inactivation: implications for fatigue, J. Appl. Physiol. 104 (1) (2008) 288–295.
[52] A. Ammar, et al., Effects of pomegranate supplementation on exercise performance and post-exercise recovery in healthy adults: a systematic review, Br. J. Nutr. 120 (11) (2018) 1201–1216.
[53] A.A. Boldyrev, E.R. Bulygina, Na/K-ATPase and oxidative stress, Ann. N.Y. Acad. Sci. 834 (1) (1997) 666–668.
[54] M.-T. García-Conesa, et al., Meta-analysis of the effects of foods and derived products containing ellagitannins and anthocyanins on cardiometabolic biomarkers: analysis of factors influencing variability of the individual responses, Int. J. Mol. Sci. 19 (3) (2018) 694.
[55] G. Sohrab, et al., Effects of pomegranate juice consumption on blood pressure and lipid profile in patients with type 2 diabetes: a single-blind randomized clinical trial, Clin. Nutr. ESPEN 29 (2019) 30–35.
[56] M. Aviram, et al., Pomegranate juice flavonoids inhibit low-density lipoprotein oxidation and cardiovascular diseases: studies in atherosclerotic mice and in humans, Drugs Exp. Clin. Res. 28 (2–3) (2002) 49–62.
[57] S. Arai, N. Stotts, K. Puntillo, Thirst in critically ill patients: from physiology to sensation, Am. J. Crit. Care 22 (4) (2013) 328–335.
[58] A.N. Murunga, et al., Grapefruit derived flavonoid naringin improves ketoacidosis and lipid peroxidation in type 1 diabetes rat model, PLoS One 11 (4) (2016), e0153241.
[59] A. Sivakumar, G. Singh, V. Varshney, Antioxidants supplementation on acid base balance during heat stress in goats, Asian Australas. J. Anim. Sci. 23 (11) (2010) 1462–1468.
[60] S.S. Adinoyi, O. Oluwagbamila, A. Ademola, Role of Moringa oleifera on electrolytes levels and cardiovascular function in human, Ther. Adv. Cardiol. 1 (2017) 80–86.
[61] F. Anwar, et al., Moringa oleifera: a food plant with multiple medicinal uses, Phytother. Res. 21 (1) (2007) 17–25.
[62] B. Umar, Integrating Conservation Agriculture with trees: trends and possibilities among Smallholder Zambian farmers, in: 5 th World Congress on Conservation Agriculture, 2011.
[63] P. Chumark, et al., The in vitro and ex vivo antioxidant properties, hypolipidaemic and antiatherosclerotic activities of water extract of Moringa oleifera Lam. leaves, J. Ethnopharmacol. 116 (3) (2008) 439–446.
[64] R. Pullakhandam, M.L. Failla, Micellarization and intestinal cell uptake of β-carotene and lutein from drumstick (Moringa oleifera) leaves, J. Med. Food 10 (2) (2007) 252–257.

[65] A.H. Gilani, et al., Pharmacological studies on hypotensive and spasmolytic activities of pure compounds from Moringa oleifera, Phytother. Res. 8 (2) (1994) 87–91.
[66] S. Faizi, et al., Novel hypotensive agents, niazimin A, niazimin B, niazicin A and niazicin B from Moringa oleifera: Isolation of first naturally occurring carbamates, J. Chem. Soc., Perkin Trans. 1 (20) (1994) 3035–3040.
[67] M.M. Ahmed, et al., Diuretic and serum electrolyte regulation potential of aqueous methanolic extract of Solanum surattense fruit validates its folkloric use in dysuria, BMC Complement. Altern. Med. 16 (1) (2016) 1–8.
[68] P. Patel, et al., Antiurolithiatic effects of Solanum xanthocarpum fruit extract on ethylene-glycol-induced nephrolithiasis in rats, J. Young Pharm. 4 (3) (2012) 164–170.
[69] G.P. Vadnere, R.S. Gaud, A.K. Singhai, Evaluation of anti-asthmatic property of Solanum xanthocarpum flower extracts, Pharmacology 1 (2008) 513–522.
[70] S. Emmanuel, et al., Antiinflammatory activity of Solanum trilobatum, Fitoterapia 77 (7–8) (2006) 611–612.
[71] S. Parmar, A. Gangwal, N. Sheth, Solanum xanthocarpum (yellow berried night shade): a review, Pharm. Lett. 2 (4) (2010) 373–383.
[72] A. Ghani, Medicinal Plants of Bangladesh: Chemical Constituents and Uses, Asiatic Society of Bangladesh, 1998.
[73] R. Mittal, et al., Urinary tract infections caused by Pseudomonas aeruginosa: a minireview, J. Infect. Public Health 2 (3) (2009) 101–111.
[74] R. Priyadarsini, et al., Antioxidant potential of the leaves and roots of Solanum surattense, Plant Archives 10 (2) (2010) 815–818.
[75] M. Ghani, M. Farooq, M. Khan, Phytochemical investigations and evaluation of antibacterial and irritant potential of different extracts of whole plant of Solanum xanthocarpum Schrad and Wendl, J. Chin. Chem. Soc. 57 (2010) 1257–1262.
[76] B. Siddiqui, S. Siddiqui, S. Faizi, Studies in the chemical constituents of the fresh berries of Solanum xanthocarpum Schrad. And Wendle, J. Chem. Soc. Pak. **5** (4) (2011) 99.
[77] D. Kar, et al., Studies on hypoglycaemic activity of Solanum xanthocarpum Schrad. & Wendl. fruit extract in rats, J. Ethnopharmacol. 108 (2) (2006) 251–256.
[78] Y. Iida, et al., Three unusual 22-β-O-23-hydroxy-(5α)-spirostanol glycosides from the fruits of Solanum torvum, Chem. Pharm. Bull. 53 (9) (2005) 1122–1125.
[79] M. Weissenberg, Isolation of solasodine and other steroidal alkaloids and sapogenins by direct hydrolysis-extraction of Solanum plants or glycosides therefrom, Phytochemistry 58 (3) (2001) 501–508.
[80] A. Gawande, et al., Isolation, purification and characterization of solasodine-A steroidal alkaloid from Solanum surattense berries, Indian Drugs 28 (3) (1990) 149–150.
[81] W. Saka, et al., Changes in serum electrolytes, urea, and creatinine in Aloe vera-treated rats, J. Young Pharm. 4 (2) (2012) 78–81.
[82] S. Shahiladevi, G. Jayanthi, M. Jegadeesan, Preliminary phytochemical studies on Solanum surattense burm. F. seeds, Anc. Sci. Life 26 (1–2) (2006) 59.
[83] D. Martin-Herrera, et al., Diuretic activity of some Withania aristata Ait. fractions, J. Ethnopharmacol. 117 (3) (2008) 496–499.
[84] A.A. Rafiu, C. Luka, Evaluation of the antidiabetic property of aqueous extract of Ipomoea batatas leaf on hyperglycemia, hyperlipidemia, blood electrolytes, and enzymatic antioxidants of streptozotocin-induced diabetic rats, J. Res. Diabetes Metab. 4 (1) (2018) 022–026.
[85] G. Liamis, H.J. Milionis, M. Elisaf, A review of drug-induced hypocalcemia, J. Bone Miner. Metab. 27 (6) (2009) 635–642.
[86] N. Sotirakopoulos, et al., Acid-base and electrolyte disorders in patients with diabetes mellitus, Saudi J. Kidney Dis. Transpl. 23 (1) (2012) 58.
[87] G.E. Anekwe, Concise Biochemistry, University Press, 2005.

[88] V. Panda, M. Sonkamble, Phytochemical constituents and pharmacological activities of Ipomoea batatas l.(Lam)–a review, Int. J. Res. Phytochem. Pharmacol. 2 (1) (2012) 25–34.

[89] I. Konczak, et al., Caffeoylquinic acids generated in vitro in a high-anthocyanin-accumulating sweet potato cell line, J. Biomed. Biotechnol. 2004 (5) (2004) 287.

[90] I.P. Ekpe, D. Amaechi, C.E. Obeleagu, Protective effect of Solanum melongena (garden egg), Solanum lycopersicum (tomatoes), Daucus carota subsp. sativus (carrot) extracts on some electrolytes and renal biomarkers of lead induced toxicity in albino wistar rats, World J. Adv. Res. Rev. 8 (3) (2020) 386–391.

[91] A. Adesuyi, et al., Nutritional and phytochemical screening of Aloe barbadensis, Curr. Res. J. Biol. Sci. 4 (1) (2012) 4–9.

[92] B. Agoreyo, E. Obansa, E. Obanor, Comparative nutritional and phytochemical analyses of two varieties of Solanum melongena, Sci. World J. 7 (1) (2012) 5–8.

[93] H. Madziga, S. Sanni, U. Sandabe, Phytochemical and elemental analysis of Acalypha wilkesiana leaf, J. Am. Sci. 6 (11) (2010) 510–514.

[94] I. Ogbuewu, et al., Evaluation of phytochemical and nutritional composition of ginger rhizome powder, Int. J. Agric. Rural. Dev. 17 (1) (2014) 1663–1670.

[95] O. Enechi, I. Odonwodo, An assessment of the phytochemical and nutrient composition of the pulverized root of Cissus quadrangularis, Bio-Research 1 (1) (2003) 63–68.

[96] H.N. Ene-Obong, H.O. Okudu, U.V. Asumugha, Nutrient and phytochemical composition of two varieties of monkey kola (Cola parchycarpa and Cola lepidota): an underutilised fruit, Food Chem. 193 (2016) 154–159.

[97] J. Jayachitra, et al., Phytochemical analysis and mineral composition of Methanolic extract of Boerhavia diffusa L, Res. J. Pharm. Technol. 13 (10) (2020) 4856–4860.

[98] C. Ceccanti, et al., Evaluation of major minerals and trace elements in wild and domesticated edible herbs traditionally used in the mediterranean area, Biol. Trace Elem. Res. (2020) 1–9.

CHAPTER 10

Therapeutic role of nutraceuticals in mitochondrial disorders

Shabnoor Iqbal[a], Muhammad Ajmal Shah[b], Azhar Rasul[a], Shahid Shah[c], Ghulam Mujtaba Shah[b,d], Muhammad Irfan[j], Uzma Saleem[e], Ifat Alsharif[f], Reem Hasaballah Alhasani[g], Norah A. Althobaiti[h], Shafiq Ur Rahman[i], and Abdul Haleem Khan[k]

[a]Department of Zoology, Faculty of Life Sciences, Government College University, Faisalabad, Pakistan
[b]Department of Pharmacy, Hazara University, Mansehra, Pakistan
[c]Department of Pharmacy Practice, Faculty of Pharmaceutical Sciences, Government College University, Faisalabad, Pakistan
[d]Department of Botany, Hazara University, Mansehra, Pakistan
[e]Department of Pharmacology, Faculty of Pharmaceutical Sciences, Government College University, Faisalabad, Pakistan
[f]Department of Biology, Jamoum University College, Umm Al-Qura University, Makkah, Saudi Arabia
[g]Department of Biology, Faculty of Applied Science, Umm Al-Qura University, Makkah, Saudi Arabia
[h]Department of Biology, College of Science and Humanities, Shaqra University, Al-Quwaiiyah, Saudi Arabia
[i]Department of Pharmacy, Shaheed Benazir Bhutto University, Sheringal, Dir Upper, Pakistan
[j]Department of Pharmaceutics, Government College University, Faisalabad, Pakistan
[k]Department of Pharmacy, Forman Christian College (A Chartered University), Lahore, Pakistan

1. Introduction

The heterogeneous category of disorders caused by defective mitochondrial function owing to change in mitochondrial DNA is referred to as primary mitochondrial disorder [1–3]. The most prevalent inborn errors of metabolism are primary mitochondrial disorders that occur in approximately 1 in 5000 individuals [1,4]. The detection, care, and prevention of these diseases are generally complex and costly [4].

Electron transport chain dysfunction decreases the production of ATP, raises anaerobic metabolism and cerebrospinal fluid, and increases the output of free radicals that induce cellular dysfunction and oxidative stress in the central nervous, spinal nerves, endocrine organs, ears, eyes, skeletal and heart muscles, liver, and the gastrointestinal tract. Multisystem or organ-specific diseases are usually found in patients [5,6]. The clinical characteristics of the primary mitochondrial disorder are distinct [6,7]. Seizures, stroke-like events, encephalopathy, diabetes, ophthalmoplegia, and auditory deficits are the main neurological disorders. Myopathy, ataxia, and peripheral neuropathy are peripheral neurological characteristics [6].

The Role of Phytonutrients in Metabolic Disorders
https://doi.org/10.1016/B978-0-12-824356-5.00013-8

The mitochondrial disorder is brought about by the inheritance of a nuclear or mitochondrial DNA mutation in the mitochondrial gene expression [8]. For any mitochondrial disorder, there is no clear, comprehensive mechanism and no such appropriate therapy was established yet. Although mitochondria's most famous physiological function is the source of adenosine triphosphate (ATP), mitochondria also play an important role in the generation and defense of reactive oxygen species (ROS), Ca^{2+} handling, nucleotide metabolism, urea cycle, and apoptosis. Several mitochondrial diseases including Friedrich's ataxia (FA), Leigh's syndrome (LS), Leber inherited optic neuropathy (LHON), mitochondrial encephalomyopathy, lactic acidosis, stroke-like episodes (MELAS), and ragged-red fiber myoclonic epilepsy (MERRF) have neurological defects or neurodegeneration [8,9].

Some dietary supplements can be of benefit in the treatment of mitochondrial disorders because they help improve the development of mitochondrial ATP as nutrients and metabolic cofactors, bypass cellular deficiencies of complexes I, II, or III [10,11].

Few randomized controlled trials have evaluated the protective effects of dietary supplements on mitochondrial disorders. The experiments suggested that few dietary supplement ingredients helped to ameliorate mitochondrial disorders in patients after individual or combination doses [6]. In comparison, most of the promising data reported regarding dietary supplementation for the treatment of mitochondrial disorders was depicted from experiments whose design may not prove [6,12,13].

Vitamins, minerals, and amino acids are categorized as nutraceuticals, as well as over 1000 other probiotic compounds were described as nutraceuticals. Indians, Chinese, and Egyptians used nutraceuticals to prevent ailments since ancient times [14]. Nutraceuticals are functional foods with enormous health effects. Accumulative studies have suggested that nutraceuticals can be used to treat numerous mitochondrial disorders [15]. Phytochemicals that are isolated from conventional drugs and their therapeutic effects to reduce pathologies are the focus of the current studies related to nutraceuticals [16]. A recent study depicted the protective role of nutraceuticals to improve neurological diseases. Throughout ancient times, medicinal plants were used all over the world to extract for therapeutic purposes to cure different diseases [17,18].

Even though data from randomized controlled trials are available to justify the usage of one or more dietary supplements for the treatment of mitochondrial disorders, nutraceuticals may be difficult to include in drugs for medical care. The explanations for this involve the complexity of the research designs, the route of dosing and experiment period tested, and variations in the clinical and biochemical criteria evaluated [5]. The research for clinical trials is difficult by using nutrients like CoQ10 in the patients with mitochondrial disorders. Sometimes patients hesitate to undergo trials that might transfer them to a placebo category and stop them from utilizing the supplements that they think will threaten the health status [19].

Clinical research on animals and humans is necessary for manufacturing medication and the findings collected to validate the therapeutic efficacy of the drug [20,21]. While no authorized techniques were used in the past to approve the medicinal effects of nutritional foods, nutraceuticals provide many benefits, including the increased value of a balanced diet and a longer life [22,23].

Our chapter aims to increase the readers' understanding of the utilization of nutraceuticals to treat mitochondrial and psychotic disorders. The current review highlights the possible role of nutraceuticals in neurological conditions and brain health.

2. Mitochondrial disorders

It is a result of insufficient mitochondria, failure to provide required substrates to mitochondria, or a deficiency of how mitochondria generate ATP. The functional state of mitochondria in a cell may be changed by boosting up undamaged components of cells to mitigate overall mitochondrial dysfunction. These events are mitigated by complex cellular processes such as depolarization of the mitochondrial membrane [24–26].

The capacity of cells to generate nearly all high-energy molecules is closely linked to the ability of mitochondria to transform energy from metabolites to the electron transport chain and then ultimately to oxygen. This mechanism produces an electrochemical gradient ($\Delta\psi m$) and transmembrane proton gradient (Δp) over the inner membrane of mitochondrial [27–29].

The reactive oxygen species (ROS) that are the by-product of electron transport chain are formed due to the oxidative phosphorylation. The mitochondria are key reservoirs of ROS and nitrogen species, which may damage cellular lipids, proteins, and DNA. The electron transport mechanism creates uncoupled proteins resulting in the release of protons through the proton gradient of the inner mitochondrial membrane into the mitochondrial matrix. This leakage of proton results in decreased ATP production [27,28,30,31].

The surplus oxygen intake and ROS production may lead to damage to mitochondrial membrane lipids especially tROS/RNS-sensitive cardiolipin that is a phospholipid of the membrane. The cardiolipin and other membrane phospholipids damage in the inner mitochondrial membrane may increase the level of proton and ion leakage into the mitochondrial matrix and reduce the electrochemical gradient. Cardiolipin is a key part of the electron transport chain, which stabilizes the cytochrome complexes [30,32–34].

The antioxidant helps to decrease the ROS/RNS levels that are regulated by protecting the cells from oxidative damage. Cellular antioxidants are endogenous and key antioxidants including superoxide dismutase, catalase, and glutathione peroxidase. Certain dietary antioxidants with a low molecular weight were used to transfer the excess concentrations of oxidative molecules to physiological levels that can be sustained by endogenous antioxidant systems [35–40] (Fig. 1).

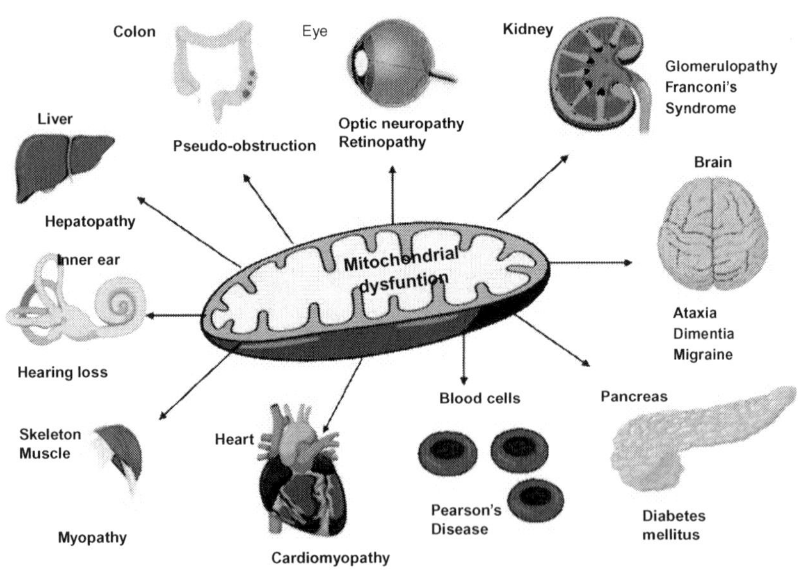

Fig. 1 Mitochondrial dysfunction are induced by various mitochondrial disorders.

3. Therapeutic nutraceuticals

3.1 Nutraceuticals

Nutraceuticals are included in various biological therapies that are used for the treatment of diseases related to mitochondrial disorders.

4. Traditional nutraceuticals

Nutraceuticals are directly derived from natural products like fruits, fish, eggs, nuts, beef, vegetables, and dairy products in their original constituents that provide dietary supplements [41].

4.1 Nutrients

The principal metabolites of compounds such as minerals, fatty acids, vitamins, and amino acids possess well-established nutritional properties. The nutrients help to improve neurological conditions owing to their antioxidant effects. The nutrient also aids to reduce fragile bones, raise hemoglobin, and increase muscle strength and synaptic transmission. Fatty acids and their metabolites assist to enhance neuron function and reduce cholesterol in the arteries to exert hypolipidemic effects [42].

4.2 Plant products

The combination of nutrients and herbs has protective effects on various illnesses such as mental health [43]. Plants that contain tannins like lavender help to reduce oxidative stress and lower blood pressure. The antioxidant properties of plant products help to reduce the risk of cardiovascular diseases, diabetes, and renal defects. Flavonoids have been scientifically proved to produce phytochemicals such as psoralen that exert carminative and diuretic effects. Terpenoid-containing chemicals like peppermint and menthol are used to improve respiratory distress. The studies found that *Aloe vera* has an antiinflammatory effect. Ephedra has bronchodilator and vasoconstriction effects and is used to treat bronchospasms [17]. Garlic and ginger are used as food additives and possess antiinflammatory effects. Garlic and ginger are also used to control blood pressure and enhance immunity [44,45]. The vegetables contain carotenoids that improve immunity, primarily killer cells, and have anticarcinogenic properties [46]. Noncarotenoid diets like chickpeas and soybeans assist to reduce cholesterol. The curcumin is derived from turmeric and possess antioxidant activity and antiinflammatory effects owing to the phenolic acids [47].

5. Plant-based nutraceuticals

5.1 Flavonoids and isoflavones

A large variety of flavonoids with varying chemical structures are linked to distinct antiinflammatory activities [48]. The most common flavones are apigenin and luteolin glycosides. Parsley, rosemary, and celery are all good sources of flavones [49]. Apigenin inhibits the synthesis of nitric oxide and prostaglandins by blocking inducible nitric oxide synthase (iNOS) and COX-2, respectively [50]. Luteolin was also shown to reduce chronic inflammation through coculture of adipocytes and macrophages as well as JNK phosphorylation in macrophages [51]. Quercetin the most researched flavonols is abundant in a variety of vegetables and fruits. Apple flavonoids have enormous antiinflammatory effects. Quercetin and its glycosides are most effective antiinflammatory drugs in sarcoidosis, arthritis, and allergic airway inflammation patients [52,53].

Flavonoids and flavones of citrus block a variety of pro-inflammatory mediators, including those produced from the arachidonic acid cascade [54]. Citrus flavanones (e.g., naringenin) exerted antiinflammatory effects in an animal model of arthritis by modulating p38 signaling cascades and STAT-1 [55,56].

Isoflavones such as glycitein, genistein, and daidzein are exclusively found in leguminous plants. Genistein was shown to reduce inflammation by downregulating the activation of NFk-B, TNF-α, IL-6, endothelin-1, and vascular cell adhesion molecule-1 expression [57]. Flavanols also exist in plants as monomers as well as oligomers or polymers. Flavan-3-ols are found in dietary plants such as *Camellia sinensis* and *Theobroma cacao*, which inhibit eicosanoid production, reduce platelet activation, and modulate proinflammatory cytokine production [58]. Anthocyanins have antiinflammatory properties, which are mediated via the mitogen-activated protein kinase pathway [59]. Mechanistic investigations showed that delphinidin, petunidin, malvidin, cyanidin, and peonidin glycosides inhibit IL-1-activation in vitro [60].

Diterpenes from *Stevia rebaudiana* leaves, which are utilized as natural sweeteners in the food industry, inhibit the production of proinflammatory cytokines [61]. Glycyrrhizin and glycyrrhetinic acid are licorice root triterpenes that have protective effect against gastritis and blood pressure owing to mineralocorticoid effects [62].

5.2 Hydroxycinnamic acid

Hydroxycinnamic acids such as p-coumaric acid, ferulic acid, sinapic acid, and caffeic acid are another class of dietary antioxidants. Hydroxycinnamic acids were shown to reduce oxidation and prevent coronary heart disease as well as atherosclerosis [63]. In a study involving human LDL as the oxidizing substrate Hydroxycinnamic acids have shown higher antioxidant activity than hydroxybenzoic acids [64].

5.3 Mulberry leaves

Mulberry is an important and its leaves have numerous cost-effective therapeutic utilizations in traditional medicine [65]; these medicinal benefits are mostly attributed to the phenolic content of the leaves, which has good antioxidant qualities [66,67]. Mulberry leaf extract scavenges free radicals such as nitric oxide and superoxide. Furthermore, lipid peroxidation reduced in erythrocyte membranes when treated with mulberry extracts. The polyphenolic components in mulberry exerted antioxidant properties in vitro as well as in vivo that helped to improve oxidative status markers in serum. Mulberry modulated underlying gene expression such as upregulation of Nrf2 and its downstream antioxidant protein as well as reduction of ROS modulator protein [68].

Regardless, it was concluded that phytochemicals of varying types and amounts exert variable "strength" in the animal body that may enhance antioxidant capacity without any damage. Furthermore, phytochemicals may be used as supplementary materials and should be included in animal diets [69].

5.4 Carotenoids

Carotenoids are one of the most common lipid-soluble phytonutrients. In addition to Xanthophyll (lutein, zeaxanthin), the most prevalent of them is carotines (beta-carotene, lycopene). As lipid peroxidation occurs, peroxyl radicals are formed. Carotenoids are known to scavenge these peroxyl radicals. Because of this protection against cell membrane disruption and damage to cellular lipids, peroxyl radical scavenging is an important strategy. Due to their peroxyl radical scavenging action, carotenoids are known to play a crucial role in protecting cellular membranes and lipoproteins from ROS [70]. Lycopene, a naturally occurring antioxidant found in many fruits and vegetables, is the most powerful antioxidant. When there are several conjugated double bonds, singlet oxygen may be quenched by lycopene. Compared to -tocopherol and -carotene, lycopene has the highest singlet oxygen quenching capacity [71]. Carotenoid -carotene is a naturally occurring orange pigment present in a wide variety of fruits and vegetables. -Carotene, like lycopene, is well known for its ability to quench singlet oxygen more effectively than -tocopherol. Another antioxidant, -carotene-15,150-dioxygenase, may split -carotene into two molecules of vitamin A [72].

5.5 Resveratrol

Resveratrol is a phytoalexin produced by a wide range of plants such as *Veratrum grandiflorum*, berry skins, and grapevines in response to stress [73,74]. According to research into resveratrol, the "French paradox," which indicates better cardiovascular effects despite a high-fat diet in French people [75–77]. Red wine contains a significant amount of resveratrol. A lot of interest in the scientific community is being focused on potential health advantages of resveratrol. Resveratrol is a polyphenolic antioxidant that belongs to the stilbene family. Resveratrol is induced in grapevine in response to pathogens attacking the precursor molecules of malonyl-coenzyme A (CoA), p-coumaroyl CoA and the enzyme stilbene synthase [78]. Resveratrol may also be present in grapes, blueberry, cranberry, and bilberry. Resveratrol was found in plum fruit, raising its natural wealth profile, especially in dietary sources [73,79]. A multitude of research suggest that dietary resveratrol supplementation had beneficial benefits on aging and numerous other age-related chronic disorders, including Alzheimer's disease and diabetes [80]. Furthermore, resveratrol was shown to increase longevity in *Saccharomyces cerevisiae* by up to 70%. Because of its antiaging qualities, resveratrol has been the topic of much research over the last two decades as a radical scavenger, a chelating agent, and having antiinflammatory properties [81].

6. Fruit- and vegetable-based nutraceuticals

6.1 Curcumin

Curcumin is the major compound found in turmeric and helps to reduce oxidative stress and modulate Nrf2 pathway to enhance antioxidant levels [82,83]. Curcumin was found to increase ARE and Nrf2 binding and activate the expression of Nrf2 as well as mRNA expression of various antioxidant elements in the liver and lung of the mice [84]. Curcumin may improve antioxidant status in chickens who fed turmeric by elevating the gene expression of SOD [85]. Ahmadi observed that supplementation of broiler diet with turmeric powder increased CAT and SOD activities. Several studies have found that curcumin disrupts the Nrf2/Keap1 complex [86–88]. Sahin et al. observed that curcumin upregulated the expression of

Nrf2 and HO-1 in heat-stressed quail [89]. The decreased MDA level could further demonstrate the positive antioxidant effects on transcription. The curcumin-induced HO-1 expression was linked to the activation of Nrf2 transcription factor [84].

6.2 Quercetin

Fruits including apples, grapes, blueberries, blackcurrants, cherries, and raspberries are high in quercetin, a polyphenolic substance found in abundance in nature [90,91]. The flavonoids and flavonols are the most potent ROS scavengers [92]. Flavonoids in H_2O_2-treated human myelogenous leukemia cells were tested for their free radical scavenging abilities [93]. The results of the experiments show that apigenin, quercetin, and luteolin provide the best protection against hydrogen peroxide-induced damage in leukemia cells. Quercetin scavenging capacity is due to two antioxidant pharmacophores within molecules with the optimal structure for free radical scavengers. Quercetin and its derivative (quercetin caprylate) regenerated human fibroblast cells and increased their viability by upregulating the proteasome [94]. As a powerful antioxidant, quercetin has a wide range of protective effects on health and medicine [95]. In addition, it may have antiinflammatory and anticancer effects. To reduce the formation of inflammatory compounds including prostaglandins and leukocytes, quercetin inhibits the production of inflammatory enzymes such as cyclooxygenase (COX) and lipoxygenase (LOX). The antiinflammatory and antioxidant properties of quercetin help to slow down the aging process by reducing inflammation and oxidative stress that are thought to be major factors in the onset of old age [75].

6.3 Tannins

Tannins have key role in distinct protective characteristics of fruits and their by-products [96]. Proanthocyanidins, which are both ellagic acid and esters of gallic acid, are included in this group. Variations in the color and tartness of the fruit are due to tannins [97]. Ellagitannins and glucosides make up about 51% of the total phenolic components as free and complex forms. Cranberries, raspberries, blackberries, strawberries, and grapes may provide health advantages owing to ellagic acid and its derivatives. The antiinflammatory, antiproliferative, and antioxidant effects of ellagic acid were observed against esophageal, pulmonary, and colon cancers [98,99]. Free ellagic acid is a minor component of the total ellagic acid in raspberries, and acid hydrolysis helps to release ellagitannin contents [100,101].

6.4 Anthocyanins

Anthocyanins are naturally occurring pigments belong to polyphenolic group [102]. Anthocyanins are present in strawberries, blackcurrants, cranberries, chokeberries, bilberries, raspberries, and blackberries [103,104]. Anthocyanins make up colorful water-soluble pigments that give different color to the fruit [3]. Anthocyanins are used as natural pigments in the food industry. About 600 anthocyanins naturally occurring have been reported [105,106]. Anthocyanins also have enormous antioxidant capacity [107]. The molecular structure of anthocyanin exerts antioxidant activity. The antioxidant capacity is owing to free hydroxyl levels around the pyrone ring [108]. Anthocyanins were shown to lower free radical generation, lower risk of several age-related disorders, and enhance memory [109]. Anthocyanins are present in the outer layer of pericarp. The most abundant anthocyanin is cyanidin-3-glucoside along with aglycones and their glycosides [110].

Anthocyanins differ in terms of the amount of hydroxyl groups. The antioxidant capacity also depend on the degree of methylation, the location, quantity of sugar molecules, aliphatic acids, and aromatic groups coupled to sugars. Anthocyanins are found in berries in various glycoside forms, such as mono-, di-, or tri- [111]. The most common sugars are sophorose, rutinose, sambubiose, galactose, arabinose, rhamnose, and glucose [112]. Anthocyanin glycoside residues are acylated through caffeic acid, ferulic, p-coumaric, malonic acid, p-hydroxybenzoic acid, and acetic [110,113].

Anthocyanins have antitumor, antiinflammatory, antioxidant, antidiabetic, anticancer, and neuroprotective effects [58]. The chemopreventive impact of anthocyanin-rich black currant skin extract was observed against diethyl nitrosamine-initiated hepatocarcinogenesis in rats [114]. The researchers observed a dose-dependent reduction in 3-nitrotyrosine, iNOS expression, and lipid peroxidation. The black currant skin extract activated the gene expression of a number of antioxidant enzymes. This therapy dramatically increased Nrf2, mRNA, and protein expression, which indicates the activation of the Nrf2-regulated antioxidant pathway which leads to the upregulation of several antioxidant genes. Furthermore, the antiinflammatory effects of anthocyanin are due to their antioxidant properties, which result in the downregulation of the redox-sensitive nuclear factor-B signaling pathway [115].

6.5 Catechin

Catechin is a polyphenolic antioxidant found in a variety of fruits such as black grapes, blueberries, strawberries, gooseberries apples, and cherries. The name catechin refers to the flavonoid class and the flavan-3-ols/flavanols subclass. Gallocatechin, epicatechin (EC), epicatechin 3-gallate (ECG), epigallocatechin 3-gallate (EGCG), and epigallocatechin (EGCG) are the most significant dietary catechins. Catechins are abundantly present in strawberries in amounts ranging from 2 to 50 mg/100 g [116]. Cherries have 5–22 mg/100 g catechins, whereas apples have 10–43 mg/100 g catechins [116]. Catechins are abundant in the peel of fruits and differ from flavonoids containing ketones, such as rutin and quercetin, which support the antioxidant defense system. Catechin of cranberries and green tea are effective for cancer prevention [100]. Catechin's antioxidant activity is beneficial in the treatment of cancer, neurological disorders, and cardiovascular diseases [117]. Epigallocatechin gallate (EGCG) inhibits an enzyme called telomerase that unlock the proliferative ability of cancer cells by repairing damaged chromosomes [118]. It is possible that another cause for catechin's anticancer action exists. Catechin's antioxidant activity was shown to reduce coronary heart disease by decreasing cytotoxicity in lung fibroblast cells [119]. Catechins also exhibit antiinflammatory properties in bowel disease in humans by influencing oxidative stress-related cell signaling pathways such as signal transducer and activator of transcription 1/3, Nrf2, mitogen-activated protein kinase, and NFk-B [120]. In an ovalbumin-induced allergic rhinitis mouse model, Pan et al. investigated the antiinflammatory effects of catechins. Catechin suppressed the production of thymic stromal lymphopoietin in epithelial cells through modulating the NF-B/TSLP pathway. It significantly reduced inflammation in allergic rhinitis. Catechins also protect neurons from degeneration by reducing oxidative stress, scavenging ROS, and boosting antioxidant enzymes [119,121].

7. Nutraceutical biocatalyst

Biocatalysts are proteins and synthesized in cells. They induce quicker metabolic processes and are primarily effective in gastrointestinal tract-related medical conditions such as gastroesophageal reflux disease, diarrhea, constipation, etc. Nutraceutical biocatalysts are easily available in supermarkets and have been shown to benefit a variety of ailments, including diabetes and cancer [44,45,122].

7.1 Probiotics

They particularly help to enhance gastric and intestinal functions. Probiotics are exerted antibiotic effect that may help to protect the gut from poisonous flora. A balanced diet results in a healthy body and brain. The stomach conditions can be enhanced by the consumption of probiotics. Probiotics are usually used as capsules and drinks to make them consumable. Therefore, modern-day probiotics are effective for various ailments such as diarrhea and neurological disorders like depression and Alzheimer's. As the literature published on the protective effect of probiotics is not sufficient it needs to be further explored. Probiotics as a therapeutic agent were able to reduce the high risk of infection in patients with weakened immune systems [123,124] (Fig. 2).

8. Nontraditional nutraceuticals

The nontraditional nutraceuticals include foods derived from agricultural products and nutrients like vitamins, calcium-fortified orange juice, and minerals in cereals. Scientists have successfully introduced new techniques that may help to improve the nutritional contents of crops [125].

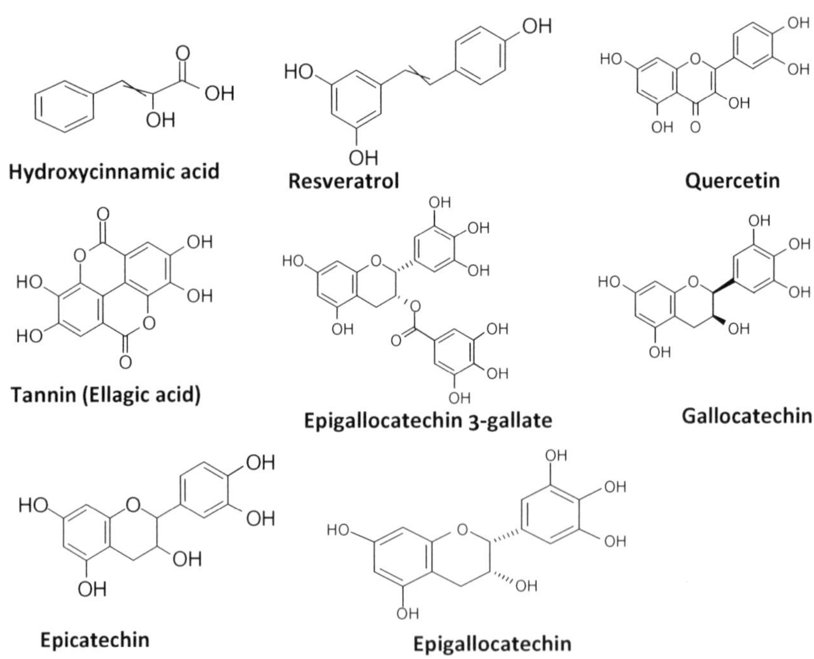

Fig. 2 Chemical structures of traditional nutraceuticals.

8.1 Recombinant nutraceuticals

Recombinant nutraceuticals are the nutraceuticals that were prepared via the use of biotechnology in food products. These nutraceuticals are among the groups that are most widely used and the extraction of nutrients from some food products, such as dairy products, cheese, and bread, to extract enzymes that are therapeutically effective when used at optimal levels [17]. Nontraditional nutraceuticals help to improve the nutrients in food products. Recombinant nutraceuticals have many benefits and some drawbacks. Regulations by the Food and Drug Administration (FDA) are now missing in the processing of nutraceuticals. Several industries synthesize low-quality nontraditional nutraceuticals to achieve larger profits and margins. Besides, the bioavailability of improved nutrients is not tracked and, in various situations, is usually low. The research of nutraceuticals is not as regulated as pharmaceuticals, with no regulations specifically indicated [126].

8.2 Alpha-lipoic acid

Alpha-lipoic acid (ALA) is naturally found in mitochondria. ALA works as cofactor for the activation of enzymes for ATP production. Dihydrolipoic acid may act as a free radical scavenger and help in the regeneration of other antioxidants such as vitamin E, vitamin C, and glutathione [127]. The body requires a sufficient amount of vitamin A that functions as an antioxidant [127,128].

ALA is produced in mitochondria endogenously. A certain quantity of this compound is present in foods like beef, liver, citrus, and vegetables, and is available as a dietary aid. Dietary supplements may contain either natural R-ALA or refined S-ALA. ALA in the range of 500–600 mg is typically utilized as oral supplements. Only 20%–40% of the oral dose of R-ALA is ingested [129].

ALA supplementation helps to decrease oxidative stress and increase mitochondrial efficacy. Many studies have reported the beneficial effects of palmitoleic acid supplementation. A case study was published in 1995 in which a patient was supplemented three times daily with 200 mg of ALA. After 7 months of supplementation, the ALA has improved the mitochondrial disorders. Supplementation can also promote higher mitochondrial function by exercise. Improved muscle activity and diminished pain after ingestion was observed in patients. Mitochondrial Medicine Society (MMS) has suggested that patients with PMDs should be instructed to take alpha-lipoic acid supplements in the absence of managed clinical trials to assess their efficacy as monotherapy in these patients. The standard dose of 50–200 mg/day is suggested [130,131]. There were no safety issues in the small clinical analysis of ALA. Taking 600 mg of $n-6$ PUFA daily for 6 months to 4 years was considered safe to treat patients with diabetic polyneuropathy. More analysis needs to be undertaken to assess the protective effect after ALA oral supplementation in PMD patients [132–135].

8.3 Arginine

Arginine is involved in a variety of metabolic processes and is an essential amino acid. Arginine assists to activate nitric oxide, a significant neurotransmitter and vasodilator. Arginine is endogenously synthesized from argininosuccinate synthase and argininosuccinate lyase [136–138].

The patients suffering from Parkinson's disease have decreased levels of nitric oxide. There are several causes for NO deficiency such as reduced endothelial function, elevated amines, or NO precursor arginine and citrulline deficiency. Owing to the inadequate availability of nitric oxide (NO), arginine supplementation is indicated for mitochondrial disorders. Arginine has a positive effect on patients with MELAS (mitochondrial encephalopathy, lactic acidosis, and stroke-like episode) due to its potential to cause vasodilation. While not specifically tested in clinical trials, arginine seems to play a significant role in alleviating the symptoms of MELAS. It is yet unsure if arginine has a role in the treatment of some types of depression. The findings of a clinical trial would likely be released next year. Results from intravenous administration of arginine to alleviate symptoms in patients with MELAS also seem to be encouraging. In certain cases, five intravenous doses of arginine (500 mg/kg) in patients with severe stroke within 30 min of the initiation of symptoms ameliorate stroke symptoms. The intravenous arginine enhances endothelial function by increasing vasodilation after 2 h [138–141].

Clinical studies have shown that arginine-rich dietary supplements help to reduce mitochondrial disorder. Accumulative studies found that arginine at concentrations in the range 50–300 mg/kg/day is effective in reducing mitochondrial disorders. Patients treated with arginine were not experienced severe stroke-like effects such as convulsions or hemiparesis, as previously reported. Accumulative studies have also shown that oral arginine supplementation has a beneficial effect on endothelial growth, which can also increase cardiac performance [140,141].

Further studies are required to evaluate the efficacy and safety of arginine for patients with mitochondrial disorders. Some experiments are expected to assess the effect of arginine supplementation on other mitochondrial disorders [142,143].

8.4 Coenzyme Q_{10}

CoQ10 is a fat-soluble quinone that transfers electrons from ATP-containing complexes I and II to complex III. It helps to reduce oxidative damage to mitochondrial DNA. It is synthesized in humans endogenously. It is also found in meats, nuts, fruit, and fish [144–146].

CoQ10 supplements tend to lower intestinal absorption rates, that is why CoQ10 is more bioavailable as compared to oxidized form and makes it suitable for supplementation. It helps to improve the absorption of the consumed food or dietary fat [130,146,147].

CoQ10 supplementations are beneficial for patients suffering from Parkinson's disease owing to their function as a coenzyme in the electron transport chain as well as an antioxidant. A significant number of patients with CoQ10 deficiency were reported to have increased severity and ataxia. There is some evidence that CoQ10 is beneficial to people with mitochondrial disease but further research is required [148,149].

Various aspects of the human effect of CoQ10 were examined in case studies; however, the studies were not reliable, so it was difficult to test them. CoQ10 supplementation at concentrations in the range of 150–1200 mg and 2 mg/kg/day helps to enhance muscle strength. The serum lactate levels were not affected before and during exercise but it improved muscle activity after supplementation [150–152].

In a randomized and placebo-controlled trial 30 patients with postural hypotension and myopathy were supplemented with CoQ10. Each patient was prescribed 1200 mg daily for 60 days and 1000 mg for 60 days. A significant increase in plasma concentration of CoQ10 was reported after administration of CoQ10 to mice [152].

In a two-armed randomized controlled crossover experiment, 160 mg/day of CoQ10 or placebo was supplemented to eight patients with CPEO, MELAS, or MERRF for 3 months. Supplementation with CoQ10 was not altered the levels of lactate and pyruvate in the blood, but the muscle density of both the upper and lower limbs continued to rise [153].

CoQ10 was shown to reduce diabetes problems such as retinopathy in subjects. In the first round, 44 patients diagnosed with MERRF received 2 mg/kg/day of CoQ10 form known as ubidecarenone in a 6-month open-label trial. The coenzyme Q10 supplementation was given to individuals to improve the mitochondrial respiratory chain enzymes in their muscles [151]. A total of 17 individuals received CoQ10 at the dose of 2mg/kg/day in a double-blind, placebo-controlled trial while 8 individuals received placebo. This study was discontinued due to the poor health condition of two participants of the placebo group. The level of serum lactate was not affected after the supplementations.

Data on clinically useful metabolic parameters were collected from an open-label study of five mitochondrial patients. The L/P ratio shows the metabolic changes in patients but overall no change in health status was found [150].

One open-label study examined the muscular activity after CoQ10 supplementations at a dose of 150mg/day for 6months in eight patients with mitochondrial disorders at rest, during, and after exercise [154]. The findings revealed the nonsignificant change in muscle function in one patient and found an increase in PCr/Pi ratio after 3months of supplementation. Improvements in biochemical parameters in patients with a mitochondrial disorder and reduced muscle weakness after CoQ10 were reported. Case reports and minimal trials show that some patients with mitochondrial disorder benefit from CoQ10 supplements. Studies have found that these antidepressants are not effective in the population. Further research is required to determine the efficacy of long-term use of CoQ10 in the treatment of these conditions. The recommended dosage range of CoQ10 is 2–8mg/kg/day. Side effects include headache, insomnia, rash, nausea, or stomach problems [130,155–157].

8.5 Folic acid

Folate plays an important role in creatine synthesis, RNA and DNA synthesis, and homocysteine remethylation. Folic acid also works as a coenzyme in the folate cycle. Folate is naturally found in different forms and the oxidized form is known as folic acid. Folic acid is most frequently used as a food supplement for fortification. There are also other types of folate supplements such as 5-methyltetrahydrofolate, L-methyl folate, and folinic acid. Folinic acid and L-methyl folate are also available as prescribed drugs to enhance fertility [158].

Folinic acid in patients with main or secondary cortical folate deficit (CFD) helps to increase the level of 5-MTHF in the brain [158,159].

The mechanism of CFD is still unknown. Patients with KSS was suggested to have cerebral folate deficiency because of the insufficient amount of ATP required for the active transport of folate to neurons via the blood-brain barrier [158,160,161]. The methylation and stabilization of myelin may be impaired by low cerebral folate levels. Consequently, myelin instability can lead to lesions of white matter in KSS patients. Folinic acid is present in varying concentrations from 400 to 1000 μg in food individual or combined supplementations along with other nutraceuticals like calcium folinate [158].

8.6 Niacin

Niacin is the precursor of the coenzymes NAD and NADP. NAD and NADP are utilized in energy metabolism and transferring electrons to complex I. Coenzyme NADP is used in the pentose phosphate pathway to synthesise fatty acid and steroid and as a hydrogen donor in the manufacture of steroid hormones [162,163].

Niacin is synthesized from the amino acid tryptophan and is also found in beef, grains, milk, and eggs [163]. Niacin is used as a dietary supplement such as nicotinic acid, inositol hexaniacinate, and nicotinamide and is also present in prescribed drug formulations like Niaspan [164].

The niacin is supplemented to patients with mitochondrial disorder to enhance the levels of NADH and NAD thereby increasing the concentrations of complex I in the electron transport chain to generate ATP [10].

Nicotinamide was used to treat patients with MELAS at 4000 mg/day for 5 months. NAD levels were increased 24 times than pretreatment levels after supplementations. Blood lactate was reduced by 40%, and blood pyruvate level reduced 50% after 3 days of supplementation [165].

8.7 Creatine

Creatine is normally found in the human body as a product of amino acids such as glycine and arginine. Creatine is usually found in meat and fish products as well as in dietary supplements that contain creatine monohydrate. High amounts of creatine are found in muscle tissue and brain tissue owing to vigorous exercise. Creatine reacts with phosphate to produce phosphocreatine in tissue. The degradation of phosphocreatine assists to produce ATP by transferring phosphate to adenosine diphosphate (ADP). The patients with mitochondrial myopathies have low creatine in muscle as well as in the brain. The creatine administration was found to increase the availability of creatine in tissues and to increase skeletal muscle energy reserve. Overall creatine and phosphocreatine levels in skeletal muscle increased up to 20% after the supplementation of creatine at a concentration of 10–20 g/day for 4–6 days [130,166,167].

Two research trials indicated that creatine supplementation could improve Parkinson's disease. The results found substantial improvements in isometric handgrip and total power relative to the placebo [168]. The second study measured the impact of a daily intake of creatine between 0.08 and 0.35 g for 9 months to 4 years in seven patients. This analysis showed a 12% rise in most people's maximum muscle strength. Self-reported signs of muscle disability increased but cognitive impairment did not increase [169].

8.8 Riboflavin

Riboflavin is a significant component of flavin mononucleotide (FMN) and flavoprotein (FAD) and is also known as vitamin B2. Electron carriers such as cytochrome *b* are active in the processing of energy and the production of fatty acids [130,162,170].

The body may extract riboflavin from food in excess like organ meat, lean meats, eggs, and milk. Riboflavin is also found in nutritional supplements and medicines. Multivitamin supplements contain 1.7 mg of riboflavin. Some multivitamins contain 400–5000 mg of riboflavin [170].

Studies show that much riboflavin is absorbed in the small intestine. The body displays no reaction to 1 or 2 higher doses and retains relatively little in the body. It is necessary to remember that excess quantities are either not consumed or a minimal portion of the excess is excreted in urine [163].

The riboflavin supplementation in people with mitochondrial disorders assists to enhance energy efficiency through electron transport pathways and improve amino acid imbalance. High doses (150 mg) of B12 vitamin was supplemented to patients with mitochondrial disorders [10]. The studies show that riboflavin supplementation assists to improve the complex I deficiency in patients with mitochondrial disorders. The riboflavin supplementation at 150 mg/day for an unspecified duration increased muscle strength and decreased plasma lactate as well as alanine concentrations in people with complex I deficiency due to acyl-coenzyme A dehydrogenase 9 (ACAD9) mutations [171]. A trial reported clinical progress after supplementation of 9 mg/day for 25 months. Riboflavin supplementation of 36 mg to the patient for 24 months helped to improve social activity, physical activity, and motor ability. Another patient taking the same dosage did not have the same beneficial effects. Compared to children with mitochondrial myopathy and complex I deficiency, those with a lower initial riboflavin intake demonstrated increased muscle strength and decreased muscle weakness. The riboflavin at the dose of 50 mg/day for 3 years assists to restore complex disability and skeletal myopathy in a woman. The patients suffered substantial clinical decline when riboflavin was discontinued for 1 month but recovered after supplementations [172–174].

Case studies also show that riboflavin supplementation can be beneficial in treating mitochondrial disorders related to complex II deficiency. In three children with riboflavin deficiency, 50–100 mg/day had beneficial effects including substantial improvements in several cognitive functions, including better communication skills, coordination, and development. In one patient, plasma lactate and pyruvate levels decreased in response to treatment [2].

The MMS advises that patients with PMDs take riboflavin supplements at a normal dosage of 50–400 mg/day [130].

Overall the case reports indicate that riboflavin might help to reduce the risk of mitochondrial disorders in people with complex I and complex II deficiencies. However, further experiments with greater sample sizes are required to validate effectiveness and protection of riboflavin.

8.9 Thiamin

Thiamin is present in several foods and is mostly found in vegetables, seafood, and meats. The compound is also found in some nutritional items and available as a dietary supplement [175]. Multivitamins contain 0.5–1 mg of thiamin but some contain 25–250 mg. The most common routes of thiamin exposure are in the form of thiamin hydrochloride and thiamin mononitrate that is stable and water soluble. Benfotiamine is a modified form of thiamin that is not water soluble, and the body transforms it into thiamin [170,176].

Thiamin helps to improve metabolism. Thiamin pyrophosphate is the metabolic form of thiamin which allows enzymes to catalyze the degradation of sugars as well as amino acids. Thiamin is an important cofactor for the decarboxylation of pyruvate to acetyl-coenzyme A where it plays a crucial role in energy production [175].

Thiamin supplementation is intended to facilitate aerobic glycolysis by increasing the rate at which pyruvate decarboxylates [10]. One study determined the impact of vitamin B1 deficiency on people with mitochondrial disorders. This study showed that the daily supplement of 900 mg thiamin hydrochloride in three split doses restored blood lactate levels in two patients, and increased the blood pyruvate levels of one patient [177]. The supplement helped boost both overall well-being and sleep in the first patient, but it made little difference in the second patient who got thiamin.

Further studies must be performed to determine the effectiveness and safety of this dietary supplement in individuals with mitochondrial disorder.

8.10 Vitamin C

Vitamin C or L-ascorbyl-6-phosphate is a water-soluble vitamin naturally found in certain foods. Most fruits and vegetables contain vitamin C.Vitamin C is added to certain diets and is available as dietary supplement. Unlike other animals, humans cannot synthesize vitamin C endogenously [178].

Vitamin C is necessary for L-carnitine production, collagen development, and neurotransmitter production. Vitamin C is involved in metabolism and electron transfer, and it is an essential source of physiological antioxidant involved in the regeneration of other antioxidants inside the body. Vitamin C also functions as a cofactor and antioxidant and assists to improve nonheme iron supply through the intestine [178–180].

For about 70%–90% of vitamin C to be completely absorbed, it must be ingested in moderate doses [180]. Data from pharmacokinetic trials suggest that the daily intake of 1.25 g ascorbic acid increase the plasma vitamin C levels by 135 μmol/L which is as high as that obtained by eating 200–300 mg/day of vitamin C-rich foods. Pharmacokinetic simulation suggests that a small amount of ascorbic acid consumed at low doses results in a low peak of vitamin C concentration in plasma [181].

Vitamins such as ascorbic acid are usually present in supplements and have the same bioavailability as that found in naturally occurring foods like broccoli and orange juice. Other vitamin C supplements include synthetic vitamin C, tablets, ascorbic acid, bioflavonoids, and combinations [10,182,183].

8.11 Vitamin E

Vitamin E is found naturally in foods. The most potassium-rich foods are nuts, beans, and vegetable oils. Many foods contain additional fat-soluble vitamins, including vitamin E, which is added to other foods and is also used as a dietary supplement.

"Vitamin E" refers to a group of fat-soluble compounds with distinctive antioxidant properties, collectively referred to as "vitamin E."Vitamin E possesses eight molecular types (gamma-, alpha-, beta-, and delta-tocopherol gamma, alpha-, beta-, and delta-tocotrienol) with varying degrees of biological activity. Tocopherols are the only type believed to give humans the necessary dose [184]. The key role of alpha-tocopherol is to provide antioxidant defense to a cell membrane against the proliferation of free radical reactions. Regeneration of vitamin E requires the use of vitamin C [185].

Vitamin E supplements are available in different forms that include alpha-tocopherol, beta-tocopherol, and other tocopherols, and also tocotrienols. It is usually applied to dietary supplements and food products to preserve its antioxidant qualities and extend shelf life. The body breaks down and consumes these esters as effectively as vitamin E. The vast majority of vitamin E supplements have at least 100 IU [185].

8.12 Vitamin K

Vitamin K is a fat-soluble vitamin and is present in green leafy vegetables [186]. A variety of vitamin K supplements such as phytonadione and phylloquinone as well as MK-7 and MK-4 are used as dietary supplements. There is a paucity of literature regarding the bioavailability of vitamin K. A research shows that MK-7 and phytonadione are assimilated with the same efficiency. MK-7 has a long half-life [163].

Many multivitamin supplements contain little or no vitamin K. Vitamin K is also used as a nutritional supplement and is used as a mixture of potassium and vitamin K. These supplements are mostly on the high side of vitamin K doses [170].

Vitamin K is used as a coenzyme for certain enzymes that perform significant roles in blood clotting and bone protection. Vitamin K3 was used in combination with vitamin C to improve complex III deficiency in patients with mitochondrial disorder [10,183,187] (Fig. 3).

9. Molecular mechanisms/targeting signaling pathway

9.1 Via Nrf2/ARE, nuclear factor (erythroid-derived 2)-like 2/ Antioxidant element response

To counteract and neutralize the harmful effects of ROS, cells evolve a variety of complex mechanisms for maintaining redox homeostasis, which may be divided into two classes of antioxidants. The antioxidants have redox activity and limited half-lives, thus they need to be supplemented [188]. Furthermore, they should be administered on a regular basis and at relatively large doses to maintain their physiological efficiency. In contrast, nutraceuticals exert indirect antioxidant activities by activating specific genes to encode antioxidant proteins via the upregulation of Nrf2 pathway that is known as a master regulator of the antioxidant response [188,189], so their physiological effects last longer than those of direct antioxidants. Furthermore, indirect antioxidants are unlikely to produce prooxidant effects, which have been seen with high-dose vitamin E treatment [190].

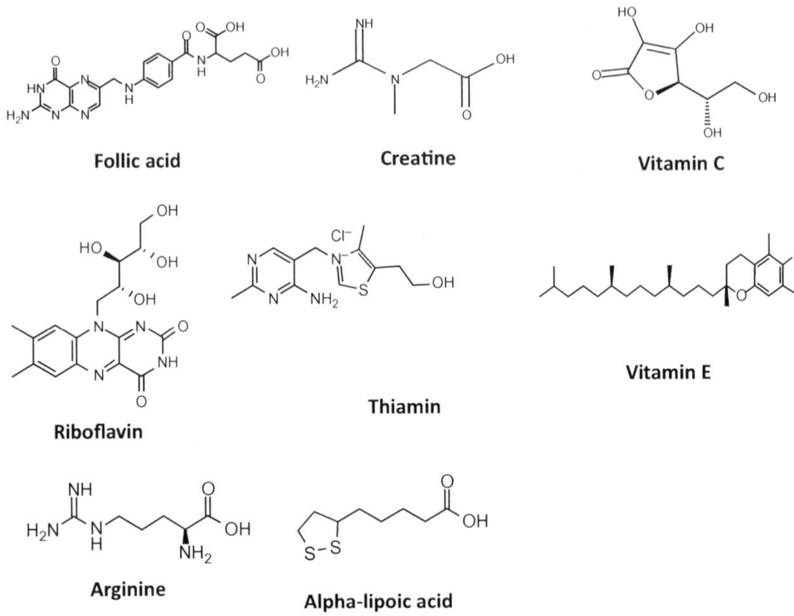

Fig. 3 Structures of nontraditional nutraceuticals.

Nrf2 activates phase II/detoxifying and many other genes via the cis-antioxidant response element (ARE), which contains a conserved core sequence (5′-A/GTGAC/GNNNGCa/c-3′) located in the promoter region. Nrf2 is sequestered in the cytoplasm by cytoskeleton binding protein Kelch-like ECH-associated protein 1 (Keap1), which then connects with Cullin 3 to create an E3 ubiquitin ligase complex that targets Nrf2 for continuous proteasomal destruction [191]. Nrf2 translocates into the nucleus where it heterodimerizes with the tiny musculoaponeurotic fibrosarcoma protein and coactivator proteins that bind to ARE, leading to the transcription of cytoprotective genes [192–195].

Many dietary phytochemicals are present in vegetables, fruits, spices, and herbal medications that activate Nrf2 and increase the production of antioxidant or phase II detoxification enzymes [189,196,197]. Epigallocatechin gallate, lycopene, and resveratrol have recently become the focus of research in animals [189,198,199]. Further research revealed that various phytochemicals may interfere with different cell-signaling pathways and might be employed in higher dosages in their natural form to alleviate stress in animals [200] (Fig. 4).

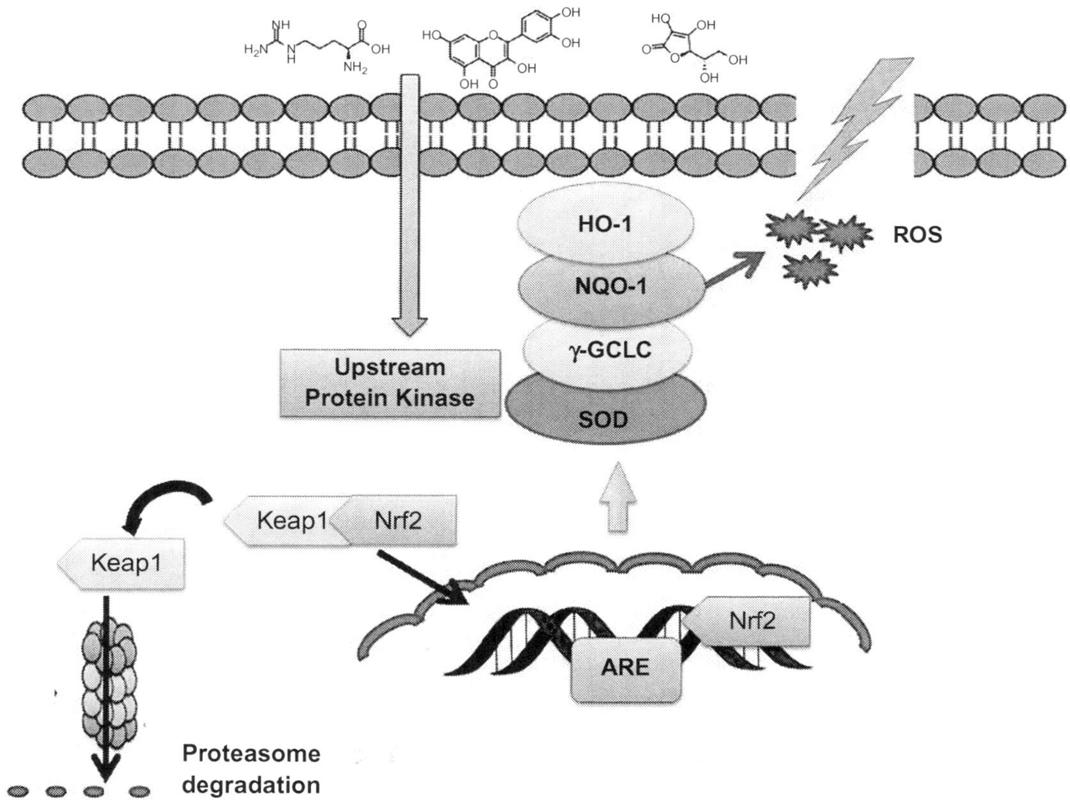

Fig. 4 The molecular mechanism of nutraceuticals activate Nrf2/ARE pathway along with downstream protein related to antioxidant.

9.2 Mechanism of action of nutraceuticals to mitigate mitochondrial dysfunction

The oxidative stress and free radicals are the main cause of mitochondria dysfunction which leads to malfunctioning of energy homeostasis and neuronal metabolism. This improves brain function and mitigates neurodegenerative diseases like Parkinson's disease. However, it is unclear if mitochondria dysfunction induces neurodegeneration. The degeneration of dopamine-producing neurons and the change in the respiratory system were speculated to bring about mitochondrial dysfunction in Parkinson's patients. The mitochondria in cells control the supply of adenosine triphosphate (ATP) and calcium to release accumulated neuropeptides into the synaptic cleft and depolarize neurons to protect cell splitting. The α-synuclein aggregates upregulate the generation of reactive oxygen species, which results in the apoptosis of brain cells. The dopaminergic neurons protect against oxidative stress. Neuromelanin helps to chelate various metals such as iron and zinc to maintain homeostasis and equilibrium within the redox system. The fluctuation of iron levels in the brain can induce Parkinson's disease and high iron levels can aggravate various neurotoxic events. These events contribute to the autooxidation of dopamine and cause neuroinflammation. Nutraceuticals as the components of food are capable of maintaining mitochondrial functioning and mitigate major pathologies related to Parkinson's disease. Nutritional supplements, phytochemicals, or synthetic compounds may help retain metabolic activities by restoring optimum mitochondrial activity. Fish oil and CoQ10 can efficiently lessen Parkinson's disease as they play an important role in ATP production and are involved in electron transfer between complex 1 and complexes II, III, and IV. The polyphenols often exert multidimensional properties to improve Parkinson's disease as they can quickly cross the blood-brain barrier and exhibit protective effect by shielding dopaminergic neurons from oxidative damage. Lycopene is a lipid-soluble acyclic carotenoid that exerts an antioxidant effect. Lycopene was found to exert neuroprotective activity in MPTP-induced neurodegeneration in mice. The beneficial effects of lycopene are due to antioxidant function that assists to lower the neurological deficiencies and improve the levels of superoxide dismutase and NADH dehydrogenase. Fish oil contains surplus amount of omega-3 fatty acids including docosahexaenoic and eicosapentaenoic acids and exert protective effects against neuronal degeneration. Epigallocatechin gallate, a polyphenol in green tea, exhibits neuroprotective effects by crossing the blood-brain barrier. The phytoconstituent of epigallocatechin gallate is scavenged free radical and has iron chelating activity. Epigallocatechin gallate effectively improved muscle activity and decreased neurotoxicity by increasing the levels of dopamine in brain striatum. Ginseng and its derivatives proved neuroprotective effects through numerous experiments on Parkinson's disease. The antioxidant function of ginsenoside helps to enhance levels of glutathione and reduce ROS generation through NF-kB pathway and modulate iron transport which minimizes the iron storage in the brain. Vincamine, an alkaloid present in vinca, was evaluated for its anti-Parkinson's disease action through several pathways. It induces vasodilation and weakens muscle tone in capillaries, allowing increased blood supply to the brain and an increase in energy output through the Krebs cycle. Likewise, oxidative stress and iron are attacked by vincamine thus increasing the production of dopamine while decreasing the deleterious effects of iron. Therefore, the function of vincamine and its derivatives, vinpocetine, is to inhibit the formation of free radicals and chelating agents. Another synthetic agent including mito Q is used to enhance Parkinson's symptoms. Mito Q is composed of a lipophilic molecule called triphenylphosphine, which renders the compound an antioxidant and the respiratory chain functioning. An endogenous phytoestrogen similar to coumarin is being studied for its ability to protect against Parkinson's disease [201–203].

10. Nutraceuticals interact with protein misfolding and endoplasmic reticulum stress pathway

When proteins are misfolded, this causes ER stress and contributes to unfolded protein reaction and autophagy. The primary purpose of drugs that target the endogenous antioxidants is to suppress the development of misfolded proteins. The protein aggregates induce necrosis and provoke neurodegeneration. The most consistently consumed nutrients are vitamins among people afflicted with Parkinson's. However, CoQ10, vitamin A, and beta-carotene are all have antifibrillogenic effects. Vitamin A stops the aggregation of α-Syn in the cell. Crocin exerts neuroprotective properties and can be used to treat central nervous system diseases. The carotenoid impairs the expression of CHOP and the binding of immunoglobulin protein (BIP)/Grp78. Thus, downregulate the activation of several proapoptotic factors such as caspase-12, which is responsible for apoptosis. Bicalein is a molecule isolated from the roots of a plant derived from Iran. This compound downregulates fibrillation and neurodegeneration by inhibiting

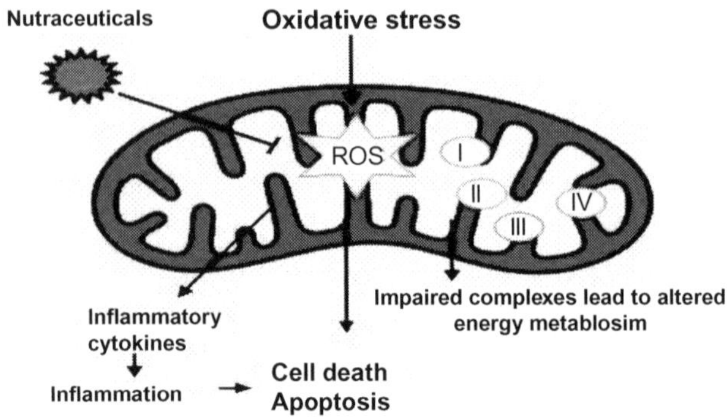

Fig. 5 General mechanism of mitochondrial dysfunction and nutraceutical protection.

the production of α-synuclein oligomers. This flavone controls autophagy, reduces inflammation and inflammatory cytokines, and prevents apoptosis, thereby restoring the levels of dopamine in a mice model of Parkinson's disease. Resveratrol is a potent medicinal agent because of its solubility and stability. It stimulates microflora in the intestine and promotes mitochondrial turnover. This behavior enhances the bioavailability of polyphenols in the brain [202,204] (Fig. 5).

11. Combined effects of nutraceuticals

Vitamins and other compounds are frequently used in combination to treat mitochondrial disorders even though the research found no data about their protection and effectiveness in this sense. A study of the present clinical treatment of mitochondria diseases demonstrated that 14 out of 32 doctors used vitamins in combination rather than prescribing each individually. Of note, 79% of physicians prescribe specific formulations while 13% of physicians use carnitine and CoQ10. Finally, 9% of physicians use a mixture of B-complex vitamins, creatine, and CoQ10 [205].

A few published articles and case reports have discussed the consequences of combinations doses (Table 1).

12. Interaction of nutraceuticals with medicines

Dietary supplements and some drugs may interfere with one another, thereby causing adverse effects on one's diet. A few basic examples are given. Patients on these and other drugs should check with their physicians for more management orders (Table 2).

Table 1 The combine nutraceutical protective effect against mitochondrial disorders.

Combination of nutraceuticals	Study design/patients	Doses/day	Duration	Mitochondrial disorder	Ref.
Creatine, ALA, CoQ_{10}	Randomzized double blind/18	CoQ_{10} (120 mg/twice a day) Creatine (3 g/twice a day) ALA (300 mg/twice a day)	2 months	MELAS, CPEO, KSS, MNGIE, LHON	[132]
Riboflavin and Carnitine	Randomized/6 year old	L-carnitine (2 g) Riboflavin (9 mg/)	7 months	Myopathy	[206]
CoQ_{10}, Carnitine, vitamin C, vitamin B complex, vitamin K1	Open-labeled trial/12	CoQ_{10} 5 mg/kg Vitamin B Complex Carnitine 500 mg pantothenic acid 25 mg Vitamin K1 0.4 mg Riboflavin 25 mg/day Thiamin 25 mg Niacin 25 mg Vitamin C 1000 mg Pyridoxine 25 mg Biotin 25 μg Folic acid 1 mg Cyanocobalamin 25 μg Riboflavin (25)	12 month	LHON, MELAS, CPEO, NARP, oxidase cytochrome *c*	[187]
Combination of nutraceuticals	Study design/patients	Doses	Duration	Mitochondrial disorder	Ref.

Continued

Table 1 The combine nutraceutical protective effect against mitochondrial disorders—cont'd

Combination of nutraceuticals	Study design/patients	Doses/day	Duration	Mitochondrial disorder	Ref.
Carnitine, vitamin C, CoQ_{10}, riboflavin vitamin E, vitamin K3	Openlabel/13	Carnitine (100–200 mg/kg) Vitamin E (80–300 mg/kg) Vitamin C (2 g) Vitamin K3 (80–160 mg) CoQ_{10} (50–100 mg)	8 moths	CPEO KSS	[207]
CoQ_{10}, vitamin C, vitamin K3, vitamin E	Open label/16	CoQ_{10} (30–120 mg) Vitamin E (400 IU) Vitamin K3 (20–60 mg) Vitamin C (20 g)	–	KSS MERRF MELAS	[208]
CoQ_{10}, vitamin C, niacin, thiamin vitamin K3, riboflavin,	Open label/16	CoQ_{10} (300 mg) Vitamin C (2 g) Vitamin K3 (60 mg) Or Supplements of Riboflavin (25 mg) Thiamin (100 mg) Niacin (200 mg) Vitamin C (500 mg)	Almost 2 months	KSS demyelinating neuropathy Myopathy MERRF	[209]
Vitamin C Vitamin K3	–	Vitamin C (4 g) Vitamin K 3 (40 mg)	Within 2 days of supplementations	Complex III deficiency	[210]

Table 2 Various side effects due to nutraceutical and medicine interaction.

Nutraceutical	Medicine nutraceutical interact	Side effects	Ref.
Carnitine	Yclosporine, Levofloxacin Pivampicillin, Valproate Etoposide, Actinomycin D, Vinblastine Omeprazole	• Impaired transport of carnitine in across the plasma membrane	[211]
CoQ_{10}	Statins Propranolol Metoprolol Glyburide Tolazamide	• Inhibit 3-hydroxy-3-methylglutaryl-CoA reductase and lower the level of mevalonic acid • Inhibit CoQ_{10}-dependent enzymes • Decrease CoQ_{10}	[143,212–214]
Folinic acid	5-Fluorouracil	• Promoted 5-FU's toxicity	[215]
Niacin	Aspirin	• Aspirin was lowered the flushing related to niacin supplementation	[216–218]
Vitamin C	Simvastatin (Zocor)	• Lowered the high-density lipoprotein levels	[219,220]
Thiamin	Furosemide (Lasix)	• Furosemide lowers the thiamin level up to deficient levels that lead to urinary thiamin loss	[221,222]
Vitamin E	Warfarin (Coumadin)	• Increase the risk of bleeding	[223]
Vitamin K	Warfarin (Coumadin)	• These medications interact with vitamin K synthesis, causing vitamin K deficits due to bleeding. People using warfarin and other anticoagulant medications need to regularly eat vitamin K from diet and supplements to prevent unnecessary improvements in anticoagulant effects	[224]

13. Regulatory challenges of nutraceuticals

Once clinical study is conducted evaluating the efficacy of dietary supplements in helping patients with mitochondrial disorder and some significant hurdles occur, translating research findings into clinical care choices, particularly though higher causality from randomized control study after a specific dietary supplement for mitochondrial disorder is troublesome owing to the heterogeneity of study designs and outcome.

A clinical trial was examined the efficacy of a nutraceutical in several mitochondrial disorder but stop without differentiating the degree of reaction between various mitochondrial disorder that lead to a false impression of effectiveness.

There is a lack of specificity in the measurements of outcomes used in the study, which greatly restricts the capacity to evaluate the reproducibility. The mitochondrial specialists have contributed to efforts to define common data for mitochondrial disorder to help with potential clinical trial designs.

Patients' baseline state cannot be entirely determined until they started supplementation, so we do not know whether the intervention fixed any residual deficits. It is impossible to determine if recorded changes in biochemical tests without biomarkers for particular health effects such as blood lactate concentration or PCr/Pi ratio that might help to evaluate clinically meaningful change in health and function.

By boosting undamaged components of cells to reduce overall mitochondrial dysfunction, the functional status of mitochondria in a cell may be modified. Mitochondria can transfer energy through the electron transport chain from metabolites to NADH and then eventually to molecular oxygen. A transmembrane proton gradient and an electrochemical gradient are created through the mitochondrial inner membrane by this mechanism. In order to drive adenosine diphosphate (ADP) to ATP, the energy from this process is used. The reactive oxygen species (ROS), which are highly reactive free radicals, are produced by oxidative phosphorylation process as a by-product of electron transport. Excess oxygen consumption and the resulting development of ROS will lead to improper damage to lipids of the mitochondrial membrane, such as tROS/RNS-sensitive cardiolipin, a phospholipid of the inner mitochondrial membrane. At concentrations that prevent oxidative damage to cellular entities, the antioxidant ROS/R NS levels are maintained. Specific biochemical drugs that are used to cure mitochondrial diseases are involved in nutraceuticals. Because of their antioxidant impact, the nutrients are urged to enhance neurological disorders.

The therapeutic effects of plant products and herbs on various disorders such as mental wellbeing are protective. Probiotics have an antibiotic activity that can help shield the intestines from toxic flora. In a stable body and brain, a good diet results. Stomach symptoms can be changed with the application of probiotics. Since it was last published on September 10, 2013, the content of this article has been updated. In order to represent the recent trends in Nutr Pharmaceuticals, the scope of the article has now been revised. Back to the pages that were on the first page. It was adapted with new details from the original edition. We are glad to clarify that the information found in this report was amended on September 13, 2013 to reflect the fact that the new research is based on a revised and modified analysis released by the National Institutes of Health.

Nutraceuticals that have been prepared by the application of biotechnology in food products are called recombinants. In the production of Nutr Pharmaceuticals, rules by the Food and Drug Administration (FDA) are still missing. Nutr Raceuticals' study is not as regulated as pharmaceuticals, with no strict legislation explicitly stated. Alpha-lipoic acid (ALA) is found naturally in mitochondria and mitochondria. ALA acts as a cofactor for the activation of ATP production enzymes. In the limited clinical review of ALA, there were no safety concerns. For patients with diabetic polyneuropathy, taking 600 mg of $n-6$ PUFA per day for 6 months to 4 years was considered safe. In order to determine the preventive effect after oral supplementation with ALA in PMD patients, further research needs to be carried out. For those with PMDs, the normal dosage of 50–200 mg/day is recommended. Foods obtained from agricultural produce and nutrients such as vitamins, calcium-fortified orange juice and minerals in cereals are included in nontraditional dietary pharmaceuticals. New techniques which can help to increase the nutritional quality of crops have been successfully developed by scientists.

A variety of metabolic pathways and essential amino acids are involved in arginine. Due to its ability to induce vasodilation, arginine has a beneficial effect on MELAS (mitochondrial encephalopathy, lactic acidosis, and stroke-like episode) patients. Scientific trials have shown that dietary supplements high in arginine tend to alleviate mitochondrial disorders. CoQ10 is a fat-soluble quinone which transfers electrons to complex III from ATP-containing complexes I and II. It is also present in beef, nuts, fruit, and fish and tends to enhance nutritional or dietary fat absorption. The results of a clinical trial on the management of certain types of depression are expected to be revealed next year. If arginine is used to treat any form of depression or not is still unknown. It may also help to decrease mitochondrial DNA oxidative damage and increase intestinal absorption. It has a positive effect on the development of endothelia, and can improve cardiac output as well. It improves the heart's effectiveness and decreases the chance of having a heart attack. It also raises the levels of blood pressure and creatinine in the body. It increases the rate of blood clotting and lowers blood pressure.

CoQ10 is a coenzyme and an antioxidant within the electron transport chain. There is some evidence that people with mitochondrial disease may find CoQ10 beneficial. In one study, serum lactate levels were not altered before and during exercise, but after supplementation, muscle function increased. In another study, CoQ10 was shown to alleviate diabetes issues such as retinopathy in subjects with MERRF. Metabolic improvements in patients were seen in the L/P ratio, but no improvement in health status was observed overall. The study was stopped when, after 3 months of supplementation, poor health condition of two members of the placebo group was reported. After the vitamins, the serum lactate level was not affected. The results showed a nonsignificant improvement in one patient's muscle function and observed an increase in the PCr/Pi ratio after 3 months of CoQ10 supplementation. Studies also show that in the population, these antidepressants are not effective. CoQ10's indicated dosage range is 2–8 mg/kg/day. Headaches, insomnia, rash, fatigue, or trouble with the stomach are the side effects of CoQ10 supplementation. As a nutritional supplement for fortification, folic acid is most commonly used. The precursors of nicotinic acid, inositol hexaniacinate, and nicotinamide coenzymes are niacin. It is also present in beef, grains, milk, and eggs, as well as in prescription medicine formulations such as Niaspan [88]. Owing to the lack of cerebral folate levels, methylation and stabilization of myelin can be compromised in CFD patients and this may lead to white matter lesions in KSS patients. The CFD function is still unclear. In patients with mitochondrial dysfunction, niakin is applied to increase the levels of NADH and NAD, thus increasing the concentrations of complex I in the electron transport chain to create ATP. Creatine is usually present as a product of amino acids including glycine and arginine in the human body. Due to strenuous exercise, high levels of creatine are present in muscle tissue and brain tissue. Patients of mitochondrial myopathy include reduced amounts of creatine in both muscle and brain activity. Creatine administration was found to increase the tissue supply of creatine and to increase the energy reserve of skeletal muscle. Creatine supplementation has been shown to enhance Parkinson's disease in two clinical trials. Excess foods such as organ meat, lean meats, eggs, and milk can extract riboflavin from the body. Multivitamin supplements include 1.7 mg of lavin rib [96]. Some multivitamins hold between 400 and 5000 mg of riboflavin. The overall muscle strength in certain individuals has been improved by 12% in seven patients after a consumption of creatine between 0.08 and 0.35 g for 9 months to 4 years. This study indicates a 12% increase in the overall muscle strength in most individuals. Self-reported symptoms of muscle disability rose, but there was no rise in neurological dysfunction.

Patients with mitochondrial abnormalities were supplemented with high doses (150 mg) of the B12 vitamin. The findings found that supplementation of riboflavin helps to strengthen the deficit of complex I. Thiamin is present in a variety of foods, mainly in vegetables, fish, and poultry. Thiamin is converted by the body into the more energy-efficient form of vitamin thiamine. The MMS suggests that patients with PMD can take a regular dose of 50–400 mg/day of riboflavin supplements. A study showed that in people with complexes I and II defects, riboflavin could help reduce the risk of mitochondrial disorders. However, to verify efficacy and safety, more studies with higher sample sizes are needed. The study discovered that riboflavin could help reduce the risk of mitochondrial dysfunction.

For the decarboxylation of pyruvate to acetyl-coenzyme A, thiamin is an essential cofactor. Supplementation of thiamin is meant to promote aerobic glycolysis. One research determined the effect of thiamin on people with mitochondrial abnormalities of vitamin B1 deficiency. This study found that the blood lactate level was restored in two patients with a daily supplement of 900 mg of thiamine hydrochloride in three split doses.

Nutraceuticals are complex products, and the bioavailability and bioactivity of their ingredients can differ greatly depending on the manufacturing process. The structure of drugs developed by pharmaceutical and biotech firms may be very different from the products marketed to the public. The studies do not have much the information required to compare what is available on the market and suitable for consumer. Various vitamin products labeled with the same ingredient may have different shapes, strengths, and chemical varieties. Unfortunately, reporting on the essential characteristics of products and procedures of scientific experiments is frequently insufficient for the reader to conclude on the essence of the intervention [225,226].

The Food and Drug Administration (FDA) rules for pharmaceutical and over-the-counter food supplements are more stringent than for nutraceuticals. Unlike nutraceuticals which do not need approval by the FDA, medications require premarket approval by the FDA. The organization must show that their goods are secure and that their argument is truthful in order to preserve its reputation.

The FDA developed Good Manufacturing Practices (GMPs) for nutraceuticals to process, package, and store in an acceptable, safe, and sanitary manner. Many nongovernmental organizations have managed GMP audits and product review services. Nutraceutical goods that carry the seals from these independent certification programs provide customers with a greater degree of certainty about the use of organic ingredients and no hazardous contaminants.

14. Conclusions

Mitochondria are energy-producing organelles that transfer energy through the electron transport chain from metabolites to NADH and then eventually to molecular oxygen. A transmembrane proton gradient and an electrochemical gradient are created through the mitochondrial inner membrane by this mechanism. The reactive oxygen species (ROS), which are highly reactive free radicals, are produced by the oxidative phosphorylation process as a by-product of electron transport. Excess oxygen consumption and ROS lead to mitochondrial membrane damage such as cardiolipin, a phospholipid of the inner mitochondrial membrane. The nutraceuticals are used to cure mitochondrial disorders. Probiotics have an antibiotic effect that helps to shield the intestines from toxic flora.

Nature has sent us useful, high-potential herbal molecules to treat and avoid life-threatening illnesses and lifestyle-related diseases, including neurodegeneration. Nutraceuticals that are prepared by the application of biotechnology in food products are known as recombinants. Alpha-lipoic acid (ALA) is found naturally in mitochondria. ALA acts as a cofactor for the activation of ATP production enzymes. Foods obtained from agricultural products and nutrients such as vitamins, calcium-fortified orange juice, and minerals in cereals are included in nontraditional dietary pharmaceuticals.

The healing effects of nutraceuticals may be due to their hypolipidemic, antiinflammatory, neuroprotective, antioxidant, and healing properties that stimulate protein synthesis by targeting numerous ligands and receptors, eventually contributing to neuroprotection. It is possible to prevent the folding of proteins and their breakdown that lead to improved nervous system disorder. Without intake of antioxidants can disrupt the defense system to scavenge free oxygen radicals to reduced oxidative stress thereby inducing chronic human diseases. Antioxidant-containing materials, such as vitamins, function intrinsically by scavenging free radicals and promoting the body's antioxidant synthesis. The current review highlights the benefits and demerits of nutraceutical treatment in neurological diseases and its vulnerability to preventing disease development. While nutraceuticals were shown to exhibit extraordinary properties, the reaction varies from individual to individual. It encourages healthy neurological well-being and illnesses can be kept at bay by drinking them in appropriate and prescribed dosages; thus, they are the best choices for treating lifestyle-related mental illnesses, such as depression.

References

[1] J. Chao, Y. Leung, M. Wang, R.C. Chang, Nutraceuticals and their preventive or potential therapeutic value in Parkinson's disease, Nutr. Rev. 70 (7) (2012) 373–386.
[2] M. Bugiani, E. Lamantea, F. Invernizzi, I. Moroni, A. Bizzi, M. Zeviani, et al., Effects of riboflavin in children with complex II deficiency, Brain Dev. 28 (9) (2006) 576–581.
[3] B. Olas, Berry phenolic antioxidants—implications for human health? Front. Pharmacol. 9 (2018) 78.
[4] R.H. Haas, S. Parikh, M.J. Falk, R.P. Saneto, N.I. Wolf, N. Darin, et al., Mitochondrial disease: a practical approach for primary care physicians, Pediatrics 120 (6) (2007) 1326–1333.
[5] A. Goldstein, L.A. Wolfe, The elusive magic pill: finding effective therapies for mitochondrial disorders, Neurotherapeutics 10 (2) (2013) 320–328.
[6] G. Pfeffer, K. Majamaa, D.M. Turnbull, D. Thorburn, P.F. Chinnery, Treatment for mitochondrial disorders, Cochrane Database Syst. Rev. (4) (2012), CD004426.
[7] G. Hayashi, G. Cortopassi, Oxidative stress in inherited mitochondrial diseases, Free Radic. Biol. Med. 88 (Pt. A) (2015) 10–17.
[8] W.J. Koopman, P.H. Willems, J.A. Smeitink, Monogenic mitochondrial disorders, N. Engl. J. Med. 366 (12) (2012) 1132–1141.
[9] J.R. Small, P.K. Thomas, A.H. Schapira, Dorsal root ganglion proteins in Friedreich's ataxia, Neurosci. Lett. 163 (2) (1993) 182–184.
[10] B. Marriage, M.T. Clandinin, D.M. Glerum, Nutritional cofactor treatment in mitochondrial disorders, J. Am. Diet. Assoc. 103 (8) (2003) 1029–1038.
[11] M.A. Tarnopolsky, S. Raha, Mitochondrial myopathies: diagnosis, exercise intolerance, and treatment options, Med. Sci. Sports Exerc. 37 (12) (2005) 2086–2093.
[12] J. Besen, S.D. Gan, A critical evaluation of clinical research study designs, J. Investig. Dermatol. 134 (3) (2014) 1–4.
[13] B. Petrisor, M. Bhandari, The hierarchy of evidence: levels and grades of recommendation, Indian J. Orthopaed. 41 (1) (2007) 11–15.
[14] J.M. Orlando, Behavioral nutraceuticals and diets, Vet. Clin. North Am. Small Anim. Pract. 48 (3) (2018) 473–495.
[15] C. Gupta, D. Prakash, Nutraceuticals for geriatrics, J. Tradit. Complement. Med. 5 (1) (2015) 5–14.
[16] W.L. Wang, Contamination of tissue sections with acid-fast bacilli as detected by fluorescence microscopy, Am. J. Clin. Pathol. 51 (1) (1969) 71–75.
[17] R.J. Williams, K.P. Mohanakumar, P.M. Beart, Neuro-nutraceuticals: the path to brain health via nourishment is not so distant, Neurochem. Int. 89 (2015) 1–6.
[18] N.A. Georgiou, J. Garssen, R.F. Witkamp, Pharma-nutrition interface: the gap is narrowing, Eur. J. Pharmacol. 651 (1–3) (2011) 1–8.

[19] P.W. Stacpoole, T.J. deGrauw, A.S. Feigenbaum, C. Hoppel, D.S. Kerr, S.E. McCandless, et al., Design and implementation of the first randomized controlled trial of coenzyme CoQ(1)(0) in children with primary mitochondrial diseases, Mitochondrion 12 (6) (2012) 623–629.
[20] D. Granato, F.J. Barba, D. Bursac Kovacevic, J.M. Lorenzo, A.G. Cruz, P. Putnik, Functional foods: product development, technological trends, efficacy testing, and safety, Annu. Rev. Food Sci. Technol. 11 (2020) 93–118.
[21] C.P. Champagne, A.G. da Cruz, M. Daga, Strategies to improve the functionality of probiotics in supplements and foods, Curr. Opin. Food Sci. 22 (2018) 160–166.
[22] C.F. Casey, D.C. Slawson, L.R. Neal, VItamin D supplementation in infants, children, and adolescents, Am. Fam. Physician 81 (6) (2010) 745–748.
[23] H.L. Nicastro, S.A. Ross, J.A. Milner, Garlic and onions: their cancer prevention properties, Cancer Prev. Res. 8 (3) (2015) 181–189.
[24] G. Twig, O.S. Shirihai, The interplay between mitochondrial dynamics and mitophagy, Antioxid. Redox Signal. 14 (10) (2011) 1939–1951.
[25] M. Priault, B. Salin, J. Schaeffer, F.M. Vallette, J.P. di Rago, J.C. Martinou, Impairing the bioenergetic status and the biogenesis of mitochondria triggers mitophagy in yeast, Cell Death Differ. 12 (12) (2005) 1613–1621.
[26] J. Lee, S. Giordano, J. Zhang, Autophagy, mitochondria and oxidative stress: cross-talk and redox signalling, Biochem. J. 441 (2) (2012) 523–540.
[27] P.R. Rich, A. Marechal, The mitochondrial respiratory chain, Essays Biochem. 47 (2010) 1–23.
[28] C. Richter, J.W. Park, B.N. Ames, Normal oxidative damage to mitochondrial and nuclear DNA is extensive, Proc. Natl. Acad. Sci. U. S. A. 85 (17) (1988) 6465–6467.
[29] A.S. Divakaruni, M.D. Brand, The regulation and physiology of mitochondrial proton leak, Physiology 26 (3) (2011) 192–205.
[30] A.A. Spector, M.A. Yorek, Membrane lipid composition and cellular function, J. Lipid Res. 26 (9) (1985) 1015–1035.
[31] M.R. Duchen, G. Szabadkai, Roles of mitochondria in human disease, Essays Biochem. 47 (2010) 115–137.
[32] G. Spiteller, Is lipid peroxidation of polyunsaturated acids the only source of free radicals that induce aging and age-related diseases? Rejuvenation Res. 13 (1) (2010) 91–103.
[33] A.J. Chicco, G.C. Sparagna, Role of cardiolipin alterations in mitochondrial dysfunction and disease, Am. J. Physiol. Cell Physiol. 292 (1) (2007) C33–C44.
[34] R.H. Houtkooper, F.M. Vaz, Cardiolipin, the heart of mitochondrial metabolism, Cell. Mol. Life Sci. 65 (16) (2008) 2493–2506.
[35] D.A. Barber, S.R. Harris, Oxygen free radicals and antioxidants: a review, Am. Pharm. NS34 (9) (1994) 26–35.
[36] Y. Sun, Free radicals, antioxidant enzymes, and carcinogenesis, Free Radic. Biol. Med. 8 (6) (1990) 583–599.
[37] I. Fridovich, Superoxide radical and superoxide dismutases, Annu. Rev. Biochem. 64 (1995) 97–112.
[38] G. Chandra Jagetia, G.K. Rajanikant, S.K. Rao, B.M. Shrinath, Alteration in the glutathione, glutathione peroxidase, superoxide dismutase and lipid peroxidation by ascorbic acid in the skin of mice exposed to fractionated gamma radiation, Clin. Chim. Acta 332 (1–2) (2003) 111–121.
[39] J.L. Schwartz, The dual roles of nutrients as antioxidants and prooxidants: their effects on tumor cell growth, J. Nutr. 126 (4 Suppl) (1996) 1221S–1227S.
[40] K.N. Prasad, W.C. Cole, B. Kumar, K.C. Prasad, Scientific rationale for using high-dose multiple micronutrients as an adjunct to standard and experimental cancer therapies, J. Am. Coll. Nutr. 20 (5 Suppl) (2001) 450S–463S. discussion 73S-75S.

[41] Z.F. Bhat, H. Bhat, Milk and dairy products as functional foods: a review, Int. J. Dairy Sci. 6 (2011) 1–11.

[42] N. Ramalingum, M.F. Mahomoodally, The therapeutic potential of medicinal foods, Adv. Pharmacol. Sci. 2014 (2014), 354264.

[43] D.D. Dohrmann, P. Putnik, D. Bursac Kovacevic, J. Simal-Gandara, J.M. Lorenzo, F.J. Barba, Japanese, Mediterranean and Argentinean diets and their potential roles in neurodegenerative diseases, Food Res. Int. 120 (2019) 464–477.

[44] P. Putnik, D. Gabric, S. Roohinejad, F.J. Barba, D. Granato, K. Mallikarjunan, et al., An overview of organosulfur compounds from Allium spp.: from processing and preservation to evaluation of their bioavailability, antimicrobial, and anti-inflammatory properties, Food Chem. 276 (2019) 680–691.

[45] M.M. Poojary, P. Putnik, D.B. Kovačević, F.J. Barba, J.M. Lorenzo, D.A. Dias, et al., Stability and extraction of bioactive sulfur compounds from Allium genus processed by traditional and innovative technologies, J. Food Compos. Anal. 61 (2019) 28–39.

[46] D. Montesano, G. Rocchetti, P. Putnik, L. Lucini, Bioactive profile of pumpkin: an overview on terpenoids and their health-promoting properties, Curr. Opin. Food Sci. 22 (2018) 81–87.

[47] J.L. Pillitteri, S. Shiffman, J.M. Rohay, A.M. Harkins, S.L. Burton, T.A. Wadden, Use of dietary supplements for weight loss in the United States: results of a national survey, Obesity 16 (4) (2008) 790–796.

[48] J. Wang, R. Zhang, Y. Xu, H. Zhou, B. Wang, S. Li, Genistein inhibits the development of atherosclerosis via inhibiting NF-kappaB and VCAM-1 expression in LDLR knockout mice, Can. J. Physiol. Pharmacol. 86 (11) (2008) 777–784.

[49] H. King, Phenolic compounds of commercial wheat germ, J. Food Sci. 27 (5) (1962) 446–454.

[50] G.M. Raso, R. Meli, G. Di Carlo, M. Pacilio, R. Di Carlo, Inhibition of inducible nitric oxide synthase and cyclooxygenase-2 expression by flavonoids in macrophage J774A.1, Life Sci. 68 (8) (2001) 921–931.

[51] S. Hirai, N. Takahashi, T. Goto, S. Lin, T. Uemura, R. Yu, et al., Functional food targeting the regulation of obesity-induced inflammatory responses and pathologies, Mediat. Inflamm. 2010 (2010), 367838.

[52] A.W. Boots, M. Drent, V.C. de Boer, A. Bast, G.R. Haenen, Quercetin reduces markers of oxidative stress and inflammation in sarcoidosis, Clin. Nutr. 30 (4) (2011) 506–512.

[53] R.A. Oliveira, I.M. Fierro, New strategies for patenting biological medicines used in rheumatoid arthritis treatment, Expert Opin. Ther. Patent. 28 (8) (2018) 635–646.

[54] K. Vafeiadou, D. Vauzour, H.Y. Lee, A. Rodriguez-Mateos, R.J. Williams, J.P. Spencer, The citrus flavanone naringenin inhibits inflammatory signalling in glial cells and protects against neuroinflammatory injury, Arch. Biochem. Biophys. 484 (1) (2009) 100–109.

[55] M. Hämäläinen, R. Nieminen, P. Vuorela, M. Heinonen, E. Moilanen, Anti-inflammatory effects of flavonoids: genistein, kaempferol, quercetin, and daidzein inhibit STAT-1 and NF-κB activations, whereas flavone, isorhamnetin, naringenin, and pelargonidin inhibit only NF-κB activation along with their inhibitory effect on iNOS expression and NO production in activated macrophages, Mediat. Inflamm. 2007 (2007).

[56] A.P. Rogerio, C.L. Dora, E.L. Andrade, J.S. Chaves, L.F. Silva, E. Lemos-Senna, et al., Anti-inflammatory effect of quercetin-loaded microemulsion in the airways allergic inflammatory model in mice, Pharmacol. Res. 61 (4) (2010) 288–297.

[57] J. Wang, R. Zhang, Y. Xu, H. Zhou, B. Wang, S. Li, Genistein inhibits the development of atherosclerosis via inhibiting NF-κ B and VCAM-1 expression in LDLR knockout mice, Can. J. Physiol. Pharmacol. 86 (11) (2008) 777–784.

[58] H.E. Khoo, A. Azlan, S.T. Tang, S.M. Lim, Anthocyanidins and anthocyanins: colored pigments as food, pharmaceutical ingredients, and the potential health benefits, Food Nutr. Res. 61 (1) (2017) 1361779.

[59] P. Mena, R. Domínguez-Perles, A. Gironés-Vilaplana, N. Baenas, C. García-Viguera, D.Villaño, Flavan-3-ols, anthocyanins, and inflammation, IUBMB Life 66 (11) (2014) 745–758.
[60] A. Murakami, K. Ohnishi, Target molecules of food phytochemicals: food science bound for the next dimension, Food Funct. 3 (5) (2012) 462–476.
[61] A. Momtazi-Borojeni, S. Esmaeili, E. Abdollahi, A. Sahebkar, A review on the 1010 pharmacology and toxicology of steviol glycosides extracted from Stevia rebaudiana, Curr. Pharm. Res. (2017) 1616–1622.
[62] T.-C. Kao, M.-H. Shyu, G.-C. Yen, Glycyrrhizic acid and 18β-glycyrrhetinic acid inhibit inflammation via PI3K/Akt/GSK3β signaling and glucocorticoid receptor activation, J. Agric. Food Chem. 58 (15) (2010) 8623–8629.
[63] M.F. Andreasen, A.-K. Landbo, L.P. Christensen, Å. Hansen, A.S. Meyer, Antioxidant effects of phenolic rye (*Secale cereale* L.) extracts, monomeric hydroxycinnamates, and ferulic acid dehydrodimers on human low-density lipoproteins, J. Agric. Food Chem. 49 (8) (2001) 4090–4096.
[64] F. Natella, M. Nardini, M. Di Felice, C. Scaccini, Benzoic and cinnamic acid derivatives as antioxidants: structure-activity relation, J. Agric. Food Chem. 47 (4) (1999) 1453–1459.
[65] C.-H. Wu, S.-C. Chen, T.-T. Ou, C.-C. Chyau, Y.-C. Chang, C.-J. Wang, Mulberry leaf polyphenol extracts reduced hepatic lipid accumulation involving regulation of adenosine monophosphate activated protein kinase and lipogenic enzymes, J. Funct. Foods 5 (4) (2013) 1620–1632.
[66] K.C. Chan, H.H. Ho, C.N. Huang, M.C. Lin, H.M. Chen, C.J. Wang, Mulberry leaf extract inhibits vascular smooth muscle cell migration involving a block of small GT-Pase and Akt/NF-kappaB signals, J. Agric. Food Chem. 57 (19) (2009) 9147–9153.
[67] M. Gundogdu, F. Muradoglu, R.I.G. Sensoy, H.Yilmaz, Determination of fruit chemical properties of *Morus nigra* L., *Morus alba* L. and *Morus rubra* L. by HPLC, Sci. Hortic. 132 (2011) 37–41.
[68] B. Andallu, M. Shankaran, R. Ullagaddi, S. Iyer, In vitro free radical scavenging and in vivo antioxidant potential of mulberry (Morus indica L.) leaves, J. Herbal Med. 4 (1) (2014) 10–17.
[69] M.T. Lee, W.C. Lin, B.Yu, T.T. Lee, Antioxidant capacity of phytochemicals and their potential effects on oxidative status in animals—a review, Asian Australas. J. Anim. Sci. 30 (3) (2017) 299–308.
[70] W. Stahl, H. Sies, Antioxidant activity of carotenoids, Mol. Asp. Med. 24 (6) (2003) 345–351.
[71] J.G. Erhardt, C. Meisner, J.C. Bode, C. Bode, Lycopene, β-carotene, and colorectal adenomas, Am. J. Clin. Nutr. 78 (6) (2003) 1219–1224.
[72] A.V. Rao, L.G. Rao, Carotenoids and human health, Pharmacol. Res. 55 (3) (2007) 207–216.
[73] K.M. Kasiotis, H. Pratsinis, D. Kletsas, S.A. Haroutounian, Resveratrol and related stilbenes: their anti-aging and anti-angiogenic properties, Food Chem. Toxicol. 61 (2013) 112–120.
[74] M. de Ligt, S. Timmers, P. Schrauwen, Resveratrol and obesity: can resveratrol relieve metabolic disturbances? Biochim. Biophys. Acta Mol Basis Dis. 1852 (6) (2015) 1137–1144.
[75] H. Si, D. Liu, Dietary antiaging phytochemicals and mechanisms associated with prolonged survival, J. Nutr. Biochem. 25 (6) (2014) 581–591.
[76] P. Kopp, Resveratrol, a phytoestrogen found in red wine. A possible explanation for the conundrum of the'French paradox'? Eur. J. Endocrinol. 138 (6) (1998) 619–620.
[77] B. Catalgol, S. Batirel, Y. Taga, N.K. Ozer, Resveratrol: French paradox revisited, Front. Pharmacol. 3 (2012) 141.

[78] M.D. Knutson, C. Leeuwenburgh, Resveratrol and novel potent activators of SIRT1: effects on aging and age-related diseases, Nutr. Rev. 66 (10) (2008) 591–596.
[79] N. Sebastià, A. Montoro, J. Mañes, J.M. Soriano, A preliminary study of presence of resveratrol in skins and pulps of European and Japanese plum cultivars, J. Sci. Food Agric. 92 (15) (2012) 3091–3094.
[80] R. Di Franco, M. Calvanese, P. Murino, R. Manzo, C. Guida, D. Di Gennaro, et al., Skin toxicity from external beam radiation therapy in breast cancer patients: protective effects of resveratrol, lycopene, vitamin C and anthocianin (Ixor), Radiat. Oncol. 7 (1) (2012) 1–6.
[81] G. Risuleo, Nutraceuticals, 2016.
[82] H.J. He, G.Y. Wang, Y. Gao, W.H. Ling, Z.W. Yu, T.R. Jin, Curcumin attenuates Nrf2 signaling defect, oxidative stress in muscle and glucose intolerance in high fat diet-fed mice, World J. Diabetes 3 (5) (2012) 94–104.
[83] E. Tapia, Z.L. Zatarain-Barron, R. Hernandez-Pando, G. Zarco-Marquez, E. Molina-Jijon, M. Cristobal-Garcia, et al., Curcumin reverses glomerular hemodynamic alterations and oxidant stress in 5/6 nephrectomized rats, Phytomedicine 20 (3–4) (2013) 359–366.
[84] R. Garg, G. Maru, Dietary curcumin enhances benzo(a)pyrene-induced apoptosis resulting in a decrease in BPDE-DNA adducts in mice, J. Environ. Pathol. Toxicol. Oncol. 28 (2) (2009) 121–131.
[85] H. Cheng, W. Liu, X. Ai, Protective effect of curcumin on myocardial ischemia reperfusion injury in rats, J. Chin. Med. Mater. 28 (10) (2005) 920–922.
[86] E. Balogun, M. Hoque, P. Gong, E. Killeen, C.J. Green, R. Foresti, et al., Curcumin activates the haem oxygenase-1 gene via regulation of Nrf2 and the antioxidant-responsive element, Biochem. J. 371 (Pt. 3) (2003) 887–895.
[87] D.A. Dickinson, K.E. Iles, H. Zhang, V. Blank, H.J. Forman, Curcumin alters EpRE and AP-1 binding complexes and elevates glutamate-cysteine ligase gene expression, FASEB J. 17 (3) (2003) 473–475.
[88] E.O. Farombi, S. Shrotriya, H.K. Na, S.H. Kim, Y.J. Surh, Curcumin attenuates dimethylnitrosamine-induced liver injury in rats through Nrf2-mediated induction of heme oxygenase-1, Food Chem. Toxicol. 46 (4) (2008) 1279–1287.
[89] K. Sahin, C. Orhan, Z. Tuzcu, M. Tuzcu, N. Sahin, Curcumin ameloriates heat stress via inhibition of oxidative stress and modulation of Nrf2/HO-1 pathway in quail, Food Chem. Toxicol. 50 (11) (2012) 4035–4041.
[90] G. Borges, A. Degeneve, W. Mullen, A. Crozier, Identification of flavonoid and phenolic antioxidants in black currants, blueberries, raspberries, red currants, and cranberries, J. Agric. Food Chem. 58 (7) (2010) 3901–3909.
[91] G. Williamson, C. Manach, Bioavailability and bioefficacy of polyphenols in humans. II. Review of 93 intervention studies, Am. J. Clin. Nutr. 81 (1 Suppl) (2005) 243S–255S.
[92] C.B. Pocernich, M.L. Lange, R. Sultana, D.A. Butterfield, Nutritional approaches to modulate oxidative stress in Alzheimer's disease, Curr. Alzheimer Res. 8 (5) (2011) 452–469.
[93] K. Horvathova, L. Novotny, D. Tothova, A. Vachalkova, Determination of free radical scavenging activity of quercetin, rutin, luteolin and apigenin in H2O2-treated human ML cells K562, Neoplasma 51 (5) (2004) 395–399.
[94] N. Chondrogianni, S. Kapeta, I. Chinou, K. Vassilatou, I. Papassideri, E.S. Gonos, Anti-ageing and rejuvenating effects of quercetin, Exp. Gerontol. 45 (10) (2010) 763–771.
[95] M. Lesjak, I. Beara, N. Simin, D. Pintać, T. Majkić, K. Bekvalac, et al., Antioxidant and anti-inflammatory activities of quercetin and its derivatives, J. Funct. Foods 40 (2018) 68–75.
[96] A. Bautista-Ortín, P. Rodríguez-Rodríguez, R. Gil-Muñoz, E. Jiménez-Pascual, N. Busse-Valverde, A. Martínez-Cutillas, et al., Influence of berry ripeness on concentration, qualitative composition and extractability of grape seed tannins, Aust. J. Grape Wine Res. 18 (2) (2012) 123–130.

[97] R. Puupponen-Pimiä, L. Nohynek, H.-L. Alakomi, K.-M. Oksman-Caldentey, Bioactive berry compounds—novel tools against human pathogens, Appl. Microbiol. Biotechnol. 67 (1) (2005) 8–18.
[98] B.S. Bushman, B. Phillips, T. Isbell, B. Ou, J.M. Crane, S.J. Knapp, Chemical composition of caneberry (Rubus spp.) seeds and oils and their antioxidant potential, J. Agric. Food Chem. 52 (26) (2004) 7982–7987.
[99] W. Mullen, J. McGinn, M.E. Lean, M.R. MacLean, P. Gardner, G.G. Duthie, et al., Ellagitannins, flavonoids, and other phenolics in red raspberries and their contribution to antioxidant capacity and vasorelaxation properties, J. Agric. Food Chem. 50 (18) (2002) 5191–5196.
[100] S.H. Nile, S.W. Park, Edible berries: bioactive components and their effect on human health, Nutrition 30 (2) (2014) 134–144.
[101] R. Bobinaitė, P. Viškelis, P.R. Venskutonis, Variation of total phenolics, anthocyanins, ellagic acid and radical scavenging capacity in various raspberry (Rubus spp.) cultivars, Food Chem. 132 (3) (2012) 1495–1501.
[102] T. Pervaiz, J. Songtao, F. Faghihi, M.S. Haider, J. Fang, Naturally occurring anthocyanin, structure, functions and biosynthetic pathway in fruit plants, J. Plant Biochem. Physiol. 5 (2) (2017) 1–9.
[103] Q. You, B. Wang, F. Chen, Z. Huang, X. Wang, P.G. Luo, Comparison of anthocyanins and phenolics in organically and conventionally grown blueberries in selected cultivars, Food Chem. 125 (1) (2011) 201–208.
[104] F.J. Olivas-Aguirre, J. Rodrigo-Garcia, N.D. Martinez-Ruiz, A.I. Cardenas-Robles, S.O. Mendoza-Diaz, E. Alvarez-Parrilla, et al., Cyanidin-3-O-glucoside: physical-chemistry, foodomics and health effects, Molecules 21 (9) (2016).
[105] A. Smeriglio, D. Barreca, E. Bellocco, D. Trombetta, Chemistry, pharmacology and health benefits of anthocyanins, Phytother. Res. 30 (8) (2016) 1265–1286.
[106] J.-M. Kong, L.-S. Chia, N.-K. Goh, T.-F. Chia, R. Brouillard, Analysis and biological activities of anthocyanins, Phytochemistry 64 (5) (2003) 923–933.
[107] F.A. Badria, A. Ananga, M. Blumenberg, Flavonoids: A Coloring Model for Cheering Up Life, BoD–Books on Demand, 2020.
[108] M.G. Miguel, Anthocyanins: antioxidant and/or anti-inflammatory activities, J. Appl. Pharm. Sci. 1 (6) (2011) 7–15.
[109] A. Srivastava, C.C. Akoh, J. Fischer, G. Krewer, Effect of anthocyanin fractions from selected cultivars of Georgia-grown blueberries on apoptosis and phase II enzymes, J. Agric. Food Chem. 55 (8) (2007) 3180–3185.
[110] S.N. Jimenez-Garcia, R.G. Guevara-Gonzalez, R. Miranda-Lopez, A.A. Feregrino-Perez, I. Torres-Pacheco, M.A. Vazquez-Cruz, Functional properties and quality characteristics of bioactive compounds in berries: biochemistry, biotechnology, and genomics, Food Res. Int. 54 (1) (2013) 1195–1207.
[111] A. Szajdek, E.J. Borowska, Bioactive compounds and health-promoting properties of berry fruits: a review, Plant Foods Hum. Nutr. 63 (4) (2008) 147–156.
[112] M. Battino, J. Beekwilder, B. Denoyes-Rothan, M. Laimer, G.J. McDougall, B. Mezzetti, Bioactive compounds in berries relevant to human health, Nutr. Rev. 67 (Suppl 1) (2009) S145–S150.
[113] P. Viskelis, M. Rubinskiene, I. Jasutiene, A. Sarkinas, R. Daubaras, L. Cesoniene, Anthocyanins, antioxidative, and antimicrobial properties of American cranberry (*Vaccinium macrocarpon* Ait.) and their press cakes, J. Food Sci. 74 (2) (2009) C157–C161.
[114] J.R. Thoppil, D. Bhatia, F.K. Barnes, E. Haznagy-Radnai, J. Hohmann, S.A. Darvesh, et al., Black currant anthocyanins abrogate oxidative stress through Nrf2-mediated antioxidant mechanisms in a rat model of hepatocellular carcinoma, Curr. Cancer Drug Targets 12 (9) (2012) 1244–1257.
[115] S. Vendrame, D. Klimis-Zacas, Anti-inflammatory effect of anthocyanins via modulation of nuclear factor-κB and mitogen-activated protein kinase signaling cascades, Nutr. Rev. 73 (6) (2015) 348–358.

[116] A. Shukla, A. Jha, R. Kumari, K. Rawat, S. Syeda, A. Shrivastava, Role of Nutraceuticals in Cancer Chemosensitization, Academic Press, 2018.
[117] A. Zanwar, S. Badole, P. Shende, M.V. Hegde, S.L. Bodhankar, Polyphenols in human health and disease, in: Cardiovascular Effects of Hesperidin: A Flavanone Glycoside, vol. 2, 2014, pp. 989–992.
[118] I. Naasani, H. Seimiya, T. Tsuruo, Telomerase inhibition, telomere shortening, and senescence of cancer cells by tea catechins, Biochem. Biophys. Res. Commun. 249 (2) (1998) 391–396.
[119] S. Coşarcă, C. Tanase, D.L. Muntean, Therapeutic aspects of catechin and its derivatives–an update, Acta Biol. Marisiensis 2 (1) (2019) 21–29.
[120] F.-Y. Fan, L.-X. Sang, M. Jiang, Catechins and their therapeutic benefits to inflammatory bowel disease, Molecules 22 (3) (2017) 484.
[121] Z. Pan, Y. Zhou, X. Luo, Y. Ruan, L. Zhou, Q. Wang, et al., Against NF-kappaB/thymic stromal lymphopoietin signaling pathway, catechin alleviates the inflammation in allergic rhinitis, Int. Immunopharmacol. 61 (2018) 241–248.
[122] A. Tapal, P.K. Tiku, Nutritional and nutraceutical improvement by enzymatic modification of food proteins, in: Enzymes in Food Biotechnology, 2019, pp. 471–481.
[123] L. Gosalbez, D. Ramon, Probiotics in transition: novel strategies, Trends Biotechnol. 33 (4) (2015) 195–196.
[124] J. Zucko, A. Starcevic, J. Diminic, D. Oros, A.M. Mortazavian, P. Putnik, Probiotic–friend or foe? Curr. Opin. Food Sci. 32 (2020) 45–49.
[125] R. Makkar, T. Behl, S. Bungau, G. Zengin, V. Mehta, A. Kumar, et al., Nutraceuticals in neurological disorders, Int. J. Mol. Sci. 21 (12) (2020).
[126] FDA, Dietary Supplement Health and Education Act of 1994, 2020, Available online: https://ods.od.nih.gov/About/DSHEA_Wording.aspx. (Accessed 11 June 2020).
[127] G.P. Biewenga, G.R. Haenen, A. Bast, The pharmacology of the antioxidant lipoic acid, Gen. Pharmacol. 29 (3) (1997) 315–331.
[128] K.P. Shay, R.F. Moreau, E.J. Smith, A.R. Smith, T.M. Hagen, Alpha-lipoic acid as a dietary supplement: molecular mechanisms and therapeutic potential, Biochim. Biophys. Acta 1790 (10) (2009) 1149–1160.
[129] J. Teichert, J. Kern, H.J. Tritschler, H. Ulrich, R. Preiss, Investigations on the pharmacokinetics of alpha-lipoic acid in healthy volunteers, Int. J. Clin. Pharmacol. Ther. 36 (12) (1998) 625–628.
[130] S. Parikh, R. Saneto, M.J. Falk, I. Anselm, B.H. Cohen, R. Haas, et al., A modern approach to the treatment of mitochondrial disease, Curr. Treat. Options Neurol. 11 (6) (2009) 414–430.
[131] S. Parikh, A. Goldstein, M.K. Koenig, F. Scaglia, G.M. Enns, R. Saneto, et al., Diagnosis and management of mitochondrial disease: a consensus statement from the Mitochondrial Medicine Society, Genet. Med. 17 (9) (2015) 689–701.
[132] M.C. Rodriguez, J.R. MacDonald, D.J. Mahoney, G. Parise, M.F. Beal, M.A. Tarnopolsky, Beneficial effects of creatine, CoQ10, and lipoic acid in mitochondrial disorders, Muscle Nerve 35 (2) (2007) 235–242.
[133] B. Barbiroli, R. Medori, H.J. Tritschler, T. Klopstock, P. Seibel, H. Reichmann, et al., Lipoic (thioctic) acid increases brain energy availability and skeletal muscle performance as shown by in vivo 31P-MRS in a patient with mitochondrial cytopathy, J. Neurol. 242 (7) (1995) 472–477.
[134] D. Ziegler, P.A. Low, W.J. Litchy, A.J. Boulton, A.I. Vinik, R. Freeman, et al., Efficacy and safety of antioxidant treatment with alpha-lipoic acid over 4 years in diabetic polyneuropathy: the NATHAN 1 trial, Diabetes Care 34 (9) (2011) 2054–2060.
[135] D. Ziegler, M. Hanefeld, K.J. Ruhnau, H. Hasche, M. Lobisch, K. Schutte, et al., Treatment of symptomatic diabetic polyneuropathy with the antioxidant alpha-lipoic acid: a 7-month multicenter randomized controlled trial (ALADIN III study). ALADIN III study group. Alpha-lipoic acid in diabetic neuropathy, Diabetes Care 22 (8) (1999) 1296–1301.

[136] A.W. El-Hattab, L.T. Emrick, W.J. Craigen, F. Scaglia, Citrulline and arginine utility in treating nitric oxide deficiency in mitochondrial disorders, Mol. Genet. Metab. 107 (3) (2012) 247–252.
[137] A.W. El-Hattab, J.W. Hsu, L.T. Emrick, L.J. Wong, W.J. Craigen, F. Jahoor, et al., Restoration of impaired nitric oxide production in MELAS syndrome with citrulline and arginine supplementation, Mol. Genet. Metab. 105 (4) (2012) 607–614.
[138] D.S. Kerr, Treatment of mitochondrial electron transport chain disorders: a review of clinical trials over the past decade, Mol. Genet. Metab. 99 (3) (2010) 246–255.
[139] Y. Koga, M. Ishibashi, I. Ueki, S. Yatsuga, R. Fukiyama, Y. Akita, et al., Effects of L-arginine on the acute phase of strokes in three patients with MELAS, Neurology 58 (5) (2002) 827–828.
[140] Y. Koga, Y. Akita, J. Nishioka, S. Yatsuga, N. Povalko, Y. Tanabe, et al., L-arginine improves the symptoms of strokelike episodes in MELAS, Neurology 64 (4) (2005) 710–712.
[141] Y. Koga, Y. Akita, N. Junko, S. Yatsuga, N. Povalko, R. Fukiyama, et al., Endothelial dysfunction in MELAS improved by l-arginine supplementation, Neurology 66 (11) (2006) 1766–1769.
[142] J.R. Brooks, H. Oketch-Rabah, T. Low Dog, D.K. Gorecki, M.L. Barrett, L. Cantilena, et al., Safety and performance benefits of arginine supplements for military personnel: a systematic review, Nutr. Rev. 74 (11) (2016) 708–721.
[143] J.M. Gerard, A. Luisiri, A fatal overdose of arginine hydrochloride, J. Toxicol. Clin. Toxicol. 35 (6) (1997) 621–625.
[144] M.A. Tarnopolsky, The mitochondrial cocktail: rationale for combined nutraceutical therapy in mitochondrial cytopathies, Adv. Drug Deliv. Rev. 60 (13–14) (2008) 1561–1567.
[145] L. Ernster, G. Dallner, Biochemical, physiological and medical aspects of ubiquinone function, Biochim. Biophys. Acta 1271 (1) (1995) 195–204.
[146] H.N. Bhagavan, R.K. Chopra, Plasma coenzyme Q10 response to oral ingestion of coenzyme Q10 formulations, Mitochondrion 7 (Suppl) (2007) S78–S88.
[147] H.N. Bhagavan, R.K. Chopra, Coenzyme Q10: absorption, tissue uptake, metabolism and pharmacokinetics, Free Radic. Res. 40 (5) (2006) 445–453.
[148] O. Musumeci, A. Naini, A.E. Slonim, N. Skavin, G.L. Hadjigeorgiou, N. Krawiecki, et al., Familial cerebellar ataxia with muscle coenzyme Q10 deficiency, Neurology 56 (7) (2001) 849–855.
[149] S. Zierz, G. Jahns, F. Jerusalem, Coenzyme Q in serum and muscle of 5 patients with Kearns-Sayre syndrome and 12 patients with ophthalmoplegia plus, J. Neurol. 236 (2) (1989) 97–101.
[150] A. Chan, H. Reichmann, A. Kogel, A. Beck, R. Gold, Metabolic changes in patients with mitochondrial myopathies and effects of coenzyme Q10 therapy, J. Neurol. 245 (10) (1998) 681–685.
[151] N. Bresolin, C. Doriguzzi, C. Ponzetto, C. Angelini, I. Moroni, E. Castelli, et al., Ubidecarenone in the treatment of mitochondrial myopathies: a multi-center double-blind trial, J. Neurol. Sci. 100 (1–2) (1990) 70–78.
[152] E.I. Glover, J. Martin, A. Maher, R.E. Thornhill, G.R. Moran, M.A. Tarnopolsky, A randomized trial of coenzyme Q10 in mitochondrial disorders, Muscle Nerve 42 (5) (2010) 739–748.
[153] R.S. Chen, C.C. Huang, N.S. Chu, Coenzyme Q10 treatment in mitochondrial encephalomyopathies. Short-term double-blind, crossover study, Eur. Neurol. 37 (4) (1997) 212–218.
[154] R. Gold, P. Seibel, G. Reinelt, R. Schindler, P. Landwehr, A. Beck, et al., Phosphorus magnetic resonance spectroscopy in the evaluation of mitochondrial myopathies: results of a 6-month therapy study with coenzyme Q, Eur. Neurol. 36 (4) (1996) 191–196.

[155] K. Hosoe, M. Kitano, H. Kishida, H. Kubo, K. Fujii, M. Kitahara, Study on safety and bioavailability of ubiquinol (Kaneka QH) after single and 4-week multiple oral administration to healthy volunteers, Regulat. Toxicol. Pharmacol. 47 (1) (2007) 19–28.
[156] H. Ikematsu, K. Nakamura, S. Harashima, K. Fujii, N. Fukutomi, Safety assessment of coenzyme Q10 (Kaneka Q10) in healthy subjects: a double-blind, randomized, placebo-controlled trial, Regulat. Toxicol. Pharmacol. 44 (3) (2006) 212–218.
[157] T. Hidaka, K. Fujii, I. Funahashi, N. Fukutomi, K. Hosoe, Safety assessment of coenzyme Q10 (CoQ10), Biofactors 32 (1–4) (2008) 199–208.
[158] A. Ormazabal, M. Casado, M. Molero-Luis, J. Montoya, S. Rahman, S.B. Aylett, et al., Can folic acid have a role in mitochondrial disorders? Drug Discov. Today 20 (11) (2015) 1349–1354.
[159] P. Quijada-Fraile, M. O'Callaghan, E. Martin-Hernandez, R. Montero, A. Garcia-Cazorla, A.M. de Aragon, et al., Follow-up of folinic acid supplementation for patients with cerebral folate deficiency and Kearns-Sayre syndrome, Orphanet J. Rare Dis. 9 (2014) 217.
[160] M. Serrano, M.T. Garcia-Silva, E. Martin-Hernandez, M. O'Callaghan Mdel, P. Quijada, A. Martinez-Aragon, et al., Kearns-Sayre syndrome: cerebral folate deficiency, MRI findings and new cerebrospinal fluid biochemical features, Mitochondrion 10 (5) (2010) 429–432.
[161] B. Perez-Duenas, A. Ormazabal, C. Toma, B. Torrico, B. Cormand, M. Serrano, et al., Cerebral folate deficiency syndromes in childhood: clinical, analytical, and etiologic aspects, Arch. Neurol. 68 (5) (2011) 615–621.
[162] F. Depeint, W.R. Bruce, N. Shangari, R. Mehta, P.J. O'Brien, Mitochondrial function and toxicity: role of the B vitamin family on mitochondrial energy metabolism, Chem. Biol. Interact. 163 (1–2) (2006) 94–112.
[163] Institute of Medicine, Dietary Reference Intakes for Thiamin, Riboflavin, Niacin, Vitamin B6, Folate, Vitamin B12, Pantothenic Acid, Biotin, and Choline, The National Academies Collection: Reports Funded by National Institutes of Health, National Academies Press, Washington (DC), 1998.
[164] H.M. Abourjaily, A review of Niaspan, an extended-release niacin, Nutr. Clin. Care 4 (5) (2001) 250–255.
[165] K. Majamaa, H. Rusanen, A.M. Remes, J. Pyhtinen, I.E. Hassinen, Increase of blood NAD+ and attenuation of lactacidemia during nicotinamide treatment of a patient with the MELAS syndrome, Life Sci. 58 (8) (1996) 691–699.
[166] R.C. Harris, K. Soderlund, E. Hultman, Elevation of creatine in resting and exercised muscle of normal subjects by creatine supplementation, Clin. Sci. 83 (3) (1992) 367–374.
[167] E. Hultman, K. Soderlund, J.A. Timmons, G. Cederblad, P.L. Greenhaff, Muscle creatine loading in men, J. Appl. Physiol. 81 (1) (1996) 232–237.
[168] M.A. Tarnopolsky, B.D. Roy, J.R. MacDonald, A randomized, controlled trial of creatine monohydrate in patients with mitochondrial cytopathies, Muscle Nerve 20 (12) (1997) 1502–1509.
[169] K. Komura, E. Hobbiebrunken, E.K. Wilichowski, F.A. Hanefeld, Effectiveness of creatine monohydrate in mitochondrial encephalomyopathies, Pediatr. Neurol. 28 (1) (2003) 53–58.
[170] Office of Dietary Supplements, National Institutes of Health, Dietary Supplement Label Databaseexternal Link Disclaimer, 2021.
[171] C. Garone, M.A. Donati, M. Sacchini, B. Garcia-Diaz, C. Bruno, S. Calvo, et al., Mitochondrial encephalomyopathy due to a novel mutation in ACAD9, JAMA Neurol. 70 (9) (2013) 1177–1179.
[172] P.L. Bernsen, F.J. Gabreels, W. Ruitenbeek, H.L. Hamburger, Treatment of complex I deficiency with riboflavin, J. Neurol. Sci. 118 (2) (1993) 181–187.

[173] R.F. Ogle, J. Christodoulou, E. Fagan, R.B. Blok, D.M. Kirby, K.L. Seller, et al., Mitochondrial myopathy with tRNA(Leu(UUR)) mutation and complex I deficiency responsive to riboflavin, J. Pediatr. 130 (1) (1997) 138–145.
[174] V. Griebel, I. Krageloh-Mann, W. Ruitenbeek, J.M. Trijbels, W. Paulus, A mitochondrial myopathy in an infant with lactic acidosis, Dev. Med. Child Neurol. 32 (6) (1990) 528–531.
[175] L.R. Gray, S.C. Tompkins, E.B. Taylor, Regulation of pyruvate metabolism and human disease, Cell. Mol. Life Sci. 71 (14) (2014) 2577–2604.
[176] Authority EFS, Benfotiamine, thiamine monophosphate chloride and thiamine pyrophosphate chloride, as sources of vitamin B1 added for nutritional purposes to food supplements—scientific opinion of the panel on food additives and nutrient sources added to food (ANS), EFSA J. 6 (11) (2008) 864.
[177] H.C. Lou, Correction of increased plasma pyruvate and plasma lactate levels using large doses of thiamine in patients with Kearns-Sayre syndrome, Arch. Neurol. 38 (7) (1981) 469.
[178] Y. Li, H.E. Schellhorn, New developments and novel therapeutic perspectives for vitamin C, J. Nutr. 137 (10) (2007) 2171–2184.
[179] B. Frei, L. England, B.N. Ames, Ascorbate is an outstanding antioxidant in human blood plasma, Proc. Natl. Acad. Sci. U. S. A. 86 (16) (1989) 6377–6381.
[180] R.A. Jacob, G. Sotoudeh, Vitamin C function and status in chronic disease, Nutr. Clin. Care 5 (2) (2002) 66–74.
[181] S.J. Padayatty, H. Sun, Y. Wang, H.D. Riordan, S.M. Hewitt, A. Katz, et al., Vitamin C pharmacokinetics: implications for oral and intravenous use, Ann. Intern. Med. 140 (7) (2004) 533–537.
[182] A.R. Mangels, G. Block, C.M. Frey, B.H. Patterson, P.R. Taylor, E.P. Norkus, et al., The bioavailability to humans of ascorbic acid from oranges, orange juice and cooked broccoli is similar to that of synthetic ascorbic acid, J. Nutr. 123 (6) (1993) 1054–1061.
[183] A. Toscano, M.C. Fazio, G. Vita, S. Cannavo, N. Bresolin, L. Bet, et al., Early-onset cerebellar ataxia, myoclonus and hypogonadism in a case of mitochondrial complex III deficiency treated with vitamins K3 and C, J. Neurol. 242 (4) (1995) 203–209.
[184] W.S. Blaner, Vitamin E: the enigmatic one! J. Lipid Res. 54 (9) (2013) 2293–2294.
[185] Institute of Medicine, Dietary Reference Intakes for Vitamin C, Vitamin E, Selenium, and Carotenoids, Washington (DC), 2000.
[186] S.L. Booth, Vitamin K: food composition and dietary intakes, Food Nutr. Res. 56 (2012).
[187] B.J. Marriage, M.T. Clandinin, I.M. Macdonald, D.M. Glerum, Cofactor treatment improves ATP synthetic capacity in patients with oxidative phosphorylation disorders, Mol. Genet. Metab. 81 (4) (2004) 263–272.
[188] K.A. Jung, M.K. Kwak, The Nrf2 system as a potential target for the development of indirect antioxidants, Molecules 15 (10) (2010) 7266–7291.
[189] K. Sahin, C. Orhan, M. Tuzcu, S. Ali, N. Sahin, A. Hayirli, Epigallocatechin-3-gallate prevents lipid peroxidation and enhances antioxidant defense system via modulating hepatic nuclear transcription factors in heat-stressed quails, Poult. Sci. 89 (10) (2010) 2251–2258.
[190] A.C. Mamede, S.D. Tavares, A.M. Abrantes, J. Trindade, J.M. Maia, M.F. Botelho, The role of vitamins in cancer: a review, Nutr. Cancer 63 (4) (2011) 479–494.
[191] L.F. Cardozo, L.M. Pedruzzi, P. Stenvinkel, M.B. Stockler-Pinto, J.B. Daleprane, M. Leite Jr., et al., Nutritional strategies to modulate inflammation and oxidative stress pathways via activation of the master antioxidant switch Nrf2, Biochimie 95 (8) (2013) 1525–1533.
[192] Y.J. Surh, Cancer chemoprevention with dietary phytochemicals, Nat. Rev. Cancer 3 (10) (2003) 768–780.

[193] L. Baird, A.T. Dinkova-Kostova, The cytoprotective role of the Keap1-Nrf2 pathway, Arch. Toxicol. 85 (4) (2011) 241–272.

[194] A. Kobayashi, M.I. Kang, Y. Watai, K.I. Tong, T. Shibata, K. Uchida, et al., Oxidative and electrophilic stresses activate Nrf2 through inhibition of ubiquitination activity of Keap1, Mol. Cell. Biol. 26 (1) (2006) 221–229.

[195] K. Takaya, T. Suzuki, H. Motohashi, K. Onodera, S. Satomi, T.W. Kensler, et al., Validation of the multiple sensor mechanism of the Keap1-Nrf2 system, Free Radic. Biol. Med. 53 (4) (2012) 817–827.

[196] H.K. Na, Y.J. Surh, Modulation of Nrf2-mediated antioxidant and detoxifying enzyme induction by the green tea polyphenol EGCG, Food Chem. Toxicol. 46 (4) (2008) 1271–1278.

[197] C.L. Saw, A.Y. Yang, D.C. Cheng, S.S. Boyanapalli, Z.Y. Su, T.O. Khor, et al., Pharmacodynamics of ginsenosides: antioxidant activities, activation of Nrf2, and potential synergistic effects of combinations, Chem. Res. Toxicol. 25 (8) (2012) 1574–1580.

[198] K. Sahin, C. Orhan, F. Akdemir, M. Tuzcu, C. Iben, N. Sahin, Resveratrol protects quail hepatocytes against heat stress: modulation of the Nrf2 transcription factor and heat shock proteins, J. Anim. Physiol. Anim. Nutr. 96 (1) (2012) 66–74.

[199] M. Tuzcu, N. Sahin, M. Karatepe, G. Cikim, U. Kilinc, K. Sahin, Epigallocatechin-3-gallate supplementation can improve antioxidant status in stressed quail, Br. Poult. Sci. 49 (5) (2008) 643–648.

[200] K. Sahin, C. Orhan, M.O. Smith, N. Sahin, Molecular targets of dietary phytochemicals for the alleviation of heat stress in poultry, World Poult. Sci. J. 69 (1) (2013) 113–124.

[201] A. Navarro, A. Boveris, Brain mitochondrial dysfunction and oxidative damage in Parkinson's disease, J. Bioenerg. Biomembr. 41 (6) (2009) 517–521.

[202] A. Lama, C. Pirozzi, C. Avagliano, C. Annunziata, M.P. Mollica, A. Calignano, et al., Nutraceuticals: an integrative approach to starve Parkinson's disease, Brain Behav. Immun. Health 2 (2020), 100037.

[203] E. Ceskova, P. Silhan, Novel treatment options in depression and psychosis, Neuropsychiatr. Dis. Treat. 14 (2018) 741–747.

[204] K. Fodor, D.M. Tit, B. Pasca, C. Bustea, D. Uivarosan, L. Endres, et al., Long-term resveratrol supplementation as a secondary prophylaxis for stroke, Oxidative Med. Cell. Longev. 2018 (2018) 4147320.

[205] S. Parikh, A. Goldstein, M.K. Koenig, F. Scaglia, G.M. Enns, R. Saneto, et al., Practice patterns of mitochondrial disease physicians in North America. Part 2: treatment, care and management, Mitochondrion 13 (6) (2013) 681–687.

[206] P.L. Bernsen, F.J. Gabreels, W. Ruitenbeek, R.C. Sengers, A.M. Stadhouders, W.O. Renier, Successful treatment of pure myopathy, associated with complex I deficiency, with riboflavin and carnitine, Arch. Neurol. 48 (3) (1991) 334–338.

[207] R. Artuch, M.A. Vilaseca, M. Pineda, Biochemical monitoring of the treatment in paediatric patients with mitochondrial disease, J. Inherit. Metab. Dis. 21 (8) (1998) 837–845.

[208] P.L. Peterson, The treatment of mitochondrial myopathies and encephalomyopathies, Biochim. Biophys. Acta 1271 (1) (1995) 275–280.

[209] P.M. Matthews, B. Ford, R.J. Dandurand, D.H. Eidelman, D. O'Connor, A. Sherwin, et al., Coenzyme Q10 with multiple vitamins is generally ineffective in treatment of mitochondrial disease, Neurology 43 (5) (1993) 884–890.

[210] S. Eleff, N.G. Kennaway, N.R. Buist, V.M. Darley-Usmar, R.A. Capaldi, W.J. Bank, et al., 31P NMR study of improvement in oxidative phosphorylation by vitamins K3 and C in a patient with a defect in electron transport at complex III in skeletal muscle, Proc. Natl. Acad. Sci. U. S. A. 81 (11) (1984) 3529–3533.

[211] A.W. El-Hattab, F. Scaglia, Disorders of carnitine biosynthesis and transport, Mol. Genet. Metab. 116 (3) (2015) 107–112.

[212] M. Banach, C. Serban, S. Ursoniu, J. Rysz, P. Muntner, P.P. Toth, et al., Statin therapy and plasma coenzyme Q10 concentrations—a systematic review and meta-analysis of placebo-controlled trials, Pharmacol. Res. 99 (2015) 329–336.
[213] P.H. Langsjoen, A.M. Langsjoen, The clinical use of HMG CoA-reductase inhibitors and the associated depletion of coenzyme Q10. A review of animal and human publications, Biofactors 18 (1–4) (2003) 101–111.
[214] A.M. Moreno-Fernandez, M.D. Cordero, J. Garrido-Maraver, E. Alcocer-Gomez, N. Casas-Barquero, M.I. Carmona-Lopez, et al., Oral treatment with amitriptyline induces coenzyme Q deficiency and oxidative stress in psychiatric patients, J. Psychiatr. Res. 46 (3) (2012) 341–345.
[215] C.L. van der Wilt, H.M. Pinedo, K. Smid, J. Cloos, P. Noordhuis, G.J. Peters, Effect of folinic acid on fluorouracil activity and expression of thymidylate synthase, Semin. Oncol. 19 (2 Suppl 3) (1992) 16–25.
[216] J.K. Wilkin, O. Wilkin, R. Kapp, R. Donachie, M.E. Chernosky, J. Buckner, Aspirin blocks nicotinic acid-induced flushing, Clin. Pharmacol. Ther. 31 (4) (1982) 478–482.
[217] P.W. Jungnickel, P.A. Maloley, E.L. Vander Tuin, T.E. Peddicord, J.R. Campbell, Effect of two aspirin pretreatment regimens on niacin-induced cutaneous reactions, J. Gen. Intern. Med. 12 (10) (1997) 591–596.
[218] H.E. Bays, C.A. Dujovne, Drug interactions of lipid-altering drugs, Drug Saf. 19 (5) (1998) 355–371.
[219] M.C. Cheung, X.Q. Zhao, A. Chait, J.J. Albers, B.G. Brown, Antioxidant supplements block the response of HDL to simvastatin-niacin therapy in patients with coronary artery disease and low HDL, Arterioscler. Thromb. Vasc. Biol. 21 (8) (2001) 1320–1326.
[220] B.G. Brown, X.Q. Zhao, A. Chait, L.D. Fisher, M.C. Cheung, J.S. Morse, et al., Simvastatin and niacin, antioxidant vitamins, or the combination for the prevention of coronary disease, N. Engl. J. Med. 345 (22) (2001) 1583–1592.
[221] S.A. Hanninen, P.B. Darling, M.J. Sole, A. Barr, M.E. Keith, The prevalence of thiamin deficiency in hospitalized patients with congestive heart failure, J. Am. Coll. Cardiol. 47 (2) (2006) 354–361.
[222] H. Seligmann, H. Halkin, S. Rauchfleisch, N. Kaufmann, M. Motro, Z. Vered, et al., Thiamine deficiency in patients with congestive heart failure receiving long-term furosemide therapy: a pilot study, Am. J. Med. 91 (2) (1991) 151–155.
[223] C. Tikiz, Z. Unlu, A. Sener, M. Efe, C. Tuzun, Comparison of the efficacy of lower and higher molecular weight viscosupplementation in the treatment of hip osteoarthritis, Clin. Rheumatol. 24 (3) (2005) 244–250.
[224] Drug-Nutrient Interaction Task Force CC, National Institutes of Health, Important Information to Know When You Are Taking: Warfarin (Coumadin) and Vitamin K, 2012.
[225] K.M. Camp, D. Krotoski, M.A. Parisi, K.A. Gwinn, B.H. Cohen, C.S. Cox, et al., Nutritional interventions in primary mitochondrial disorders: developing an evidence base, Mol. Genet. Metab. 119 (3) (2016) 187–206.
[226] A. Karaa, S. Rahman, A. Lombes, P. Yu-Wai-Man, M.K. Sheikh, S. Alai-Hansen, et al., Common data elements for clinical research in mitochondrial disease: a National Institute for Neurological Disorders and Stroke project, J. Inherit. Metab. Dis. 40 (3) (2017) 403–414.

CHAPTER 11

Phytonutrients in regulation of malabsorption disorders

Giuseppe Annunziata[a] and Gian Carlo Tenore[a]
[a]Department of Pharmacy, University of Naples Federico II, Naples, Italy

1. Summary

Malabsorption is a common clinical condition affecting a large number of people of different age groups worldwide. This condition is generally due to functional and/or structural abnormalities of the intestinal mucosa that become unable to absorb the nutrients introduced with the diet. It is mainly secondary to various diseases (including bacterial or viral infections, or autoimmune diseases) or physiological conditions, such as aging. Malabsorption causes a large variety of gastrointestinal symptoms, including diarrhea, constipation, steatorrhea, abdominal pain, or malnutrition. Not recently, both scientific research and clinical practice focused attention on the identification of alternative remedies for the management of malabsorption, in terms of symptom treatments. Among these, phytonutrients (plant-derived bioactive compounds able to exert biological effects in humans) are emerging as promising and useful tool for a nutraceutical treatment of intestinal symptoms. The purpose of this chapter is to provide a general overview on the main phytonutrients with reported efficacy on gastrointestinal symptoms secondary to malabsorption.

2. Introduction

The term "malabsorption" refers to a peculiar clinical condition where digestion, absorption, and transport of nutrients at the intestinal level are affected. In particular, after food ingestion, nutrients are subjected to: (i) intraluminal hydrolysis, (ii) enzymatic digestion (operated by enzymes on the brush-border membrane of small intestine enterocytes), and (iii) absorption across the intestinal mucosa. Generally, the term malabsorption is improperly used when one of these three steps is affected, but it more specifically refers to point (iii) [1,2].

The Role of Phytonutrients in Metabolic Disorders
https://doi.org/10.1016/B978-0-12-824356-5.00005-9

Several disorders and/or functional abnormalities, such as celiac disease, pancreatic insufficiency, and bacterial or viral infections, are among the leading causes of malabsorption. In particular, they can alter the physiological structure of the gastrointestinal (GI) epithelium or the normal release of digestive enzymes, resulting in impaired absorption of macronutrients (i.e., fats, carbohydrates, proteins), micronutrients (i.e., vitamins and minerals), or both. When nonabsorbed, nutrients transit toward the lower gut to be excreted, causing the characteristic intestinal symptomatology, including malnutrition, diarrhea, constipation, steatorrhea, and abdominal pain [1–3]. More specifically:

- bacterial overgrowth causes bile salts deconjugation and dehydroxylation, resulting in impaired fat absorption. Nonabsorbed fats and bile salts in turn cause water secretion into the colon, resulting in diarrhea. Moreover, nonabsorbed fats bind liposoluble vitamins, causing their deficit
- nonabsorbed carbohydrates are fermented by the colon microbiota, producing (i) gases (including H_2, methane, carbon dioxide) that cause bloating, abdominal distension, and abdominal pain, and (ii) short-chain fatty acids (i.e., butyrate, propionate, acetate) that cause diarrhea
- nonabsorbed macro- and micronutrients can cause malnutrition [1,4].

Malabsorption-related GI disorders are frequently associated with and exacerbated by pharmacological treatments [5], cultural habits [6], and socioeconomic factors [7]. In this regard, since the majority of pharmacological treatments are not free of undesirable effects involving the GI system, both research and clinical practice focused attention on identification of alternative options for the treatment of malabsorption-related GI disorders [8]. Among these, phytonutrients and phytochemicals are the most promising ones [8,9]. These are chemical constituents of both vegetable and medical plants, whose efficacy in regulation of GI symptoms has been widely reported.

In the following section of the present chapter, we will provide an overview on malabsorption, analyzing its different features. In addition, the role of the most representative phytonutrients in the management of malabsorption-related GI disorders will be presented.

3. Pathophysiology of malabsorption

3.1 Leading causes of malabsorption

3.1.1 Giardiasis

Giardiasis is a common GI parasitic infection with a high prevalence [2,10,11], estimated at about 200 million people in the world, according to the World Health Organization [11]. It is caused by *Giardia intestinalis*, a flagellated protozoan parasite that colonizes the upper GI tract of many vertebrates, including humans [2,11].

Although most patients are asymptomatic [2], giardiasis is associated with a large number of GI symptoms, including diarrhea, nausea, steatorrhea, abdominal pain, and weight loss [11] for malabsorption [2], especially in children [12–22]. More specifically, malabsorption is caused by histological alteration at the small intestinal mucosal level, such as villous atrophy with crypt hyperplasia and intraepithelial lymphocyte infiltration [23]. This in turn severely impairs both the activity of such enzymes (i.e., disaccharidases) and the fluid electrolytes absorption [24]. Also, *Giardia intestinalis* infection causes alteration in various luminal factors (including bile salt deconjugation, enzyme inhibition, bacterial overgrowth) that can contribute to both morphological abnormalities and malabsorption development [25].

3.1.2 Celiac disease

Celiac disease (CD) is a unique autoimmune disorder characterized by a peculiar histological and serological profile, triggered by ingestion of gluten in genetically predisposed individuals [26]. The prevalence in the world is about 0.5%–1%, with increasing cases in Western countries [27–34]. The diagnosis of CD is more frequent in women than in men (women-to-men ratio ranged from 2:1 to 3:1) [26,35]. It has been well established that both genetic (human leukocyte antigen (HLA)-DQ2 and HLA-DQ8), the auto-antigen involved in tissue transglutaminase) and environmental (gluten) factors concur in the development of CD [36].

CD is associated with a plethora of both intestinal and extraintestinal symptoms [2,36] that share the same etiology based on an immune-mediated intestinal mucosa atrophy that results in impaired absorption of nutrients [2,36]. More specifically, intestinal symptoms include diarrhea, abdominal distension, bloating constipation, and abdominal pain [37,38]; moreover, irritable bowel syndrome- and dyspepsia-like symptoms are frequently associated with CD [35]. It appears clear that, due to the CD Pathophysiology, these GI symptoms are related to malabsorption as the main leading cause. This in turn causes weight loss, asthenia, cachexia, sarcopenia, hypoalbuminemia, and failure to thrive in children [36]. Similarly, other extraintestinal symptoms include iron deficiency and microcytic anemia (caused by iron, folate, and vitamin B12 malabsorption), osteopenia and osteoporosis (caused by calcium and vitamin D3 malabsorption) [36].

3.1.3 Whipple's disease

Whipple's disease is a chronic, multisystemic disorder caused by *Tropheryma whipplei* infection [39] which involves various organs, mainly the GI tract [2]. It is a rare disease with a prevalence of about 1 per 1 million [40]; the incidence is associated with poor hygienic habits and/or attitudes and related to oral-fecal route transmission [39]. In addition to other symptoms, Whipple's disease presents a classical GI symptomatology characterized by diarrhea, abdominal pain, weight loss [39].

3.1.4 Tropical sprue

Tropical sprue is a syndrome with unknown etiology considered as a primary diagnosis in patients with severe GI symptoms (more frequently diarrhea) resident in or returning from tropical or subtropical areas. The leading cause of tropical sprue is the intestinal colonization with fecal flora or other protozoan parasites (*including Isospora belli, Cryptosporidium parvus, Cyclospora cayetanensis*) causing structural and/or functional abnormalities at the intestinal level, resulting in malabsorption of several nutrients (i.e., xylose, folate, and vitamin B12) [2].

3.1.5 Aging

With aging, most GI functions suffer a progressive decline, resulting in onset of digestive problems. This is mostly referred to as the globally reduced absorptive capacity of the small intestine, mainly due to structural and/or functional alterations of the GI mucosa. This results in malabsorption of various micro- and macronutrients [2]. More specifically, it is mainly caused by gastric hypochlorhydria, dysmotility, or chronic intestinal ischemia [41]. As the main consequences of aging-related malabsorption, malnutrition, weight loss, and cachexia occur frequently in the elderly, contributing to morbidity and mortality [2].

3.2 Single macronutrient malabsorption

As mentioned earlier, malabsorption may involve both micro- and macronutrients, causing various symptoms or pathological conditions. Here we focused attention on malabsorption of carbohydrates and fats, contributing to the development of a severe GI symptomatology.

3.2.1 Oligosaccharides and monosaccharides malabsorption

To be absorbed, carbohydrates need to be previously digested. This is a preliminary luminal digestion operated by specific enzymes producing oligosaccharides. These in turn are further hydrolyzed by disaccharidases, a class of digestive enzymes produced by epithelial cells and localized in the brush border of enterocytes. Once digested, the hydrolysis products can be absorbed across the mucosal microvillous membrane. Several diseases (i.e., gastroenteritis, celiac diseases) may cause a chronic deficiency of these enzymes, resulting in carbohydrates malabsorption [2]. One of the most common hydrolase deficiencies is related to lactase, the enzyme hydrolyzing lactose into glucose and galactose. A lactase deficiency (constitutional, secondary, or congenital) induces lactose intolerance [2]. Congenital hydrolase deficiencies (i.e., sucrase-isomaltase deficiency) are rare genetic mutations causing production of an incomplete enzyme or of a complete enzyme that is not transported to the brush border [2]. Also, malabsorption of monosaccharides (i.e., fructose) may be caused by factors that modulate the functional capability of their transporters (i.e., GLUT5) [42,43]. Malabsorption of oligosaccharides and monosaccharides mainly causes abdominal distension, flatulence, cramps, and diarrhea [42,43].

3.2.2 Bile acid malabsorption

Bile acids are synthesized in the liver, stored in the gallbladder, and excreted into the small intestine, where they play a central role in the correct absorption of dietary fats and sterols. In particular, bile acids emulsify the triglycerides and form micelles with monoglycerides and fatty acids that will be absorbed across the intestinal mucosa. In the distal intestine, more than 90% of bile acids are reabsorbed through the enterohepatic recirculation. The nonreabsorption of bile acids firstly causes malabsorption of fats. On the other hand, the malabsorption of both bile acids and fats causes diarrhea and steatorrhea [1,2].

3.3 Assessment of intestinal malabsorption

The most relevant tests for the diagnosis of intestinal malabsorption [3] are reported in Table 1.

4. The role of phytonutrients in management of malabsorption-related disorders

As largely discussed in the previous section of this chapter, malabsorption represents a disabling pathological condition, due to its related GI symptoms. A considerable amount of evidence reported the efficacy of several phytonutrients in the treatment of GI symptoms, consistent with the popular

Table 1 Diagnostic tests for diagnosis of intestinal malabsorption.

Disorder	Test	Procedure	Reference
Carbohydrate malabsorption	Benedict's test	This test is based on the ability of sugar to act as reducing agents. A specific chemical reaction is performed on stool samples, obtaining a peculiar colored precipitate that is used for a semi-quantitative determination of reducing sugars. This test has poor sensitivity and specificity.	[44]
	Hydrogen breath test	This test is based on the concept that colon microbiota fermentation produces gases (N_2, O_2, CO_2, H_2, and CH_4) that diffuse in the blood and are exhaled by breath. This test measures the amount of H_2 in breath after ingestion of 25 g of lactose (children: 1 g/kg). Samples are collected each 30 min for 3 h. Sensitivity: 77.5%–Specificity: 97.6%	[45,46]
	Genetic investigation	Identification of specific mutations (C/T-13910 and G/A-22018) in gene encoding lactase-pholiriz hydrolase.	[47]
	Lactose tolerance test	Measurement of serum glucose levels after integestion of 50 g lactose within 3 h. Low sensitivity and specificity.	[48,49]
	Urine galactose	Measurement of urine levels of galactose after ingestion of 50 g of lactose. High urinary galactose levels indicate optimal intestinal lactase activity; low urinary galactose levels indicate lactase deficiency.	[50–52]
	Intestine biopsy	Biochemical assay for evaluation of the disaccharidase enzymatic activity. Golden standard for diagnosis of lactase deficiency.	[45,53]
	D-xylose absorption test	This test is based on the concept that D-xylose is a monosaccharide absorbed unchanged at duodenum and jejunum level and minimally metabolized. Serum and urinary concentration of D-xylose are measured after ingestion of 25 g of D-xylose after 1 and 5 h, respectively.	[54]
	Bacterial overgrowth	Small intestinal bacterial overgrowth is defined when the bacterial load in jejuna aspirate is more than 10^5 CFU/mL. This test has low sensitivity (30%–40%) and good specificity (80%).	[55]

Fat malabsorption	Fecal fat test	Determination of fecal fat levels with dietary fat control in 72-h stool samples.	[56]
	Fecal fat globules	Microscopy determination of fat globules in stool samples. The test allows detecting triglycerides and fatty acids (of dietary origin) and phospholipids and cholesterol (from intestinal epithelial cell turnover).	[57]
	Breath test	Measurement of breath $^{13}CO_2$ after ingestion of ^{13}C-mixed-chain triglycerides added to a standard fatty meal. Sensitivity: 89%, specificity: 81%.	[58–60]
	Serum retinyl palmitate	This test is based on the concept that, as a fat-soluble vitamin, retinol (vitamin A) follows the same metabolic fate of dietary lipids. It measures serum levels of retinyl palmitate (an equivalent of retinol).	[61]
	Pancreatic exocrine insufficiency test	Aspiration and analysis of the pancreatic content during administration of secretin-CCK/cerulean or secretin.	[62]
	Fecal elastase-1	This is a monoclonal antibody test performed on stool sample. It has good sensitivity (ranged from 73% to 100%) only in severe exocrine pancreatic insufficiency patients.	[62,63]
Bile salt malabsorption	Four tests are available for direct measure of bile acids: • Measurement of ^{14}C-glycocholate in breath and stool • Measurement of fecal bile acid levels • ^{75}Selenium HomotauroCholic Test • Measurement of 7α-hydroxy-4-cholesten-3-one serum levels.		[64–69]
Vitamin B12 malabsorption	Schilling test	Measurement of vitamin B12 urine levels after administration of radiolabelled vitamin B12 with or without intrinsic factor.	[70]

phytotherapy. It represents a valid alternative for a general management of malabsorption-associated GI disturbances. In this section, we summarized the most relevant evidence on the use of phytonutrients for these medical scopes [8].

Dietary fibers are indigestible carbohydrates that are metabolized by gut microbiota. They include nonstarch polysaccharides (NSP) (i.e., cellulose, hemicelluloses, gum, pectin, resistant starch, resistant dextrin, and lignin). Dietary fibers are classified into two groups: soluble (β-glucans, pectins, gums, mucilages, and hemicelluloses) and insoluble (celluloses, some hemicelluloses, and lignins) [8]. In contrast with soluble fibers that undergo colonic fermentation producing short-chain fatty acids (SCFAs) (i.e., propionate, acetate, and butyrate), insoluble fibers are minimally fermented and increase fecal mass, accelerating the colonic transit [71–73]. Thus, regular consumption of this class of fiber may be useful in the treatment of constipation. In addition, SCFAs produced by colonic fermentation of soluble fiber (in particular, butyrate) have been reported to increase the colonic water absorption, which thus may prevent diarrhea [74]. Fibers from Psyllium have been demonstrated to both increase the frequency and improve the consistency of stool [75].

In addition to dietary fiber, evidence reported the efficacy of various medical herbs in the treatment of GI disorders. More specifically, herbs such as Senna, *Aloe vera*, Frangula, Cascara, and Rhubarb have been demonstrated to relieve constipation [76].These herbs contain within their phytocomplex anthraquinones, a specific class of bioactive compounds (present in the form of glucoside derivatives of anthracene) that act as important botanic laxatives [77]. In particular, anthraquinones exert their anticonstipation effects by increasing the fluid content in the colon and altering the intestinal motility. At the intestinal level, anthraquinones stimulate the chloride release from intestinal mucosa, determining an osmotic effect with conveying water and sodium that accumulate in the intestinal lumen, increasing the volume and fluidity of feces. Moreover, anthraquinones cause an irritation of the intestinal smooth muscle cells, increasing muscle contraction and peristalsis [78]. The anti-constipation effects of herbs containing anthraquinones have been reported in several clinical trials [77,79,80].

5. Conclusions

In summary, as widely discussed, several factors and/or pathological conditions can severely affect both the function and structure of the GI tract, causing malabsorption of different micro- and macronutrients. This in turn results in the onset of GI symptoms that may be efficiently treated with phytonutrients from various plants and medical herbs. Further studies and clinical trials will be necessary to produce specific guidelines aimed to provide official nutraceutical treatment schemes for these disabling disorders.

References

[1] J. Keller, P. Layer, The pathophysiology of malabsorption, Viszeralmedizin 30 (2014) 150–154, https://doi.org/10.1159/000364794.

[2] J.C. Bai, Malabsorption syndromes, Digestion 5 (1998) 530–546, https://doi.org/10.1159/000007529.

[3] K. Nikaki, G.L. Gupte, Assessment of intestinal malabsorption, Best Pr. Res. Clin. Gastroenterol. 30 (2016) 225–235, https://doi.org/10.1016/j.bpg.2016.03.003.

[4] J. Keller, Gastrointestinal digestion and absorption, in: W.L. Lennarz, M.D. Lane (Eds.), Encycl. Biol. Chem., second ed., Elsevier, 2013, https://doi.org/10.1016/B978-0-12-378630-2.00106-7.

[5] E. Myasoedova, N.J. Talley, N.J. Manek, C.S. Crowson, Prevalence and risk factors of gastrointestinal disorders in patients with rheumatoid arthritis: results from a population-based survey in Olmsted County, Minnesota, Gastroenterol. Res. Pr. 2011 (2011) 745829, https://doi.org/10.1155/2011/745829.

[6] K.H. Chuah, S. Mahadeva, Cultural factors influencing functional gastrointestinal disorders in the east, J. Neurogastroenterol. Motil. 24 (2018) 536–543, https://doi.org/10.5056/jnm18064.

[7] D.G. Ribaldone, R. Pellicano, G.C. Actis, Inflammation in gastrointestinal disorders: prevalent socioeconomic factors, Clin. Exp. Gastroenterol. 12 (2019) 321–329, https://doi.org/10.2147/CEG.S210844.

[8] A. De Filippis, H. Ullah, A. Baldi, M. Dacrema, C. Esposito, E.U. Garzarella, C. Santarcangelo, A. Tantipongpiradet, M. Daglia, Gastrointestinal disorders and metabolic syndrome: Dysbiosis as a key link and common bioactive dietary components useful for their treatment, Int. J. Mol. Sci. 21 (2020) 4929, https://doi.org/10.3390/ijms21144929.

[9] K. Gul, A.K. Singh, R. Jabeen, Nutraceuticals and functional foods: the foods for the future world, Crit. Rev. Food Sci. Nutr. 56 (2016) 2617–2627, https://doi.org/10.1080/10408398.2014.903384.

[10] J. Ankarklev, J. Jerlström-Hultqvist, E. Ringqvist, K. Troell, S.G. Svärd, Behind the smile: cell biology and disease mechanisms of Giardia species, Nat. Rev. Microbiol. 8 (2010) 413–422, https://doi.org/10.1038/nrmicro2317.

[11] V. Vivancos, I. González-Alvarez, M. Bermejo, M. Gonzalez-Alvarez, Giardiasis: characteristics, pathogenesis and new insights about treatment, Curr. Top. Med. Chem. 18 (2018) 1287–1330, https://doi.org/10.2174/1568026618666181002095314.

[12] F.A. Carvalho-Costa, A.Q. Gonçalves, S.L. Lassance, L.M. Da Silva Neto, C.A.A. Salmazo, M.N. Bóia, *Giardia lamblia* and other intestinal parasitic infections and their relationships with nutritional status in children in Brazilian Amazon, Rev. Inst. Med. Trop. Sao Paulo 49 (2007) 147–153, https://doi.org/10.1590/s0036-46652007000300003.

[13] M.M. Ahmed, H.M. el Hady, A preliminary survey of parasitic infections and nutritional status among school children in Riyadh, Saudi Arabia, Egypt Soc. Parasitol. 19 (1989) 101–105.

[14] W.M. Wilson, D.L. Dufour, L.K. Staten, M. Barac-Nieto, J.C. Reina, G.B. Spurr, Gastrointestinal parasitic infection, anthropometrics, nutritional status, and physical work capacity in Colombian boys, Am. J. Hum. Biol. 11 (1999) 763–771, https://doi.org/10.1002/(SICI)1520-6300(199911/12)11:6<763::AID-AJHB6>3.0.CO;2-M.

[15] S. Awasthi, V.K. Pande, Prevalence of malnutrition and intestinal parasites in preschool slum children in Lucknow, Indian Pediatr. 34 (1997) 599–605.
[16] R. Loewenson, P.R. Mason, B.A. Patterson, Giardiasis and the nutritional status of Zimbabwean school children, Ann. Trop. Paediatr. 6 (1986) 73–78, https://doi.org/10.1080/02724936.1986.11748415.
[17] M.I. Muniz-Junqueira, E.F.O. Queiroz, Relationship between protein-energy malnutrition, vitamin A, and parasitoses in living in Brasília, Rev. Soc. Bras. Med. Trop. 35 (2002) 133–141, https://doi.org/10.1590/s0037-86822002000200002.
[18] M.A. Rodrigues, M.F. De-Carvalho, M.R. Montenegro, Effects of protein deficiency and natural intestinal infection with *Giardia lamblia* on jejunal intraepithelial lymphocytes in rats of different ages, Braz. J. Med. Biol. Res. 27 (1994) 1347–1353.
[19] M.E. Sackey, M.M. Weigel, R.X. Armijos, Predictors and nutritional consequences of intestinal parasitic infections in rural Ecuadorian children, J. Trop. Pediatr. 49 (2003) 17–23, https://doi.org/10.1093/tropej/49.1.17.
[20] N.W. Solomons, Giardiasis: nutritional implications, Rev. Infect. Dis. 4 (1982) 859–869, https://doi.org/10.1093/4.4.859.
[21] D.S. Berkman, A.G. Lescano, R.H. Gilman, S.L. Lopez, M.M. Black, Effects of stunting, diarrhoeal disease, and parasitic infection during infancy on cognition in late childhood: a follow-up study, Lancet 359 (2002) 564–571, https://doi.org/10.1016/S0140-6736(02)07744-9.
[22] F.T. Cordingley, G.P. Crawford, Giardia infection causes vitamin B12 deficiency, Aust. N. Z. J. Med. 16 (1986) 78–79, https://doi.org/10.1111/j.1445-5994.1986.tb01127.x.
[23] G. Oberhuber, N. Kastner, M. Stolte, Giardiasis: a histologic analysis of 567 cases, Scand. J. Gastroenterol. 32 (1997) 48–51, https://doi.org/10.3109/00365529709025062.
[24] A.M. Cevallos, S. Carnaby, M. James, M.J.G. Farthing, Small intestinal injury in a neonatal rat model of giardiasis is strain dependent, Gastroenterology 109 (1995) 766–773, https://doi.org/10.1016/0016-5085(95)90383-6.
[25] M.J.G. Farthing, The molecular pathogenesis of giardiasis, J. Pediatr. Gastroenterol. Nutr. 24 (1997) 79–88, https://doi.org/10.1097/00005176-199701000-00018.
[26] A. Fasano, C. Catassi, Clinical practice Celiac Disease, N. Engl. J. Med. 367 (2012) 2419–2426, https://doi.org/10.1056/NEJMcp1113994.
[27] G.R. Corazza, M.L. Andreani, F. Biagi, G. Corrao, S. Pretolani, G. Giulianelli, G. Ghironzi, G. Gasbarrini, The smaller size of the "coeliac iceberg" in adults, Scand. J. Gastroenterol. 32 (1997) 917–919, https://doi.org/10.3109/00365529709011202.
[28] A. Ivarsson, L.Å. Persson, P. Juto, M. Peltonen, O. Suhr, O. Hernell, High prevalence of undiagnosed coeliac disease in adults: a Swedish population-based study, J. Intern. Med. 245 (1999) 63–68, https://doi.org/10.1046/j.1365-2796.1999.00403.x.
[29] S. Riestra, E. Fernández-Rodriguez, L. Rodrigo, S. Garcia, G. Ocio, Prevalence of coeliac disease in the general population of northern Spain: strategies of serologic screening, Scand. J. Gastroenterol. 35 (2000) 398–402, https://doi.org/10.1080/003655200750023967.
[30] U. Volta, S. Bellentani, F.B. Bianchi, G. Brandi, L. De Franceschi, L. Miglioli, A. Granito, F. Balli, C. Tiribelli, High prevalence of celiac disease in Italian general population, Dig. Dis. Sci. 46 (2001) 1500–1505, https://doi.org/10.1023/A:1010648122797.
[31] K. Mustalahti, C. Catassi, A. Reunanen, E. Fabiani, M. Heier, S. McMillan, L. Murray, M.H. Metzger, M. Gasparin, E. Bravi, M. Mki, The prevalence of celiac disease in Europe: results of a centralized, international mass screening project, Ann. Med. 42 (2010) 587–595, https://doi.org/10.3109/07853890.2010.505931.
[32] A. Rubio-Tapia, J.F. Ludvigsson, T.L. Brantner, J.A. Murray, J.E. Everhart, The prevalence of celiac disease in the United States, Am. J. Gastroenterol. 107 (2012) 1538–1544, https://doi.org/10.1038/ajg.2012.219.

[33] P. Singh, S. Arora, A. Singh, T.A. Strand, G.K. Makharia, Prevalence of celiac disease in Asia: a systematic review and meta-analysis, J. Gastroenterol. Hepatol. 31 (2016) 1095–1101, https://doi.org/10.1111/jgh.13270.

[34] C. Catassi, D. Kryszak, B. Bhatti, C. Sturgeon, K. Helzlsouer, S.L. Clipp, D. Gelfond, E. Puppa, A. Sferruzza, A. Fasano, Natural history of celiac disease autoimmunity in a USA cohort followed since 1974, Ann. Med. 42 (2010) 530–538, https://doi.org/10.3109/07853890.2010.514285.

[35] U. Volta, G. Caio, V. Stanghellini, R. De Giorgio, The changing clinical profile of celiac disease: a 15-year experience (1998–2012) in an Italian referral center, BMC Gastroenterol. 14 (2014) 194, https://doi.org/10.1186/s12876-014-0194-x.

[36] G. Caio, U. Volta, A. Sapone, D.A. Leffler, R. De Giorgio, C. Catassi, A. Fasano, Celiac disease: a comprehensive current review, BMC Med. 17 (2019) 142, https://doi.org/10.1186/s12916-019-1380-z.

[37] S. Vivas, J.M. Ruiz De Morales, M. Fernandez, M. Hernando, B. Herrero, J. Casqueiro, S. Gutierrez, Age-related clinical, serological, and histopathological features of celiac disease, Am. J. Gastroenterol. 103 (2008) 2360–2365, https://doi.org/10.1111/j.1572-0241.2008.01977.x.

[38] N.R. Reilly, K. Aguilar, B.G. Hassid, J. Cheng, A.R. Defelice, P. Kazlow, G. Bhagat, P.H. Green, Celiac disease in normal-weight and overweight children: clinical features and growth outcomes following a gluten-free diet, J. Pediatr. Gastroenterol. Nutr. 53 (2011) 528–531, https://doi.org/10.1097/MPG.0b013e3182276d5e.

[39] R. El-Abassi, M.Y. Soliman, F. Williams, J.D. England, Whipple's disease, J. Neurol. Sci. 377 (2017) 197–206, https://doi.org/10.1016/j.jns.2017.01.048.

[40] J.C. Sieracki, Whipple's disease-observation on systemic involvement. I. Cytologic observations, A.M.A. Arch. Pathol. 66 (1958) 464–467.

[41] R.C. Barker, Malabsorption syndrome associated with ulcération of the stomach and small bowel caused by chronic intestinal ischemia in a patient with hyperhomocysteinemia, Mayo Clin. Proc. 72 (1997) 546–550, https://doi.org/10.4065/72.6.546.

[42] F. Fernández-Bañares, M. Esteve, J.M. Viver, Fructose-sorbitol malabsorption, Curr. Gastroenterol. Rep. 11 (2009) 368–374, https://doi.org/10.1007/s11894-009-0056-9.

[43] M. Montalto, A. Gallo, V. Ojetti, A. Gasbarrini, Fructose, trehalose and sorbitol malabsorption, Eur. Rev. Med. Pharmacol. Sci. 17 (2013) 26–29.

[44] S.R. Benedict, A reagent for the detection of reducing sugars, J. Biol. Chem. 277 (2002) e5.

[45] A. Gasbarrini, G.R. Corazza, G. Gasbarrini, M. Montalto, M. Di Stefano, G. Basilisco, A. Parodi, P.U. Satta, P. Vernia, C. Anania, M. Astegiano, G. Barbara, L. Benini, P. Bonazzi, G. Capurso, M. Certo, A. Colecchia, L. Cuoco, A.D.I. Sario, D. Festi, C. Lauritano, E. Miceli, G. Nardone, F. Perri, P. Portincasa, R. Risicato, M. Sorge, A. Tursi, Methodology and indications of H2-breath testing in gastrointestinal diseases: The Rome consensus conference, Aliment. Pharmacol. Ther. 29 (2009) 1–49, https://doi.org/10.1111/j.1365-2036.2009.03951.x.

[46] M.D. Levitt, R.M. Donaldson, Use of respiratory hydrogen (H2) excretion to detect carbohydrate malabsorption, J. Lab. Clin. Med. 75 (1970) 937–945, https://doi.org/10.5555/uri:pii:0022214370901939.

[47] N.S. Enattah, T. Sahi, E. Savilahti, J.D. Terwilliger, L. Peltonen, I. Järvelä, Identification of a variant associated with adult-type hypolactasia, Nat. Genet. 30 (2002) 233–237, https://doi.org/10.1038/ng826.

[48] M. Pimentel, Y. Kong, S. Park, Breath testing to evaluate lactose intolerance in irritable bowel syndrome correlates with lactulose testing and may not reflect true lactose malabsorption, Am. J. Gastroenterol. 98 (2003) 2700–2704, https://doi.org/10.1111/j.1572-0241.2003.08670.x.

[49] G. Metz, T.J. Peters, D.J.A. Jenkins, A. Newman, L.M. Blendis, Breath hydrogen as a diagnostic method for hypolactasia, Lancet 1 (1975) 1155–1157, https://doi.org/10.1016/S0140-6736(75)93135-9.

[50] J. Alvarez-Coca, M. Pérez-Miranda, M. Iritia, H. Escobar, I. Jiménez-Alonso, J.M. Pajares, Usefulness of urinary galactose for the diagnosis of hypolactasia, J. Clin. Gastroenterol. 23 (1996) 79–80, https://doi.org/10.1097/00004836-199607000-00026.

[51] J.D. Grant, J.A. Bezerra, S.H. Thompson, R.J. Lemen, O. Koldovsky, J.N. Udall, Assessment of lactose absorption by measurement of urinary galactose, Gastroenterology 97 (1989) 895–899, https://doi.org/10.1016/0016-5085(89)91494-7.

[52] H. Arola, H. Jokela, T. Koivula, M. Isokoski, Simple urinary test for lactose malabsorption, Lancet 2 (1982) 524–525, https://doi.org/10.1016/S0140-6736(82)90602-X.

[53] A.D. Newcomer, D.B. McGill, P.J. Thomas, A.F. Hofmann, Prospective comparison of indirect methods for detecting lactase deficiency, N. Engl. J. Med. 293 (1975) 1232–1236, https://doi.org/10.1056/nejm197512112932405.

[54] R.M. Craig, A.J. Atkinson, D-xylose testing: a review, Gastroenterology 95 (1988) 223–231, https://doi.org/10.1016/0016-5085(88)90318-6.

[55] U.C. Ghoshal, How to interpret hydrogen breath tests, J. Neurogastroenterol. Motil. 17 (2011) 312–317, https://doi.org/10.5056/jnm.2011.17.3.312.

[56] J.H. Van De Kamer, H. Ten Bokkel Huinink, H.A. Weyers, Rapid method for the determination of fat in feces, J. Biol. Chem. 177 (1949) 347–355, https://doi.org/10.1016/s0021-9258(18)57092-7.

[57] M.R. Khouri, G. Huang, Y.F. Shiau, Sudan stain of fecal fat: new insight into an old test, Gastroenterology 92 (1989) 421–427, https://doi.org/10.1016/0016-5085(89)91566-7.

[58] S. Amarri, M. Harding, W.A. Coward, T.J. Evans, L.T. Weaver, 13Carbon mixed triglyceride breath test and pancreatic enzyme supplementation in cystic fibrosis, Arch. Dis. Child. 76 (1997) 349–351, https://doi.org/10.1136/adc.76.4.349.

[59] K. Van Dijk-Van Aalst, M. Van Den Driessche, S. Van Der Schoor, S. Schiffelers, T. Van't Westeinde, Y. Ghoos, G. Veereman-Wauters, 13C mixed triglyceride breath test: a non-invasive method to assess lipase activity in children, J. Pediatr. Gastroenterol. Nutr. 32 (2001) 579–585, https://doi.org/10.1097/00005176-200105000-00017.

[60] G.R. Vantrappen, P.J. Rutgeerts, Y.F. Ghoos, M.I. Hiele, Mixed triglyceride breath test: a noninvasive test of pancreatic lipase activity in the duodenum, Gastroenterology 94 (1989) 1126–1134, https://doi.org/10.1016/0016-5085(89)91632-6.

[61] M. Raman, T. Fenton, P. Crotty, S. Ghosh, K. Rioux, R. Hundal, A novel method to identify fat malabsorption: the serum Retinyl palmitate test, Clin. Chim. Acta 438 (2015) 103–106, https://doi.org/10.1016/j.cca.2014.08.001.

[62] R. Pezzilli, A. Andriulli, C. Bassi, G. Balzano, M. Cantore, G. Delle Fave, M. Falconi, L. Frulloni, Exocrine pancreatic insufficiency in adults: a shared position statement of the Italian association for the study of the pancreas, World J. Gastroenterol. 19 (2013) 7930–7946, https://doi.org/10.3748/wjg.v19.i44.7930.

[63] P.G.S. Lankisch, Fecal elastase 1 is not the indirect pancreatic function test we have been waiting for, Dig. Dis. Sci. 45 (2000) 166–167, https://doi.org/10.1023/a:1005486032702.

[64] P. Vijayvargiya, M. Camilleri, A. Shin, A. Saenger, Methods for diagnosis of bile acid malabsorption in clinical practice, Clin. Gastroenterol. Hepatol. 11 (2013) 1232–1239, https://doi.org/10.1016/j.cgh.2013.04.029.

[65] L. Wedlake, R. A'Hern, D. Russell, K. Thomas, J.R.F. Walters, H.J.N. Andreyev, Systematic review: the prevalence of idiopathic bile acid malabsorption as diagnosed by SeHCAT scanning in patients with diarrhoea-predominant irritable bowel syndrome, Aliment. Pharmacol. Ther. 30 (2009) 707–717, https://doi.org/10.1111/j.1365-2036.2009.04081.x.

[66] R. Riemsma, M. Al, I.C. Ramos, S.N. Deshpande, N. Armstrong, Y.C. Lee, S. Ryder, C. Noake, M. Krol, M. Oppe, J. Kleijnen, H. Severens, SeHCAT [tauroselcholic (selenium-75) acid] for the investigation of bile acid malabsorption and measurement of bile acid pool loss: a systematic review and cost-effectiveness analysis, Health Technol. Assess. (Rockv). 17 (2013) 1–236, https://doi.org/10.3310/hta17610.
[67] F. Gothe, F. Beigel, C. Rust, M. Hajji, S. Koletzko, F. Freudenberg, Bile acid malabsorption assessed by 7 alpha-hydroxy-4-cholesten-3-one in pediatric inflammatory bowel disease: correlation to clinical and laboratory findings, J. Crohns Colitis 8 (2014) 1072–1078, https://doi.org/10.1016/j.crohns.2014.02.027.
[68] W.G. Brydon, H. Nyhlin, M.A. Eastwood, M.V. Merrick, Serum 7α-hydroxy-4-cholesten-3-one and selenohomocholyltaurine (SeHCAT) whole body retention in the assessment of bile acid induced diarrhoea, Eur. J. Gastroenterol. Hepatol. 8 (1996) 117–123, https://doi.org/10.1097/00042737-199602000-00005.
[69] F. Freudenberg, F. Gothe, F. Beigel, C. Rust, S. Koletzko, Serum 7-alpha-hydroxy-4-cholesten-3-one as a marker for bile acid loss in children, J. Pediatr. 163 (2013) 1367–1371, https://doi.org/10.1016/j.jpeds.2013.06.083.
[70] L.S. Zuckier, L.R. Chervu, Schilling evaluation of pernicious anemia: current status, J. Nucl. Med. 25 (1984) 1032–1039.
[71] J.W. Anderson, P. Baird, R.H. Davis, S. Ferreri, M. Knudtson, A. Koraym, V. Waters, C.L. Williams, Health benefits of dietary fiber, Nutr. Rev. 67 (2009) 188–205, https://doi.org/10.1111/j.1753-4887.2009.00189.x.
[72] N.G. Asp, C.G. Johansson, H. Hallmer, M. Siljeström, Rapid enzymatic assay of insoluble and soluble dietary fiber, J. Agric. Food Chem. 31 (1983) 476–482, https://doi.org/10.1021/jf00117a003.
[73] I.T. Johnson, Fiber: physiological and functional effects, in: Encycl. Hum. Nutr., Elsevier Inc., 2012, pp. 240–245, https://doi.org/10.1016/B978-0-12-375083-9.00105-7.
[74] O.C. Velázquez, H.M. Lederer, J.L. Rombeau, Butyrate and the colonocyte: production, absorption, metabolism, and therapeutic implications, Adv. Exp. Med. Biol. 427 (1997) 123–134, https://doi.org/10.1007/978-1-4615-5967-2_14.
[75] S. Noureddin, J. Mohsen, A. Payman, Effects of psyllium vs. placebo on constipation, weight, glycemia, and lipids: a randomized trial in patients with type 2 diabetes and chronic constipation, Complement. Ther. Med. 40 (2018) 1–7, https://doi.org/10.1016/j.ctim.2018.07.004.
[76] X. Gao, J. Liu, L. Li, W. Liu, M. Sun, A brief review of nutraceutical ingredients in gastrointestinal disorders: evidence and suggestions, Int. J. Mol. Sci. 21 (2020) 1822, https://doi.org/10.3390/ijms21051822.
[77] C. Cirillo, R. Capasso, Constipation and botanical medicines: an overview, Phyther. Res. 19 (2015) 1488–1493, https://doi.org/10.1002/ptr.5410.
[78] H. Mao, C. Wang, Y. Wang, Synthesis of polymeric dyes based on waterborne polyurethane for improved color stability, New J. Chem. 182 (2015) 1953–1965, https://doi.org/10.1039/c4nj02222j.
[79] M. Gordon, J.K. Macdonald, C.E. Parker, A.K. Akobeng, A.G. Thomas, Osmotic and stimulant laxatives for the management of childhood constipation, Cochrane Database Syst. Rev. 2016 (2016), https://doi.org/10.1002/14651858.CD009118.pub3, CD009118.
[80] C.W. Sobrado, I.J.F.C. Neto, R.A. Pinto, L.F. Sobrado, S.C. Nahas, I. Cecconello, Diagnosis and treatment of constipation: a clinical update based on the Rome IV criteria, J. Coloproctology 38 (2018) 134–144, https://doi.org/10.1016/j.jcol.2018.02.003.

CHAPTER 12

Skin metabolic syndrome and phytonutrients

Antoni Sureda[a] and Silvia Tejada[b]
[a]Research Group on Community Nutrition and Oxidative Stress (NUCOX), Department of Fundamental Biology and Health Sciences, Health Research Institute of the Balearic Islands (IdISBa), and CIBEROBN (Physiopathology of Obesity and Nutrition CB12/03/30038), University of the Balearic Islands, Palma, Spain
[b]Laboratory of Neurophysiology, Department of Biology, Health Research Institute of the Balearic Islands (IdISBa), and CIBEROBN (Physiopathology of Obesity and Nutrition CB12/03/30038), University of the Balearic Islands, Palma, Spain

1. Introduction

The multifaceted metabolic syndrome (MetS) or syndrome X, originally described by Reaven in 1988, is a disorder characterized by the presence of a cluster of conditions including central obesity, hyperglycemia, dyslipidemia (hypertriglyceridemia, low plasma HDL-cholesterol), and hypertension [1]. According to the revised National Cholesterol Education Program Adult Treatment Panel III, the presence of three of the five risk factors confirms the diagnosis of MetS (Table 1) [2]. An untreated and persistent state of MetS is directly related to an increased risk of developing chronic diseases, including cardiovascular diseases (coronary heart disease, cardiac failure, and stroke), diabetes and hepatic steatosis [3,4]. In addition, MetS is also associated with high mortality risk and elevated economic healthcare costs [5]. Although the etiology of MetS is largely unknown and complex, it is believed to derive from an interaction between genetic predisposition and metabolic and environmental factors [6]. In developed countries, MetS already affects more than 25% of the entire population, exceeding values of 35% in the US and Mexican populations [7,8]. Furthermore, its prevalence is increasing rapidly and throughout the world, in line with the increasing prevalence of diabetes and obesity rates in recent decades, so that it has become a major public health problem [9].

Increasing evidence suggests the existence of a strong relationship between MetS and skin diseases, mainly psoriasis, acne vulgaris, hidradenitis suppurativa, and acanthosis nigricans [10]. The skin is the main organ exposed to external environmental variations, but it also communicates with the internal environment. In addition, many internal diseases can present cutaneous manifestations and serve as a marker for an underlying internal

The Role of Phytonutrients in Metabolic Disorders
https://doi.org/10.1016/B978-0-12-824356-5.00001-1

Table 1 The five main risk factors related to metabolic syndrome.

Main risk factors	Values attending to the NCEP ATP III criteria
Obesity: waist circumference	>88 cm for women >102 cm for men
HDL cholesterol	<50 mg/dL for women <40 mg/dL for men
Triglycerides	> or equal 150 mg/dL
Blood pressure	> or equal 130/85 mmHg
Glycaemia (fasting sample)	> or equal 110 mg/dL

HDL, High-density lipoprotein; *NCEP ATP III*, National Cholesterol Education Program Adult Treatment Panel III.

disease [11]. In this sense, the skin is one of the main organs affected by alterations associated with MetS through a complex interaction of hormones, chronic inflammation (adipokines and proinflammatory cytokines), and impaired insulin signaling [12].

2. Metabolic syndrome and skin diseases

MetS comprises a number of risk factors that predispose people to develop type 2 diabetes and cardiovascular disease. Diverse dermatological diseases are also associated with MetS or its components; nevertheless, the mechanisms by which these disorders are related to MetS are not fully elucidated. What is known is that of all the mechanisms involved, resistance to insulin, the alteration in the production and release of physiologically active peptides, known as adipocytokines, chronic inflammation and oxidative stress, appear to be the main factors in the appearance and progression of MetS [13,14]. Specifically, visceral fat accumulation has been shown to be a major element for most of the pathways and mechanisms associated with MetS. This excess of visceral fat increases the levels of circulating free fatty acids (FFA) and leads to reduced insulin-mediated glucose uptake in the muscle and liver [15]. As a result, blood glucose levels rise and higher levels of insulin are required to promote glucose uptake. In addition, insulin resistance alters the antilipolytic activity of the hormone itself, further contributing to the release of more fatty acids into the circulation [16,17]. Adipose tissue-derived adipocytokines participate in the control of metabolism and have been evidenced to be related to MetS and cardiovascular disease [18]. These adipocytokines include leptin, adiponectin, and the inflammatory cytokines tumor necrosis factor alpha (TNF-α) and interleukin-6 (IL-6). Leptin, which favors the T cell shifting toward the proinflammatory Th1 phenotype, and the inflammatory cytokines are elevated in obese subjects, whereas the antiinflammatory and antiatherogenic adiponectin is reduced [13,19]. In addition, subjects with MetS present lower activities of antioxidant enzymes and higher levels of oxidative damage markers with respect to healthy individuals, which could contribute to the instauration of an oxidative stress condition [20]. This situation of oxidative stress also contributes to the progression of MetS, inducing the establishment of a chronic low-grade inflammation and favoring thrombosis, atherosclerosis, and vascular disease [21].

2.1 Psoriasis

Psoriasis is an immune-mediated inflammatory disease characterized by the expansion and activation of different T cell subsets, mainly Th-1, Th-17, and Th-22T cells, and the production of proinflammatory cytokines in the skin. Altogether induces angiogenesis and epidermal hyperproliferation, mainly of keratinocytes [22]. The hyperproliferation and abnormal differentiation of keratinocytes, as a secondary phenomenon induced by the immune response, leads to epidermal thickening and expansion toward the papillary dermis. In turn, these activated keratinocytes contribute to the stimulation of immune cell infiltration. The main clinical manifestations of psoriasis are the presence of delimited papulosquamous plaques from the surrounding normal skin [23]. These plaques are pinkish lesions covered by white or silver scales, which are usually distributed symmetrically and principally in the elbows and knees, scalp, and lumbosacral region. Inflammatory mediators produced in the skin lesions can be released into the systemic circulation contributing to vascular alterations [24]. In this sense, though psoriasis is a disease that affects the skin, patients are at increased risk of developing cardiovascular disease, MetS, and diabetes [24]. In addition, several epidemiological studies have shown that obesity or metabolic diseases lead to an increased risk of developing psoriasis and a worse long-term clinical outcome of the disease [25,26]. The presence of chronic low-grade inflammation in obesity influences the pathogenesis of psoriasis by promoting a proinflammatory state, which raises the susceptibility to the development of the disorder or the severity of skin lesions in an established psoriasis. An interesting report evidenced that normal glucose-tolerant patients with psoriasis had significantly reduced insulin sensitivity with respect to healthy subjects, suggesting that psoriasis may contribute to a prediabetic condition [27]. Besides these data, a reduction in the weight of patients with psoriasis helps reduce relapses of the disease and the severity of symptoms [28,29].

2.2 Acne vulgaris

Acne is the most common skin condition and is often overlooked as a simple, self-limiting disorder of adolescents. Acne consists of a chronic inflammation of the folliculopilosebaceous unit—hair follicles in the skin associated with an oil gland—due to hyperkeratosis and related to sebaceous hypersecretion [30]. In addition, the release of lipid mediators in the skin and the follicular colonization by *Cutibacterium acnes* (previously known as *Propionibacterium acnes*) also play a role in the formation of acne lesions [31]. It is a more frequent pathology in adolescence and in the female gender and is generally located where there is a greater density of pilosebaceous units (on the face, shoulders, back, and chest). The clinical features of acne include lesions ranging from excess fat seborrhea, noninflammatory open or closed comedones, inflammatory lesions that can be papules, pustules, or nodules to various degrees of scarring [32,33].

Among the different mechanisms involved in acne, it has been suggested that a diet rich in hyperglycemic carbohydrates and insulinotropic products associated with overweight and insulin resistance could contribute to this pathology [34,35]. These characteristics of the Western diet could increase androgen release, activate the mammalian target of rapamycin complex 1 (mTORC1) pathway, which can alter the sebaceous gland homeostasis and stimulate insulin/insulin-like growth factor (IGF-1) signaling [36]. Specifically, mTORC1 increases sebaceous lipogenesis, sebaceous gland hyperplasia, and hyperproliferation of keratinocytes. Also, subjects with acne present higher levels of serum IGF-1 and increased expression of IGF-1 and its receptor in the epidermis [37]. The excessive activation of this pathway leads to uncontrolled lipogenesis inducing lipotoxicity and inflammation [38]. In this sense, a low-glycemic-load diet has been evidenced to improve the acne lesions together with a reduction in the weight and an improvement in the insulin sensitivity [39,40].

2.3 Hidradenitis suppurativa

Hidradenitis suppurativa or acne inversa is a chronic and inflammatory disorder, characterized by recurrent abscesses, deep-seated nodules, and sinus tracts with suppuration which can result in hypertrophic scarring [41]. This pathology mainly affects adults, appearing between the ages of 20–30 with a higher prevalence among women [42]. Hidradenitis suppurativa mainly appears in the intertriginous areas, such as the axillae, inguinal area, infra- and intermammary areas, perineal and perianal regions, and the nape [43]. The etiology of the disease has not been fully elucidated yet but genetic, hormonal, and microbial factors are involved, as well as risk factors such as obesity, tobacco, or alterations of the epithelial immune system [42,44]. In the progression of the disease, the first signal that is observed is an increased keratinocyte proliferation in the infundibular area of the terminal hair follicle leading to follicular duct occlusion. This process is followed by the subsequent rupture of the follicle and release of the contents into the surrounding dermis causing the activation and infiltration of cells of the immune system [45].

Different studies have shown the existence of a direct relationship between hidradenitis suppurativa and MetS [46–48]. In fact, it has been observed that subjects with hidradenitis suppurativa have a higher risk of developing diabetes, obesity, and hyperlipidemia [47,49]. Moreover, it has been shown that treatments against MetS or its components can contribute to a reduced hidradenitis suppurativa pathology. What is more, it has been shown that treatments against MetS or its components such as metformin, an insulin-sensitizing agent, as well as weight loss can help reduce HS activity [50,51].

2.4 Acanthosis nigricans

Acanthosis nigricans is a cutaneous condition characterized by the presence of symmetrical, hyperpigmented, dark and velvety plaques that may occur in almost any location but mainly in the intertriginous areas and the posterior neck [52]. The pathogenesis of this disease is complex and is not fully understood, including the classifications mainly based on the etiologic factors that are unclear and confusing [53]. A classification according to severity depending on the number of affected areas is possibly the clearest way with high interobserver reliability [54,55]. It is not only the excessive proliferation of dermal fibroblasts but also the epidermal keratinocytes induced by certain growth factors that could play a central role in the pathogenesis of acanthosis nigricans. In this sense, alterations in the signaling of insulin and IGF and consequently obesity, hyperinsulinemia, and insulin resistance have been correlated with this disease [53,56]. In obese patients, hyperinsulinemia induces a decrease in the levels of IGF binding proteins (IGFBPs), which increases the IGF-1 half-life. Thus, a local increase in free IGF-1 levels can occur, facilitating the development of hyperkeratosis and papillomatosis, characteristics of the illness [57,58]. In addition, genetic mutations that affect some genes such as insulin receptors or fibroblast growth factor receptors are known to cause acanthosis nigricans [59,60]. It has been reported that weight loss with improvement in both insulin resistance and compensatory hyperinsulinemia associated with MetS leads to an improvement of acanthosis nigricans [61,62]. The use of insulin sensitizers, mainly metformin, to increase peripheral insulin responsiveness is also a promising strategy against the disease [63,64].

3. Phytochemicals in metabolic syndrome

The first-line strategy to deal with MetS focuses on a comprehensive lifestyle intervention, promoting a balanced low-energy diet and regular physical activity, also being the most cost-effective approach for this pathology. Diverse evidence has shown the relationship between the incidence and prevention of MetS and modifiable lifestyle factors, particularly the dietary habits. In this sense, a systematic review and meta-analysis reported the beneficial effects of different dietary approaches on inflammatory biomarkers in patients with MetS [65]. Similarly, another meta-analysis indicated the protective effects of the promotion of healthy dietary patterns in the prevention of MetS [66]. The characteristic dietary pattern of the Mediterranean diet and other dietary patterns rich in plant-derived products make the prevention or reversion of MetS possible [67,68]. It has been suggested that the favorable effects of these diets are associated with the presence of bioactive compounds and of mono- and polyunsaturated fatty acids [69,70]. In addition to this improvement in lifestyle, some phytochemicals could be useful tools in the treatment of one or more components of MetS and contribute to the improvement of the patients' status [71,72].

A bioactive compound can be defined as a secondary metabolite found in foods, mainly of plant origin, and with the capacity to modulate some metabolic processes or pathways in the body. Among these bioactive compounds, the group of polyphenols stands out, with about 10,000 different described structures (Fig. 1). Phenolic compounds have a very diverse structure from a simple molecule to complex polymers with high molecular weight, although they all possess an aromatic ring with at least one hydroxyl group [73]. In general, these compounds are subdivided into two large groups: flavonoids (anthocyanins, flavanols, flavanones, flavonols, flavonones, and isoflavones) and nonflavonoid polyphenols (phenolic acids, stilbenes, and lignans) [74]. In addition, some terpenoids and sterols, antioxidant vitamins, vitamin D, omega 3 fatty acids, or dietary fiber supplements have shown the ability to improve some of the MetS factors [71,75,76].

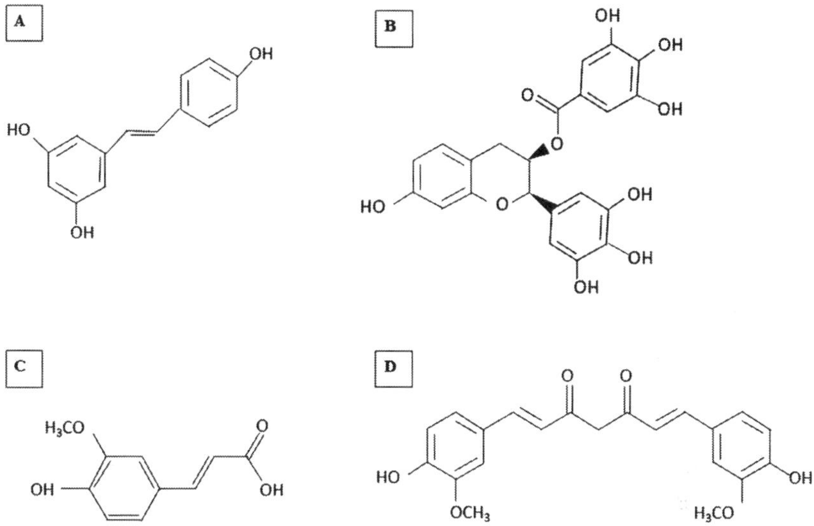

Fig. 1 Structures of some natural polyphenols studied in skin pathologies in animal models and human studies. Chemical structures of (A) resveratrol, (B) (−)-epigallocatechin-3-gallate, (C) ferulic acid, and (D) curcumin.

3.1 Phytochemicals and psoriasis

Conventional treatments for psoriasis are very varied, ranging from topical treatments (such as steroids, vitamin D analogues, retinoids, fumaric acid esters) to systemic drugs (methotrexate, cyclosporine, retinoids, new developed agents including adalimumab, etanercept, infliximab) or phototherapy [77,78]. Although most of these conventional treatments reduce the symptoms of psoriasis, they cannot recover it and they also have significant side effects, including skin alterations and infection, toxicity, immunosuppression, and even carcinogenicity, which limit their long-term application. Thus, the use of phytonutrients can be an alternative or coadjuvant therapy for psoriasis with fewer side effects.

Numerous studies have observed potentially beneficial effects not only against psoriasis from topical application but also from ingestion of numerous isolated bioactive compounds or plant extracts [79,80]. The main targets of phytonutrients are based on reducing keratinocyte hyperproliferation or inducing apoptosis, regulating keratinocyte differentiation, and reducing the proinflammatory state (Fig. 2). In in vitro studies, remarkable effects of bioactive compounds have been observed using keratinocyte cell models. For example, resveratrol, a stilbene polyphenol, is capable

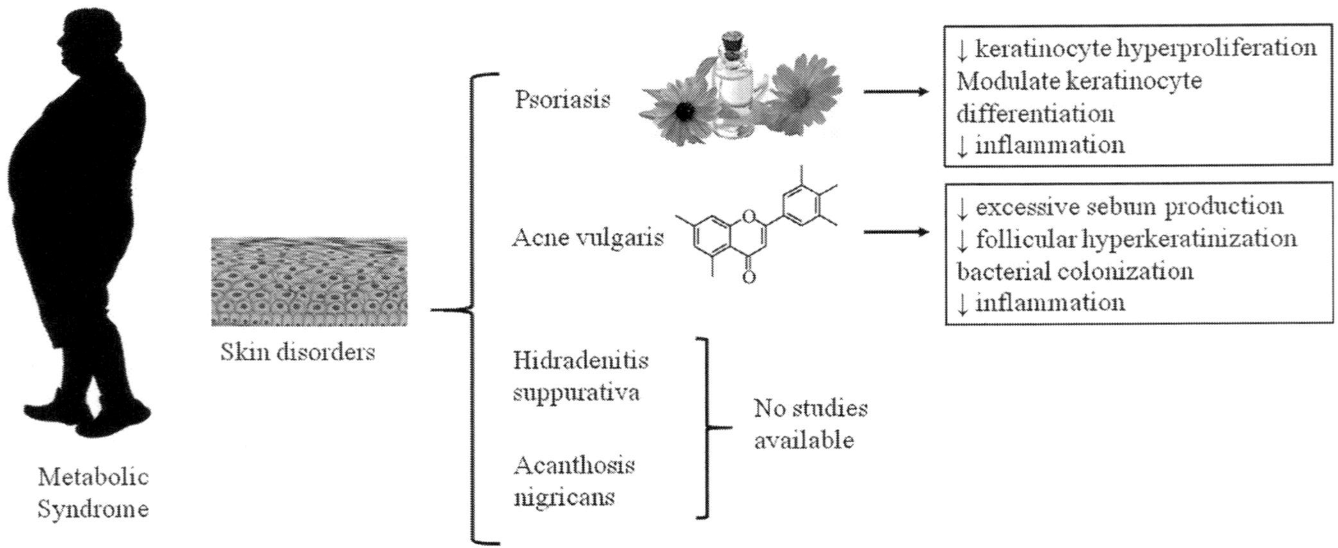

Fig. 2 Summary of the main cutaneous manifestations associated with metabolic syndrome and beneficial effects of treatment with bioactive compounds or plant extracts.

of inhibiting the proliferation of normal human epidermal keratinocytes in a dose-dependent manner by decreasing the expression of aquaporin 3 (AQP3) whose overexpression contributes to hyperplastic epidermal disorders [81]. The mechanism of action was dependent on the sirtuin 1 (Sirt1)/aryl hydrocarbon receptor nuclear translocator (ARNT)/extracellular-regulated kinase (ERK1/2) pathway since the blockage of Sirt1 avoided the effects of resveratrol. Similarly, it has been reported that resveratrol inhibited cell proliferation and induced apoptosis in human HaCaT keratinocytes in a process mediated by Akt signaling inhibition by inducing Sirt1 expression [82]. Curcumin, a polyphenol derived from the golden spice turmeric (*Curcuma longa*), induced apoptosis in HaCaT cells stimulated with tumor necrosis factor alpha (TNFα) by upregulating the TRAIL receptor 1/2 expression and inhibiting the expression of antiapoptotic proteins [83]. In addition, curcumin exerted antiinflammatory effects decreasing the synthesis of IL-6 and IL-8 induced by TNFα. Other studies have shown that the combined treatment of curcumin with exposure to ultraviolet or visible light significantly increased keratinocyte apoptosis, reduced proliferation, and inhibited the activity of nuclear factor κB (NFκB) [84,85]. In another study, the effects of an extract of *Lavandula angustifolia* Mill. (Lamiaceae) rich in rosmarinic acid were assayed in HaCaT keratinocytes stimulated with several cytokines in order to mimic a psoriasis-like inflammatory environment [86]. The results evidenced that the extract reduced psoriasis-like inflammation by inhibiting diverse signaling pathways including the Janus kinase/signal transducer and activator of transcription (JAK/STAT), phosphoinositide-3-kinase-protein kinase B/Akt (PI3K-PKB/Akt) and NF-κB. Among nonphenolic compounds with beneficial effects on psoriasis is the triterpene celastrol. This compound was evidenced to inhibit the NFκB signaling pathway to induce apoptosis in HaCaT cells by activating both the mitochondrial and the death receptor pathways [87].

Many naturally occurring compounds or plant extracts have been tested in animal models of psoriasis induced mainly by treatment with the endosomal toll-like receptor 7 (TLR7) agonist imiquimod. Oral administration of resveratrol in an imiquimod-induced mouse model of psoriasis significantly reduced the severity of skin inflammation, skinfold thickening, and erythema and downregulated the expression of IL-17A and IL-19, both contributing mediators in the progression of the disease [88]. The phenolic compound rottlerin through gavage administration was capable of reducing keratinocyte and vascular proliferation, infiltration of inflammatory cells, and the expression of proinflammatory cytokines in a psoriatic mouse model [89].

The polyphenol (−)-epigallocatechin-3-gallate (EGCG), mainly present in green tea, topically applied as a chitosan-based polymeric nanoparticle formulation improved psoriasiform markers more effectively than EGCG alone in a mouse model of psoriasis [90]. Treatment with the nanoformulation diminished skin thickness and erythema, keratinocyte proliferation, and immune cell infiltration. The steroidal compounds withanolides, extracted from *Datura metel* L. (Solanaceae), intragastrically administered also reduced epidermal hyperplasia and the infiltration of inflammatory cell in imiquimod-treated mice [91]. The mechanism of action was associated with the suppression of the activation of the signal transducer and the activator of transcription 3 (STAT3), ERK1/2, and P38 mitogen-activated protein kinase signaling pathways. Recent studies have evaluated the effects of several triterpenes in a murine model of imiquimod-induced psoriasis-like symptoms. The beneficial effects of two derivatives of ursolic acid, randialic acid B, and tomentosolic acid isolated from *Ilex kaushue* S.Y.Hu (Aquifoliaceae) were reported against psoriatic symptoms in mice [92]. Both compounds significantly reduced imiquimod-induced psoriasis-like symptoms as well as neutrophil ROS production, elastase release, and CD11b expression. The mechanism of action was related to the inhibition of formyl peptide receptor 1 which triggers neutrophil activation and the downstream signaling pathways. Using the same mouse model, Tian et al. [93] evidenced the antipsoriasis effects of a cream composed of three pentacyclic triterpenes—uvaol, oleanolic acid, and methyl corosolate—obtained from *Eriobotrya japonica* (Thunb.) Lindl. (Rosaceae). After 7 days, the cream significantly reduced skin inflammation, keratinocyte proliferation, and Th17 cells cytokine expression suppressing the retinoid-related orphan receptor γt (RORγt) transcription activity. Regarding plant extracts, it has been shown that the treatment with extracts of *Terminalia chebula* Retzius (Combretaceae) exerted notable antipsoriatic effects in a mouse model of psoriasis [94]. The extract, intragastrically administered, ameliorated skin inflammation and keratinocyte proliferation in a mechanism mediated by heme oxygenase (HO)-1 inhibition of the NFκB pathway. In another study, oral administration water-boiled rosin, an exudate of *Pinus masscnlana* (Pinaceae), was investigated in a mouse model of imiquimod-induced psoriasis [95]. Rosin significantly improved the psoriasis-like dermatitis restoring the normal keratinization, reduced the proliferation of Th1/Th17 cells and the production of proinflammatory cytokines. *Melissa officinalis* L., (Lamiaceae) gel formulations—using plant decoction or dichloromethane extract—notably reduced epidermal hyperplasia and scaling and ameliorated the inflammatory state [96].

Regarding clinical trials, they are still scarce and the published ones did not focus on patients with MetS. In a double-blind, placebo-controlled trial, a hydrophilic cream containing *Aloe vera* (L.) Burm.f. (Asphodelaceae) extract was assayed in subjects with slight to mild psoriasis vulgaris [97]. The treatment with the cream during 16 weeks had no side effects and led to a significant clearance of psoriatic plaques and a decrease in the Psoriasis Area and Severity Index (PASI) score. In another clinical trial, patients with mild-to-moderate psoriasis were treated with a topical cream with *Mahonia aquifolium* (Pursh) Nutt. (Berberidaceae) extract during 12 weeks [98]. The treatment significantly improved the PASI and the Quality of Life Index (QLI) with respect to the control group with no evidence of notable side effects. An interesting cross-sectional, case-control observational study investigated the antiinflammatory effects of coffee consumption and the severity of psoriasis [99]. The results evidenced a negative association between coffee drinking, prevalence of MetS, and severity of psoriasis. Topical administration of silver and gold nanoparticles with *Cornus mas* L. (Cornaceae) was evaluated in patients with psoriasis for 6 weeks [100]. The treatment with the nanoparticles improved psoriasis plaques by reducing the plaque thickness, erythema, and scaling and suppressed the infiltration of inflammatory cells. Beneficial effects were also observed in patients with mild-to-moderate scalp psoriasis after 9-week treatment with turmeric tonic [101]. The tonic improved the PASI and QLI indexes and reduced the erythema and scaling compared to the placebo group. A topical botanical complex, named herbal antiinflammatory treatment (HAT1) with more than 20 plant extracts in its composition, was evaluated in a 10-week, open-label, pilot clinical trial [102]. The treatment with HAT1 significantly improved the severity and extent of psoriasis and reduced desquamation and erythema in patients with mild-to-moderate psoriasis. In another clinical trial, the effects of *Gracilaria* red algae topical cream 3% were investigated in the treatment of psoriasis using clobetasol cream 0.05% as control [103]. After 8 weeks, the modified PASI score was significantly more reduced in the *Gracilaria* group with respect to the clobetasol group and also obtained a higher degree of satisfaction from the patients in favor of algae cream. Also, the efficacy of *M. officinalis* L. (Lamiaceae) syrup was assayed in patients with mild-to-moderate psoriasis in a randomized clinical trial [104]. The consumption of the syrup during 12 weeks significantly reduced pruritus and PASI scores and improved quality of life when compared with the placebo group. However, not all the studies have shown clear effects against psoriasis. In this sense, the *Abies alba* Mill. (Pinaceae) bark extract resulted in a slight but not significant improvement in the disease in elbows of adult patients with mild psoriasis applied as topical cream [105].

3.2 Phytochemicals and acne vulgaris

Acne is one of the most common dermatological diseases affecting many people both in adolescence and in adulthood, which results in a large number of studies becoming available. There are abundant acne treatments that allow a large number of possible therapeutic combinations. These treatments are aimed at reducing some of the factors that contribute to the disorder such as excessive sebum production, follicular hyperkeratinization, bacterial colonization, and inflammation [35]. Many of these treatments have side effects and cause initial skin irritation during their first applications. Thus, plant-based agents can be a good, safe, and effective alternative to treat acne.

Many of the in vitro studies focus on the antibacterial properties, especially against *C. acnes*, and the antiinflammatory properties of some compounds or plant extracts. Among the phenolic compounds that have shown efficacy in vitro are curcumin, EGCG, gallic acid, myricetin or resveratrol, and also some terpenoids such as lupeol or ursolic acid and alkaloids such as berberine [106,107]. Regarding plant extracts, examples that can be mentioned are green tea, *Humulus lupulus* L. (Cannabaceae), *Rosmarinus officinalis* Spenn. (Lamiaceae), *Inula helenium* L. (Asteraceae), *Saponaria officinalis* L. (Caryophyllaceae), and genus *Santalum* (Santalaceae) and *Thymus* (Lamiaceae) [108–110]. Animal studies are based on models generated by intradermal injection of *C. acnes*, usually in the ear, which mimics inflammatory acne on human skin. In an interesting approach, the effects of Jumihaidokuto, a mixture rich in polyphenols used in the traditional Japanese medicine, made from aqueous extracts of 10 crude plants including *Quercus* cortex (Fagaceae), *Schizonepetae* spica (Lamiaceae), and *Glycyrrhizae* radix (Fabaceae) were investigated in a rat model of acne [111]. The mixture orally administered significantly reduced inflammation and ear thickness similarly to the effects of prednisolone, used as a reference drug. The effects of diverse polyphenols—resveratrol, quercetin, gallic acid—and benzoyl peroxide as the reference drug were assayed in a mouse model of acne induced by *C. acnes* [112]. All polyphenols significantly reduced ear edema, levels of lipid peroxidation and inflammatory mediators such as IL-1β and myeloperoxidase, and increased catalase and superoxide dismutase activities in comparison with benzoyl peroxide. *Rosa davurica* Pall. (Rosaceae) significantly improved the inflammatory response in a mouse model of acne and reduced the growth of skin bacteria, *C. acnes*, *Staphylococcus aureus*, and *Staphylococcus epidermidis* [113]. The extract inhibited the production of proinflammatory cytokines, TNFα, IL-1β, and IL-8 via downregulation of the NFκβ pathway. In another study, the topical administration of EGCG reduced the magnitude of comedones and sebaceous glands in rabbit ears, comparable to the treatment with all-trans-retinoic acid, a recognized anti-comedonic agent [114].

Different clinical trials have shown the beneficial effects of several plant extracts against acne vulgaris. In most of these trials, subjects with symmetrical acne are usually recruited, so that the treatment to be studied is topically applied to one-half of the face and the placebo or vehicle is applied to the other one. In contrast, clinical trials analyzing the effects of some plant extracts after ingestion are scarce. The effects of a gel containing resveratrol was investigated in adult patients with facial acne vulgaris during 4 weeks in a single-blind, pilot study [115]. The treatment induced a decrease in the Global Acne Grading System (GAGS) score and reduced the average area of micro-comedones with respect to the vehicle alone. In another randomized clinical trial, topical application of EGCG significantly improved acne by reducing inflammatory and noninflammatory lesions after 8 weeks [116]. EGCG also reduced the levels of the proinflammatory proteins IL-8, NFκB, sterol regulatory element binding protein (SREBP)-1 and phospho-c-Jun N-terminal kinase (JNK) in active acne lesions and increased the number of TUNEL-positive nuclei sebocytes, suggesting an antiproliferative effect. In another study, oral consumption of the decaffeinated green tea extract, rich in EGCG, reduced the number of acne lesions in the nose, mouth, and chin after 4 weeks of treatment in adult women compared to the control group [117]. Additionally, various studies have shown that the topical application of green tea extracts reduces sebum secretion and inflammatory and noninflammatory lesions (see review by Saric et al. [118]). The suggested mechanisms of action are based on the antibacterial and proapoptotic action of the extract, the reduction of the SREBP-1 signaling pathway, which leads to a reduction in lipogenesis, and of NFκB that in turn reduces inflammation. In another study, *Berberis vulgaris* L. (Berberidaceae) extract orally consumed during 4 weeks as gelatin capsules in a double-blind, randomized, placebo-controlled clinical trial significantly reduced acne lesions in patients with moderate-to-severe acne vulgaris [119]. The topical application of *Copaifera langsdorffii* Desf. (Fabaceae) essential oil incorporated in a gel for 21 days significantly reduced the surface area affected by mild acne [120]. In another study, the application of the hydrophobic fraction *Panax ginseng* C.A. Meyer (Araliaceae) ethanolic extract rich in the polyacetylenes panaxynol and panaxydol during 4 weeks exhibited antimicrobial activity on *C. acnes* and reduced the sebum content and redness of the skin [121]. The treatment with a gel containing *Centella asiatica* (L.) Urban (Apiaceae) applied after the laser skin resurfacing procedure reduced the erythema and improved the wound appearance after 3 months in patients with facial acne scars [122]. *Cirsium eriophorum* (L.) Scop. (Asteraceae) extract topically applied during 28 days significantly reduced the sebum production, reduced the pore size, and reduced the transepidermal water loss in volunteers with acne-prone skin [123]. A herbal cream containing *I. helenium, S. Officinalis,* and *Solanum nigrum* L. (Solanaceae) extracts exerted notable antisebum, antimicrobial, and antiinflammatory activities in patients with facial acne vulgaris after 6 weeks of treatment [109]. In another randomized clinical trial, a hydrogel containing *Nigella sativa* L. (Ranunculaceae) was assayed in patients with mild-to-moderate acne vulgaris [106,107]. After 2 months, the treatment with *N. sativa* significantly reduced the amount of comedones, pustules, and papules and the acne disability index without evidence of adverse events. Another study investigated the effects of tea tree, *Melaleuca alternifolia*, Maiden & Betche ex Cheel (Myrtaceae), oil nanoemulsion in patients with acne for 12 weeks [124]. The topical application of the emulsion significantly reduced the inflammatory and noninflammatory acne lesions and the mean acne severity index (ASI) with respect to the placebo group. Another study investigated the effects of a herbal formulation composed of four plant extracts (*Garcinia mangostana* L. (Clusiaceae), *Houttuynia cordata* Thunb. (Saururaceae), *Lithospermum officinale* L. (Boraginaceae), *Tribulus terrestris* L. (Zygophyllaceae)) during 8 weeks as a cleanser formulation [125]. The treatment significantly reduced the number of acne lesions with respect to the vehicle group. In addition, the immunohistochemistry results of biopsy specimens from the face showed a reduction in IL-1α, IL-8, and keratin 16 in the group using the herbal extracts.

Although clinical trials focus on observing the evolution of the main symptoms of acne, in vitro studies have evaluated the possible underlying mechanisms of action. The mechanisms of action associated with the different compounds, although diverse, are usually mediated by the downregulation of the expression of mitogen-activated protein kinases (MAPKs), such as p38, ERK1/2, PI3K-PKB/Akt, and JNK suppressing NFκB activation and inflammation [106,107]. Furthermore, the decrease in the production of sebum is related to the inhibition of the expression of SREBP and enzymes related to sebum production and pore enlargements such as 5α-reductase and kallikrein 5, leading to a decrease in the production of lipids [123].

3.3 Phytochemicals and hidradenitis suppurativa

Hidradenitis suppurativa is a disease that does not have a simple treatment due to its unknown pathogenesis and is mainly based on antimicrobial and antiinflammatory approaches [126]. In advanced cases, where fibrosis appears as a consequence of the chronic inflammation, its treatment may require surgery to reduce the area of damaged tissue and to increase the functionality of the affected areas. Although it has been suggested that some dietary interventions focused on limiting carbohydrate intake, especially simple ones, eliminating dairy products, and avoiding brewer's yeast and vegetables from the Solanaceae family, may be beneficial as adjuvant therapy, there are practically no studies with specific phytonutrients [127,128]. In one study, a relationship between less adherence to the Mediterranean diet and the severity of hidradenitis suppurativa has been evidenced. This association has been attributed to the high content of bioactive compounds with antiinflammatory properties in the Mediterranean diet [129]. Another interesting work evaluated the foods that worsen or improve hidradenitis suppurativa [130]. A total of 728 patients participated in the study, of which 32% reported foods that exacerbated symptoms and only 12% that alleviated them. The foods that most often worsened symptoms were sweets followed by bread/pasta/rice and dairy products (reported by more than 50% of participants) and foods high in fat (44% of partients). On the contrary, the foods reported that gave a feeling of relief were mainly vegetables and fruits. The authors conclude that more studies are required to evaluate the molecular basis that relates diet and hidradenitis suppurativa.

3.4 Phytochemicals and acanthosis nigricans

To date, there is no clear and completely effective treatment for acanthosis nigricans. Due to its direct relationship with MetS, the first strategy is to correct the underlying disease pathology, mainly weight loss with a dietary and lifestyle intervention [131]. Hyperpigmentation of the skin can be treated with keratolytic agents like salicylic acids or α-hydroxy acids that can be combined with depigmenting agents like hydroquinone. Other treatments such as retinoids or vitamin D analogues can help normalize epidermal turnover, inhibit keratinocyte proliferation, and correct hyperkeratosis [53]. Some studies have shown the beneficial effects of herbal extracts such as *Glycyrrhiza glabra*, *Moringa oleifera*, or *N. sativa* in patients with polycystic ovary syndrome, among whose clinical manifestations is acanthosis nigricans (see review by Kamble et al. [132]). However, there are no studies that have specifically evaluated the potentially beneficial effects of bioactive plant compounds on acanthosis nigricans.

4. Conclusions

MetS is a metabolic disorder directly related to an increased risk of cardiovascular disease and diabetes, but it is also associated with several dermatological pathological conditions and diverse cutaneous manifestations. The progressive increase in obesity mainly due to the loss of traditional dietary patterns due to less healthy diets and processed foods and an increasingly sedentary lifestyle has caused its significant increase. Pharmacological treatments for MetS-associated skin manifestations, mainly acne vulgaris, psoriasis, hidradenitis suppurativa, and acanthosis nigricans, are not fully effective and are associated with various long-term side effects. Thus, the use of natural compounds or plant extracts as dietary supplements or applied topically, due to their great diversity of biological activities and low toxicity, can be considered as alternative therapies and contribute to the improvement of patient care. For psoriasis, the targets of the tested compounds seek to reduce keratinocyte hyperproliferation, modulate keratinocyte differentiation, and reduce inflammation. In relation to acne vulgaris, treatments are aimed at reducing excessive sebum production, follicular hyperkeratinization, bacterial load, and inflammation. On the contrary, to date, there are no studies that analyze the effects of phytonutrients against hidradenitis suppurativa and acanthosis nigricans. Although the mechanisms of action are very diverse and depend on each compound or extract, most act on the MAPK pathways leading to the suppression of NFκB activation and inflammation. Furthermore, some compounds induce apoptosis by activating both the intrinsic mitochondrial and extrinsic death receptor pathways; they inhibit the SREBP-1 signaling pathway, which leads to a reduction in sebum accumulation, and exert antibacterial effects against *C. acnes*, *Staphylococcus* spp. The use of natural bioactive compounds such as resveratrol or curcumin and plant extracts with the ability to improve or reverse various dermatological disorders complementary to a dietary intervention and healthy lifestyle can contribute to the treatment and/or prevention of these pathologies. In addition, as many of these compounds also have beneficial effects against the MetS components, their use could contribute to improving this condition and its skin manifestations.

Acknowledgment

This work was supported by the Spanish Ministry of Economy and Competitiveness, Instituto de Salud Carlos III (CIBEROBN—CB12/03/30038).

References

[1] G.M. Reaven, Banting lecture 1988. Role of insulin resistance in human disease, Diabetes 37 (12) (1988) 1595–1607.
[2] NCEP, Third report of the national cholesterol education program (NCEP) expert panel on detection, evaluation, and treatment of high blood cholesterol in adults (adult treatment panel III) final report, Circulation 106 (25) (2002) 3143–3421.
[3] F. Aberg, J. Helenius-Hietala, P. Puukka, M. Farkkila, A. Jula, Interaction between alcohol consumption and metabolic syndrome in predicting severe liver disease in the general population, Hepatology 67 (6) (2018) 2141–2149.
[4] M. Mongraw-Chaffin, M.C. Foster, C.A.M. Anderson, G.L. Burke, N. Haq, R.R. Kalyani, P. Ouyang, C.T. Sibley, R. Tracy, M. Woodward, D. Vaidya, Metabolically healthy obesity, transition to metabolic syndrome, and cardiovascular risk, J. Am. Coll. Cardiol. 71 (17) (2018) 1857–1865.
[5] A.S. Gami, B.J. Witt, D.E. Howard, P.J. Erwin, L.A. Gami, V.K. Somers, V.M. Montori, Metabolic syndrome and risk of incident cardiovascular events and death: a systematic review and meta-analysis of longitudinal studies, J. Am. Coll. Cardiol. 49 (4) (2007) 403–414.
[6] P. Mirmiran, N. Noori, F. Azizi, A prospective study of determinants of the metabolic syndrome in adults, Nutr. Metab. Cardiovasc. Dis. 18 (8) (2008) 567–573.
[7] K.G. Alberti, R.H. Eckel, S.M. Grundy, P.Z. Zimmet, J.I. Cleeman, K.A. Donato, J.C. Fruchart, W.P. James, C.M. Loria, S.C. Smith Jr., Harmonizing the metabolic syndrome: a joint interim statement of the International Diabetes Federation Task Force on Epidemiology and Prevention; National Heart, Lung, and Blood Institute; American Heart Association; World Heart Federation; International Atherosclerosis Society; and International Association for the Study of Obesity, Circulation 120 (16) (2009) 1640–1645.
[8] R. Salas, M. Bibiloni Mdel, E. Ramos, J.Z. Villarreal, A. Pons, J.A. Tur, A. Sureda, Metabolic syndrome prevalence among Northern Mexican adult population, PLoS One 9 (8) (2014), e105581.
[9] A. Spalding, J. Kernan, W. Lockette, The metabolic syndrome: a modern plague spread by modern technology, J. Clin. Hypertens (Greenwich) 11 (12) (2009) 755–760.
[10] A.S. Karadag, E. Ozlu, M.J. Lavery, Cutaneous manifestations of diabetes mellitus and the metabolic syndrome, Clin. Dermatol. 36 (1) (2018) 89–93.
[11] D. Rigopoulos, G. Larios, A. Katsambas, Skin signs of systemic diseases, Clin. Dermatol. 29 (5) (2011) 531–540.
[12] E. McCracken, M. Monaghan, S. Sreenivasan, Pathophysiology of the metabolic syndrome, Clin. Dermatol. 36 (1) (2018) 14–20.
[13] Y. Rochlani, N.V. Pothineni, S. Kovelamudi, J.L. Mehta, Metabolic syndrome: pathophysiology, management, and modulation by natural compounds, Ther. Adv. Cardiovasc. Dis. 11 (8) (2017) 215–225.
[14] R. Vona, L. Gambardella, C. Cittadini, E. Straface, D. Pietraforte, Biomarkers of oxidative stress in metabolic syndrome and associated diseases, Oxidative Med. Cell. Longev. 2019 (2019) 8267234.
[15] D. Leroith, Pathophysiology of the metabolic syndrome: implications for the cardiometabolic risks associated with type 2 diabetes, Am J Med Sci 343 (1) (2012) 13–16.

[16] G. Boden, G.I. Shulman, Free fatty acids in obesity and type 2 diabetes: defining their role in the development of insulin resistance and beta-cell dysfunction, Eur. J. Clin. Investig. 32 (Suppl. 3) (2002) 14–23.
[17] A.B. Engin, What is lipotoxicity? in: A. Engin, A. Engin (Eds.), Obesity and Lipotoxicity, Advances in Experimental Medicine and Biology, vol. 960, 2017, pp. 197–220.
[18] A. Sureda, M.D.M. Bibiloni, A. Julibert, C. Bouzas, E. Argelich, I. Llompart, A. Pons, J.A. Tur, Adherence to the Mediterranean diet and inflammatory markers, Nutrients 10 (1) (2018).
[19] R. Cancello, K. Clement, Is obesity an inflammatory illness? Role of low-grade inflammation and macrophage infiltration in human white adipose tissue, BJOG 113 (10) (2006) 1141–1147.
[20] M. Monserrat-Mesquida, M. Quetglas-Llabres, X. Capo, C. Bouzas, D. Mateos, A. Pons, J.A. Tur, A. Sureda, Metabolic syndrome is associated with oxidative stress and proinflammatory state, Antioxidants (Basel) 9 (3) (2020).
[21] G. Grandl, C. Wolfrum, Hemostasis, endothelial stress, inflammation, and the metabolic syndrome, Semin. Immunopathol. 40 (2) (2018) 215–224.
[22] B.B. Davidovici, N. Sattar, J. Prinz, L. Puig, P. Emery, J.N. Barker, P. van de Kerkhof, M. Stahle, F.O. Nestle, G. Girolomoni, J.G. Krueger, Psoriasis and systemic inflammatory diseases: potential mechanistic links between skin disease and co-morbid conditions, J. Invest. Dermatol. 130 (7) (2010) 1785–1796.
[23] C.E. Griffiths, J.N. Barker, Pathogenesis and clinical features of psoriasis, Lancet 370 (9583) (2007) 263–271.
[24] Y. Liu, J.G. Krueger, A.M. Bowcock, Psoriasis: genetic associations and immune system changes, Genes Immun. 8 (1) (2007) 1–12.
[25] J.H. Han, J.H. Lee, K.D. Han, H.N. Kim, C.H. Bang, Y.M. Park, J.Y. Lee, T.Y. Kim, Increased risk of psoriasis in subjects with abdominal obesity: a nationwide population-based study, J. Dermatol. 46 (8) (2019) 695–701.
[26] I. Snekvik, T.I.L. Nilsen, P.R. Romundstad, M. Saunes, Metabolic syndrome and risk of incident psoriasis: prospective data from the HUNT study, Norway, Br. J. Dermatol. 180 (1) (2019) 94–99.
[27] M. Gyldenlove, H. Storgaard, J.J. Holst, T. Vilsboll, F.K. Knop, L. Skov, Patients with psoriasis are insulin resistant, J. Am. Acad. Dermatol. 72 (4) (2015) 599–605.
[28] E. Klingberg, A. Bilberg, S. Bjorkman, M. Hedberg, L. Jacobsson, H. Forsblad-d'Elia, H. Carlsten, B. Eliasson, I. Larsson, Weight loss improves disease activity in patients with psoriatic arthritis and obesity: an interventional study, Arthritis Res. Ther. 21 (1) (2019) 17.
[29] M. Wolters, Diet and psoriasis: experimental data and clinical evidence, Br. J. Dermatol. 153 (4) (2005) 706–714.
[30] S. Titus, J. Hodge, Diagnosis and treatment of acne, Am. Fam. Physician 86 (8) (2012) 734–740.
[31] D. Thiboutot, H. Gollnick, V. Bettoli, B. Dreno, S. Kang, J.J. Leyden, A.R. Shalita, V.T. Lozada, D. Berson, A. Finlay, C.L. Goh, M.I. Herane, A. Kaminsky, R. Kubba, A. Layton, Y. Miyachi, M. Perez, J.P. Martin, E.S.M. Ramos, J.A. See, N. Shear, J. Wolf Jr., New insights into the management of acne: an update from the Global Alliance to Improve Outcomes in Acne group, J. Am. Acad. Dermatol. 60 (5 Suppl) (2009) S1–50.
[32] Y.J. Bhat, I. Latief, I. Hassan, Update on etiopathogenesis and treatment of acne, Indian J. Dermatol. Venereol. Leprol. 83 (3) (2017) 298–306.
[33] K. Degitz, M. Placzek, C. Borelli, G. Plewig, Pathophysiology of acne, J. Dtsch. Dermatol. Ges. 5 (4) (2007) 316–323.
[34] M.P. Canale, A. Noce, M. Di Lauro, G. Marrone, M. Cantelmo, C. Cardillo, M. Federici, N. Di Daniele, M. Tesauro, Gut dysbiosis and western diet in the pathogenesis of essential arterial hypertension: a narrative review, Nutrients 13 (4) (2021) 1162.

[35] H.C. Williams, R.P. Dellavalle, S. Garner, Acne vulgaris, Lancet 379 (9813) (2012) 361–372.

[36] B.C. Melnik, C.C. Zouboulis, Potential role of FoxO1 and mTORC1 in the pathogenesis of Western diet-induced acne, Exp. Dermatol. 22 (5) (2013) 311–315.

[37] O. Isard, A.C. Knol, M.F. Aries, J.M. Nguyen, A. Khammari, N. Castex-Rizzi, B. Dreno, *Propionibacterium acnes* activates the IGF-1/IGF-1R system in the epidermis and induces keratinocyte proliferation, J. Invest. Dermatol. 131 (1) (2011) 59–66.

[38] S. Briganti, E. Flori, A. Mastrofrancesco, M. Ottaviani, Acne as an altered dermato-endocrine response problem, Exp. Dermatol. 29 (9) (2020) 833–839.

[39] J.S. Barbieri, Diet and acne-challenges of translating nutritional epidemiologic research into clinical practice, JAMA Dermatol. 156 (8) (2020) 841–843.

[40] R.N. Smith, N.J. Mann, A. Braue, H. Makelainen, G.A. Varigos, A low-glycemic-load diet improves symptoms in acne vulgaris patients: a randomized controlled trial, Am. J. Clin. Nutr. 86 (1) (2007) 107–115.

[41] T. Ergun, Hidradenitis suppurativa and the metabolic syndrome, Clin. Dermatol. 36 (1) (2018) 41–47.

[42] A. Alikhan, P.J. Lynch, D.B. Eisen, Hidradenitis suppurativa: a comprehensive review, J. Am. Acad. Dermatol. 60 (4) (2009) 539–561. quiz 562-533.

[43] C. Dessinioti, A. Katsambas, C. Antoniou, Hidradenitis suppurrativa (acne inversa) as a systemic disease, Clin. Dermatol. 32 (3) (2014) 397–408.

[44] G. Kelly, C.M. Sweeney, A.M. Tobin, B. Kirby, Hidradenitis suppurativa: the role of immune dysregulation, Int. J. Dermatol. 53 (10) (2014) 1186–1196.

[45] M. von Laffert, P. Helmbold, J. Wohlrab, E. Fiedler, V. Stadie, W.C. Marsch, Hidradenitis suppurativa (acne inversa): early inflammatory events at terminal follicles and at interfollicular epidermis, Exp. Dermatol. 19 (6) (2010) 533–537.

[46] I.M. Miller, C. Ellervik, G.R. Vinding, K. Zarchi, K.S. Ibler, K.M. Knudsen, G.B. Jemec, Association of metabolic syndrome and hidradenitis suppurativa, JAMA Dermatol. 150 (12) (2014) 1273–1280.

[47] G. Shalom, T. Freud, I. Harman-Boehm, I. Polishchuk, A.D. Cohen, Hidradenitis suppurativa and metabolic syndrome: a comparative cross-sectional study of 3207 patients, Br. J. Dermatol. 173 (2) (2015) 464–470.

[48] T. Tzellos, C.C. Zouboulis, W. Gulliver, A.D. Cohen, P. Wolkenstein, G.B. Jemec, Cardiovascular disease risk factors in patients with hidradenitis suppurativa: a systematic review and meta-analysis of observational studies, Br. J. Dermatol. 173 (5) (2015) 1142–1155.

[49] D.A. Gold, V.J. Reeder, M.G. Mahan, I.H. Hamzavi, The prevalence of metabolic syndrome in patients with hidradenitis suppurativa, J. Am. Acad. Dermatol. 70 (4) (2014) 699–703.

[50] J. Boer, Resolution of hidradenitis suppurativa after weight loss by dietary measures, especially on frictional locations, J. Eur. Acad. Dermatol. Venereol. 30 (5) (2016) 895–896.

[51] R. Verdolini, N. Clayton, A. Smith, N. Alwash, B. Mannello, Metformin for the treatment of hidradenitis suppurativa: a little help along the way, J. Eur. Acad. Dermatol. Venereol. 27 (9) (2013) 1101–1108.

[52] R.A. Schwartz, Acanthosis nigricans, J. Am. Acad. Dermatol. 31 (1) (1994) 1–19. quiz 20-12.

[53] A.S. Karadağ, Y. You, R. Danarti, S. Al-Khuzaei, W. Chen, Acanthosis nigricans and the metabolic syndrome, Clin. Dermatol. 36 (1) (2018) 48–53.

[54] J.P. Burke, D.E. Hale, H.P. Hazuda, M.P. Stern, A quantitative scale of acanthosis nigricans, Diabetes Care 22 (10) (1999) 1655–1659.

[55] A.S. Karadağ, T.K. Uzuncakmak, E. Ozlu, M. Takir, R. Karadag, O. Kostek, M. Simsek, N. Akdeniz, U. Wollina, W. Chen, Introduction of a novel quantitative scoring system

for acanthosis nigricans and its validation in a pilot study, Dermatol. Ther. 33 (6) (2020), e14450.
[56] T. Ayaz, S. Baydur Sahin, O.Z. Sahin, Relation of Acanthosis nigricans to metabolic syndrome in overweight and obese women, Metab. Syndr. Relat. Disord. 12 (6) (2014) 320–323.
[57] S.R. Edmondson, S.P. Thumiger, P. Kaur, B. Loh, R. Koelmeyer, A. Li, J.V. Silha, L.J. Murphy, C.J. Wraight, G.A. Werther, Insulin-like growth factor binding protein-3 (IGFBP-3) localizes to and modulates proliferative epidermal keratinocytes in vivo, Br. J. Dermatol. 152 (2) (2005) 225–230.
[58] S.M. Rudman, M.P. Philpott, G.A. Thomas, T. Kealey, The role of IGF-I in human skin and its appendages: morphogen as well as mitogen? J. Invest. Dermatol. 109 (6) (1997) 770–777.
[59] R. Fonseca, M.A. Costa-Lima, V. Cosentino, I.M. Orioli, Second case of Beare-Stevenson syndrome with an FGFR2 Ser372Cys mutation, Am. J. Med. Genet. A 146A (5) (2008) 658–660.
[60] A. Stears, S. O'Rahilly, R.K. Semple, D.B. Savage, Metabolic insights from extreme human insulin resistance phenotypes, Best Pract. Res. Clin. Endocrinol. Metab. 26 (2) (2012) 145–157.
[61] R. Novotny, J. Davis, J. Butel, C.J. Boushey, M.K. Fialkowski, C.R. Nigg, K.L. Braun, R.T. Leon Guerrero, P. Coleman, A. Bersamin, A.A.R. Areta, L.R. Barber Jr., T. Belyeu-Camacho, J. Greenberg, T. Fleming, E. Dela Cruz-Talbert, A. Yamanaka, L.R. Wilkens, Effect of the children's healthy living program on young child overweight, obesity, and acanthosis Nigricans in the us-affiliated pacific region: a randomized clinical trial, JAMA Netw. Open 1 (6) (2018), e183896.
[62] S. Sinha, R.A. Schwartz, Juvenile acanthosis nigricans, J. Am. Acad. Dermatol. 57 (3) (2007) 502–508.
[63] D. Giri, H. Alsaffar, R. Ramakrishnan, Acanthosis Nigricans and its response to metformin, Pediatr. Dermatol. 34 (5) (2017) e281–e282.
[64] A. Sett, S. Pradhan, K. Sancheti, D. Basu, A. Datta, L. Biswas, S. Das, S.K. Pal, N. Gupta, A. Sil, N.K. Das, Effectiveness and safety of metformin versus canthex in patients with acanthosis nigricans: a randomized, double-blind controlled trial, Indian J. Dermatol. 64 (2) (2019) 115–121.
[65] N. Steckhan, C.D. Hohmann, C. Kessler, G. Dobos, A. Michalsen, H. Cramer, Effects of different dietary approaches on inflammatory markers in patients with metabolic syndrome: a systematic review and meta-analysis, Nutrition 32 (3) (2016) 338–348.
[66] J. Godos, G. Zappala, S. Bernardini, I. Giambini, M. Bes-Rastrollo, M. Martinez-Gonzalez, Adherence to the Mediterranean diet is inversely associated with metabolic syndrome occurrence: a meta-analysis of observational studies, Int. J. Food Sci. Nutr. 68 (2) (2017) 138–148.
[67] N. Babio, M. Bullo, J. Salas-Salvado, Mediterranean diet and metabolic syndrome: the evidence, Public Health Nutr. 12 (9A) (2009) 1607–1617.
[68] Q. Qi, M. Xu, H. Wu, L. Liang, C.M. Champagne, G.A. Bray, F.M. Sacks, L. Qi, IRS1 genotype modulates metabolic syndrome reversion in response to 2-year weight-loss diet intervention: the POUNDS LOST trial, Diabetes Care 36 (11) (2013) 3442–3447.
[69] S. Castro-Barquero, A.M. Ruiz-Leon, M. Sierra-Perez, R. Estruch, R. Casas, Dietary strategies for metabolic syndrome: a comprehensive review, Nutrients 12 (10) (2020).
[70] M.A. Martínez-González, J. Salas-Salvado, R. Estruch, D. Corella, M. Fito, E. Ros, Benefits of the Mediterranean diet: insights from the PREDIMED study, Prog. Cardiovasc. Dis. 58 (1) (2015) 50–60.
[71] A.F. Cicero, A. Colletti, Role of phytochemicals in the management of metabolic syndrome, Phytomedicine 23 (11) (2016) 1134–1144.

[72] A. Mahdavi, M. Bagherniya, M.S. Mirenayat, S.L. Atkin, A. Sahebkar, Medicinal plants and phytochemicals regulating insulin resistance and glucose homeostasis in type 2 diabetic patients: a clinical review, Adv. Exp. Med. Biol. 1308 (2021) 161–183.
[73] H. El Gharras, Polyphenols: food sources, properties and applications. A review, Int. J. Food Sci. Technol. 44 (12) (2009) 2512–2518.
[74] A. Durazzo, M. Lucarini, E.B. Souto, C. Cicala, E. Caiazzo, A.A. Izzo, E. Novellino, A. Santini, Polyphenols: a concise overview on the chemistry, occurrence, and human health, Phytother. Res. 33 (9) (2019) 2221–2243.
[75] N. Beukes, R.A. Levendal, C.L. Frost, Selected terpenoids from medicinal plants modulate endoplasmic reticulum stress in metabolic disorders, J. Pharm. Pharmacol. 66 (11) (2014) 1505–1525.
[76] B.L. Graf, I. Raskin, W.T. Cefalu, D.M. Ribnicky, Plant-derived therapeutics for the treatment of metabolic syndrome, Curr. Opin. Investig. Drugs 11 (10) (2010) 1107–1115.
[77] M. Daniyal, M. Akram, R. Zainab, N. Munir, S.M.A. Shah, B. Liu, W. Wang, M. Riaz, F. Jabeen, Progress and prospects in the management of psoriasis and developments in phyto-therapeutic modalities, Dermatol. Ther. 32 (3) (2019), e12866.
[78] T.L. Timis, I.A. Florian, S.C. Vesa, D.R. Mitrea, R.I. Orasan, An updated guide in the management of psoriasis for every practitioner, Int. J. Clin. Pract. 75 (8) (2021), e14290.
[79] A. Herman, A.P. Herman, Topically used herbal products for the treatment of psoriasis—mechanism of action, drug delivery, clinical studies, Planta Med. 82 (17) (2016) 1447–1455.
[80] T.H. Huang, C.F. Lin, A. Alalaiwe, S.C. Yang, J.Y. Fang, Apoptotic or antiproliferative activity of natural products against keratinocytes for the treatment of psoriasis, Int. J. Mol. Sci. 20 (10) (2019).
[81] Z. Wu, H. Uchi, S. Morino-Koga, W. Shi, M. Furue, Resveratrol inhibition of human keratinocyte proliferation via SIRT1/ARNT/ERK dependent downregulation of aquaporin 3, J. Dermatol. Sci. 75 (1) (2014) 16–23.
[82] J.H. Lee, J.S. Kim, S.Y. Park, Y.J. Lee, Resveratrol induces human keratinocyte damage via the activation of class III histone deacetylase, Sirt1, Oncol. Rep. 35 (1) (2016) 524–529.
[83] J. Sun, J. Han, Y. Zhao, Q. Zhu, J. Hu, Curcumin induces apoptosis in tumor necrosis factor-alpha-treated HaCaT cells, Int. Immunopharmacol. 13 (2) (2012) 170–174.
[84] E. Maioli, G. Valacchi, Rottlerin: bases for a possible usage in psoriasis, Curr. Drug Metab. 11 (5) (2010) 425–430.
[85] T. Niu, Y. Tian, Q. Cai, Q. Ren, L. Wei, Red light combined with blue light irradiation regulates proliferation and apoptosis in skin keratinocytes in combination with low concentrations of curcumin, PLoS One 10 (9) (2015), e0138754.
[86] I.K. Koycheva, L.V. Vasileva, K.M. Amirova, A.S. Marchev, Z.P. Balcheva-Sivenova, M.I. Georgiev, Biotechnologically produced *Lavandula angustifolia* Mill. Extract rich in rosmarinic acid resolves psoriasis-related inflammation through Janus kinase/signal transducer and activator of transcription signaling, Front. Pharmacol. 12 (2021) 940.
[87] L.L. Zhou, Z.X. Lin, K.P. Fung, C.H. Cheng, C.T. Che, M. Zhao, S.H. Wu, Z. Zuo, Celastrol-induced apoptosis in human HaCaT keratinocytes involves the inhibition of NF-kappaB activity, Eur. J. Pharmacol. 670 (2–3) (2011) 399–408.
[88] T.N. Kjær, K. Thorsen, N. Jessen, K. Stenderup, S.B. Pedersen, Resveratrol ameliorates imiquimod-induced psoriasis-like skin inflammation in mice, PLoS One 10 (5) (2015), e0126599.
[89] M. Min, B.X. Yan, P. Wang, L. Landeck, J.Q. Chen, W. Li, S.Q. Cai, M. Zheng, X.Y. Man, Rottlerin as a therapeutic approach in psoriasis: evidence from in vitro and in vivo studies, PLoS One 12 (12) (2017), e0190051.

[90] J.C. Chamcheu, I.A. Siddiqui, V.M. Adhami, S. Esnault, D.J. Bharali, A.S. Babatunde, S. Adame, R.J. Massey, G.S. Wood, B.J. Longley, S.A. Mousa, H. Mukhtar, Chitosan-based nanoformulated (-)-epigallocatechin-3-gallate\ (EGCG) modulates human keratinocyte-induced responses and alleviates imiquimod-induced murine psoriasiform dermatitis, Int. J. Nanomedicine 13 (2018) 4189–4206.

[91] T. Li, Z. Wei, Y. Sun, Q. Wang, H. Kuang, Withanolides, extracted from *Datura Metel* L. inhibit keratinocyte proliferation and imiquimod-induced psoriasis-like dermatitis via the STAT3/P38/ERK1/2 pathway, Molecules 24 (14) (2019).

[92] M. Korinek, P.S. Hsieh, Y.L. Chen, P.W. Hsieh, S.H. Chang, Y.H. Wu, T.L. Hwang, Randialic acid B and tomentosolic acid block formyl peptide receptor 1 in human neutrophils and attenuate psoriasis-like inflammation in vivo, Biochem. Pharmacol. 190 (2021), 114596.

[93] X. Tian, L. Tang, F. Wei, H. Chen, L. Sheng, Y. Yang, X. Zhou, Y. Li, X. Xu, B. Zhang, Z. Liu, Y. Lei, B. You, C. Bai, X. He, Z. Huang, Pentacyclic triterpene compounds from loquat leaves reduce skin inflammation and epidermal hyperplasia in psoriasis via inhibiting the Th17 cells, Mol. Immunol. 132 (2021) 30–40.

[94] J. An, T. Li, Y. Dong, Z. Li, J. Huo, Terminalia chebulanin attenuates psoriatic skin lesion via regulation of heme oxygenase-1, Cell. Physiol. Biochem. 39 (2) (2016) 531–543.

[95] X.Q. Li, Y. Chen, H.M. Zhou, H.L. Shi, X.N. Yan, L.P. Lin, R.X. Tan, Anti-psoriasis effect of water-processed rosin in mice, J. Ethnopharmacol. 242 (2019), 112073.

[96] D. Dimitris, T. Ekaterina-Michaela, K. Christina, S. Ioannis, S.K. Ioanna, L. Aggeliki, H. Sophia, R. Michael, S. Helen, *Melissa officinalis* ssp. altissima extracts: a therapeutic approach targeting psoriasis in mice, J. Ethnopharmacol. 246 (2020) 112208.

[97] T.A. Syed, S.A. Ahmad, A.H. Holt, S.H. Ahmad, M. Afzal, Management of psoriasis with *Aloe vera* extract in a hydrophilic cream: a placebo-controlled, double-blind study, Tropical Med. Int. Health 1 (4) (1996) 505–509.

[98] S. Bernstein, H. Donsky, W. Gulliver, D. Hamilton, S. Nobel, R. Norman, Treatment of mild to moderate psoriasis with Relieva, a *Mahonia aquifolium* extract- -a double-blind, placebo-controlled study, Am. J. Ther. 13 (2) (2006) 121–126.

[99] L. Barrea, G. Muscogiuri, C. Di Somma, G. Annunziata, M. Megna, A. Falco, A. Balato, A. Colao, S. Savastano, Coffee consumption, metabolic syndrome and clinical severity of psoriasis: good or bad stuff? Arch. Toxicol. 92 (5) (2018) 1831–1845.

[100] D. Crisan, K. Scharffetter-Kochanek, M. Crisan, S. Schatz, A. Hainzl, L. Olenic, A. Filip, L.A. Schneider, A. Sindrilaru, Topical silver and gold nanoparticles complexed with *Cornus mas* suppress inflammation in human psoriasis plaques by inhibiting NF-kappaB activity, Exp. Dermatol. 27 (10) (2018) 1166–1169.

[101] P. Bahraini, M. Rajabi, P. Mansouri, G. Sarafian, R. Chalangari, Z. Azizian, Turmeric tonic as a treatment in scalp psoriasis: a randomized placebo-control clinical trial, J. Cosmet. Dermatol. 17 (3) (2018) 461–466.

[102] P. Alex, S. Williams, L. Sutton, T. Yesudas, C. Sutton, S. Thomas, M. Centola, Efficacy and safety of HAT1 compared with calcipotriol in the treatment of patients with mild to moderate chronic plaque psoriasis: results from an open-label randomized comparative pilot clinical study, Clin. Exp. Dermatol. 45 (3) (2020) 318–322.

[103] M.A. Shatalebi, S. Bokaie Jazi, A. Yegdaneh, F. Iraji, A.H. Siadat, P. Noorshargh, Comparative evaluation of *Gracilaria* algae 3% cream vs Clobetasol 0.05% cream in treatment of plaque type psoriasis: a randomized, split-body, triple-blinded clinical trial, Dermatol. Ther. 33 (6) (2020), e14317.

[104] A. Yargholi, L. Shirbeigi, R. Rahimi, P. Mansouri, M.H. Ayati, The effect of *Melissa Officinalis* syrup on patients with mild to moderate psoriasis: a randomized, double-blind placebo-controlled clinical trial, BMC Res. Notes 14 (2021) 253.

[105] M.S. Zorko, B. Strukelj, U. Svajger, S. Kreft, T. Lunder, Efficacy of a polyphenolic extract from silver fir (*Abies alba*) bark on psoriasis: a randomised, double-blind, placebo-controlled trial, Pharmazie 73 (1) (2018) 56–60.

[106] S. Soleymani, M.H. Farzaei, A. Zargaran, S. Niknam, R. Rahimi, Promising plant-derived secondary metabolites for treatment of acne vulgaris: a mechanistic review, Arch. Dermatol. Res. 312 (1) (2020) 5–23.
[107] S. Soleymani, A. Zargaran, M.H. Farzaei, A. Iranpanah, F. Heydarpour, F. Najafi, R. Rahimi, The effect of a hydrogel made by *Nigella sativa* L. on acne vulgaris: a randomized double-blind clinical trial, Phytother. Res. 34 (11) (2020) 3052–3062.
[108] J. Hoffmann, F. Gendrisch, C.M. Schempp, U. Wolfle, New herbal biomedicines for the topical treatment of dermatological disorders, Biomedicine 8 (2) (2020).
[109] O. Said, I. Khamaysi, A. Kmail, S. Fulder, B. AboFarekh, R. Amin, J. Daraghmeh, B. Saad, In vitro and randomized, double-blind, placebo-controlled trial to determine the efficacy and safety of nine antiacne medicinal plants, Evid. Based Complement. Alternat. Med. 2020 (2020) 3231413.
[110] W.J. Winkelman, Aromatherapy, botanicals, and essential oils in acne, Clin. Dermatol. 36 (3) (2018) 299–305.
[111] T. Matsumoto, Y. Matsubara, Y. Mizuhara, K. Sekiguchi, J. Koseki, K. Tsuchiya, H. Nishimura, J. Watanabe, A. Kaneko, K. Maemura, T. Hattori, Y. Kase, Plasma pharmacokinetics of polyphenols in a traditional Japanese medicine, Jumihaidokuto, which Suppresses *Propionibacterium acnes*-induced dermatitis in rats, Molecules 20 (10) (2015) 18031–18046.
[112] Z.M.Q. Dos Santos, M.Q. Dos Santos, V. Zancanaro, E.H. Bellaver, G.M. Nardi, J.M.L. Gelinski, C. Locatelli, Topical application of phenolic compounds suppresses *Propionibacterium acnes*-induced inflammatory responses in mice with ear edema, Naunyn Schmiedeberg's Arch. Pharmacol. 392 (5) (2019) 529–540.
[113] D.H. Hwang, D.Y. Lee, P.O. Koh, H.R. Yang, C. Kang, E. Kim, *Rosa davurica* Pall. improves *Propionibacterium acnes*-induced inflammatory responses in mouse ear edema model and suppresses pro-inflammatory chemokine production via MAPK and NF-kappaB pathways in HaCaT cells, Int. J. Mol. Sci. 21 (5) (2020).
[114] M. Im, S.Y. Kim, K.C. Sohn, D.K. Choi, Y. Lee, Y.J. Seo, C.D. Kim, Y.L. Hwang, C.C. Zouboulis, J.H. Lee, Epigallocatechin-3-gallate suppresses IGF-I-induced lipogenesis and cytokine expression in SZ95 sebocytes, J. Invest. Dermatol. 132 (12) (2012) 2700–2708.
[115] G. Fabbrocini, S. Staibano, G. De Rosa, V. Battimiello, N. Fardella, G. Ilardi, M.I. La Rotonda, A. Longobardi, M. Mazzella, M. Siano, F. Pastore, V. De Vita, M.L. Vecchione, F. Ayala, Resveratrol-containing gel for the treatment of acne vulgaris: a single-blind, vehicle-controlled, pilot study, Am. J. Clin. Dermatol. 12 (2) (2011) 133–141.
[116] J.Y. Yoon, H.H. Kwon, S.U. Min, D.M. Thiboutot, D.H. Suh, Epigallocatechin-3-gallate improves acne in humans by modulating intracellular molecular targets and inhibiting P. acnes, J. Invest. Dermatol. 133 (2) (2013) 429–440.
[117] P.H. Lu, C.H. Hsu, Does supplementation with green tea extract improve acne in post-adolescent women? A randomized, double-blind, and placebo-controlled clinical trial, Complement. Ther. Med. 25 (2016) 159–163.
[118] S. Saric, M. Notay, R.K. Sivamani, Green tea and other tea polyphenols: effects on sebum production and acne vulgaris, Antioxidants (Basel) 6 (1) (2016).
[119] R.F. Fouladi, Aqueous extract of dried fruit of Berberis vulgaris L. in acne vulgaris, a clinical trial, J. Diet Suppl. 9 (4) (2012) 253–261.
[120] A.G. da Silva, F. Puziol Pde, R.N. Leitao, T.R. Gomes, R. Scherer, M.L. Martins, A.S. Cavalcanti, L.C. Cavalcanti, Application of the essential oil from copaiba (Copaifera langsdori Desf.) for acne vulgaris: a double-blind, placebo-controlled clinical trial, Altern. Med. Rev. 17 (1) (2012) 69–75.
[121] J.H. Hou, H. Shin, K.H. Jang, C.K. Park, B. Koo, H. Shin, S.H. Yuk, K.Y. Lee, Anti-acne properties of hydrophobic fraction of red ginseng (*Panax ginseng* C.A. Meyer) and its active components, Phytother. Res. 33 (3) (2019) 584–590.

[122] W. Damkerngsuntorn, P. Rerknimitr, R. Panchaprateep, N. Tangkijngamvong, C. Kumtornrut, S.J. Kerr, P. Asawanonda, M.H. Tantisira, P. Khemawoot, The effects of a standardized extract of *Centella asiatica* on postlaser resurfacing wound healing on the face: a split-face, double-blind, randomized, placebo-controlled trial, J. Altern. Complement. Med. 26 (6) (2020) 529–536.

[123] S. Laneri, I. Dini, A. Tito, R. Di Lorenzo, M. Bimonte, A. Tortora, C. Zappelli, M. Angelillo, A. Bernardi, A. Sacchi, M.G. Colucci, F. Apone, Plant cell culture extract of Cirsium eriophorum with skin pore refiner activity by modulating sebum production and inflammatory response, Phytother. Res. 35 (1) (2021) 530–540.

[124] R. Najafi-Taher, V.E. Farsani, N.M. Rayeni, H.R. Moghimi, A. Ehsani, A. Amani, A topical gel of tea tree oil nanoemulsion containing adapalene versus adapalene marketed gel in patients with acne vulgaris: a randomized clinical trial, Arch. Dermatol. Res. (2021) 1–7.

[125] J.H. Yang, E.J. Hwang, J. Moon, J.Y. Yoon, J.W. Kim, S. Choi, S.I. Cho, D.H. Suh, Clinical efficacy of herbal extracts in treatment of mild to moderate acne vulgaris: an 8-week, double-blinded, randomized, controlled trial, J. Dermatol. Treat. 32 (3) (2021) 297–301.

[126] R.K. Andersen, G.B. Jemec, Treatments for hidradenitis suppurativa, Clin. Dermatol. 35 (2) (2017) 218–224.

[127] A.J. Hendricks, P.A. Hirt, S. Sekhon, A.R. Vaughn, H.A. Lev-Tov, J.L. Hsiao, V.Y. Shi, Non-pharmacologic approaches for hidradenitis suppurativa—a systematic review, J. Dermatol. Treat. 32 (1) (2021) 11–18.

[128] A. Silfvast-Kaiser, R. Youssef, S.Y. Paek, Diet in hidradenitis suppurativa: a review of published and lay literature, Int. J. Dermatol. 58 (11) (2019) 1225–1230.

[129] L. Barrea, G. Fabbrocini, G. Annunziata, G. Muscogiuri, M. Donnarumma, C. Marasca, A. Colao, S. Savastano, Role of nutrition and adherence to the Mediterranean diet in the multidisciplinary approach of hidradenitis suppurativa: evaluation of nutritional status and its association with severity of disease, Nutrients 11 (1) (2018).

[130] J.M. Fernandez, K.D. Marr, A.J. Hendricks, K.N. Price, C.M. Ludwig, M. Maarouf, J.L. Hsiao, V.Y. Shi, Alleviating and exacerbating foods in hidradenitis suppurativa, Dermatol. Ther. 33 (6) (2020), e14246.

[131] A. Das, D. Datta, M. Kassir, U. Wollina, H. Galadari, T. Lotti, M. Jafferany, S. Grabbe, M. Goldust, Acanthosis nigricans: a review, J. Cosmet. Dermatol. 19 (8) (2020) 1857–1865.

[132] A.V. Kamble, S.P. Dhamane, A.S. Kulkarni, V.V. Potnis, Review on effects of herbal extract for the treatment of polycystic ovarian syndrome (PCOS), Plant Arch. 20 (1) (2020) 1189–1195.

CHAPTER 13

Cachexia and phytonutrients

Sajad Fakhri[a,*], Sana Piri[a,*], and Haroon Khan[b]
[a]Pharmaceutical Sciences Research Center, Health Institute, Kermanshah University of Medical Sciences, Kermanshah, Iran
[b]Department of Pharmacy, Abdul Wali Khan University Mardan, Mardan, Pakistan

1. Introduction

Muscle and fat loss is a pathological condition in several diseases interconnected to cachexia [1]. The word cachexia is obtained from "kakos" and "hexis" which mean bad and condition/habit, respectively [2]. With the prevalence of 60%–80%, cachexia reduces muscle mass, followed by fatigue, declined life quality, and decreased survival [3,4]. Cachexia could be the result of several diseases, including cancer, chronic obstructive pulmonary disease (COPD), chronic kidney disease (CKD), and chronic heart failure (CHF) [5]. Studies have indicated several dysregulated signaling pathways behind cachexia [6]. Evidence also has shown that cachexia induces dysregulated levels of inflammatory mediators, including nuclear factor-kappa B (NF-κB), tumor necrosis factor-alpha (TNF-α), interleukin-1 (IL-1), and IL-6. Additionally, transforming growth factor type beta (TGF-β), myostatin, glucocorticoids, and angiotensin II (Ang-II) encountered changes [7]. Besides, downstream muscle mechanisms are also involved including, muscle-specific RING finger-1 (MuRF 1), muscle atrophy F-box (MAFbx), ubiquitin-proteasome system (UPS), and phosphoinositide 3-kinases (PI3K)/protein kinase B (Akt)/mammalian target of rapamycin (mTOR) [8,9]. Considering several side effects in the use of existing drugs in combating cachexia [10], increasing studies are trying to find novel treatments with higher potency and lower side effects. Previously, different nutrients, including amino acids (e.g., arginine, glutamine) and fatty acids (e.g., omega-3) were recommended in combating cachexia [11,12]. In recent decades, plant-derived natural products have shown critical roles in the treatment of diseases [13–17]. Due to the complexity of dysregulated pathways behind cachexia, phytonutrients could employ their multitargeting potential toward a simultaneous modulation of several signaling mediators.

*The authors, as the first authors, have contributed equally to this chapter.

The Role of Phytonutrients in Metabolic Disorders
https://doi.org/10.1016/B978-0-12-824356-5.00007-2

Of those secondary metabolites, phenolic compounds, polyphenols, flavonoids, and alkaloids seem to be promising candidates in the prevention and treatment of skeletal muscle atrophy as well as symptoms of cachexia in cancer, heart failure, kidney disease, and other associated disorders.

Here in this chapter, more precise dysregulated signaling pathways have been revealed in cachexia, which was ignored previously. Additionally, the role of natural products in the modulation of cachexia-associated signaling pathways has been highlighted in several disorders.

2. Cachexia and molecular mechanisms: Targeted signaling pathways

During the human life span, muscle growth occurs in size and number, although muscle fibers are declined with aging and other reasons [18]. Cachexia is a disorder of wasting muscle and adipose tissues [19] as well as a reduction of body function, declined endurance for treatment, and increased death ratio [20]. It is a complex syndrome that occurs during the end phase of several diseases such as cancer, COPD, kidney disease, cystic fibrosis, liver cirrhosis, and many neurodegenerative diseases, stroke, malaria, tuberculosis, multiple sclerosis, and CHF. The properties associated with cachexia, include reducing weight in adults, growth imperfect in children as well as anorexia, inflammation, insulin resistance, increased muscle protein decomposition, decreased protein synthesis, nausea, immune-depression, anemia, stomatitis, vomiting, constipation, dyspnea, depression, pain, fatigue, increased energy metabolism, and accelerated lipolysis. Studies have indicated the role of different pathways in cachexia-associated muscle loss such as PI3K/Akt, NF-κB, myostatin pathway, apoptosis, and oxidative stress [6,18]. PI3K/Akt/mTOR is an important pathway in muscle that is modulated by insulin-like growth factor-1 (IGF-1). In this regard, the serine/threonine kinase Akt increases protein synthesis. Consequently, in muscle, PI3K can activate Akt and then induce receptor binding or integrin-mediated activation of focal adhesion kinase (FAK) [21]. Besides, mTOR is the latter downstream mediator composed of two complexes, mTORC1 and mTORC2. It has been shown that mTORC1 regulates different processes such as protein synthesis, ribosome/mitochondrial biogenesis, and also autophagy [21]. NF-κB, as an inflammatory transcription factor, is increased under cachexia conditions [22]. Besides, cytokines activate NF-κB, which transfers to the nucleus and binds to the MuRF1 promoter regarding initiating muscle breakdown. In cachexia, TNF-α also activates NF-κB by triggering IκB kinase (IKK) and then phosphorylating and degrading the NF-κB inhibitor protein. Studies have shown that inflammation and inflammatory cytokines such as IL-1, TNF-α, and IL-6 play an important function in cachexia through inducing myofibrillar decomposition with activation of the ubiquitin proteasome pathway, via the NF-κB pathway [23]. Indeed, activation of inflammatory cytokines and imbalance between IL-1, TNF-α, IL-6, IL-4, interferon gamma (IFN-γ), IL-12, and IL-15 have important functions in the pathophysiology of cachexia [24,25]. Based on consistent studies, the level of IL-15 increased according to the changes in body weight [24]. Evidence has shown that cytokines increase the release of cortisol and adrenergic hormones, through which increase fat oxidation/atrophy [23]. Moreover, cytokines and associated inflammation can decline mitochondrial biogenesis with reduced activation of peroxisome proliferator-activated receptor gamma coactivator 1-alpha (PGC-1α), NRF-1, and sirtuin-1 (Sirt-1) as well as increased autophagy in cachectic muscle via inducing LC3 and Beclin-1. Furthermore, dysregulating dynamics shown by elevated FIS-1/Drp-1 and reduced MFN-2, MFN-1, and OPA-1 are associated with the reduction of mitochondrial function and ATP synthesis [26].

From the myostatin pathway point of view, as a negative regulator of muscle growth, it activates and phosphorylates Smad2/3 transcription factors by the Activin IIB membrane receptor, and modulating the transcription of genes such as MyoD. Myostatin levels also increase muscle atrophy in cachexia situation. Along with the myostatin pathway, the apoptotic pathway is important in cachexia and there is a relationship between reactive oxygen species (ROS) with immobilization and unloading atrophy as well as DNA fragmentation. In muscle, there is a controlled generation of reactive oxidant species such as hydrogen peroxide (H_2O_2), superoxide anion (O_2^-), and hydroxyl radical (OH) with the major share of the former [6,27]. Besides, there are several antioxidant enzymes, such as glutathione peroxidase (GPx), catalase (CAT), and superoxide dismutase (SOD). The latter antioxidant has three isoforms of SOD1/2/3. SOD1, 2, and 3 are respectively presented in intracellular cytoplasmic, mitochondria, and extracellular matrix. SOD has an important function and research evidence indicated that SOD1 has a function in the maintenance of muscle fibers [28,29]. Besides, CAT catalyzes the H_2O_2 conversion in the cytoplasmic reticulum and mitochondria in muscles. Altogether, inflammation, oxidative stress, apoptosis, and autophagy seem to play critical roles in cachexia which should be modulated.

2.1 Cachexia in cancer

Cancer cachexia is a complex syndrome with a relationship between the host condition and tumor stage. Related manifestations of cancer cachexia are weight loss, anorexia, and anemia in 50%–80% of cancer patients [30]. Studies have shown three types of cancer cachexia, including precachexia, cachexia, and refractory cachexia [31]. Precachexia is observed in the first stage of cancer with metabolic anomalies, such as glucose intolerance, anorexia, and weight loss. During the phase of cancer cachexia, patients have a rapid development of tumors with limited efficacy of treatment. The last, refractory cachexia, is difficult to be reversed owing to the presence of active catabolism [32]. Evidence has suggested excessive consumption of glucose by tumors, leading to the reduction of blood glucose. At the end phase of tumor development, a decrease of saved glycogen in the liver as well as glycogen reduction by muscle degradation and depletion of adipose tissue is termed cachexia and leads to poor response to chemotherapy, fatigue, and declined life quality in cancer patients [33]. Accordingly, evidence indicates that cachexia is more widespread in cancer patients, although tumor type and stage of progression are important. Among the cancers, the rate of cachexia prevalence is highest in pancreatic and gastric cancer compared to other cancers [34]. There are several hormones and mediators affecting cancer cachexia. Ghrelin is a hormone generated by enteroendocrine cells in the colon, pituitary, placenta, endocrine pancreas, hypothalamus, cardiomyocytes, lung, ovaries, and testes. Evidence has also indicated that ghrelin is expressed in many cancers and tumors. Ghrelin has important functions such as stimulating appetite and inhibiting energy consumption [35]. There is a direct relationship between reduced appetite in cancer patients and the ghrelin level in the body. Evidence suggests that there is a high level of ghrelin and acylated ghrelin in cancer patients, as ghrelin reduces the levels of IL-1β, IL-6, and TNF-α while increasing IL-10 [34,36,37].

In addition to ghrelin, leptin is another hormone involved in the pathogenesis of cachexia generated in adipose tissue and several other tissues. It plays an important function in the regulation of body mass and energy consumption [38]. In cancer cachexia, there is a reduced level of leptin in fat mass. Research indicates that there is a hypoxic condition in solid tumors that induces hypoxia-induced factor-1 (HIF-1), then triggers the promoter gene of leptin in fibroblasts and human adipocytes. Studies have shown that HIF-1, in turn, increases the expression of IL-6, TNF-α, leptin, and angiopoietin 4 involved in the increase of cachexia and metastasis [39,40]. In general, there are two types of cytokines in cachexia such as procachectic

(TNF-α, IL-6, IL-1, INF-γ, and PIF) or anticachectic (IL-4, IL-10, IL-12, IL-15, INF-α, and IGF-I) factors [41]. There is a close relationship between these factors and the control of cachexia [42]. Kemik et al. surveyed the level of proteins, cytokines, and hormones in cachectic patients and observed that there are increased concentrations of TNF-α and IL-6, in patients with different types of cancers [43]. Accordingly, studies indicated that IL-6 plays functional roles in tumor growth metastasis and promotion of cancer cachexia. Guyer and Macara showed that IL-6 could induce STAT3 in mammary epithelial cells [44]. Batista et al. investigated the relationship between ILs in cachectic and noncachectic patients. They observed a higher level of IL-6 in the cachectic cancer group [45]. Also, Kim et al. evaluated the role of proinflammatory cytokines in patients with lung and colorectal cancers and cachexia. They found that patients with high levels of IL-6 encountered weight loss after 6 months and suggested that IL-6 induces the maintenance of cancer cachexia [46]. IL-1β as a proinflammatory cytokine has several functions such as regulating inflammatory and immune responses, induction of muscle wasting by increasing hypothalamic serotonergic activity and declining food intake [2].

TNF-α is a crucial inflammatory mediator found in the tumor, especially in the late phase [47]. Interestingly, the levels of TNF-α correlated to the cancer phase, which reflects the size of the tumor. Studies have shown that TNF-α is involved in the progression of cancer cachexia. TNF-α can elevate the expression of ubiquitin and promote the accumulation of ubiquitinated proteins, which possess a functional role in the atrophy of muscle mass [48,49]. Evidence indicates that TNF-α stimulates the p38 mitogen-activated protein kinase (MAPK) pathway and NF-κB to increase the expression of E3 ligases MuRF1 and MAFbx genes, to inhibit protein synthesis and lead to muscle atrophy [50,51]. It has been shown that NF-κB induces muscle wasting via an increase in the ubiquitin-proteasome pathway (UPP) and inducible nitric oxide synthase (iNOS). Accordingly, there are several genes in protein degradation such as polyubiquitins, Ub fusion proteins, the Ub ligases atrogin-1/MAFbx, MuRF-1 and cathepsin L [52], increasing the rate of muscle protein degradation in cachexia [52]. Evidence has shown that there is insulin resistance in cancer patients. When insulin bind to a receptor, it leads to the activation of PI3K and Akt. The activation of the PI3K/Akt pathway causes the suppression of Forkhead box protein O (FoxO) and caspase-3 activity, and then reduces atrogin-1 and MuRF-1, 2. This pathway indicates that insulin can reduce the proteolysis of skeletal muscle [53]. It has been shown that in cachexia patients there is a reduction of circulating anabolic hormones such as testosterone through reducing muscle protein synthesis [52].

Coletti et al. indicated that cachexia is associated with the increased level of Pax7 in satellite cell cancer and other C26 colon carcinoma myogenic precursors of mice as well as pancreatic cancer patients. It indicated that Pax7 inhibits the differentiation of muscle stem cells [54].

Alves et al. indicated that cachectic patients with gastrointestinal cancer showed morphological rearrangement in adipose tissue, leading to a reduction of adipocyte size [55]. Evidence has shown that there are atrophy adipocytes and increased collagen fibril content, as well as each collagen isoform being modified in cancer cachexia. There is also an increased level of TGFβ1 in cancer cachexia [55,56]. Evidence indicates a correlation between adipose tissue fibrosis in cachectic cancer and the TGFβ pathway. TGFβ, as a cytokine, can activate cellular functions such as Rho-like signaling. Rho-Rho-kinase signaling is associated with deregulated adipocytokine expression [57]. In cachexia patients, there is loss of adipose tissue and then reductions in skeletal muscle mass and food intake [58]. There is also an increased in lipid catabolism with hormone-sensitive lipase and lipolytic response to catecholamines, which cause the loss of adipose tissue. Lipid-mobilizing factor (LMF) is an important agent in the urine of cachectic cancer patients that leads to lipolysis via cyclic AMP (c-AMP) interacting with the beta3-adreno receptor [42,59]. It has been shown that mitochondrial uncoupling proteins (UCPs) have an important function in brown adipose tissue and are found in mitochondria, lipid droplets, and rich vascularization. Besides, evidence indicated that there is an elevated level of UCP1, Pbe, and Cpt-1α associated with high brown adipose tissue temperature in cachectic mice [60,61]. Recent evidence indicates that in cancer cachexia there is fat loss and then triacylglycerol (TAG) depletion, which leads to decreased lipogenesis, reduced fatty acid (FA) transport, and increased lipolysis [62]. Studies have shown that white adipose tissue (WAT) shrinkage represents one of the symptoms in cachexia and is caused by β-adrenergic activation or inflammatory cytokine and interconnected lipolysis [63].

Studies indicated that TNF-α and IFN-γ could reduce the expression of myosin in the muscles, thereby activating muscle atrophy. Adiponectin is a protein found in adipocytes associated with body weight. In different types of cancer such as breast and colon neoplasia as well as cancer cachexia adiponectine has low levels [64].

2.2 Cachexia in heart failure

Heart failure (HF) occurs when the heart is unable to maintain cardiac function [65], and has been considered a serious disorder with high mortality increased with aging [66]. Cachexia, spontaneously leads to loss of body mass, and affects several patients with HF [67]. Cachexia occurs in 10%–15% of patients with HF [66]. It has been shown that muscle damage in cardiac cachexia causes decreased fat tissue, lean tissue, and bone tissue [66]. There are several symptoms in cardiac cachexia, including breathlessness, fatigue, and exercise intolerance [68]. Evidence has shown that cardiac cachexia has several symptoms such as decreased muscle strength, fatigue, anorexia, low fat-free mass index, and abnormal biochemistry, which is identified by increased inflammatory mediators [69]. Levine et al. observed that the levels of TNF-α are elevated in cachectic patients with HF. Evidence has shown that epicardial adipose tissue (EAT) is in close contact with the coronary artery [69]. In addition to the inflammatory mediators involved in cardiac cachexia, the level of adiponectin is increased in HF in patients of cachexia. There is a relationship between increased serum adiponectin and reduced peripheral muscle mass and muscle strength, which occurs in HF patients [70]. Several protein degradation pathways are the cause of HF, which makes protein loss and atrophy of the heart. In this line, IL-6 binds to the receptor and leads to the activation of MAPK and caspases, as well as activation of the IKK and NF-κB toward apoptosis. NF-κB, in turn, transfers to the nucleus and leads to protein degradation. Evidence has also suggested TNF-α as another activator of NF-κB in cancer [71,72].

In cachexia patients, an elevated level of angiotensin II (Ang II) plays an important function. It has been shown that Ang II has important functions such as regulation of blood pressure and salt/water balance and also controlling the effects of the adrenal gland, vasculature, kidney, and cardiovascular disease, ranging from early endothelial dysfunction to target-organ damage [73]. Interestingly, Ang II elevated the levels of TNF-α, IL-6, and myostatin which, in turn, induces protein degradation through activation of the NF-κB pathway. Myostatin inhibits Akt phosphorylation, which leads to decreased protein synthesis and increased protein degradation. In this line, IL-6 activates SOCS-3, and prevents IGF-1 signaling that causes decreased protein synthesis [74,75]. From another point of view, myostatin also binds to the ActRIIB receptor to activate Smad2/3, toward inhibiting protein synthesis via blocking the functional role of Akt to the nucleus and leads to the expression of genes that cause protein degradation [71,72].

Doehner et al. also indicated that in patients with HF there is insulin resistance in both cachectic and noncachectic patients [76].

2.3 Cachexia in chronic obstructive pulmonary disease

COPD is a lung-associated disease with the obstruction of airflow leading to inflammation and emphysema in the airways [77]. It has been shown that there are symptoms of cachexia in COPD patients with the prevalence of 20%–40% [77]. During the COPD cachexia, several symptoms are highlighted, including reduction of appetite, declined body mass, reduced concentration of testosterone, loss of muscle mass, and functional status. Inflammatory mediators play a critical role in COPD cachexia. In this line, NF-κB is increased in muscle, as well as an increased level of muscle protein decomposition in cachectic patients with COPD [52]. Besides, evidence indicates that UPS is an important system in muscle atrophy. In a UPS system, there are important mediators such as the muscle-specific E3 ligases atrogin-1 and MuRF1, which is controlled by fork-head transcription factors FoxO-1 and 3 [78].

Research indicates that the rate of MuRF1 mRNA, protein ubiquitination, atrogin-1 mRNA, Nedd4 (another E3 ubiquitin-protein ligase) and level of FoxO-1 and FoxO-3 are dysregulated in the muscle of COPD patients with cachexia [79]. Similar studies reported an increased level of atrogin-1 protein in COPD patients correlated with increased MAPK activation (p38, ERK1/2, and JNK). Studies have shown that the IGF-1/Akt signaling pathway is an important pathway in muscle anabolism and hypertrophy. Accordingly, it is observed that the level of IGF-1 decreases in cachectic COPD patients [80], while apoptosis is increased in COPD patients [79,80].

Evidence indicates that the level of muscle myogenin protein decreases in cachectic patients and also that MyoD protein was remarkably reduced in cachexia [81]. As mentioned above, myostatin as a negative regulator of muscle growth induces muscle atrophy via myoblast proliferation inhibition by suppressing MyoD, and down regulating anabolic signaling via the IGF/Akt pathway in COPD patients [82]. Studies indicate elevated levels of TNF-α, TNF-α receptors, C-reactive protein (CRP), IL-1β, and IL-6 in COPD patients with cachexia [83]. As TNF receptors are involved, apoptosis is important in COPD cachexia. In this line, several signaling mediators are engaged via Akt to inhibit mTORC1 in cachexia. Also, unc-51 like autophagy activating kinase 1 (ULK1) is engaged in the muscles of COPD patients [84,85]. So, Akt is suppressed to increase muscle loss and cachexia in COPD patients. On the other hand, the levels of mitochondrial oxidative enzymes decreased in muscles of COPD patients [86]. Additionally, peroxisome proliferator-activated receptors (PPAR)-α and -δ and also PGC-1α play functional roles in mitochondrial biogenesis, and are decreased in COPD patients [22,87].

2.4 Cachexia in kidney diseases

CKD patients have encountered increased levels of proinflammatory cytokines, decreased renal function, oxidative or carbonyl stress, reduced levels of antioxidants, and also increased susceptibility to infection in uremia [88]. The aforementioned dysregulated inflammatory and oxidative pathways resulted in cachexia in patients with CKD leading to end-stage renal disease (ESRD) [89]. Among those inflammatory pathways, IL-6 and TNF-α have an important function in CKD and related cachexia. Researchers showed a remarkable increase in the level of IL-6 in ESRD patients. It has been demonstrated that mitochondrial UCP-1 and UCP-3 play an important function toward energy consumption in the pathogenesis of elevated energy expenditure in patients with CKD [90]. Inflammation in CKD patients can cause muscle loss via increased protein catabolism, decreased protein synthesis, or impaired muscle progenitor and cell proliferation [88]. Several proteolytic pathways, such as lysosomal, Ca^{2+}-dependent, matrix metalloproteinases, and ubiquitin-proteasome-dependent pathways, are involved in muscle loss. This system plays a pivotal role in metabolic acidosis and muscle wasting of CKD patients [91]. Research also suggests that muscle loss in CKD patients and dialysis patients is mediated by the activation of caspase-3. Caspase-3 breaks actomyosin, which lead to the generation of actin fragments and the accumulation of actin fragments observed in CKD patients [91].

Studies suggested that abnormal IGF-I signaling can promote muscle wasting in patients with CKD and also observed that increased proteolysis of muscle is correlated with cachexia in CKD patients. Insulin resistance can cause muscle atrophy in CKD patients via the IRS-1/PI3K/Akt pathway. The renin-angiotensin system (RAS) system and the inflammatory pathway have a function in renal and cardiovascular disease [92].

3. Effect of natural products on cachexia

Nutrition plays a critical role in decreasing protein breakdown and ameliorating muscle function. Natural products are promising agents in human health and contribute to the protection of diseases. In recent years, evidence indicated that natural products play hopeful roles in the prevention of neurodegenerative diseases, skeletal muscle atrophy, cancer, and related disorders [93,94]. Several studies are conducted on the effects of phenolic compounds, polyphenols, catechins, lignans, and alkaloids in combating cachexia and muscle atrophy during diseases. Reports have shown that benzoic acids (e.g., gallic acid) and cinnamic acid (e.g., caffeic acid and p-coumaric acid) derivatives as phenolic compounds have beneficial effects on skeletal muscle [93]. In this regard, Pierno et al. indicated the effects of gallic acid and homovanillic acid on preventing skeletal muscle dysfunction by reducing aging-associated oxidative stress [95]. As another phenolic compound, urolithin B increased protein synthesis by activating mTORC1 and inhibiting AMPK phosphorylation. It also decreased protein degradation by reducing the ubiquitin-proteasome system [96]. Curcumin as a phenolic compound increased PGC-1α, to regulate the expression of various genes in mitochondrial metabolism and biogenesis [97] and prevented myotube protein degradation [98]. An important part of the anticachectic effects of some phytonutrients is exerted through their potential in the inhibition of NF-κB [99]. Curcumin also reduced ROS production by decreasing NF-κB, which has an important function in muscle development, maintenance, regeneration, and preventing against muscle proteolytic activities [100]. Chaudhary et al. indicated that curcumin prevents the reduction of myofibrillar protein degradation in hypobaric hypoxia [101]. Studies have shown that curcumin in combination with caffeic acid can increase the expression of SMN2, regarding modulating the severity and treatment of motor abilities and decreasing neurodegeneration and maintenance of muscle functions [102]. In another study by da Costa et al., curcumin limited weight loss and rutin (a flavonoid) preserved muscle mass during cancer cachexia [103]. Combination therapy of curcumin and green tea extract attenuated weight loss and muscle wasting by reducing MuRF1, MAFbx, PIF, and TNF-α [104].

Hydroxycinnamic acid is another phenolic compound in fruits and coffee and have shown antioxidant, antiinflammatory, antimetastatic, and antitumor properties. It could be a useful agent in ameliorating muscular atrophy, lipid metabolism, and glucose uptake via the AMP-activated protein kinase pathway [93,105].

Of polyphenols, quercetin and myricetin as flavonols protect dystrophic skeletal muscle from cell damage [106]. Chan et al. indicated that quercetin might suppress gene-1 and MURF-1 level, which are promoters in muscle loss [107]. Davis et al. suggested that quercetin increased the level of genes that correlated to mitochondrial biogenesis such as SIRT1, PGC-1α, cytochrome *c* concentration, and mitochondrial DNA content, which is found in muscle and brain, also blocked the elevated level of IL-6 activation by inhibiting glycoprotein, janus kinase (JAK) 1, and STAT3 phosphorylation [108,109]. In a recent study by Otsuka et al., quercetin reduced Akt, MuRF, and atrogin-1 in cachexia [110]. Consistently, quercetin also prevented loss of mass and muscle atrophy [111]. Of flavonols, dihydromyricetin, is a flavonoid with biological and pharmacological effects such as antiinflammatory, antitumor, antioxidant, neuroprotective, and hepatoprotective effects [112] and also can reverse skeletal muscle-associated mitochondrial dysfunction [113]. It also showed modulatory effects on myotube diameter, and Akt, mTOR, atrogin-1, and PGC-1α to be promising agents in combating cachexia [114]. Licorice is another flavonoid to decrease the expression of MuRF1 and atrogin-1; the markers function in muscle atrophy [115]. Ampelopsin, as another natural flavonoid, has functions such as antiinflammatory, antioxidative, and hepatoprotective functions, which declined ubiquitin and atrogin-1/MAFbx [116]. Oligonol, as another polyphenol, has antiobesity and antidiabetic effects, and also modulating diabetes-related muscle loss. Accordingly, Liu et al. indicated that oligonol can inhibit MuRF1 and atrogin-1 activation, thereby suppressing muscle atrophy [117]. Evidence have shown that delphinidin, as an anthocyanidin, plays anticancer and antiinflammatory effects, and also suppresses MuRF1expression to inhibit muscle atrophy in cachexia [118]. Catechins as another flavonoid found in green tea and cacao consisting of epigallocatechin gallate, gallocatechin gallate, and epicatechin gallate, play cardioprotective, antiatherogenic, antioxidant, antiinflammatory, and anticarcinogenic effects [119,120]. In a report by Wang et al., epigallocatechin 3-gallate (EGCG) potentially modulated skeletal muscle atrophy in cancer cachexia by regulating NF-κB and downstream mediators MAFbx and MuRF 1 [121]. A recent study also confirmed the nutraceutical potential of flavonoids in counteracting muscle atrophy [122]. Increasing myotube formation and myogenin, protein synthesis, fiber size, muscle mass, NRF1, SOD, Akt, PGC-1α, while decreasing Bax and caspase-3 are other protective mechanisms of EGCG and derivatives against cachexia. In an in vivo study, baicalin (a flavonoid) ameliorated anorexia, weight loss and muscle atrophy through reducing MURF1, atrogin-1, p65, NF-κB, TNF-α, and IL-6 [123].

Resveratrol is one of the polyphenols found in berries, grapes, wine, other fruits and vegetables [124]. Momken et al. indicated that resveratrol reduced muscle disuse atrophy [125] as well as decreasing the atrogin-1-dependent system and ameliorating the autophagic defects via AMPK activation [93].

Grape extract and some others rich in procyanidines, anthocyanes, catechins, and resveratrol also limited tibialis anterior muscle wasting [126] through suppressing inflammation (e.g., NF-κB), apoptosis (e.g., caspase-3 and -9), and ROS [127]. Lignans as natural products have a function in preventing wasting skeletal muscle. Studies have shown that magnolol, as a lignan, plays critical roles against inflammation, angiogenesis, and cancer growth [128,129]. Chen et al. indicated that magnalol ameliorated atrophic phenotype in rats [130]. Magnolol also increased IGF-1 through inhibition of myostatin formation and inflammation. In this line, schisandrin A and C as other lignins can reduce ROS, attenuate mitochondria biogenesis and support their functionality [131,132].

In addition to phenolic compounds, catechins, and lignans, alkaloids are another class of phytochemicals in combating cachexia and related muscle atrophy. Piperlongumine (PL) as an alkaloid has a tumor-associated cytotoxic activity through the accumulation of ROS, C/EBP homologous protein (CHOP) activation, and EBV-encoded oncogene (LMP-1) suppression. It also triggers NF-κB inhibition, AMPK phosphorylation, activation of ERK, autophagy development, GADD45α induction, suppressing telomerase reverse transcriptase and PI3K/Akt/mTOR pathway inhibition [133]. Other evidence indicates that EGCG as a main catechin found in green tea showed broad biological effects. EGCG has an antiangiogenic activity and also anticytokine synthesis, such as inhibiting NF-κB, IL-6, IL-1β, and TNF-α [121,134,135].

The evidence has shown that cannabinoid (Δ-9-tetrahydrocannabinol and cannabidiol) can be useful for improving the appetite, body fat level, body weight, mood, caloric intake, and life quality in several kinds of diseases. Growing well-documented studies are indicating the appetite-stimulating properties of cannabis [136].

Silibinin [137], apigenin [138], luteolin [139], icaritin [140], morin [141], daidzein [142], and genistein [143] are other auspicious plant-derived secondary metabolites, which employ the aforementioned mechanisms to combat cachexia. Altogether, phytonutrients seem to be potential agents in modulating cachexia through targeting inflammation, oxidative stress, and apoptosis.

4. Conclusions

Cachexia is a pathological condition leading to the reduction of body function, decreased endurance for treatment, and increased death as well as reduction of muscle mass. Several dysregulated pathways are behind the

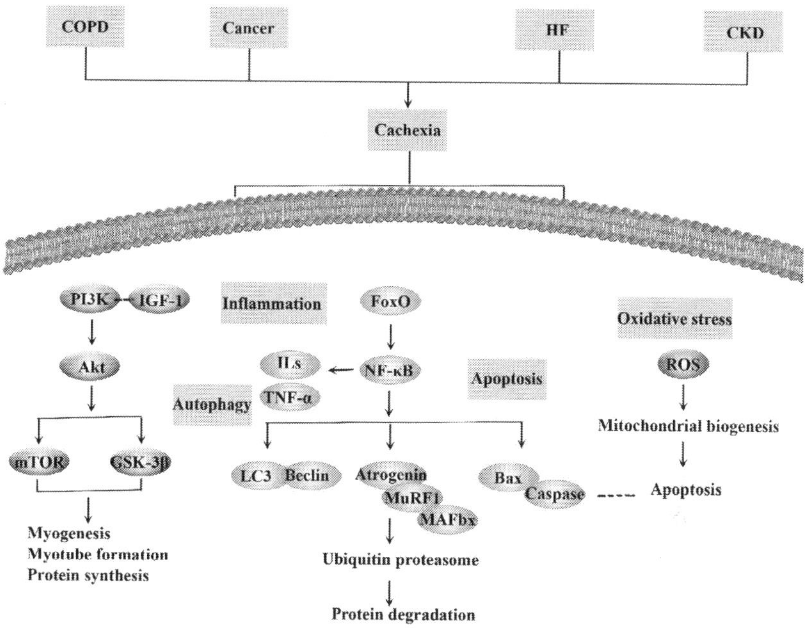

Fig. 1 Major dysregulated pathways in cachexia modulated by phytonutrients. CKD: chronic kidney disease, COPD: chronic obstructive pulmonary disease, FoxO: Forkhead box protein O, GSK-3: glycogen synthase kinase 3, HF: heart failure, ILs: interleukins, LC3: light chain3, mTOR: mammalian target of rapamycin, MAFbx: mediators including muscle atrophy F-box, MuRF1: muscle-specific RING finger-1, PI3K: phosphoinositide 3-kinases, ROS: reactive oxygen species, TNF-α: tumor necrosis factor-alpha.

development of skeletal muscle atrophy, such as inflammation, UPS overactivation, autophagy deregulation, protein synthesis pathway, increased myonuclear oxidative stress, and apoptosis (Fig. 1). So, there is a need to develop multitarget agents possessing higher potency/efficacy and fewer side effects. Natural entities have shown the potential of simultaneous targeting of altered signaling pathways in cachexia with fewer side effects. Such effects have presented phytonutrients as hopeful candidates for cachexia therapy through modulating the aforementioned dysregulated pathways.

This chapter underscores the major dysregulated pathways during cachexia. It also provides the promising effects of natural products on cachexia toward indicating a new prospect in the prevention and treatment of cachexia symptoms. Further reports on the pathophysiological mechanisms behind cachexia will pave the road for investigating novel therapies in the treatment of muscle damages. More experimental research followed by well-controlled clinical trials will help to reveal novel ways in treating cachexia.

Author contributions

Conceptualization S·F. and H.K.; drafting the chapter, S.F., and S.P.; software, S.F.; review and editing the chapter, S.F, and H.K.

References

[1] B. Sishi, B. Loos, B. Ellis, W. Smith, E.F. du Toit, A.M. Engelbrecht, Diet-induced obesity alters signalling pathways and induces atrophy and apoptosis in skeletal muscle in a prediabetic rat model, Exp. Physiol. 96 (2) (2011) 179–193.

[2] P. Mondello, M. Mian, C. Aloisi, F. Fama, S. Mondello, V. Pitini, Cancer cachexia syndrome: pathogenesis, diagnosis, and new therapeutic options, Nutr. Cancer 67 (1) (2015) 12–26.

[3] S. Al-Majid, D.O. McCarthy, Cancer-induced fatigue and skeletal muscle wasting: the role of exercise, Biol. Res. Nurs. 2 (3) (2001) 186–197.

[4] M.L. Winningham, L.M. Nail, M.B. Burke, L. Brophy, B. Cimprich, L.S. Jones, S. Beck (Eds.), Fatigue and the cancer experience: the state of the knowledge, Oncol. Nurs. Forum 21 (1994) 23–36.

[5] J.E. Morley, D.R. Thomas, M.-M.G. Wilson, Cachexia: pathophysiology and clinical relevance, Am. J. Clin. Nutr. 83 (4) (2006) 735–743.

[6] J. Ábrigo, A.A. Elorza, C.A. Riedel, C. Vilos, F. Simon, D. Cabrera, L. Estrada, C. Cabello-Verrugio, Role of oxidative stress as key regulator of muscle wasting during cachexia, Oxid. Med. Cell. Longev. 2018 (2018).

[7] J.M. Argilés, S. Busquets, B. Stemmler, F.J. López-Soriano, Cancer cachexia: understanding the molecular basis, Nat. Rev. Cancer 14 (11) (2014) 754–762.

[8] A. Fanzani, V.M. Conraads, F. Penna, W. Martinet, Molecular and cellular mechanisms of skeletal muscle atrophy: an update, J. Cachexia. Sarcopenia Muscle 3 (3) (2012) 163–179.

[9] P. Sanders, S. Russell, M. Tisdale, Angiotensin II directly induces muscle protein catabolism through the ubiquitin-proteasome proteolytic pathway and may play a role in cancer cachexia, Br. J. Cancer 93 (4) (2005) 425–434.

[10] N.P. Gullett, V. Mazurak, G. Hebbar, T.R. Ziegler, Nutritional interventions for cancer-induced cachexia, Curr. Probl. Cancer 35 (2) (2011) 58.

[11] R. Siddiqui, D. Pandya, K. Harvey, G.P. Zaloga, Nutrition modulation of cachexia/proteolysis, Nutr. Clin. Pract. 21 (2) (2006) 155–167.

[12] S.A. Pötgens, M. Sboarina, L.B. Bindels, Polyunsaturated fatty acids, polyphenols, amino acids, prebiotics: can they help to tackle cancer cachexia and related inflammation? Curr. Opin. Clin. Nutr. Metab. Care 21 (6) (2018) 458–464.

[13] S. Fakhri, M. Pesce, A. Patruno, S.Z. Moradi, A. Iranpanah, M.H. Farzaei, E. Sobarzo-Sánchez, Attenuation of Nrf2/Keap1/ARE in Alzheimer's disease by plant secondary metabolites: a mechanistic review, Molecules 25 (21) (2020) 4926.

[14] F. Abbaszadeh, S. Fakhri, H. Khan, Targeting apoptosis and autophagy following spinal cord injury: therapeutic approaches to polyphenols and candidate phytochemicals, Pharmacol. Res. (2020) 105069.

[15] S. Fakhri, F. Abbaszadeh, M. Jorjani, M.H. Pourgholami, The effects of anticancer medicinal herbs on vascular endothelial growth factor based on pharmacological aspects: a review study, Nutr. Cancer (2019) 1–15.

[16] S. Fakhri, M. Khodamorady, M. Naseri, M.H. Farzaei, H. Khan, The ameliorating effects of anthocyanins on the cross-linked signaling pathways of cancer dysregulated metabolism, Pharmacol. Res. (2020).

[17] S. Fakhri, S.Z. Moradi, M.H. Farzaei, A. Bishayee (Eds.), Modulation of dysregulated cancer metabolism by plant secondary metabolites: a mechanistic review, in: Seminars in Cancer Biology, Elsevier, 2020.

[18] M. Romanick, L.V. Thompson, H.M. Brown-Borg, Murine models of atrophy, cachexia, and sarcopenia in skeletal muscle, Biochim. Biophys. Acta (BBA) - Mol. Basis Dis. 1832 (9) (2013) 1410–1420.

[19] M.J. Puppa, J.P. White, S. Sato, M. Cairns, J.W. Baynes, J.A. Carson, Gut barrier dysfunction in the ApcMin/+ mouse model of colon cancer cachexia, Biochim. Biophys. Acta (BBA) - Mol. Basis Dis. 1812 (12) (2011) 1601–1606.

[20] S.T. Arthur, J.M. Noone, B.A. Van Doren, D. Roy, C.M. Blanchette, One-year prevalence, comorbidities and cost of cachexia-related inpatient admissions in the USA, Drugs Context 3 (2014).

[21] K. Sakuma, W. Aoi, A. Yamaguchi, Molecular mechanism of sarcopenia and cachexia: recent research advances, Arch. Eur. J. Physiol. 469 (5–6) (2017) 573–591.

[22] A. Remels, H. Gosker, P. Schrauwen, P. Hommelberg, P. Sliwinski, M. Polkey, J. Galdiz, E. Wouters, R. Langen, A. Schols, TNF-α impairs regulation of muscle oxidative phenotype: implications for cachexia? FASEB J. 24 (12) (2010) 5052–5062.

[23] S. Ali, J.M. Garcia, Sarcopenia, cachexia and aging: diagnosis, mechanisms and therapeutic options-a mini-review, Gerontology 60 (4) (2014) 294–305.

[24] N. Ebner, C.G. Werner, W. Doehner, S.D. Anker, S. von Haehling, Recent Developments in the Treatment of Cachexia: Highlights From the 6th Cachexia Conference, Springer, 2012.

[25] M. Muscaritoli, S. Anker, J. Argiles, Z. Aversa, J. Bauer, G. Biolo, Y. Boirie, I. Bosaeus, T. Cederholm, P. Costelli, Consensus definition of sarcopenia, cachexia and pre-cachexia: joint document elaborated by Special Interest Groups (SIG)"cachexia-anorexia in chronic wasting diseases" and "nutrition in geriatrics", Clin. Nutr. 29 (2) (2010) 154–159.

[26] B.N. VanderVeen, D.K. Fix, J.A. Carson, Disrupted skeletal muscle mitochondrial dynamics, mitophagy, and biogenesis during cancer cachexia: a role for inflammation, Oxid. Med. Cell. Longev. 2017 (2017).

[27] W. Droge, Free radicals in the physiological control of cell function, Physiol. Rev. 82 (1) (2002) 47–95.

[28] I.N. Zelko, T.J. Mariani, R.J. Folz, Superoxide dismutase multigene family: a comparison of the CuZn-SOD (SOD1), Mn-SOD (SOD2), and EC-SOD (SOD3) gene structures, evolution, and expression, Free Radic. Biol. Med. 33 (3) (2002) 337–349.

[29] F.L. Muller, W. Song, Y. Liu, A. Chaudhuri, S. Pieke-Dahl, R. Strong, T.-T. Huang, C.J. Epstein, L.J. Roberts II, M. Csete, Absence of CuZn superoxide dismutase leads to elevated oxidative stress and acceleration of age-dependent skeletal muscle atrophy, Free Radic. Biol. Med. 40 (11) (2006) 1993–2004.

[30] J. Wang, Y. Wang, M. Tong, H. Pan, D. Li, Medical cannabinoids for cancer cachexia: a systematic review and meta-analysis, Biomed. Res. Int. 2019 (2019).

[31] M.N. Khatib, A. Gaidhane, S. Gaidhane, Z.S. Quazi, Ghrelin as a promising therapeutic option for cancer cachexia, Cell. Physiol. Biochem. 48 (5) (2018) 2172–2188.

[32] K.C. Fearon, The 2011 ESPEN Arvid Wretlind lecture: cancer cachexia: the potential impact of translational research on patient-focused outcomes, Clin. Nutr. 31 (5) (2012) 577–582.

[33] S.K. Shukla, T. Gebregiworgis, V. Purohit, N.V. Chaika, V. Gunda, P. Radhakrishnan, K. Mehla, I.I. Pipinos, R. Powers, F. Yu, Metabolic reprogramming induced by ketone bodies diminishes pancreatic cancer cachexia, Cancer Metab. 2 (1) (2014) 1–19.

[34] N. Inácio Pinto, J. Carnier, L.M. Oyama, J.P. Otoch, P.S. Alcântara, F. Tokeshi, C.M. Nascimento, Cancer as a proinflammatory environment: metastasis and cachexia, Mediators Inflamm. 2015 (2015), 791060.

[35] L.K. Chopin, I. Seim, C.M. Walpole, A.C. Herington, The ghrelin axis—does it have an appetite for cancer progression? Endocr. Rev. 33 (6) (2012) 849–891.

[36] M. Kojima, K. Kangawa, Ghrelin discovery: a decade after, in: The Ghrelin System, vol. 25, Karger Publishers, 2013, pp. 1–4.

[37] J.M. Argilés, B. Stemmler, The potential of ghrelin in the treatment of cancer cachexia, Expert Opin. Biol. Ther. 13 (1) (2013) 67–76.

[38] S. Margetic, C. Gazzola, G. Pegg, R. Hill, Leptin: a review of its peripheral actions and interactions, Int. J. Obes. (Lond) 26 (11) (2002) 1407–1433.

[39] P. González-Muniesa, C. de Oliveira, F.P. de Heredia, M.P. Thompson, P. Trayhurn, Fatty acids and hypoxia stimulate the expression and secretion of the adipokine ANGPTL4 (angiopoietin-like protein 4/fasting-induced adipose factor) by human adipocytes, J. Nutrigenet. Nutrigenomics 4 (3) (2011) 146–153.

[40] P. Trayhurn, Hypoxia and adipocyte physiology: implications for adipose tissue dysfunction in obesity, Annu. Rev. Nutr. 34 (2014) 207–236.

[41] J.K. Onesti, D.C. Guttridge, Inflammation based regulation of cancer cachexia, Biomed. Res. Int. 2014 (2014).

[42] R. Gorjao, C.M.M. Dos Santos, T.D.A. Serdan, V.L.S. Diniz, T.C. Alba-Loureiro, M.F. Cury-Boaventura, E. Hatanaka, A.C. Levada-Pires, F.T. Sato, T.C. Pithon-Curi, New insights on the regulation of cancer cachexia by N-3 polyunsaturated fatty acids, Pharmacol. Ther. 196 (2019) 117–134.

[43] O. Kemik, A.S. Kemik, H. Begenik, F.M. Erdur, H. Emre, A. Sumer, S. Purisa, S. Tuzun, C. Kotan, The relationship among acute-phase responce proteins, cytokines, and hormones in various gastrointestinal cancer types patients with cachectic, Hum. Exp. Toxicol. 31 (2) (2012) 117–125.

[44] R.A. Guyer, I.G. Macara, Loss of the polarity protein PAR3 activates STAT3 signaling via an atypical protein kinase C (aPKC)/NF-κB/interleukin-6 (IL-6) axis in mouse mammary cells, J. Biol. Chem. 290 (13) (2015) 8457–8468.

[45] M.L. Batista Jr., M. Olivan, P.S. Alcantara, R. Sandoval, S.B. Peres, R.X. Neves, R. Silverio, L.F. Maximiano, J.P. Otoch, M. Seelaender, Adipose tissue-derived factors as potential biomarkers in cachectic cancer patients, Cytokine 61 (2) (2013) 532–539.

[46] H.J. Kim, H.J. Kim, J. Yun, K.H. Kim, S.H. Kim, S.C. Lee, S.B. Bae, C.K. Kim, N.S. Lee, K.T. Lee, S.K. Park, J.H. Won, H.S. Park, D.S. Hong, Pathophysiological role of hormones and cytokines in cancer cachexia, J. Korean Med. Sci. 27 (2) (2012) 128–134.

[47] G. Landskron, M. De la Fuente, P. Thuwajit, C. Thuwajit, M.A. Hermoso, Chronic inflammation and cytokines in the tumor microenvironment, J. Immunol. Res. 2014 (2014), 149185.

[48] L.G. Melstrom, K.A. Melstrom Jr., X.Z. Ding, T.E. Adrian, Mechanisms of skeletal muscle degradation and its therapy in cancer cachexia, Histol. Histopathol. 22 (7) (2007) 805–814.

[49] L. Zhang, H. Tang, Y. Kou, R. Li, Y. Zheng, Q. Wang, X. Zhou, L. Jin, MG132-mediated inhibition of the ubiquitin-proteasome pathway ameliorates cancer cachexia, J. Cancer Res. Clin. Oncol. 139 (7) (2013) 1105–1115.

[50] C.M. Liu, Z. Yang, C.W. Liu, R. Wang, P. Tien, R. Dale, L.Q. Sun, Myostatin antisense RNA-mediated muscle growth in normal and cancer cachexia mice, Gene Ther. 15 (3) (2008) 155–160.

[51] J.M. Argiles, F.J. Lopez-Soriano, S. Busquets, Counteracting inflammation: a promising therapy in cachexia, Crit. Rev. Oncog. 17 (3) (2012) 253–262.

[52] W.J. Evans, Skeletal muscle loss: cachexia, sarcopenia, and inactivity, Am. J. Clin. Nutr. 91 (4) (2010) 1123S–1127S.

[53] J.A. Norton, M. Maher, R. Wesley, D. White, M.F. Brennan, Glucose intolerance in sarcoma patients, Cancer 54 (12) (1984) 3022–3027.

[54] D. Coletti, P. Aulino, E. Pigna, F. Barteri, V. Moresi, D. Annibali, S. Adamo, E. Berardi, Spontaneous physical activity downregulates Pax7 in cancer cachexia, Stem Cells Int. 2016 (2016).

[55] M.J. Alves, R.G. Figuerêdo, F.F. Azevedo, D.A. Cavallaro, N.I.P. Neto, J.D.C. Lima, E. Matos-Neto, K. Radloff, D.M. Riccardi, R.G. Camargo, Adipose tissue fibrosis in human cancer cachexia: the role of TGFβ pathway, BMC Cancer 17 (1) (2017) 190.

[56] K. Flanders, M. Sato, A. Ooshima, A. Russo, A. Roberts, Smad-3 as a mediator of the fibrotic response, Int. J. Exp. Pathol. 85 (1) (2004) A13-A.

[57] Y.E. Zhang, Non-Smad signaling pathways of the TGF-β family, Cold Spring Harb. Perspect. Biol. 9 (2) (2017), a022129.

[58] S. Dalal, Lipid metabolism in cancer cachexia, Ann. Palliat. Med. 8 (1) (2019) 13.

[59] M.J. Tisdale, Cancer cachexia, Langenbecks Arch. Surg. 389 (4) (2004) 299–305.

[60] D. Richard, F. Picard, Brown fat biology and thermogenesis, Front. Biosci. 16 (2011) 1233–1260.

[61] M. Tsoli, M. Moore, D. Burg, A. Painter, R. Taylor, S.H. Lockie, N. Turner, A. Warren, G. Cooney, B. Oldfield, Activation of thermogenesis in brown adipose tissue and dysregulated lipid metabolism associated with cancer cachexia in mice, Cancer Res. 72 (17) (2012) 4372–4382.

[62] S.K. Das, G. Hoefler, The role of triglyceride lipases in cancer associated cachexia, Trends Mol. Med. 19 (5) (2013) 292–301.

[63] M. Petruzzelli, M. Schweiger, R. Schreiber, R. Campos-Olivas, M. Tsoli, J. Allen, M. Swarbrick, S. Rose-John, M. Rincon, G. Robertson, R. Zechner, E.F. Wagner, A switch from white to brown fat increases energy expenditure in cancer-associated cachexia, Cell Metab. 20 (3) (2014) 433–447.

[64] O. Kemik, A. Sumer, A.S. Kemik, I. Hasirci, S. Purisa, A.C. Dulger, B. Demiriz, S. Tuzun, The relationship among acute-phase response proteins, cytokines and hormones in cachectic patients with colon cancer, World J. Surg. Oncol. 8 (2010) 85.

[65] A. Rahman, S. Jafry, K. Jeejeebhoy, A.D. Nagpal, B. Pisani, R. Agarwala, Malnutrition and cachexia in heart failure, J. Parenter. Enteral Nutr. 40 (4) (2016) 475–486.

[66] M. Zamboni, A.P. Rossi, F. Corzato, C. Bambace, G. Mazzali, F. Fantin, Sarcopenia, cachexia and congestive heart failure in the elderly, Endocr. Metab. Immune Disord. Drug Targets 13 (1) (2013) 58–67.

[67] M. Valentova, S. von Haehling, J. Bauditz, W. Doehner, N. Ebner, T. Bekfani, S. Elsner, V. Sliziuk, N. Scherbakov, J. Murín, Intestinal congestion and right ventricular dysfunction: a link with appetite loss, inflammation, and cachexia in chronic heart failure, Eur. Heart J. 37 (21) (2016) 1684–1691.

[68] M. Saitoh, J. Ishida, W. Doehner, S. von Haehling, M.S. Anker, A.J. Coats, S.D. Anker, J. Springer, Sarcopenia, cachexia, and muscle performance in heart failure: review update 2016, Int. J. Cardiol. 238 (2017) 5–11.

[69] K. Selthofer-Relatić, A. Kibel, D. Delić-Brkljačić, I. Bošnjak, Cardiac obesity and cardiac cachexia: is there a pathophysiological link? J. Obes. 2019 (2019).

[70] G. Loncar, J. Springer, M. Anker, W. Doehner, M. Lainscak, Cardiac cachexia: hic et nunc, J. Cachexia. Sarcopenia Muscle 7 (3) (2016) 246–260.

[71] K.T. Murphy, The pathogenesis and treatment of cardiac atrophy in cancer cachexia, Am. J. Physiol. Heart Circ. Physiol. 310 (4) (2016) H466–H477.

[72] K. Sakuma, A. Yamaguchi, Sarcopenia and cachexia: the adaptations of negative regulators of skeletal muscle mass, J. Cachexia. Sarcopenia Muscle 3 (2) (2012) 77–94.

[73] C. Werner, J. Pöss, M. Böhm, Optimal antagonism of the renin-angiotensin-aldosterone system, Drugs 70 (10) (2010) 1215–1230.

[74] M.N. Goodman, Interleukin-6 induces skeletal muscle protein breakdown in rats, Proc. Soc. Exp. Biol. Med. 205 (2) (1994) 182–185.

[75] A.U. Trendelenburg, A. Meyer, D. Rohner, J. Boyle, S. Hatakeyama, D.J. Glass, Myostatin reduces Akt/TORC1/p70S6K signaling, inhibiting myoblast differentiation and myotube size, Am. J. Physiol. Cell Physiol. 296 (6) (2009) C1258–C1270.
[76] W. Doehner, M. Rauchhaus, I.F. Godsland, K. Egerer, J. Niebauer, R. Sharma, M. Cicoira, V.G. Florea, A.J. Coats, S.D. Anker, Insulin resistance in moderate chronic heart failure is related to hyperleptinaemia, but not to norepinephrine or TNF-alpha, Int. J. Cardiol. 83 (1) (2002) 73–81.
[77] A. Remels, H.R. Gosker, R.C. Langen, A.M. Schols, The mechanisms of cachexia underlying muscle dysfunction in COPD, J. Appl. Physiol. 114 (9) (2013) 1253–1262.
[78] D.J. Glass, Skeletal muscle hypertrophy and atrophy signaling pathways, Int. J. Biochem. Cell Biol. 37 (10) (2005) 1974–1984.
[79] B.B. Lemire, R. Debigaré, A. Dubé, M.-E. Thériault, C.H. Côté, F. Maltais, MAPK signaling in the quadriceps of patients with chronic obstructive pulmonary disease, J. Appl. Physiol. 113 (1) (2012) 159–166.
[80] I. Vogiatzis, D.C. Simoes, G. Stratakos, E. Kourepini, G. Terzis, P. Manta, D. Athanasopoulos, C. Roussos, P.D. Wagner, S. Zakynthinos, Effect of pulmonary rehabilitation on muscle remodelling in cachectic patients with COPD, Eur. Respir. J. 36 (2) (2010) 301–310.
[81] C. Fermoselle, R. Rabinovich, P. Ausín, E. Puig-Vilanova, C. Coronell, F. Sanchez, J. Roca, J. Gea, E. Barreiro, Does oxidative stress modulate limb muscle atrophy in severe COPD patients? Eur. Respir. J. 40 (4) (2012) 851–862.
[82] P.J. Plant, D. Brooks, M. Faughnan, T. Bayley, J. Bain, L. Singer, J. Correa, D. Pearce, M. Binnie, J. Batt, Cellular markers of muscle atrophy in chronic obstructive pulmonary disease, Am. J. Respir. Cell Mol. Biol. 42 (4) (2010) 461–471.
[83] Y. Nussbaumer-Ochsner, K.F. Rabe, Systemic manifestations of COPD, Chest 139 (1) (2011) 165–173.
[84] Y. Guo, H.R. Gosker, A.M. Schols, S. Kapchinsky, J. Bourbeau, M. Sandri, R.T. Jagoe, R. Debigaré, F. Maltais, T. Taivassalo, S.N. Hussain, Autophagy in locomotor muscles of patients with chronic obstructive pulmonary disease, Am. J. Respir. Crit. Care Med. 188 (11) (2013) 1313–1320.
[85] C. Mammucari, S. Schiaffino, M. Sandri, Downstream of Akt: FoxO3 and mTOR in the regulation of autophagy in skeletal muscle, Autophagy 4 (4) (2008) 524–526.
[86] T. Crul, D. Testelmans, M.A. Spruit, T. Troosters, R. Gosselink, I. Geeraerts, M. Decramer, G. Gayan-Ramirez, Gene expression profiling in vastus lateralis muscle during an acute exacerbation of COPD, Cell. Physiol. Biochem. 25 (4-5) (2010) 491–500.
[87] A.H. Remels, P. Schrauwen, R. Broekhuizen, J. Willems, S. Kersten, H.R. Gosker, A.M. Schols, Peroxisome proliferator-activated receptor expression is reduced in skeletal muscle in COPD, Eur. Respir. J. 30 (2) (2007) 245–252.
[88] W.W. Cheung, K.H. Paik, R.H. Mak, Inflammation and cachexia in chronic kidney disease, Pediatr. Nephrol. 25 (4) (2010) 711–724.
[89] R. Pecoits-Filho, L.C. Sylvestre, P. Stenvinkel, Chronic kidney disease and inflammation in pediatric patients: from bench to playground, Pediatr. Nephrol. 20 (6) (2005) 714–720.
[90] E.S. Hansen, J. Knudsen, Parallel measurements of heat production and thermogenin content in brown fat cells during cold acclimation of rats, Biosci. Rep. 6 (1) (1986) 31–38.
[91] V. Rajan, W.E. Mitch, Ubiquitin, proteasomes and proteolytic mechanisms activated by kidney disease, Biochim. Biophys. Acta (BBA) - Mol. Basis Dis. 1782 (12) (2008) 795–799.
[92] E. Siew, L. Pupim, K. Majchrzak, A. Shintani, P. Flakoll, T. Ikizler, Insulin resistance is associated with skeletal muscle protein breakdown in non-diabetic chronic hemodialysis patients, Kidney Int. 71 (2) (2007) 146–152.

[93] S. Salucci, E. Falcieri, Polyphenols and their potential role in preventing skeletal muscle atrophy, Nutr. Res. 74 (2020) 10–22.
[94] J. Lee, M.I. Jeong, H.-R. Kim, H. Park, W.-K. Moon, B. Kim, Plant extracts as possible agents for sequela of cancer therapies and cachexia, Antioxidants 9 (9) (2020) 836.
[95] S. Pierno, D. Tricarico, A. Liantonio, A. Mele, C. Digennaro, J.-F. Rolland, G. Bianco, L. Villanova, A. Merendino, G.M. Camerino, An olive oil-derived antioxidant mixture ameliorates the age-related decline of skeletal muscle function, Age 36 (1) (2014) 73–88.
[96] J. Rodriguez, N. Pierre, D. Naslain, F. Bontemps, D. Ferreira, F. Priem, L. Deldicque, M. Francaux, Urolithin B, a newly identified regulator of skeletal muscle mass, J. Cachexia. Sarcopenia Muscle 8 (4) (2017) 583–597.
[97] M. Zhang, J. Tang, Y. Li, Y. Xie, H. Shan, M. Chen, J. Zhang, X. Yang, Q. Zhang, X. Yang, Curcumin attenuates skeletal muscle mitochondrial impairment in COPD rats: PGC-1α/SIRT3 pathway involved, Chem. Biol. Interact. 277 (2017) 168–175.
[98] T. Ono, S. Takada, S. Kinugawa, H. Tsutsui, Curcumin ameliorates skeletal muscle atrophy in type 1 diabetic mice by inhibiting protein ubiquitination, Exp. Physiol. 100 (9) (2015) 1052–1063.
[99] M. Francaux, L. Deldicque, Using polyphenol derivatives to prevent muscle wasting, Curr. Opin. Clin. Nutr. Metab. Care 21 (3) (2018) 159–163.
[100] A. Sadeghi, A. Rostamirad, S. Seyyedebrahimi, R. Meshkani, Curcumin ameliorates palmitate-induced inflammation in skeletal muscle cells by regulating JNK/NF-kB pathway and ROS production, Inflammopharmacology 26 (5) (2018) 1265–1272.
[101] P. Chaudhary, Y.K. Sharma, S. Sharma, S.N. Singh, G. Suryakumar, High altitude mediated skeletal muscle atrophy: protective role of curcumin, Biochimie 156 (2019) 138–147.
[102] D. Dayangac-Erden, G. Bora-Tatar, S. Dalkara, A.S. Demir, H. Erdem-Yurter, Carboxylic acid derivatives of histone deacetylase inhibitors induce full length SMN2 transcripts: a promising target for spinal muscular atrophy therapeutics, Arch. Med. Sci. 7 (2) (2011) 230.
[103] R.M.G. da Costa, S. Aragão, M. Moutinho, A. Alvarado, D. Carmo, F. Casaca, S. Silva, J. Ribeiro, H. Sousa, R. Ferreira, HPV16 induces a wasting syndrome in transgenic mice: amelioration by dietary polyphenols via NF-κB inhibition, Life Sci. 169 (2017) 11–19.
[104] K.A. Mirza, M. Luo, S. Pereira, A. Voss, T. Das, M.J. Tisdale, In vitro assessment of the combined effect of eicosapentaenoic acid, green tea extract and curcumin C3 on protein loss in C 2 C 12 myotubes, In Vitro Cell. Dev. Biol. Anim. 52 (8) (2016) 838–845.
[105] C. Luceri, F. Guglielmi, M. Lodovici, L. Giannini, L. Messerini, P. Dolara, Plant phenolic 4-coumaric acid protects against intestinal inflammation in rats, Scand. J. Gastroenterol. 39 (11) (2004) 1128–1133.
[106] Y. Kim, C.-S. Kim, Y. Joe, H.T. Chung, T.Y. Ha, R. Yu, Quercetin reduces tumor necrosis factor alpha-induced muscle atrophy by upregulation of Heme oxygenase-1, J. Med. Food 21 (6) (2018) 551–559.
[107] S.-T. Chan, C.-H. Chuang, Y.-C. Lin, J.-W. Liao, C.-K. Lii, S.-L. Yeh, Quercetin enhances the antitumor effect of trichostatin A and suppresses muscle wasting in tumor-bearing mice, Food Funct. 9 (2) (2018) 871–879.
[108] J.M. Davis, E.A. Murphy, M.D. Carmichael, B. Davis, Quercetin increases brain and muscle mitochondrial biogenesis and exercise tolerance, Am. J. Physiol. Regul. Integr. Comp. Physiol. 296 (4) (2009) R1071–R1077.
[109] K.T. Velázquez, R.T. Enos, A.A. Narsale, M.J. Puppa, J.M. Davis, E.A. Murphy, J.A. Carson, Quercetin supplementation attenuates the progression of cancer cachexia in ApcMin/+ mice, J. Nutr. 144 (6) (2014) 868–875.
[110] Y. Otsuka, K. Egawa, N. Kanzaki, T. Izumo, T. Rogi, H. Shibata, Quercetin glycosides prevent dexamethasone-induced muscle atrophy in mice, Biochem. Biophys. Rep. 18 (2019), 100618.

[111] R. Mukai, N. Matsui, Y. Fujikura, N. Matsumoto, D.-X. Hou, N. Kanzaki, H. Shibata, M. Horikawa, K. Iwasa, K. Hirasaka, Preventive effect of dietary quercetin on disuse muscle atrophy by targeting mitochondria in denervated mice, J. Nutr. Biochem. 31 (2016) 67–76.

[112] P. Liu, D. Zou, K. Chen, Q. Zhou, Y. Gao, Y. Huang, J. Zhu, Q. Zhang, M. Mi, Dihydromyricetin improves hypobaric hypoxia-induced memory impairment via modulation of SIRT3 signaling, Mol. Neurobiol. 53 (10) (2016) 7200–7212.

[113] D. Zou, K. Chen, P. Liu, H. Chang, J. Zhu, M. Mi, Dihydromyricetin improves physical performance under simulated high altitude, Med. Sci. Sports Exerc. 46 (11) (2014) 2077–2084.

[114] Y. Huang, K. Chen, Q. Ren, L. Yi, J. Zhu, Q. Zhang, M. Mi, Dihydromyricetin attenuates dexamethasone-induced muscle atrophy by improving mitochondrial function via the PGC-1α pathway, Cell. Physiol. Biochem. 49 (2) (2018) 758–779.

[115] Y. Yoshioka, Y. Yamashita, H. Kishida, K. Nakagawa, H. Ashida, Licorice flavonoid oil enhances muscle mass in KK-Ay mice, Life Sci. 205 (2018) 91–96.

[116] X. Kou, J. Li, X. Liu, X. Yang, J. Fan, N. Chen, Ampelopsin attenuates the atrophy of skeletal muscle from d-gal-induced aging rats through activating AMPK/SIRT1/PGC-1α signaling cascade, Biomed. Pharmacother. 90 (2017) 311–320.

[117] H.W. Liu, Y.J. Chen, Y.C. Chang, S.J. Chang, Oligonol, a low-molecular weight polyphenol derived from lychee, alleviates muscle loss in diabetes by suppressing atrogin-1 and MuRF1, Nutrients 9 (9) (2017).

[118] M. Murata, H. Nonaka, S. Komatsu, M. Goto, M. Morozumi, S. Yamada, I.C. Lin, S. Yamashita, H. Tachibana, Delphinidin prevents muscle atrophy and upregulates miR-23a expression, J. Agric. Food Chem. 65 (1) (2017) 45–50.

[119] P.C. Chen, D.S. Wheeler, V. Malhotra, K. Odoms, A.G. Denenberg, H.R. Wong, A green tea-derived polyphenol, epigallocatechin-3-gallate, inhibits IkappaB kinase activation and IL-8 gene expression in respiratory epithelium, Inflammation 26 (5) (2002) 233–241.

[120] J. Qin, Y. Wang, Y. Bai, K. Yang, Q. Mao, Y. Lin, D. Kong, X. Zheng, L. Xie, Epigallocatechin-3-gallate inhibits bladder cancer cell invasion via suppression of NF-κB-mediated matrix metalloproteinase-9 expression, Mol. Med. Rep. 6 (5) (2012) 1040–1044.

[121] H. Wang, Y.-J. Lai, Y.-L. Chan, T.-L. Li, C.-J. Wu, Epigallocatechin-3-gallate effectively attenuates skeletal muscle atrophy caused by cancer cachexia, Cancer Lett. 305 (1) (2011) 40–49.

[122] C. Kim, J.-K. Hwang, Flavonoids: nutraceutical potential for counteracting muscle atrophy, Food Sci. Biotechnol. 29 (12) (2020) 1619–1640.

[123] B. Li, L. Wan, Y. Li, Q. Yu, P. Chen, R. Gan, Q. Yang, Y. Han, C. Guo, Baicalin, a component of Scutellaria baicalensis, alleviates anorexia and inhibits skeletal muscle atrophy in experimental cancer cachexia, Tumour Biol. 35 (12) (2014) 12415–12425.

[124] E.J. Park, J.M. Pezzuto, The pharmacology of resveratrol in animals and humans, Biochim. Biophys. Acta 1852 (6) (2015) 1071–1113.

[125] I. Momken, L. Stevens, A. Bergouignan, D. Desplanches, F. Rudwill, I. Chery, A. Zahariev, S. Zahn, T.P. Stein, J.L. Sebedio, E. Pujos-Guillot, M. Falempin, C. Simon, V. Coxam, T. Andrianjafiniony, G. Gauquelin-Koch, F. Picquet, S. Blanc, Resveratrol prevents the wasting disorders of mechanical unloading by acting as a physical exercise mimetic in the rat, FASEB J. 25 (10) (2011) 3646–3660.

[126] K. Lambert, M. Coisy-Quivy, C. Bisbal, P. Sirvent, G. Hugon, J. Mercier, A. Avignon, A. Sultan, Grape polyphenols supplementation reduces muscle atrophy in a mouse model of chronic inflammation, Nutrition 31 (10) (2015) 1275–1283.

[127] J. Rodriguez, O. Caille, D. Ferreira, M. Francaux, Pomegranate extract prevents skeletal muscle of mice against wasting induced by acute TNF-α injection, Mol. Nutr. Food Res. 61 (4) (2017) 1600169.

[128] Y.J. Lee, Y.M. Lee, C.K. Lee, J.K. Jung, S.B. Han, J.T. Hong, Therapeutic applications of compounds in the Magnolia family, Pharmacol. Ther. 130 (2) (2011) 157–176.

[129] M.C. Chen, C.F. Lee, W.H. Huang, T.C. Chou, Magnolol suppresses hypoxia-induced angiogenesis via inhibition of HIF-1α/VEGF signaling pathway in human bladder cancer cells, Biochem. Pharmacol. 85 (9) (2013) 1278–1287.

[130] M.C. Chen, Y.L. Chen, C.F. Lee, C.H. Hung, T.C. Chou, Supplementation of magnolol attenuates skeletal muscle atrophy in bladder cancer-bearing mice undergoing chemotherapy via suppression of FoxO3 activation and induction of IGF-1, PLoS One 10 (11) (2015), e0143594.

[131] Y.H. Choi, Schisandrin A prevents oxidative stress-induced DNA damage and apoptosis by attenuating ROS generation in C2C12 cells, Biomed. Pharmacother. 106 (2018) 902–909.

[132] J.S. Kim, H.K. Yi, Schisandrin C enhances mitochondrial biogenesis and autophagy in C2C12 skeletal muscle cells: potential involvement of anti-oxidative mechanisms, Naunyn Schmiedebergs Arch. Pharmacol. 391 (2) (2018) 197–206.

[133] S. Kumar, N. Agnihotri, Piperlongumine, a piper alkaloid targets Ras/PI3K/Akt/mTOR signaling axis to inhibit tumor cell growth and proliferation in DMH/DSS induced experimental colon cancer, Biomed. Pharmacother. 109 (2019) 1462–1477.

[134] Y.-L. Lin, J.-K. Lin, (−)-Epigallocatechin-3-gallate blocks the induction of nitric oxide synthase by down-regulating lipopolysaccharide-induced activity of transcription factor nuclear factor-κB, Mol. Pharmacol. 52 (3) (1997) 465–472.

[135] S. Ahmed, H. Marotte, K. Kwan, J.H. Ruth, P.L. Campbell, B.J. Rabquer, A. Pakozdi, A.E. Koch, Epigallocatechin-3-gallate inhibits IL-6 synthesis and suppresses transsignaling by enhancing soluble gp130 production, Proc. Natl. Acad. Sci. 105 (38) (2008) 14692–14697.

[136] J. Wang, Y. Wang, M. Tong, H. Pan, D. Li, New prospect for cancer cachexia: medical cannabinoid, J. Cancer 10 (3) (2019) 716.

[137] S.K. Shukla, A. Dasgupta, K. Mehla, V. Gunda, E. Vernucci, J. Souchek, G. Goode, R. King, A. Mishra, I. Rai, Silibinin-mediated metabolic reprogramming attenuates pancreatic cancer-induced cachexia and tumor growth, Oncotarget 6 (38) (2015) 41146.

[138] W.H. Choi, Y.J. Jang, H.J. Son, J. Ahn, C.H. Jung, T.Y. Ha, Apigenin inhibits sciatic nerve denervation-induced muscle atrophy, Muscle Nerve 58 (2) (2018) 314–318.

[139] S. Hedya, N. Hawila, A. Abdin, A.E. Maaly, Luteolin attenuates dexamethasone-induced skeletal muscle atrophy in male albino rats, Med. J. Cairo Univ. 87 (September) (2019) 3365–3374.

[140] Z.-K. Zhang, L. Jie, L. Jin, G. Baosheng, A. Leung, G. Zhang, B.-T. Zhang, Icaritin requires Phosphatidylinositol 3 kinase (PI3K)/Akt signaling to counteract skeletal muscle atrophy following mechanical unloading, Sci. Rep. 6 (2016) 20300.

[141] T. Yoshimura, K. Saitoh, L. Sun, Y. Wang, S. Taniyama, K. Yamaguchi, T. Uchida, T. Ohkubo, A. Higashitani, T. Nikawa, Morin suppresses cachexia-induced muscle wasting by binding to ribosomal protein S10 in carcinoma cells, Biochem. Biophys. Res. Commun. 506 (4) (2018) 773–779.

[142] S.-J. Lee, T.A. Vuong, G.-Y. Go, Y.-J. Song, S. Lee, S.-Y. Lee, S.-W. Kim, J. Lee, Y.K. Kim, D.-W. Seo, An isoflavone compound daidzein elicits myoblast differentiation and myotube growth, J. Funct. Foods 38 (2017) 438–446.

[143] W. Zheng, M.L. Hemker, M. Xie, S.T. Soukup, P. Diel, Anabolic activity of a soy extract and three major isoflavones in C2C12 myotubes, Planta Med. 84 (14) (2018) 1022–1029.

Index

Note: Page numbers followed by *f* indicate figures and *t* indicate tables.

D

H

I

N

O

T

Made in the USA
Monee, IL
13 September 2026

63138374R00249